Diploma in Dental Nursing, Level 3

Diploma in Dental Nursing, Level 3

Third Edition

Carole Hollins, BDS

General Dental Practitioner
Former Chairman and Member of the Panel of Examiners, National Examining Board for Dental Nurses

WILEY Blackwell

Registered Office
John Wiley & Sons, Ltd, The Atrium, Southern Gate, Chichester, West Sussex, PO19 8SQ, UK

Editorial Offices
9600 Garsington Road, Oxford, OX4 2DQ, UK
The Atrium, Southern Gate, Chichester, West Sussex, PO19 8SQ, UK
1606 Golden Aspen Drive, Suites 103 and 104, Ames, Iowa 50010, USA

For details of our global editorial offices, for customer services and for information about how to apply for permission to reuse the copyright material in this book please see our website at www.wiley.com/wiley-blackwell

Library of Congress Cataloging-in-Publication Data

Hollins, Carole, author.
[NVQs for dental nurses]
Diploma in dental nursing, level 3 / Carole Hollins. – Third edition.
    1 online resource.
  Preceded by NVQs for dental nurses / Carole Hollins. 2nd ed. 2009.
  Includes bibliographical references and index.
  Description based on print version record and CIP data provided by publisher; resource not viewed.
  ISBN 978-1-118-62945-1 (Adobe PDF) – ISBN 978-1-118-62947-5 (ePub) – ISBN 978-1-118-62948-2 (paper)
I. Title.
[DNLM: 1. Dental Assistants–Examination Questions.   2. Dental Care–methods–Examination Questions.   WU 18.2]
  RK60
  617.60076–dc23
                                              2014021565

A catalogue record for this book is available from the British Library.

Wiley also publishes its books in a variety of electronic formats. Some content that appears in print may not be available in electronic books.

Cover image: iStock © hidesy
Cover design by Steve Thompson

Set in 9/11 pt Vectora by SPi Publisher Services, Pondicherry, India
Printed and bound in Malaysia by Vivar Printing Sdn Bhd

1   2014

Contents

Introduction to the Third Edition

Since the last edition was written, dental nurses have joined other members of the dental team to become registered professionals with the General Dental Council (GDC) and have at last been elevated to their well-deserved status as invaluable dental care professionals. With this professional recognition comes the necessity for set standards of attitude and behaviour outside the workplace, as well as suitable qualification, ethical work practices, and the requirement for lifelong learning and continuous professional development during their careers.

This edition provides the underpinning knowledge required to cover the curriculum contents of the City & Guilds Level 3 Diploma in Dental Nursing. A similar textbook is available to cover the National Examining Board for Dental Nurses' curriculum for their new Diploma in Dental Nursing qualification, which has recently replaced the National Certificate. Although the same registerable qualification is awarded to successful candidates following either route to registration, the training and assessment methods involved for each are quite different.

The revised and updated text of this latest edition embraces all the numerous legislative and regulatory changes of the last 5 years, including issues around health and safety, infection control, information governance, quality assurance requirements and the expansion of the concept of continuous professional development into that of team members becoming "reflective practitioners". The book is set out into 15 chapters, with the first 11 detailing the practical aspects of those units that are assessed through completion of the workplace-based portfolio requirement of the qualification. The final four chapters cover Units 312 to 315, which provide the theory and underpinning knowledge required to understand the holistic role of the dental nurse in the modern dental workplace. The information in these final four chapters is assessed by the written examination component of the qualification, as a set of one of four multiple choice questions (MCQs). The interactive companion website to this book (www.wiley.com/go/hollins/dentalnursinglevel3) provides similar test questions for the readership to use as an additional learning tool for their studies, as well as including a glossary of terms. A separate Question & Answers revision book will soon be available for use by dental nurses studying for the City & Guilds qualification, with a wide range of MCQs providing comprehensive coverage of the full curriculum.

Where necessary, website addresses are included to allow readers to access further information on many topics covered throughout the text – especially links to various websites covering legal and ethical issues, and to more information on subject topics with national variations, such as infection control.

It is hoped that the increased use of photographs and illustrations, as well as of bullet points to highlight key facts throughout the text, will make this edition particularly user-friendly and easy to understand for all readers, without detracting from the high standards now expected of dental nurse students as they evolve into fully fledged dental professionals. Finally, and as always, I sincerely hope that this text stimulates at least some readers into becoming sufficiently inspired during their studies to continue their careers beyond their initial qualification, and consider extended duties, post-registration qualifications and further dental professional careers too.

Carole Hollins

Acknowledgements

Once again, I must extend my grateful thanks to the patients and staff of Kidsgrove dental practice for their modelling skills, and give sincere thanks also to my sister (yet again!) for her technical and computer-related wizardry – thank goodness she knows what she's doing!

In updating this edition, I am very grateful to the General Dental Council and the Department of Health for their permissions to reproduce various documents and booklets throughout the text, and I hope I have done justice to their content. I must also express great appreciation for the continued support of previous illustrators.

Finally, a huge "thank you" to the various staff of Wiley Blackwell (past and present) for their superb help and support throughout the updating and publishing process, and especially the speedy professionalism with which they work.

About the Companion Website

This book is accompanied by a companion website:

www.wiley.com/go/hollins/dentalnursinglevel3

The website includes:

- More than 150 interactive multiple choice questions
- Glossary of terms

1

Unit 301: Ensure Your Own Actions Reduce Risks to Health and Safety

Learning outcomes

1. Be able to identify the hazards in the workplace
2. Be able to act upon hazards in the workplace
3. Be able to reduce the risks to health and safety in the workplace

Outcome 1 assessment criteria
The learner can:
- Identify which workplace procedures are relevant to their job
- Identify those working practices in the job that could harm them or others
- Identify those aspects of the workplace that could harm them or others
- Outline any differences between workplace legislation and supplier's or manufacturer's instructions

Outcome 2 assessment criteria
The learner can:
- Report hazards to the identified responsible person
- Demonstrate the ability to deal with hazards in the workplace

Outcome 3 assessment criteria
The learner can:
- Carry out their work in accordance with workplace legislation or manufacturer's instructions
- Behave in a way that does not endanger their health and safety or that of others, or of the materials in the workplace

Diploma in Dental Nursing, Level 3, Third Edition. Carole Hollins.
© 2014 John Wiley & Sons, Ltd. Published 2014 by John Wiley & Sons, Ltd.
Companion website: www.wiley.com/go/hollins/dentalnursinglevel3

- Contribute to health and safety improvements within the workplace
- Follow guidelines for environmentally friendly working practices
- Ensure personal presentation protects their health and safety and that of others in line with instructions

This unit is assessed by:
- Observation in the workplace, with examples included in the learner's portfolio
- An appropriate alternative method

Details of various elements of theory and underpinning knowledge are included in Chapter 12, and these are assessed within the written paper.

The theory and underpinning knowledge required to understand the need to act responsibly in the workplace, to understand and follow all the health and safety policies and protocols in place, and to recognise which particular workplace activities may be hazardous to the dental team are discussed in detail in Chapters 12, 14 and 15. The actions that the dental nurse will need to take in the event of a medical emergency occurring on the premises are discussed in detail in Chapter 13.

This chapter explains the dental nurses' roles and responsibilities in relation to identifying and dealing with risks and hazards in the dental workplace. Those responsibilities are to themselves and any other person on the workplace premises. In the dental workplace, "any other person" includes patients and their guardians or escorts, visiting utility workers, such as postal workers and meter readers, and visitors such as repair and maintenance personnel.

The relevant workplace procedures that may pose a risk or hazard to the dental nurse are:

- Use of some occupational equipment and items
- Use of some hazardous occupational substances
- Moving and handling of heavy items or hazardous substances
- Disposal of hazardous substances

Overview of responsibilities

All dental workplaces, their staff and patients are covered by the provisions of the Health and Safety at Work Act (1974), as is any other workplace. In addition, other legislation is relevant to the dental workplace, due to the potentially harmful nature of the equipment and chemicals used, as well as the occupational hazards associated with delivering dental treatment or working in the dental environment.

The health and safety legislation seeks to protect staff and patients while on the premises by making staff aware of any potential hazards at work and encouraging them to find the best ways of making their particular premises safer for all concerned. In legal terms, the employer has a statutory duty to ensure that, as far as is reasonably practicable, the health, safety and welfare at work of all employees and all visitors (including patients) are protected at all times. To do this, all of the potential hazards first need to be identified, and then the likelihood of them actually causing harm to anyone must be determined. The chance that a particular workplace hazard could cause harm to someone is known as its risk, and the correct procedure to be followed by the employer (and the staff) to identify those hazards in the dental workplace that could cause harm is called a risk assessment.

Compliance with the Health and Safety at Work Act is overseen and regulated by the Health and Safety Executive (HSE). This is a government body that provides guidance to employers on the correct enforcement of the Act and investigates any serious incidents that occur in any workplace where someone suffers serious harm or is killed. Every dental workplace is required to be registered with the HSE. Compliance with the additional legislation specific to the dental workplace is also a requirement by the General Dental Council (GDC), under their *Standards for the Dental Team* documentation.

3

In the dental workplace, normal procedures that are carried out on a day-to-day basis include the assessment of a patient's oral health, the diagnosis of oral disease, and performing the necessary dental treatment required to cure that disease. In addition, elective dental procedures are carried out to prevent or reduce the likelihood of disease developing, and an array of administrative procedures will also be necessary to support the clinical functions of the workplace.

To ensure the safety of everyone while on the premises, both the employer and employees have responsibilities to be followed.

Employers' responsibilities

All workplaces must have a current Health and Safety Law poster on display on the premises for all staff to see (Figure 1.1). This gives the name of the employer or employing organisation and states in broad terms what employees can expect from the employer (or organisation) in relation

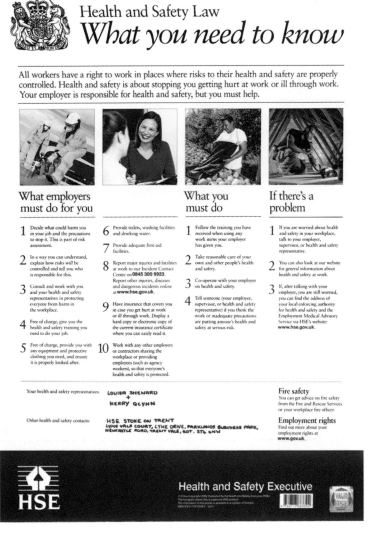

Figure 1.1   A health and safety poster.

to the safeguarding of their health and safety while on the premises, as well as what employees can do themselves. It also gives contact details for the HSE in case any problem arises with regard to the employee safety.

To comply with the basic requirements of the Health and Safety at Work Act, every employer in the dental workplace must abide by the following requirements:

- Provide a working environment for employees that is safe, without risks to health, and adequate as regards facilities and arrangements for their welfare at work
- Maintain the place of work, including the means of access and exit, in a safe condition
- Provide and maintain safe equipment, appliances and systems of work
- Ensure all staff members are trained in the safe handling and storage of any dangerous or potentially harmful items or substances
- Provide such instruction, training and supervision as is necessary to ensure health and safety
- Review the health and safety performance of all staff annually, and be aware of and investigate any failures or concerns highlighted when they occur
- Display the official health and safety poster for all staff to refer to

To comply with these statutory obligations, dentists must keep their staff informed of all the safety measures adopted. Practices with five or more employees must produce a comprehensive health and safety policy and provide all staff with a copy. The policy will classify the practice's health and safety procedures and name the persons responsible. It should also list the telephone numbers of all dental, administration and equipment maintenance contractors, the local HSE contact and the emergency services.

Under the Act, all employers must therefore ensure, as far as is reasonably possible, that the health and safety of all persons on the premises is protected – and this must be achieved by carrying out a risk assessment of the workplace activities that occur on the premises. This is a specific requirement under the Management of Health and Safety at Work Regulations 1999.

Risk assessment to identify the hazards

A risk assessment is merely a detailed examination of the normal day-to-day activities that occur in the workplace in an effort to identify those that have the potential to cause harm to anyone on the premises – these are called the **hazards**. Once the hazards have been identified, a set of **precautions** can be determined that will prevent or minimise the risk associated with each hazard, thereby ensuring the safety of all those on the premises.

The aim is not necessarily to eliminate every risk completely – this is probably impossible in most workplaces, including dental surgeries – but instead to minimise those risks identified as far as possible, so that there is little chance of them causing harm to anyone.

For example, various chemicals are used in the dental workplace to carry out dental treatment successfully, including decontamination solutions, X-ray processing solutions, and mercury in amalgam fillings – all are potentially harmful, but only if they are mishandled. Knowledge of their correct storage and usage by staff, and protection from misuse by all others are key factors in avoiding a hazardous event from occurring.

The procedure for carrying out a risk assessment on a hazard, whatever its nature, should always follow the same steps:

1. **Identify the hazard** – e.g. a chemical, a piece of equipment, a procedure that occurs in the workplace
2. **Identify who may be harmed** – e.g. certain staff, certain patients, visitors, everyone
3. **Evaluate the risk** – is there a hazard only if the item in question is misused; is there a hazard with every use; or is there a hazard only if certain precautions are not followed?

4. **Control the risk** – e.g. train all staff in correct usage, improve precautions to prevent misuse, keep hazards away from untrained persons, install health monitoring where appropriate, remove the risk where possible
5. **Record the risk assessment findings** – this is done to prove compliance, to provide a reference for all users, to ensure all staff are fully informed of the potential hazards in the dental workplace
6. **Review the assessment process** – do this on a regular basis to ensure that hazardous events or injuries do not occur

Recording the findings of the risk assessment is considered "best practice" for all workplaces, and is a legal requirement for all employers with five or more employees. As any relevant laws and regulations are updated, areas of the risk assessment may then need to be reconsidered and updated too.

Employees' responsibilities – role of the dental nurse

All employees are legally required to take reasonable care for their own and others' health and safety, and to cooperate with their employer to this effect while carrying out their normal workplace activities. Indeed, it is an offence for an employee to intentionally break the workplace rules and policies in relation to health and safety, whether or not this causes harm to themselves or others.

All dental nurses have a legal obligation to co-operate with their employers in carrying out the practice requirements in respect of these safety measures. They are designed to protect not only the staff and patients, but also anyone else using or visiting the premises. In a large dental workplace, a dental nurse may be appointed as the safety representative under the Act for the purpose of improving liaison within the practice about health and safety matters.

Many dental nurses begin their careers as young trainees in the dental environment, so the following two sets of regulations are specifically important in protecting their welfare too:

- Health and Safety (Young Persons) Regulations 1997
- Management of Health and Safety at Work Regulations 1999

These sets of regulations dictate that a risk assessment of the dental environment has to be carried out with particular regard to the protection of younger staff members, by taking into account the following points:

- The risks to young people before they start work
- The psychological or physical immaturity and inexperience of young people
- Their lack of awareness of existing or potential risks to their health and safety
- The fitting and layout of the workplace and surgery areas, with regard to the safety of young people
- The nature, degree and duration of any exposure to biological, chemical or physical agents in the work environment
- The form, range, use and handling of dental equipment
- The way in which processes and activities are organised
- Any health and safety training given, or intended to be given

A typical risk assessment summary of the types of work activities that a young dental nurse is likely to carry out in the workplace is shown in the following table. The second column identifies all of the possible hazards that the dental nurse may be exposed to when carrying out each particular activity, and the third column shows the precautions that must be taken to ensure that the hazards are reduced as far as possible.

Work activity	Potential risk	Prevention with controls
Chairside assisting	Eye injury from projectiles during treatment Inhalation of aerosols during treatment	Explanation of risks, training in activities undertaken, initial supervision Provision and use of all personal protective equipment (PPE)
Instrument decontamination	Inoculation injury (clean or dirty) Contamination splash during cleaning	Explanation of risks, training in cleaning methods, initial supervision Additional PPE – plastic apron and thick rubber gloves
Use of autoclave	Burns from hot machine or instruments Scalds from steam	Explanation of risks, training in handling methods, initial supervision
Exposure to hazardous chemicals	Inhalation of vapours, skin contact, eye contact	Explanation of risks, training in handling methods, initial supervision Provision and use of full PPE Adequate ventilation
Use of X-rays	Accidental exposure to X-rays	Explanation of risks, inform of designated control area, avoid unauthorised entry to area

Without exception, the reduction of risk for each activity relies on suitable induction training being given, where dental nurses are made aware of the hazards they face and are then trained how to carry out each activity safely. They will then be supervised by a more senior colleague until they can carry out the activity correctly and without putting themselves or others at risk. This supervision also forms the basis of the observation and assessment criteria "sign-off" that is carried out by the assessor during the Level 3 Diploma qualification, where student dental nurses are formally observed during their training and gradually build up their portfolio of evidence.

There are also everyday activities and events in the dental workplace that may present a hazard to people on the premises and that are not exclusive to the dental workplace but may occur anywhere. The risk assessment process must consider them as well, rather than focusing solely on the particular hazards of the dental workplace, and must then produce a list of methods to avoid or control them too. Obvious examples of these commonplace events and the sensible actions to take to avoid them are shown in the following table, but the list is not exhaustive and will vary greatly between dental workplaces.

Scenario of potential hazard	Common-sense actions to avoid harm
Injury sustained by falling down on the premises	Keep all access routes clear of debris and blockages Maintain floor covering adequately Avoid cleaning during work time Clear all spillages immediately Use hazard signs to highlight potential sources of injury (Figure 1.2)

Scenario of potential hazard	Common-sense actions to avoid harm
Child drinking harmful chemical	Keep harmful chemicals out of reach Keep chemicals in locked storage area Keep children out of storage area Keep children under control at all times
Person falling out of window on premises	Install window locks Install restricted opening device Keep staff-only areas locked
Injury sustained from slammed door	Keep doors locked when rooms are not in use Install slow-closure devices to prevent slamming Install safety glass

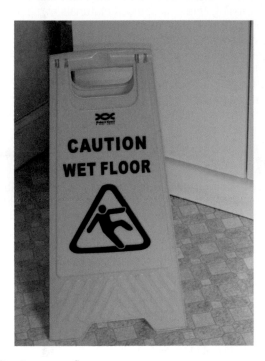

Figure 1.2   Hazard sign indicating a wet floor.

If the simple common-sense actions have not been carried out initially, then the employer is to blame if someone is harmed as a direct result of these failings. If, however, a risk assessment has resulted in the necessary preventative measures being put into place, and someone else has flouted them – such as by leaving a door or cupboard unlocked to avoid the inconvenience of having to keep unlocking it – then that person is to blame instead.

Dental nurses will be required to carry out the following tasks within their own workplace, and provide evidence to their assessor of having done so in their workplace portfolio:

- Identify the workplace procedures that are relevant to their role as a dental nurse
- Identify the working practices in their role as a dental nurse that may cause harm to themselves or others (these are shown in the preceding table)

- Identify the aspects of their particular workplace that may cause harm to themselves or others (these will vary between workplaces)
- Outline any differences between workplace legislation and suppliers'/manufacturers' instructions

All members of staff have a legal obligation under the Health and Safety at Work Act to co-operate with their employer by following the policies and procedures put in place to protect all persons while on the premises. They must also take reasonable care for their own and others' health and safety while on the premises. Failure to do so, as indicated earlier, will result in their possible investigation and prosecution by the HSE and a "fitness to practise" hearing with the GDC, for those who are registrants.

The level of reasonable care expected to be taken for their own health and safety as employees (and in line with fitness to practise requirements by the GDC) requires dental nurses to abide by the following when in the dental workplace:

- Undergo suitable training in the use of dental materials and equipment items
- Always follow that training when using those materials and equipment items
- Always follow all policies in relation to health, safety and welfare issues
- Never misuse any materials or equipment on the premises
- In particular, never misuse or fail to use any materials or equipment that are specifically meant to reduce or eliminate hazardous risks
- Always report any faults in procedures or equipment to a senior colleague immediately
- Never enter certain designated "hazardous" areas unless authorised to do so
- Always report any suspected health problem that will impact on their normal work to a senior colleague as soon as possible

Personal presentation

In the dental workplace the emphasis is often very much on the avoidance of cross-infection from patients to staff, especially by following "standard precautions" in relation to infection control (see Chapters 4 and 12). However, patients may also be at risk of cross-infection from staff members if the latter's basic personal hygiene is inadequate or if they fail to apply the relevant health and safety actions when dealing with patients.

Consequently, a certain standard of personal presentation is required of the dental nurse when in the workplace, under the following three areas:

- Personal hygiene
- Use of PPE
- Suitable clothing and accessories when in the workplace

Personal hygiene

A good standard of personal hygiene by any healthcare worker could be considered to be a professional obligation by some, and the dental nurse working in close proximity to patients on a daily basis is no exception. It is therefore reasonable for patients to expect the following standards from dental nurses:

- Body washed to avoid odours, and the sensible use of anti-perspirant/deodorants
- Clean hair, with long hair tied back while working so that it does not fall across the face or onto any surrounding items
- Clean hands and nails, with no nail varnish or false nails present and hands washed to a clinical/hygienic standard when working at the chairside (see later)
- Clean and well-restored teeth, and the sensible use of oral health products
- Sensible use of any facial make-up

- Minimal evidence of any facial piercings or tattoos – some employers may request the removal of various facial jewellery if they are considered to be a health and safety issue, and tattoos may have to be kept covered if they may cause offence

Hand washing is the most important method of preventing cross-infection, and the technique used should be that stipulated by the Health and Safety Council. The three recognised levels of hand hygiene are as follows:

- **Social** – to become physically clean from socially acquired microorganisms, using general purpose liquid soap
- **Clinical/hygienic** – to destroy microorganisms, maintain cleanliness and avoid direct cross-infection, using an approved antibacterial hand cleanser
- **Surgical** – to significantly reduce the numbers of normally resident microorganisms on the hands, before an invasive surgical procedure is carried out, using an approved antibacterial hand cleanser

Generally, hand hygiene of a socially acceptable standard is adequate, but when working at the chairside the dental nurse will need to achieve a clinical standard of hand hygiene instead. The correct procedure for **hygienic hand washing** should be displayed in poster form at each dedicated hand washing sink in the workplace, and the instructions are as follows (Figure 1.3):

- Turn on the tap using the foot or elbow control, to prevent contamination of the tap
- Wet both hands under running water of a suitable temperature
- Apply a suitable antibacterial liquid soap from the specially operated dispenser and wash all areas of both hands and wrists thoroughly – this should take up to 30 seconds to carry out correctly
- Nail brushes are not advised unless they are autoclavable, as they can become contaminated with repeated use
- Rinse both hands under running water, holding them up so that the water does not flow back over the fingers
- Dry the hands thoroughly, using single-use disposable paper towels
- Heavy-duty gloves must be worn whenever the cleaning of dirty instruments is being carried out
- Clinical gloves must be worn whenever patients are being treated, and discarded between patients – these should be non-powdered and of a non-latex material, such as nitrile or vinyl, to avoid the development of skin sensitisation conditions

Use of PPE

This is worn to prevent staff from coming into contact with blood and other bodily fluids, and its correct use should be stipulated in the infection control policy. If the dental nurse has any wounds present on the hands or fingers, they should be covered with waterproof dressings beneath the PPE. It is a legal requirement for dental employers to provide the following protective clothing for their staff:

- **Gloves** of varying quality (clinical or household)
- High-temperature-washed **uniform**, to be worn in the work area only
- **Plastic apron** to be worn over the uniform when soiling may occur during surgical procedures or while cleaning the surgery
- **Safety glasses** or goggles, to prevent contaminated material from entering the eyes
- Prescription glasses should be further protected by wearing a **visor** or face shield
- Visors or face shields alone do not provide adequate protection to the eyes, or prevent the inhalation of aerosol contaminants without the use of a **face mask** too

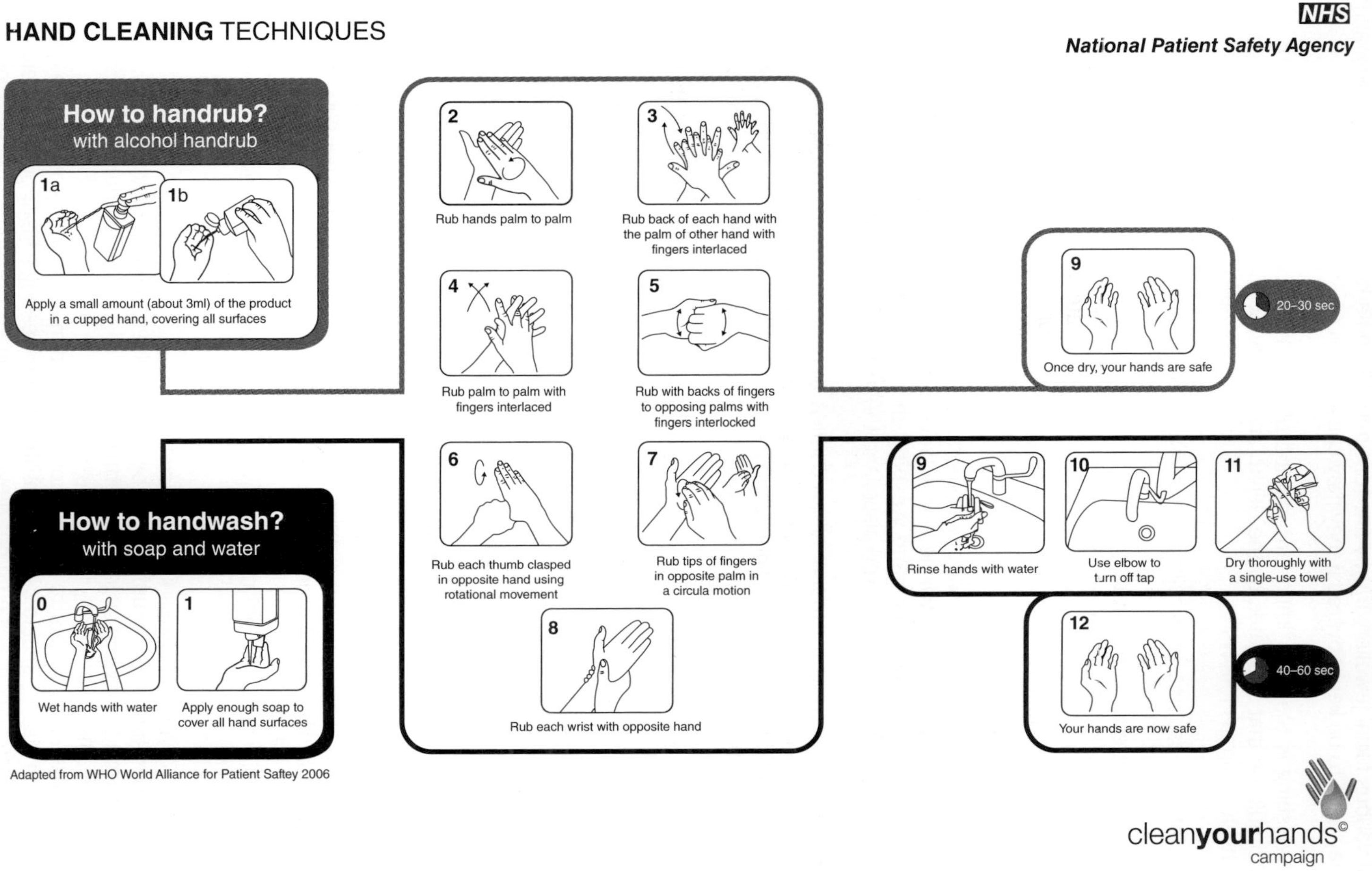

Figure 1.3 A hand washing poster.

- **Face masks** of surgical quality should be worn whenever dental hand pieces or ultrasonic equipment are in use, to prevent the inhalation of aerosol contamination and pieces of flying debris

Alcohol-based hand gels should not be used with clinical gloves, as they can damage the nitrile or vinyl material, allowing leakage to occur. Household gloves can be safely washed with detergent and hot water, and then left to dry naturally.

Suitable clothing and accessories

When working at the chairside, dental nurses must wear the uniform provided by their employer. This can then be removed before leaving the workplace so that contaminants from the surgery area are not transferred into the wider community. Suitable footwear is provided by some employers, too, and is usually a style of surgical clog which provides adequate coverage and protection of the toes. Alternatively, personal footwear is worn and must be flat or minimally heeled and also provide full coverage of the toes. Ideally the shoes worn should not have a patterned surface or a lace-up design, so that they can be cleaned more easily if they become contaminated by spillages and so on.

If dental nurses are carrying out administrative duties rather than clinical duties, some employers may allow their attendance without a uniform, so their attire should be smart and sensible. In particular, denims and T-shirts bearing logos should be avoided in these instances, as should party-style or casual clothing and footwear. The dental nurse should always give the impression of being a professional member of staff when working in the dental workplace.

Any jewellery worn should be discreet – dangling earrings or necklaces must be removed during work time. To reduce the risk of cross-infection, it is ideal for all rings, bracelets and watches to be removed when the dental nurse is working at the chairside, but this is not necessary when only performing administrative duties.

Summary of health and safety requirements

Full compliance with health and safety legislation for all dental workplaces, be that is a practice, a clinic or a hospital department, involves all of the following:

- Fire Precaution (Workplace) Regulations (1999)
- Health and Safety (First Aid) Regulations (1981) – see Chapter 3 for full details
- COSHH – Control of Substances Hazardous to Health (1994)
- RIDDOR – Reporting of Injuries, Diseases and Dangerous Occurrences (1995)
- Environmental Protection Act (1990)
- Special Waste and Hazardous Waste Regulations (2005)
- Ionising radiation legislation (IRR 99 and IR(ME)R 2000) – see Chapter 7 for full details
- Occupational hazards – inoculation injury
- General safety measures – moving and handling

Dental nurses must understand and demonstrate how each area of legislation and regulation impacts on them and their daily duties in the dental workplace.

Fire Precaution (Workplace) Regulations

These became law in 2006 and state the following:

- Employer/owner of the premises must take reasonable steps to:
  - Reduce the risk of fire
  - Ensure adequate means of safe escape from a fire
- They must therefore risk assess their premises to determine the fire precautions required

The fire precautions required will vary from one workplace to another; for example, a ground floor practice will be considered less dangerous to staff and patients in the event of a fire than one that is in a multi-storey building.

A typical fire risk assessment should consider the following points, in the order shown:

1. **Identify the fire hazards on the premises** – these will include flammable materials (liquids, vapours, textiles, paper products), heating appliances with naked flames, electrical equipment, static sparks from electrical equipment, flammable sedation gases, flammable rubbish
2. **Identify who may be harmed** – consider anyone on the premises, paying special attention to children and vulnerable adults who may be attending, and where they may be on the premises
3. **Evaluate the risk of a fire occurring** – consider the amount of various flammable materials on the premises, and where they are used or stored, the number of heating appliances and items of electrical equipment, any sedation gases, the amount of flammable rubbish at any time
4. **Control the risk by taking precautions** – reduce the amount of flammable materials used where possible, and ensure they are stored away from heat sources; replace naked flame heat sources with safer alternatives (the only likely exception will be portable burners used for denture work); ensure electrical appliances are properly serviced and maintained; use and store sedation gas cylinders away from heat sources; avoid storing flammable waste near heat sources; consider whether or not current fire detection methods, firefighting equipment and evacuation procedures are adequate
5. **Record the risk assessment findings** – in particular, record all findings and details of the actions taken to improve precautions; ensure all staff are notified of the findings and any new actions to be followed
6. **Review the risk assessment periodically** – annually is adequate, recording the date of the review and whether or not any revisions were made

All dental workplaces then undergo a fire safety inspection, so that the premises can be formally recorded as having carried out the necessary risk assessment. Although several companies provide the means for this to be carried out by post, a visit by a suitably qualified inspector from the Fire Service will hold more weight if a fire does occur, and the practice is held to account for its level of compliance.

The inspection will give advice with regard to the following:

- The number and positioning of smoke detectors
- The number and positioning of fire extinguishers
- Written records of staff training in the use of fire extinguishers
- The types of fire extinguishers to be provided, with at least two types present in all workplaces
- The presence of any obvious fire risks that must be removed, such as the use of open-flame gas heaters to warm a room

Fire detection

Fires are detected by some type of alarm system, operated either manually by an individual when a fire has been discovered or automatically by smoke or heat detection. The larger the workplace premises, the more sophisticated the detection system tends to be. The types of premises that require an electrical fire alarm system and/or an automatic detection system are large workplaces, perhaps over several levels, where a fire breaking out in one area could go undetected by an ordinary smoke alarm or unnoticed by a person for some time. Hospital departments and health clinics are likely examples where these additional fire detection methods would be required.

In smaller workplaces (the majority of dental practices), a fire risk assessment should determine that adequate fire detection is provided by the use of strategically placed, battery-operated smoke alarms around the premises (Figure 1.4). These should be tested on a regular basis to ensure they are functioning correctly, and a record kept of these test dates and results. Obviously the battery should be changed as soon as it begins to fail, or the alarm changed if any malfunctions occur.

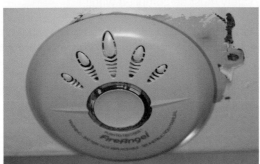

Figure 1.4   A smoke alarm.

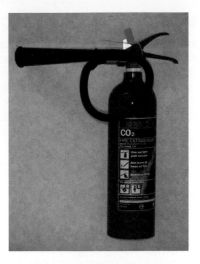

Figure 1.5   A fire extinguisher.

Firefighting

The main equipment available for use in firefighting is the fire extinguisher (Figure 1.5), although some premises will have additional equipment such as fire blankets, water sprinklers and hoses. To decide what firefighting equipment should be available, the classification of fires is considered to determine which products are the most likely to pose a fire risk in the workplace:

- **Class A fire** – caused by the ignition of carbon-containing items, such as paper, wood and textiles
- **Class B fire** – caused by flammable liquids, such as oils, solvents and petrol
- **Class C fire** – caused by flammable gases, such as domestic gas, butane, liquefied petroleum gas (LPG)
- **Class D fire** – caused by reactive metals that oxidise in air, such as sodium and magnesium
- **Class E fire** – caused by electrical components and equipment
- **Class F fire** – caused by liquid fats, such as used in kitchens and restaurants

In the dental workplace, the likeliest causes of fire suggest that extinguishers to fight classes A, B, C and E should be available. The content of each fire extinguisher varies depending on its recommended use, and is identifiable by a coloured label or specific wording on the label of the extinguisher. All extinguishers are coloured red so that they are easily visible, while the label and its wording describe the fire classification it is suitable for, as follows:

- Red (water) extinguisher – for use on all except electrical fires
- Black (carbon dioxide) extinguisher – for use on all fires
- Blue (dry powder) extinguisher – for use on all fires

The extinguishers must all be inspected and certificated by a competent person on an annual basis, and replaced as necessary. The dental nurse will receive induction training with regard to the health and safety in the workplace, and this should include the location of all firefighting equipment and instruction in its use. The extinguishers should be located:

- Within easy reach, ideally along escape routes
- Placed in conspicuous positions (e.g. not hidden by surrounding cupboards)
- On wall mountings and signposted
- In a similar position on each level of the premises

Evacuation and escape routes

During the risk assessment process, consideration will be given to whether, in the event of a fire, all persons on the premises could leave safely and reach a place of safety. There should be no possibility of anyone being cut off from escaping from the premises by either smoke or flames.
  In particular, the following areas of fire safety must be complied with:

- Escape routes must be kept free from all obstructions to allow immediate evacuation from the premises if necessary – in particular, key-operated outer doors must be kept **unlocked** during normal working hours
- In large dental workplaces such as a hospital, security is maintained during normal working hours by having fire exits that cannot be opened from the outside of the building but can be opened from inside the premises by activating an alarmed "lift bar" device
- Fire exits must lead directly to a place of safety, usually outside the building itself
- They must be clearly marked by green "fire exit" signs, with an accompanying pictogram of a running man (Figure 1.6)
- Emergency lighting should be provided if necessary – this applies to hospitals rather than smaller workplaces, and their need will have been identified during the fire risk assessment
- Emergency doors should open manually in the direction of escape and should **not** be operated electrically
- Sliding or revolving doors should **not** be used as fire exits
- All staff must be aware of the fire safety and evacuation process, and the procedure for evacuation should be practised at least annually
- In addition, some staff should be charged with certain actions during the evacuation procedure, such as checking certain areas are clear, or closing certain doors to contain the fire
- Special consideration also needs to be given to the needs of disabled persons, and in small workplaces they should only be treated in ground floor surgeries so that they can be easily evacuated from the premises

The culmination of the findings from the fire risk assessment will ultimately be the development of a written fire policy, or an emergency plan. This is a legal requirement in workplaces with more than five employees and it must be available to all employees and to the fire inspector. It should detail what action everyone on the premises should take in the event of a fire, and may be covered by a simple "fire action" poster displayed in the reception area (Figure 1.7).

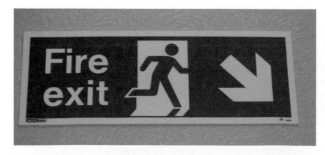

Figure 1.6   A fire exit pictogram.

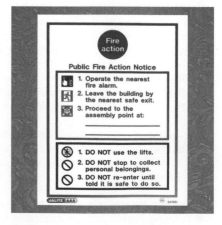

Figure 1.7   A fire action poster.

Larger dental workplaces (hospitals, clinics and large multi-surgery premises) will be expected to provide more detail still, and a suitable emergency plan should cover the following points:

- Action to take in the event of a fire
- Alarm warnings (klaxon, whistle, bell, etc.)
- How to call the rescue services
- Evacuation arrangements, including details for disabled persons
- Assembly point
- Method of accounting for all persons (e.g. use of the day list)
- Key escape routes
- Location and use of firefighting equipment
- Responsibilities of nominated persons
- Power shutdown methods
- Staff training

Whatever the size and layout of the particular dental workplace, the dental nurse must be fully aware of the following:

- The fire alarm system in use on the premises and when a test drill is being carried out
- The location of all firefighting equipment and its correct use
- The escape routes available and the assembly point(s)
- How to open any fire exits along the escape route taken
- The method to be used to account for all persons on the premises

Smoking in the workplace

Smoking in all enclosed workplaces is now prohibited throughout the UK. All enclosed workplaces, which include all types of dental workplace, must display a "no smoking" sign at each entrance to the premises, and they must contain the following wording: "No smoking. It is against the law to smoke in these premises."

Before the ban, careless disposal of cigarettes was a significant cause of fires in the workplace. As a member of staff, the dental nurse must abide by this ban and actively assist the employer in enforcing it, by reporting all breaches to a senior colleague, whether another staff member or any other individual is involved.

First aid regulations

In the dental workplace, a health and safety policy will have been developed after a risk assessment has been carried out for the premises, usually by the employer. The dental nurse must follow this policy when on the premises at all times, as should all other personnel, to avoid the potential for accidents to occur.

Specifically, dental nurses must ensure they are not responsible for any acts or omissions in relation to the health and safety policy that would put themselves, their colleagues or any other individuals in the workplace at risk of harm, at any time. Obvious examples of poor practice would be a failure to follow ionising radiation regulations, failure to wash their hands and wear PPE when dealing with patients, or failure to take adequate precautions when using cleaning chemicals.

Dental nurses must therefore ensure that they are familiar with the following:

- Where the health and safety policy is kept
- Its contents
- The details of any updates or amendments to the policy
- The changes required in their actions following the updates or amendments

When dental nurses are called upon to act as emergency first aiders away from the dental workplace (such as coming upon the scene of a car crash), the knowledge and skills they have in relation to health and safety must be adapted accordingly. They must use their common sense in the emergency situation to ensure that no one else is put at risk while attempting to help any casualties.

Knowledge and use of emergency equipment

All dental workplaces should have first aid provision available for their employees, in the form of a first aid box (Figure 1.8) that is in an easily accessible position and highlighted with a typical poster showing a white cross on a green background (Figure 1.9).

In a workplace of five or more employees, at least one person should be trained as an emergency first aider, although having as many trained staff as possible is ideal so that holiday periods and sick leave are covered too. The contents of the first aid box will have been chosen in light of the risk assessment carried out on the premises, and should include all of the following items in the dental workplace as a minimum:

- Emergency first aid booklet – as a quick reference guide
- Assorted waterproof plasters
- Eye pads
- Assorted medium and large dressings, with scissors
- Triangular bandage and safety pins to secure once applied
- Sealed cleansing wipe packets
- Face shield for non-contact mouth-to-mouth resuscitation
- Burn shield
- Finger dressings
- Space blanket to maintain body temperature
- "Micropore" tape
- Non-latex clinical gloves

Suitable first aid training will cover the use of each item. When the dental nurse has received training it is advisable to maintain a similar first aid box for personal use away from the dental workplace; it could be stored in the car, for example. Some of the items will have "use by" dates,

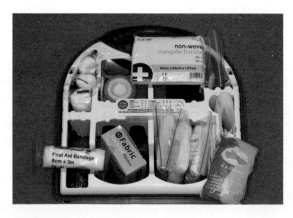

Figure 1.8   A first aid box.

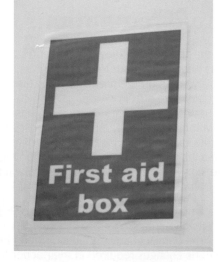

Figure 1.9   A first aid box location poster.

and there must be a simple process in place to ensure that they are checked on a regular basis so that items can be replaced as necessary. This should be a duty of the first aider and must be delegated within the workplace accordingly.

In addition to the first aid kit, the dental workplace must also have certain specialist resuscitation equipment available on the premises and in good working order, and all personnel must be regularly trained in its use. The management of medical emergencies is a verifiable continuing professional development requirement for all staff in the dental workplace. Medical emergencies and their management are discussed in detail in Chapter 13.

Control of Substances Hazardous to Health (COSHH)

Many of the chemicals and other hazardous substances used in the dental workplace on a day-to-day basis can be harmful to a person's health if they are misused or if adequate precautions are not taken to prevent access by unauthorised persons. However, without these substances, the business of dentistry could not be carried out, so the continued use of the chemicals under safe conditions is the desired outcome.

Again, the determination of the level of risk from any of the chemicals or substances involved, those who may be harmed and the necessary precautions to take are all determined by carrying out a risk assessment.

The risk assessment process to be followed in this case is determined by the COSHH regulations, which require all dental workplaces to carry out a risk assessment of all the chemicals and potentially hazardous substances used on the premises, to identify those that could harm or injure staff members. Hazardous substances include any that have been labelled as **dangerous** by the manufacturer, and these are easily recognised by the use of a universal system of symbols indicating the specific hazard of the substance (Figure 1.10) – they may be classed as "toxic", "harmful", "corrosive", "irritant", and so on.

Harm may be caused if an accident occurs to expose personnel to an unusually large amount of a chemical, or if a chemical accidentally gains entry to the body (e.g. by being inhaled), or merely just by the dangerous nature of even small amounts of a chemical (e.g. mercury).

The risk assessment process follows the usual steps (as detailed previously), but the written report produced must include every potential chemical hazard found and the following specific information:

- The hazardous ingredient(s) it contains
- The nature of the risk, ideally by indicating the risk category using recognised symbols
- The possible health effects of the hazardous ingredient(s)
- The precautions required for the safe handling of the product
- Any additional hazard control methods required for its safe use
- All necessary first aid measures required in the event of an accident involving the product

The reports are then kept in a COSHH file for quick reference as necessary, and updated regularly. They should be available to the whole dental team for reference, and all staff members should sign to say they have read and understood the information. An example of a COSHH assessment sheet is shown in Figure 1.11.

The risk assessment follows the usual steps, with pertinent points to be determined as detailed in the following for each substance used in the dental practice – ranging from specific dental materials through to general cleaning agents:

- **Identify those substances that are hazardous** – by reading the manufacturer's leaflets and instruction sheets enclosed with the product, or shown on the label
- **Identify who may be harmed** – this is likely to be anyone who uses the substance, although potential public access must be taken into consideration too

Know your hazardous chemical products. Below are the four health categories:

TOXIC
– can cause damage to health at low levels
for example, mercury is toxic by inhalation

HARMFUL
– can cause damage to health
for example, some disinfectants /tray adhesives are harmful by inhalation

CORROSIVE
– may destroy living tissue on contact
for example, phosphoric acid (etchant) causes burns in contact with skin

IRRITANT
– may cause inflammation to skin and/or eyes, nose and throat
for example, some disinfectants and x-ray developer can irritate the eyes and skin

Note:
For packaged hazardous chemical products, the label (depending on the size) should contain a symbol (as above) and simple information about the hazard and the precautions required. The Safety Data Sheet will provide more detailed information and the supplier is obliged to provide this if the substance is hazardous to health and is used at work.

Figure 1.10 Symbols of Control of Substances Hazardous to Health (COSHH) risk categories. Source: *Levison's Textbook for Dental Nurses*, 11th edition (Hollins), 2013. Reproduced with permission of Wiley-Blackwell.

- **Identify how they may be harmed** – e.g. is the product hazardous on skin contact, or by inhaling fumes, or an eye irritant?
- **Evaluate the risk** – is the substance only harmful if misused or is it harmful with every use?
- **Determine whether health monitoring is required** – e.g. during exposure to mercury or nitrous oxide gas used in inhalation sedation as a conscious sedation technique
- **Control the risk** – by ensuring the substance is not misused, by providing suitable PPE, or reduce the risk as far as possible if it is harmful with every use; this may involve changing the product if the potential risk is considered too great
- **Inform all staff of the risks** – by staff meetings, and introduction of the COSHH sheets to be read and signed by all team members
- **Record the risk assessment** – keep documented evidence that the assessment has been carried out, with review and update dates recorded as necessary

While the dental nurse is an integral part of the risk assessment procedure as a member of staff, more senior dental nurses may take over the role of maintaining the COSHH files and updating them as necessary, once suitable and documented training has been given. However, all student dental nurses must receive health and safety information covering these issues as part of their induction training with their employer.

Some general safety points with regard to hazardous substances likely to be found in the dental workplace are given in the following sections.

Name of Substance						
Hazardous Ingredients						
Used for						
By whom						
Frequency						
Amount						
Nature of Risks	Chemical		Flammable		Poisonous	Biological
Exposure Limits	OES (MEL if applicable)		ppm		mg m^{-3}	
	Long term (8 hr TWA)		–			
			–			
Other						
Health Effects						
Eye contact						
Skin contact						
Inhalation						
Ingestion						
Precautions for Safe Handling and Use						
Spillage						
Waste disposal						
Storage						
Control Measures						
Ventilation						
Eye protection						
Respiratory protection						
Gloves						
Health monitoring						
Staff training						
Other						
First Aid Measures						
Eye contact						
Skin contact						
Inhalation						
Ingestion						

Dentists and staff members to sign to confirm these Control Measures are carried out:

1 .... 4 .... 7 ....
2 .... 5 .... 8 ....
3 .... 6 .... 9 ....

Figure 1.11 Example of a Control of Substances Hazardous to Health (COSHH) assessment sheet. Source: *Levison's Textbook for Dental Nurses*, 11th edition (Hollins), 2013. Reproduced with permission of Wiley-Blackwell.

Storage

All chemicals should be stored in the dental workplace as follows:

- In cupboards/rooms away from public access, or in locked cupboards/rooms in areas of public access
- In separate fire-resistant locked storage facilities for inflammable substances and poisons
- At the ideal storage temperature as indicated by the manufacturer's instructions (this is usually room temperature of 20°C or less)
- Mercury must be stored in a cool cupboard in properly sealed containers
- Oxygen and nitrous oxide cylinders should ideally be stored outdoors, but if this is not possible, a well-ventilated fire-resistant storage area should be used
- Larger cylinders should be secured in an upright position so that they cannot fall over and be punctured or harm someone
- An appropriate trolley should be available for moving heavy cylinders

Exceptions to these storage requirements are emergency oxygen cylinders, which must remain in easy access locations throughout the dental workplace at all times.

Ventilation and temperature control

Suitable ventilation in the dental workplace can be achieved simply by having windows open, or by the use of extractor fans that are positioned so that they do not exhaust directly onto any passers-by. Air conditioning units may also be installed, but the correct location of their vents and adequate system maintenance are crucial to prevent the risk of passers-by contracting Legionnaires' disease. Units that use recycled air are not recommended for the dental workplace, as they will allow airborne contamination to cross-infect other persons.

Where nitrous oxide gas is used during inhalation sedation sessions, the waste gas must be removed by a suitable scavenging system to prevent the build-up of harmful levels of the gas in the surgery.

In summary, then, adequate ventilation is essential to prevent the accumulation of hazardous vapours and gases, and in this way to minimise any risk of harm from them. This is particularly relevant to dangerous or irritant vapours from mercury, some disinfectants, nitrous oxide and some laboratory chemicals.

The temperature within the dental workplace is usually maintained by the central heating system in cooler months and by adequate ventilation throughout the summer. While the minimum working temperature should be no less than 16°C, there is no maximum temperature above which work should stop.

However, higher temperatures usually allow for a greater volume of vapours, gases and fumes to develop, so in warmer periods the ideal is to maintain a temperature of around 20°C – "room temperature".

Occupational hazardous chemicals

In the dental workplace, there are three hazardous substances used on a daily basis by most staff that require special mention in relation to COSHH:

- Mercury
- Acid etchant
- Bleach (and other disinfectants)

Mercury

Mercury is a liquid metal that is mixed with various metal powders to form dental amalgam – a material used to fill teeth. Mercury is classed as a hazardous substance because it is toxic and it can enter the body in the following ways:

- **Inhalation** – toxic vapours are released from uncovered sources at room temperature and above, and are particularly hazardous because they are colourless and odourless and therefore difficult to detect
- **Absorption** – particles can be absorbed through the skin, nail beds and eye membranes, and eventually become lodged in the kidneys
- **Ingestion** – particles can contaminate foodstuffs and drinks, and be taken into the digestive system and eventually lodge in the kidneys

Dental amalgam is still the commonest material used to fill teeth, so mercury is present in significant amounts in the majority of dental workplaces. Exposure to the hazards mercury poses cannot easily be avoided, but the risks can be minimised by following simple rules designed to limit the chances of staff contact.

Inhalation

- Ensure that the workplace is adequately ventilated and kept at a reasonable working temperature, so that fumes do not build up
- Avoid placing mercury and waste amalgam near heat sources (including sunny windowsills), as more fumes are given off at higher temperatures
- Use pre-loaded amalgam capsules (Figure 1.12) so that bottles of mercury do not have to be stored on the premises
- Store all waste amalgam in special sealed tubs containing a mercury absorption chemical (Figure 1.13)
- Similarly, used amalgam capsules must be stored in special sealed tubs, as it is likely that tiny amounts of mercury will remain in them after use (Figure 1.14)
- Ensure every trace of amalgam is removed from instruments before they are sterilised in the autoclave, otherwise fumes will be released as the autoclave heats up
- If a mercury spillage occurs, wear appropriate PPE, including a face mask, to avoid inhalation

Absorption

- Always wear the correct PPE when handling amalgam capsules and waste amalgam, to avoid skin, nail and eye contact
- Open-toed shoes must not be worn in the surgery area, to avoid absorption through the feet if any amalgam or mercury is spilled

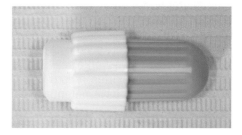

Figure 1.12   A pre-loaded amalgam capsule.

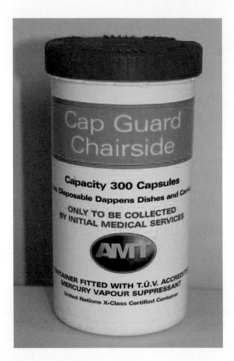

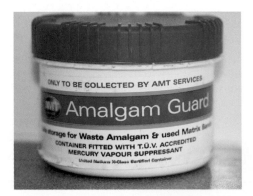

Figure 1.13 A waste amalgam tub.   **Figure 1.14** A tub for waste amalgam capsules.

- Always wear safety goggles or a face visor when old amalgam fillings are being removed, so that stray specks do not enter the eyes
- If a mercury spillage occurs, wear gloves and safety goggles to avoid skin or eye contact

Ingestion

- Food and drink must never be consumed in the surgery area
- Stocks of mercury and amalgam capsules must not be stored within the staff bathroom
- Waste amalgam containers must not be stored within the staff rest room

Handling of mercury spillages

The use of capsulated amalgam products will limit the likelihood of a large mercury spillage, but the capsules themselves can rupture during use, releasing liquid mercury into the environment, although on a much smaller scale.

All spillages of mercury, no matter how small, must be reported to the responsible person and recorded in the workplace "accident book" (Figure 1.15). The responsible person will vary between dental workplaces and may be a senior dental colleague, a line manager or supervisor, a hospital section leader or a designated health and safety person. Dental nurses will be required to be able to identify the responsible person in their own workplace.

The accident book entry will provide a written record of any accident or incident that has occurred on the premises, and which could have potentially harmed someone. It must include details of the following:

- The date and location of the accident/incident
- Who was affected
- The names of any witnesses

Once completed tear along perforation and store securely
Report Number

Accident Report Book

1 Person affected/injured
Name
Home Address
Postcode
Occupation   Works No.

2 Person reporting the incident - if other than injured person
Name
Home Address

Occupation   Postcode
Department   Date   /   /

3 Accident/incident
Date   /   /   Time
Place/Room
Equipment/machinery involved

4 Description of incident - including cause and nature of injury

Action taken/recommendations

Signed   Date   /   /

Employer please initial box if accident reportable under RIDDOR
(Reporting of Injuries, Diseases and Dangerous Occurrences Regulations 1995)

Figure 1.15   A page of an accident book.

- Details of the accident/incident
- Actions taken to assist those affected

In the unfortunate event of any long-term health effects, this report will provide valuable evidence about whether correct procedures were followed, and whether the accident/incident was unavoidable or not.

If mercury is spilled, it tends to form into liquid globules or small balls. In this shape, the liquid can easily roll around and be difficult to pick up; indeed larger globules often break into smaller ones when attempts are made to handle them. The correct actions to take after a mercury spillage are therefore very important, to prevent further contamination and spread into the workplace environment.

If there is a **small spillage**:

- Wear suitable PPE
- Suck up small globules into a disposable plastic syringe or a dedicated bulb aspirator (Figures 1.16 and 1.17)
- Put the particles into the waste amalgam special waste container
- Never use the dental suction unit, or the vacuum cleaner, to suck up spilt mercury – their use will release toxic mercury vapours into the workplace
- Alternatively, the lead foils present in intra-oral X-ray film packets can be used to gather the globules together and scoop them up, but the use of a disposable syringe is preferable

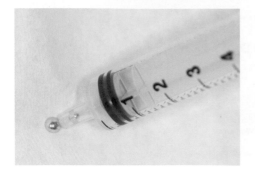

Figure 1.16 Collection of mercury droplets.

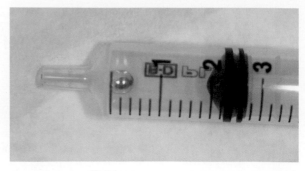

Figure 1.17 Mercury droplets collected in a syringe.

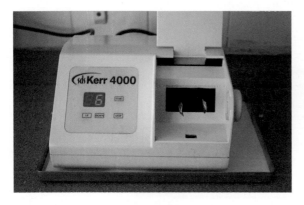

Figure 1.18 An amalgamator with a lid.

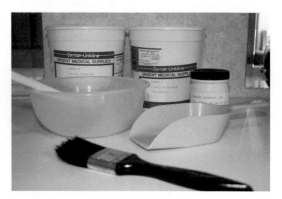

Figure 1.19 A mercury spillage kit.

To avoid the release of small globules into the workplace, the amalgamator machine should have a lid on it and be stood on a foil tray to collect any spillages without them contaminating the workplace (Figure 1.18). Any globules collected by these methods can be simply tipped into the waste amalgam store.

If there is a **larger spillage**:

- Wear suitable PPE
- Open windows to ventilate the area
- Inform the responsible person
- Use the contents of the mercury spillage kit to control the spread of the spillage (Figure 1.19)
- Mix the powders of flours of sulphur and calcium hydroxide with water to make a paste, and paint this around the spillage to contain it
- The remaining paste can be painted over the spillage
- Once dry, the contaminated paste and spillage are wiped up thoroughly with damp paper towels and disposed of in the waste amalgam store

If the size of the spillage is significant, such as a full bottle of mercury, or if globules roll into inaccessible areas, the work area must be sealed off and closed down. The HSE must be informed of the spillage, and Environmental Health will attend to clear away the contamination professionally and safely.

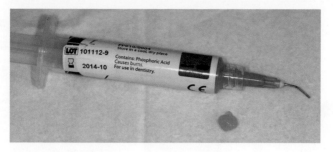

Figure 1.20 An acid etchant gel.

Acid etchant

This material is used during the placement of composite (tooth-coloured) fillings. As the name suggests, it is acidic and can therefore burn soft tissues inside the patient's mouth or the skin of those handling it. The material itself is 33% phosphoric acid and comes as either a liquid or a gel (Figure 1.20).

All staff handling the etchant must be wearing the correct PPE, and when placed within the patient's mouth it must be confined to the tooth undergoing restoration. Very careful aspiration must be used while the material is washed off the tooth, so that it does not fall elsewhere and burn the patient's oral mucosa. To help with this, the acid etchant is usually brightly coloured so that it is easily visible – some manufacturers produce a bright pink liquid, others a bright blue gel.

The manufacturer's instructions for use will show the necessary symbol indicating that it is a hazardous substance and will provide details of the first aid actions to be taken should an accident occur, in accordance with COSHH regulations.

Bleach (and other disinfectants)

With the major emphasis on robust infection control in all healthcare environments nowadays, including the dental workplace, exposure to many types of disinfectant throughout the working day is the norm for all staff. Some disinfectants can irritate the skin, the airway and the eyes when used carelessly, while others can cause irritation or initiate hypersensitivity or even allergic reactions in staff, no matter how low their exposure to the disinfectant. PPE consisting of gloves, mask and glasses should be worn when handling them and working areas must be well ventilated to avoid irritation of the airway. Manufacturers' instructions must always be followed, in particular the first aid advice recorded in the COSHH file in the event of an accident.

Having said that, all disinfectants have a huge role to play in the decontamination of work areas and fixed equipment in the dental practice. Bleach (sodium hypochlorite) is a powerful disinfectant and is used in many situations in the workplace:

- Fresh solution (10 000ppm ~ 1%) to disinfect all non-metallic, non-fabric surfaces within the surgery
- Fresh solution to disinfect impressions and removable prostheses before transferring between the patient and the laboratory
- Fresh solution to clean away blood spillages within the surgery

Other disinfectants used for surface and laboratory item decontamination include a variety of anti-microbial and isopropyl alcohol solutions, often also sold as spray solutions or pre-soaked wipes (Figure 1.21).

Bleach has an unpleasant taste and smell, and is a chemical irritant to soft tissues. It can cause tissue damage to the mouth and digestive tract, the eyes and the lungs if strong vapours are

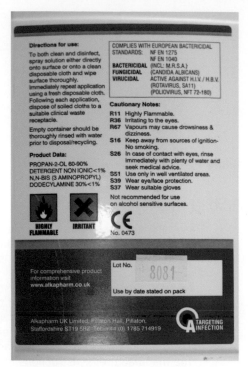

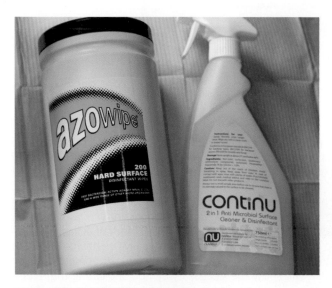

Figure 1.21   Examples of disinfectants.

Figure 1.22   Bottle label displaying hazard symbol.

inhaled. Appropriate PPE must be worn whenever it is handled and fresh solutions made daily for the uses indicated earlier should be held in lidded containers, so that the noxious chlorine vapours do not become overpowering.

Disinfectant bottles of any solutions used will show the necessary hazardous substance symbol, and give the necessary first aid actions in the event of an accident, in line with the COSHH regulations (Figure 1.22).

Reporting of Injuries, Diseases, and Dangerous Occurrences Regulations (RIDDOR)

From time to time an accident may occur within the dental workplace and the dental nurse must be aware of the correct procedure to be followed in each instance. Accidents that occur in the workplace fall into one of two categories:

- **Minor accidents** – these result in no serious injury to persons or the premises, and are dealt with "in house" and recorded in the accident book:
  - A written record of the minor accident must be made and kept by the workplace in the accident book, under the Notification of Accidents and Dangerous Occurrences Regulations (see Figure 1.15)
  - Examples of minor accidents include a trip or fall resulting in no serious injury, a clean (non-infectious) needlestick injury, or a minor mercury spillage that can be safely dealt with using the spillage kit

- **Major accidents** – these result in a serious injury to a person, or severe damage to the premises; they are classed as "significant events" and are therefore **notifiable incidents** that must be reported to the HSE under RIDDOR

Notifiable incidents do not include those occurring to a patient while undergoing dental treatment, but do cover all persons on the premises otherwise.

Once notified, the HSE will carry out an investigation into how the incident occurred, to determine whether it was purely an accident or whether the practice or a staff member was at fault. Advice will then be given on how to avoid similar incidents in future, but in serious cases prosecution may follow.

Dental nurses should remember that, once qualified and registered with the GDC, they are personally responsible for their own errors and acts of omission under health and safety law – so it may be that they are the ones who are prosecuted. While in the dental workplace as a student, the trainee dental nurse is under the supervision of a more senior colleague at any one time, and that senior person will be the one held accountable for any event under RIDDOR. The only exception to this would be if written records proved that the trainee had received the correct training in health and safety issues, but had knowingly and blatantly disregarded them, resulting in the occurrence of the notifiable incident.

The significant events covered by the regulations fall into one of three categories – injuries, diseases, or dangerous occurrences. Further information is available at www.hse.gov.uk/riddor.

As with any other workplace, the occurrence of an accidental injury while on the premises is a rare event in the dental world – but nevertheless injuries can, and do, happen. Minor injuries, as discussed earlier, are handled "in house" as they are not life-changing or do not result in serious harm. However, major injuries do result in serious harm or even death to the casualty.

The **injuries that must be reported** are:

- Fracture of the skull, spine or pelvis
- Fracture of the long bone of an arm or leg
- Amputation of a hand or foot
- Loss of sight in one eye
- Hypoxia (oxygen deprivation to the brain) severe enough to produce unconsciousness
- Any other injury requiring 24-hour hospital admission for treatment

The dental team may be exposed to common diseases in the workplace on a daily basis from patients (such as with simple colds or chest infections), or they may be exposed away from the workplace – in this case they are at risk of transmitting the infection to others in the workplace themselves. Dental personnel are also at risk of exposure to more serious pathogens by direct contact with infected blood and saliva from patients, and particularly from an inoculation injury.

The risk of infection by airborne diseases is increased significantly when the workplace is inadequately ventilated or poorly temperature-controlled, and through the possibility of cross-infection when the workplace is inadequately cleaned.

The **diseases that must be reported** under RIDDOR are any that cause acute ill health as a result of infection with dangerous pathogens or infectious materials, such as:

- Legionella – causing Legionnaires' disease
- Hepatitis B or hepatitis C infection – both linked to the development of liver cancer
- Human immunodeficiency virus (HIV) – causing acquired immune deficiency syndrome (AIDS)

In the hospital environment or in those with poor personal hygiene, dental personnel may also be exposed to, or even transmit, other dangerous pathogens, such as methicillin-resistant *Staphylococcus aureus* (MRSA – referred to as one of the "superbugs" by the lay public), or *Clostridium difficile* (an intestinal microorganism associated with diarrhoea and tetanus).

A dangerous occurrence is a significant event that could result in a serious injury or death to anyone on the premises at the time that it happens. It would result in the attendance by the emergency services (ambulance, firefighters and/or police) as well as specialists in service provision, depending on the cause (e.g. gas, electricity, service engineer, environmental health officer). The **dangerous occurrences that must be reported** are:

- Explosion, collapse or burst of a pressure vessel (an autoclave or compressor)
- Electrical short circuit or overload that causes more than a 24-hour stoppage of business
- Explosion or fire due to gases or inflammable products that causes more than a 24-hour stoppage of business
- Uncontrolled release or escape of mercury vapour due to a major mercury spillage
- Any accident involving the inhalation, ingestion or absorption of a hazardous substance that results in hypoxia that is severe enough to require medical treatment

Several of the dangerous occurrences listed involve a catastrophic failing of an electrically operated equipment item, resulting in a fire or an explosion. Fire is a daily hazard that can occur in any workplace and, as discussed previously, a risk assessment of the dental workplace will identify several specific fire hazards.

In addition to the fire potential from chemicals and gases, all dental equipment is electrically operated and may short circuit, malfunction or spark and cause a fire at any time, especially if not serviced and maintained correctly. Of equal importance is the fact that all electrical items and equipment are handled and operated correctly by all members of staff at all times, so that the risk of a dangerous occurrence is reduced to a minimum. Dental nurses have a duty to behave in a way that does not endanger the health and safety of anyone (including themselves) while on the premises, and not to use items, materials or equipment in a way that would put someone at risk of harm.

The health and safety requirements and protocols to be followed may have to vary between workplaces – those suitable for a hospital may not be relevant for a small dental practice, for example – and dental nurses must be familiar with any variations between workplaces and act accordingly. Sensible precautions to avoid accidents that should apply to all workplaces, however, include the following:

- **Surgery area** – no trailing wires from electrical equipment; good ventilation at all times; all chemicals stored away safely and securely when not in use
- **Reception and waiting room** – no trailing wires from electrical equipment; heaters surrounded with a guard to prevent burns; floor uncluttered to avoid trips; display cabinets not overloaded
- **Kitchen and staff rest room** – kept hygienically clean and tidy; no storage of stock or waste materials in food fridge; cupboards not overloaded; all equipment undergone portable appliance testing (PAT)
- **Store rooms** – no access to anyone except staff members; floors uncluttered
- **Stairs** – double hand rails for ease of use; uncluttered steps; stair covering kept in good repair

Waste disposal

The current legislation and regulations in relation to the safe disposal of hazardous waste apply to all healthcare waste producers, which includes all dental workplaces. Healthcare waste is of particular concern for environmental and personal safety because, by its nature, it is likely to be contaminated with body fluids or body parts and could therefore potentially cross-infect anyone who handles it. This may be dental personnel or waste management contractors as well as the public, if the waste is not disposed of safely. In addition, if hazardous waste is not disposed of correctly, it may also pose an environmental contamination issue, such as the incorrect disposal of amalgam waste causing mercury contamination in a landfill site.

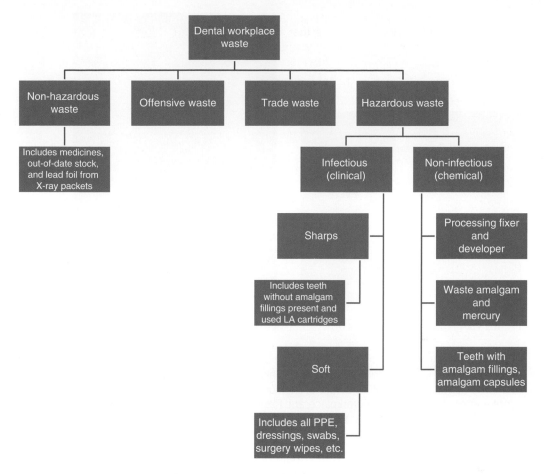

Figure 1.23   Current waste classifications relevant to the dental workplace. PPE, personal protective equipment; LA, local anaesthetic.

Some waste products in the dental workplace will pose a greater risk of cross-infection than others, while other waste products are hazardous by their chemical nature and possible toxicity. All must be correctly segregated, safely stored and then handed over to a licensed waste contractor to be disposed of in a suitable manner.

Dental workplaces produce a wide range of both hazardous and non-hazardous wastes, and in order to segregate the waste correctly, it must first be identified and then classified in line with the current regulatory guidance. The legislation that sets out which waste products must be classed as hazardous is contained in the Special Waste and Hazardous Waste Regulations (2005). The current waste classifications relevant to the dental workplace are shown in Figure 1.23.

Offensive waste is defined as "wastes which are non-infectious, do not require specialist treatment or disposal but may cause offence to those coming into contact with it". In the dental workplace this will include any PPE, cleaning towels, X-ray films and other similar items that have not been contaminated with body fluids, medicines, chemicals or amalgam, as well as toilet hygiene waste. Trade waste includes items such as dental equipment (dental chairs, curing lights, portable suction units, etc.), as well as commercial electronic waste like computer screens, televisions, fluorescent lighting tubes and batteries.

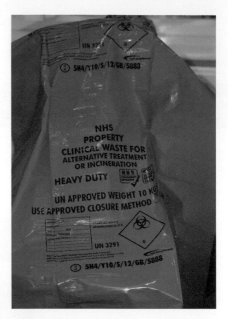

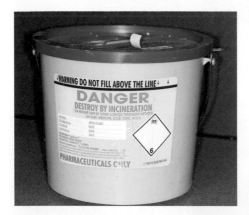

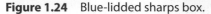

Figure 1.24   Blue-lidded sharps box.   **Figure 1.25**   An orange hazardous waste sack.

Each category of waste must be segregated and stored in the correct container, so that it is easily recognised by the waste contractors and can also be handled safely without any risk of cross-infection. The dental nurse must be aware of the correct segregation categories and the correct storage containers to be used in their workplace, and follow the waste storage and disposal policy at all times.

Details of the storage containers to be used are as follows:

- Offensive waste – yellow sack with black stripe, tied at the neck
- Non-hazardous medicines and out-of-date stock – blue-lidded yellow rigid container (Figure 1.24)
- Soft infectious (clinical) hazardous waste – orange sack, no more than three-quarters full and tied at the neck (Figure 1.25)
- Sharps infectious (clinical) hazardous waste – all yellow rigid container, no more than two-thirds full (Figure 1.26)
- Non-infectious (chemical) hazardous waste:
  - Processing chemicals – separate securely lidded, rigid containers (Figure 1.27)
  - Waste amalgam/mercury – white, securely lidded container with a mercury vapour suppressant sponge insert (see Figure 1.13)
  - Amalgam-containing teeth and spent capsules – white, securely lidded containers with a mercury vapour suppressant sponge insert (see Figure 1.14)

Dental nurses will be required to demonstrate the ability to handle waste safely and dispose of it appropriately during observation sessions with their assessor.

In accordance with the Environmental Protection Act, the duty of care is with the dental workplace to ensure that healthcare waste is managed and disposed of safely and correctly. To comply fully, managers of every dental workplace must ensure that they:

- Have a written healthcare waste policy in place which identifies a named person as responsible for waste management on the premises (referred to as the "registered manager" in HTM 01-05)
- Provide staff access to the policy and give recorded training in correct waste management methods

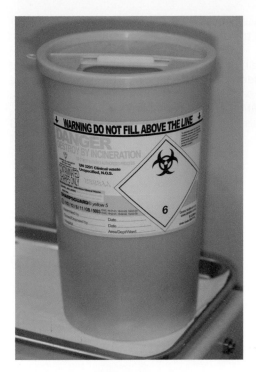

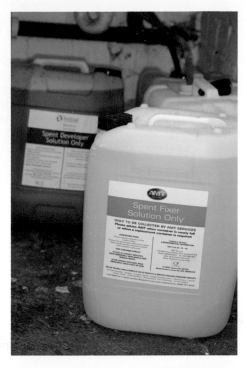

Figure 1.26   A sharps box.   **Figure 1.27**   Waste processing chemical storage drums.

- Segregate waste in accordance with Figure 1.23 and store it safely while on the premises, away from public access
- Use the correct storage containers for each waste category
- Only use licensed waste collectors for the removal from the premises and disposal of the waste at an authorised disposal site
- Accurately describe the container contents of all non-hazardous waste on transfer notes, which must be kept for a minimum of two years from the date of collection
- Accurately describe the container contents of all hazardous waste on consignment notes, which must be kept for a minimum of 3 years from the date of collection
- Receive and keep the quarterly "consignee returns" documentation, which records the final destination of the hazardous waste consignment, and its disposal details
- Register with the Environment Agency as a hazardous waste producer if more than 500 kg of hazardous waste is produced annually

Waste handling training

All dental personnel who are likely to be involved in handling any healthcare waste must be correctly trained to do so. The training should cover all of the following points:

- Risks associated with each category of waste (such as sharps injury, exposure to toxic vapours, cross-infection)
- Correct classification, segregation and storage procedures, in line with the healthcare waste policy of the workplace
- COSHH information on all non-infectious hazardous waste chemicals used on the premises
- Safe handling, including the use of appropriate PPE and moving techniques

- Correct procedures in the event of spillages or accidents
- Correct completion of relevant documentation – transfer notes and consignment notes

The avoidance of cross-infection when handling hazardous waste relies on dental nurses wearing the appropriate PPE at all times, following the infection control policy of the workplace, and ensuring that their own immunity from the relevant pathogens is up to date, through vaccination. This is especially important with regard to immunisation against hepatitis B.

The principles of infection control, including details of pathogens and immunity, are discussed in detail in Chapter 12.

Ionising radiation

Ionising radiation, in the form of X-rays, is widely used in dentistry as a diagnostic and treatment tool. However, there is no "safe" level of use of ionising radiation – every X-ray exposure can cause some amount of tissue damage in the patient, or indeed anyone else in the imaging area who is exposed to the X-ray beam. An overdose can cause serious health effects, ranging from a mild burn to leukaemia and, ultimately, death.

For this reason, specific legislation is in place to ensure full compliance with the health and safety aspects of ionising radiation by all dental workplaces, under the following regulations:

- Ionising Radiation Regulations 1999 (IRR99)
- Ionising Radiation (Medical Exposure) Regulations 2000 (IR(ME)R2000)

While IRR99 is concerned with the protection of staff and IR(ME)R with the protection of patients, the aim of both sets of regulations is to keep the numbers of X-ray exposures, and their dose levels, to the absolute minimum required for clinical necessity, at all times.

In relation to these regulations, dental nurses must be fully knowledgeable of the following:

- Actions they can take in relation to imaging procedures
- Actions they cannot take in relation to imaging procedures
- How to protect patients and others from unwanted ionising radiation exposure

The safe use of dental radiography is discussed in detail in Chapter 14, and the roles and responsibilities of dental nurses in ensuring that they reduce the risks to themselves and others during the use of ionising radiation are reiterated here.

In relation to IRR99 the dental nurse must have received documented training and then comply with the following:

- Local rules in association with each X-ray machine in the dental workplace, in particular:
  - Location of the 1.5-metre controlled area and the 2-metre safety zone (Figure 1.28)
  - Location of the isolator switch in case of malfunction
  - Contingency plan in case of malfunction
  - Name of the radiation protection supervisor (RPS) in the workplace, as the person to contact in case of malfunction
  - Methods in place to ensure that no person but the patient can enter the controlled area during exposure, and to follow them at all times
- The dental workplace requirements with regard to the use of monitoring badges
- The GDC's continuing professional development requirements with regard to ionising radiation updates, which is a core topic

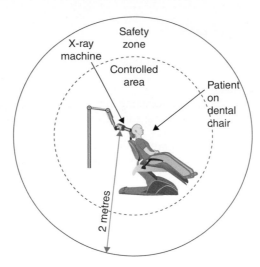

Figure 1.28   Controlled area and safety zone. Source: *Levison's Textbook for Dental Nurses*, 11th edition (Hollins), 2013. Reproduced with permission of Wiley-Blackwell.

In relation to IR(ME)R 2000, dental nurses must have received documented training and then comply with the following:

- Only carry out those duties that they are legally able to, specifically:
  - Patient identification
  - Setting up the resources to enable exposure to occur
  - Pressing the exposure button, but only when requested by the "set up" operator
  - Processing and mounting of radiographs
  - Contribute to quality assurance programmes
- Correctly store dental films so that they do not become damaged before use
- Maintain processing equipment correctly, so that re-takes are not necessary
- Use processing chemicals correctly to avoid accidents and be aware of COSHH guidelines in relation to any accident and follow them accordingly
- Maintain the security of controlled areas at all times in accordance with the workplace policies, to avoid the possibility of accidental exposures

If any processing chemicals are accidentally spilled, the following actions should be taken:

- Remove all other persons from the area, to avoid the inhalation of any fumes as well as to avoid someone slipping on the wet floor
- Erect the "wet floor" hazard sign
- Ventilate the area if possible to remove the chemical fumes – these are not harmful as such, but they are strong-smelling and may be irritant to such persons as asthmatics
- Apply appropriate PPE – rubber gloves, safety glasses, face mask, and plastic apron
- Cover the spillage with paper towels to soak up the chemicals, or mop up the excess liquid and carefully pour it into the appropriate storage drum
- Once the liquid has been removed, wash the floor area with a suitable detergent solution and leave the hazard sign in place until the area is completely dry
- Complete the accident book, if relevant, and review the incident to determine if changes are required in the handling and use of the processing chemicals, including further staff training

Occupational hazards

The three major occupational hazards in dentistry are:

- Exposure to ionising radiation
- Exposure to high levels of mercury, resulting in mercury poisoning
- Exposure to pathogens, resulting in cross-infection

All three hazards are relevant to the dental nurse, and they must be trained to be aware of the dangers and know how to avoid them. The hazards associated with ionising radiation and mercury are described earlier, and cross-infection by inoculation injury is covered in the next section.

Inoculation injury

This is an injury caused by the piercing of the skin (or other membrane) by a sharp object, and in this context the sharp object involved is usually a dental instrument or needle. Nearly all dental procedures involve the use of sharp items; these include local anaesthetic needles, sharp instruments such as probes, and scalpel blades. All must be handled with great care by staff to avoid an inoculation injury.

Every dental workplace must have a policy in place to avoid a sharps injury and it should ideally include all of the following points:

- The operator using a local anaesthetic needle should be the person responsible for its re-sheathing and safe placement in a sharps bin, so that injury to others does not occur as there is no transference of the sharp item from one person to another
- Needle guards should be used when re-sheathing needles, so that they can be placed in their plastic sheath without being held with the fingers (Figure 1.29)
- Heavy-duty rubber gloves and full PPE should be worn by any staff responsible for instrument cleaning and debridement before sterilisation

Although a sharps injury from a sterile, unused instrument may be momentarily painful, it is of no consequence save to reconsider the level of care taken by the staff member involved. However, if a contaminated inoculation injury occurs as a result of an object which has been used on a patient, the following actions must be carried out:

- Stop all treatment immediately and attend to the wound
- Squeeze the wound to encourage bleeding, but do not suck it
- Wash the area with soap and running water, then dry and cover the wound with a waterproof dressing
- Note the name, address and contact details of the source patient if a contaminated item is involved, so that their medical history can be checked immediately
- Complete the accident book
- Report the incident to the senior dentist/line manager
- The consultant microbiologist at the local hospital must be contacted immediately if the source patient is a known or suspected HIV or hepatitis C carrier, as emergency antiviral treatment must commence within 1 hour of the injury

The contact details for the consultant microbiologist should be readily available in the infection control policy documentation, and updated whenever necessary.

Dental nurses will be required to demonstrate their ability to deal with an inoculation injury during observation sessions with their assessor.

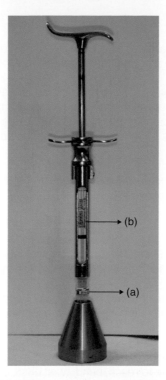

Figure 1.29   A re-sheathing device. (a) Needle guard in place. (b) Syringe re-sheathed in the device.

General safety measures

These relate to any work premises where any staff are employed to provide a service to the public, and therefore apply to all dental workplaces, whether they are practices, clinics or hospital departments. Those in the following list are all common-sense precautions aimed at preventing injury to anyone using or visiting the premises, and dental nurses should report any issues they discover to the responsible person in their workplace if they come across anything they believe to be a potential hazard.

General safety measures in the dental workplace should include all of the following:

- A safe means of entry which is adequately lit and unobstructed, including for disabled people
- Non-slip floor coverings which are secure, to prevent tripping
- No dust traps in the décor of surgical areas, such as those present with embossed wallpaper coverings
- No sharp edges on furniture and fittings
- Guards around fires and heaters to avoid burns
- No trailing electrical cables that could cause tripping
- All portable electrical appliances must be inspected yearly for wear and tear – this is called PAT testing, and may be carried out by any approved person as long as written records are kept
- All electric appliances should be disconnected overnight as a matter of routine, although this may not be possible with some items, such as a fridge or the main computer server
- A fully stocked first aid kit should be available for minor injuries

Manual handling

The other important area of general safety for the dental nurse is that involving any moving or lifting work, which may cause personal injury if not done correctly. This is collectively referred to as manual handling.

In the majority of dental workplaces, the usual manual handling that occurs is the transport of boxes containing stock items, or the movement of waste containers in and out of storage. Hospital departments and dental clinics may also require staff to be involved with the movement of disabled, sedated or unconscious patients, and separate and specific training must be given in these areas by the employer.

Lifting heavy or awkward items incorrectly can result in all kinds of injuries to staff, and employers must ensure that, as far as is reasonably practicable, they adhere to the regulations laid down in the Manual Handling Operations Regulations 1992. These were further revised in 2002, and state the following:

- All hazardous manual handling should be avoided, as far as is reasonably practicable
- Any hazardous manual handling that cannot be avoided must be correctly risk-assessed
- All efforts must then be made to reduce the risk of injury as far as possible

While carrying out the risk assessment of any manual handling and lifting that has to be carried out in the dental workplace, the following points must be considered when deciding whether the task is hazardous or not:

- The weight and dimensions of the object being moved or lifted
- The likelihood of staff having to reach, bend, twist or stoop while moving or handling the object
- The frequency of the task
- The likelihood of excessive movements being required, such as pushing or pulling
- The distance that the object has to be moved
- The need for the object to be carried up or down stairs
- The physical ability of the staff involved in moving and handling
- The existence of any medical conditions that contraindicate staff from moving or handling objects (this includes pregnancy)
- The need for any training to be given in the correct techniques of moving and handling

If each point is taken separately, it can be seen that much can be done to avoid injury to staff during moving and handling activities.

Weight and dimensions

The heavier the load and the greater its dimensions, the more difficult it will be to handle and the more likely it is that injury will occur, so consider the following:

- Split the load to make it lighter
- Ask other staff to help while lifting and moving it
- Use a trolley or other handling aids, if available

Awkward movements and frequency

Examples of these include twisting, and bending while lifting or moving a load – and the more times the move is carried out, the more likely it is to cause injury, so consider the following:

- Clear the path of travel before lifting, to avoid having to twist, etc.
- Move the feet to change direction, rather than twisting, etc.

- When precise positioning is required, put the load down then adjust its position
- When loads have to be moved frequently, use a trolley or other handling aid to avoid straining the back

Excessive movements

Pushing and pulling lighter loads do not usually cause a problem, but when heavier loads are involved, either they must be split into smaller units first or a trolley or other handling aid must be used.

In most instances, large boxes of stock can be opened and put into their place of storage individually, to avoid having to push or pull them into position.

Distance and stairs

It makes sense to move objects the minimum distance whenever possible and to avoid having to carry them up and down stairs manually. Where stock is stored should be carefully considered, to avoid repetitive strain injuries to staff, and a lift must always be used if available. Otherwise, a trolley or other handling aid needs to be provided.

Physical ability and medical conditions

Elderly or unfit staff members are more likely to injure themselves while moving and handling, by over-estimating their own capabilities, and the following must be considered:

- Elderly staff tend not to be as strong as younger staff and may have less stamina to hold a load for any length of time
- Overweight staff will find it difficult to hold loads as close to their centre of gravity as they need to for stability, and this will put unnecessary strain on their arms and back
- Short staff will find it more difficult to lift and carry loads than taller staff
- Male staff tend to be stronger than female staff, although this cannot always be assumed to be the case
- Various medical conditions will prevent some staff from being capable of moving and handling objects without risking injury to themselves, such as back problems, heart and respiratory conditions, hernias
- Pregnant staff should not be involved in moving and handling heavy objects

Training

A correct handling technique should be taught to all staff involved in moving and lifting objects in the dental workplace, and this may involve the following:

- Sending the staff (and the employer) on a well-run training course to learn the best posture to adopt while lifting and moving loads
- Acquiring trolleys and other handling aids for the premises
- Changing the location of storage rooms, to make them closer to the delivery point and ideally at ground level
- Acquiring more storage cupboards or shelves at waist height for heavier items
- Acquiring step ladders for the placement of light loads in storage spaces above shoulder level

2

Unit 302: Reflect On and Develop Your Practice

Learning outcomes

1. Be able to identify the competence requirements of the job role
2. Be able to reflect on own performance
3. Be able to implement a plan to improve performance
4. Be able to evaluate the effectiveness of the development plan
5. Be able to comply with current legislation, policy, good practice, and organisational and professional codes of practice and ethical standards

Outcome 1 assessment criteria
The learner can:
- Identify what is required for competent, effective, and safe practice
- Provide active support for individuals and key people

Outcome 2 assessment criteria
The learner can:
- Regularly review performance in the job role
- Use constructive feedback from individuals to develop practice
- Identify supervision and support required

Outcome 3 assessment criteria
The learner can:
- Identify any actions needed to improve practice
- Prioritise aspects of practice that need to be enhanced
- Prepare SMART objectives using available resources
- Utilise development opportunities

Diploma in Dental Nursing, Level 3, Third Edition. Carole Hollins.
© 2014 John Wiley & Sons, Ltd. Published 2014 by John Wiley & Sons, Ltd.
Companion website: www.wiley.com/go/hollins/dentalnursinglevel3

Outcome 4 assessment criteria

The learner can:
- Reflect on practice following implementation of the plan
- Demonstrate improvement in practice
- Regularly review the impact of the plan on working practice
- Implement identified development opportunities

Outcome 5 assessment criteria

The learner can:
- Work in accordance with the standard operating procedures at all times
- Demonstrate compliance with legal, professional and organisational requirements, guidelines and confidentiality at all times
- Keep up-to-date records of their personal and professional development

This unit is assessed by:
- Observation in the workplace, with examples included in the learner's portfolio
- An appropriate alternative method

Dental nurses are an integral member of the dental team, and following the onset of compulsory registration with the General Dental Council (GDC) in 2008, they are now referred to as dental care professionals (DCPs) along with all other dental staff besides the dentist.

All dental nurses must now undergo formal training and achieve qualification before they can become registered with the GDC, and their registration must then be renewed on an annual basis to enable them to work legally as a dental nurse in the UK. As the GDC is the regulator of the dental professions, they have set out the outcomes that dental nurses must be able to demonstrate by the end of their training period in order to become a registrant and be deemed "fit to practise". Within a training course, demonstration of these outcomes is met through education, training and assessment, and they are therefore referred to as "learning outcomes". They are derived from the GDC's own *Standards for the Dental Team* document, and include the requirements they have set for lifelong learning to be achieved.

In the UK, student dental nurses can currently meet the training requirements by completing an approved course and passing either the City & Guilds (C&G) Level 3 Diploma in Dental Nursing examination (for which this text is written) or the National Examining Board for Dental Nurses' (NEBDN) National Diploma examination.

The curricula developed by C&G and NEBDN have also been informed by the National Occupational Standards for dental nursing. These are developed by Skills for Health (www.skillsforhealth.org.uk), which has worked alongside the GDC to ensure that these standards are fit for purpose within the qualifications that may lead to GDC registration.

The National Occupational Standards for any work activity (not just dental nursing) define what a competent person should know and be able to do when carrying out that role, and are used to help in future learning and qualification development for that job role.

The GDC learning outcomes have also been developed so that students who achieve them can be said to be competent – they can practise safely, effectively and professionally as dental nurses. The learning outcomes are set out in the GDC publication, *Preparing for Practice – Dental Team Learning Outcomes for Registration*, which, once achieved, demonstrate that the student has the knowledge, skills, attitudes and behaviours required to become a GDC registrant.

To understand what is required from student dental nurses during their training, education and assessment, the following interpretations of these key terms may be useful:

- **Knowledge** – the underpinning, theoretical information gained from learning or experience, which gives the student understanding of a subject

- **Skills** – the special abilities acquired by learning and practice to be able to complete a task, often manually or verbally
- **Attitudes and behaviours** – the moral and ethical beliefs held by students, which demonstrate their values and priorities, and guide their actions

Students must exhibit all of these attributes to be considered as a professional dental nurse after qualification, and to be entered onto the GDC register. They must then maintain and improve upon these qualities throughout their working lives, in order to stay on the register.

The GDC learning outcomes are grouped into four domains for all registrants, and their specific relevance to the dental nurse is as follows:

- **Clinical** – described as the range of skills required to deliver direct care, where registrants interact with patients
- **Communication** – described as the skills involved in effectively interacting with patients, their representatives, the public and colleagues, and recording appropriate information to inform patient care
- **Professionalism** – described as the knowledge, skills and attitudes/behaviours required to practise in an ethical and appropriate way, putting patients' needs first and promoting confidence in the dental team
- **Management and leadership** – described as the skills and knowledge required to work effectively as a dental team, manage their own time and resources, and contribute to professional practices

Further details of relevant GDC publications can be found at www.gdc-uk.org.

Once qualified, however, dental nurses will be expected to develop a system of lifelong learning and continuing professional development (CPD) in line with all other registrants, so that as dentistry and dental nursing evolve and develop, new skills and information will be understood and practised by all. Qualification and compulsory registration are now the basics required by dental nurses, rather than their end goal of achievement.

To achieve this, dental nurses must be able to reflect on and develop their practice throughout their working life, and be able to demonstrate that they have done so. In effect, they must become a "reflective practitioner" by being able to achieve the following:

- Identify the competence requirements of their role as a dental nurse (see earlier)
- Reflect on their own performance in the job role
- Implement a plan to improve their own performance
- Evaluate the effectiveness of their development plan
- Comply with current legislation, policy, good practice, organisational and professional codes of practice, and ethical standards

Reflect on performance

Learning can occur on a regular basis in the workplace as dental nurses reflect on their work performance – constantly analysing, constructively criticising and evaluating themselves. The aim is to recognise their own shortcomings and act upon them to improve their overall work performance. In this way, dental nurses become **reflective practitioners**.

However, it is human nature to be subjective and tend towards being either overly critical or overly lenient when reflecting on one's own performance, as one's ideas are based on the perception one has of oneself. More constructive analysis is that carried out by others, especially more experienced colleagues who have previously gone through the learning and reflection process themselves. This is the basis for an appraisal system within the workplace, where a senior colleague acts as a mentor for a more junior colleague, and gives verbal and written feedback on their performance (see later).

This can be carried out on a daily basis initially, with new employees being "shadowed" by senior colleagues so that problems and shortfalls can be identified and addressed early in the learning process through the use of constructive criticism. This is the term used to describe feedback that has been carefully considered and given to help someone improve their performance. It can be given verbally or in written or electronic format. Dental nurse students will receive various forms of feedback from their employers or senior work colleagues, from their tutor and from their assessor throughout their training course.

The two main types of reflection that occur are:

- **Reflection in action** – occurs as a situation happens
- **Reflection on action** – occurs after the event and is also referred to as "hindsight"

Reflection enables dental nurses to think about how learning occurs, especially from experience, so that their work performance becomes more effective. In particular, reflection in action should produce a thinking professional who can react effectively and appropriately to changing circumstances at the time, to produce a successful outcome for the patient and the dental team. An example of a reflection on action learning event is given here.

Compare the competence of a dental nurse when nursing for a certain procedure for the first time with what it will be when nursing for the same procedure for the fourth or fifth time. Obviously nurses will feel more comfortable as experience is gained, because subconsciously their own techniques are bettered after each event. In other words, "practice makes perfect".

So, for instance, **when aspirating for an oral surgery procedure the first time**, the following may occur:

- The nurse is unsure of all the instrument identifications, as some may be being handled for the first time
- Aspiration is not fully effective, as there is uncertainty about when to intervene without blocking the dentist's vision
- The nurse is hesitant when handling some instruments, because of a lack of familiarity
- The nurse concentrates so much on the procedure that the patient is forgotten

However, when nursing for the procedure for **the fourth or fifth time**:

- Instruments are now known because they are more familiar
- Aspiration is more effective, perhaps by learning from the fact that the first patient choked and the dentist was unable to see clearly
- The nurse is confident when handling instruments because they are more familiar
- The nurse is able to monitor and reassure the patient at the same time as performing the other duties

Use of diaries or portfolios

Reflection on action occurs by being able to think back over the procedure at a later date. This allows nurses to identify what problems were encountered and then to recognise how to improve their performance next time. Most of us carry out this second type of reflection on a regular basis, for example when driving home from work and "going over" the day's events in our minds, or by discussing our day with a family member, friend or colleague. However, we often forget the full impact of our thoughts unless we write them down at the time and review them at a later date.

Therefore, it is prudent for dental nurses to keep a diary, or portfolio, on a daily or at least a weekly basis. This helps to organise and clarify their thoughts, so that the reason why problems occurred can be discovered and **action plans** can be developed to prevent their recurrence. These activities will naturally form part of the workplace portfolio that is built up during the Level 3 Diploma training course, or the "record of experience" used for the National Diploma qualification.

A suggested layout of a diary or portfolio is as follows:

- **Describe** the event
- **Record** any thoughts and emotions
- **Evaluate** the event – giving both good and bad points
- **Critically analyse** the event – why did it happen?
- Reach a **conclusion** – what could have been done differently?
- **Develop an action plan** – what will be done differently next time?

After going through this process, it is relatively easy to determine whether a gap in knowledge, skills or experience has been identified. This information can then be used to determine what supervision and support are required to fill that gap, whether they need to be given on a formal or informal basis, and whether they can be provided in the workplace or will involve a more formal training event elsewhere.

Use of personal development plans

Self-evaluation and reflection can also be recorded in more detail in the form of a personal development plan (PDP). The PDP is used to effectively look at the following points on a personal basis:

- Professionally, where am I now?
- What qualifications, knowledge and special interests helped me to achieve this position?
- What learning needs do I have now, if any?
- Do I wish to acquire new knowledge or skills?
- What is preventing me? – carry out a **SWOT analysis** (strengths, weaknesses, opportunities, threats – see later)
- What can be done to overcome any obstacles identified?
- Collate all the information to develop a personal learning/development plan, with achievable timescales if possible
- Evaluate the PDP at least annually, to determine whether, and to what extent, the development needs that were identified have been met
- Summarise the progress made and use it to determine the desired future learning and development needs
- Keep a written record of all CPD events for each year, both verifiable and non-verifiable (see later)
- Analyse the CPD events attended to ensure that the core subjects are covered, but also to determine the necessity and relevance of the others to their personal learning and development needs

A SWOT analysis is an excellent method for determining whether the obstacles to future learning and development are identified as being of a personal nature or involve external pressures. It is used as shown in Figure 2.1.

Once the relevant points have been identified and recorded, efforts can be made to determine how to overcome the obstacles to future development. In some instances, this may be as dramatic as determining that an unsupportive employer is holding you back and that a change of workplace is required.

Use of staff appraisal

Private reflection carried out using diaries, portfolios or PDPs can give a distorted view of dental nurses' needs, because by definition they are recording their own perception of themselves. Of far more value is the input of professional colleagues, such as that provided by a system of staff appraisal where the employer or a senior colleague reviews the performance of the staff member in the workplace, to achieve the following aims:

Strengths
These are personal to the individual, and may include previous achievements as well as points such as reliability or ambition

Weaknesses
These are personal, and may include a personal lack of ambition, or home circumstances that make studying difficult

Opportunities
These are beneficial external factors which will influence success, and may include a supportive employer who encourages and funds further training

Threats
These are harmful external factors, or obstacles to future success, and may include an unsupportive employer, or lack of training opportunities

---

Figure 2.1   SWOT analysis.

- Identify the strengths and weaknesses of the staff member
- Identify the strengths and weaknesses of the running of the workplace, to give valuable information for good workplace development
- Disclose any barriers to the efficient working of the dental team
- Improve communication amongst the dental team
- Encourage problem-solving
- Reduce any negative tensions between staff members
- Improve practice morale

Annual reviews in the form of staff appraisals are a requirement under the Care Quality Commission registration process, as they provide evidence of "good practice" in the workplace by the employer. Several areas of appraisal can be carried out at one time during an annual review, or just one area can be highlighted. Common areas to consider are the following:

- Personal – hygiene, attitude, punctuality, dress code
- Administrative – policies and protocols, regulations, filing, knowledge of paperwork
- Clinical – infection control, mixing techniques, nursing skills, patient management
- Teamwork – ability to function as a team member, acceptance of authority, ability to take responsibility
- Communication – interpersonal, telephone manner, patient management
- Development – self-evaluation, self-study, attendance at courses, learning by experience

Once the relevant areas to be appraised have been selected, discussed and agreed upon, an appraisal sheet can be drawn up which gives dental nurses the opportunity to self-evaluate their performance in these areas, before being compared with the recorded comments of the workplace evaluation (Figure 2.2).

Differences of opinion regarding performance can be explored and resolved, and then an action plan can be developed to determine future goals and aims. All details should be recorded on the appraisal sheet and then copied so that both the dental nurse and the practice can refer back to it in future, to assess the level of success of that appraisal. It should also serve as a record of the dental nurse's self-development and progression within the practice, and expose any areas which continue to cause problems in future appraisals.

The areas can be adjusted to suit individual workplaces as necessary. The frequency of appraisal will also differ between workplaces as well as for different staff members. Younger, less experienced staff members are likely to require more frequent appraisal while learning all the

Areas of appraisal	Self-appraisal	Practice appraisal	Notes
Personal hygiene Dress Punctuality			
NHS procedures Rules/regulations Medico-legal knowledge			
Materials techniques Infection control Patient management X-ray procedures Equipment handling			
Courses of study Self-study Experiential learning Problem-based learning Peer group learning			
Teamwork experience Innovation Originality			
Communication skills Interpersonal skills Administrative accuracy Telephone manner Complaints handling			
APPRAISAL SUMMARY Signed. Signed. Date.			

Figure 2.2 A sample staff appraisal sheet.

relevant practice policies and protocols, and how to put them into practice. More experienced staff will need to be supportive and non-judgmental during this period.

When run correctly, appraisals can be an invaluable tool for the development of the whole dental team, so that the end result is the best possible outcome for the patient. It should identify the strengths and weaknesses not only of the staff members, but also of the workplace environment itself, indicating routes that can be taken for good workplace development. By relying on feedback and constructive criticism, it should remove any inter-staff communication barriers and improve problem-solving techniques. Overall, appraisals should improve the workforce morale by providing an opportunity for discussion without recrimination.

Implement a performance improvement plan

When self-reflection or an appraisal has determined that an improvement in performance is desired or required, dental nurses will need to draw up and implement a development plan which will determine the following points:

- What actions are needed to improve their performance?
- Which particular work activity is the most important to be tackled first? What is the priority?
- Set out the improvement plan as a "do-able" event, using SMART (specific, measurable, attainable, realistic, time-based) objectives
- What development opportunities are available and how can they be accessed?

By following this ordered process, dental nurses are more likely to be successful in their efforts to improve their own performance. The help and support available from their employer are likely to vary between workplaces, ranging from obstructive, through indifference, to fairly or fully supportive. As shown earlier, a SWOT analysis may already have determined that the dental nurse's biggest threat to success in self-improvement and career prospects is their own employer or employing organisation.

Actions needed

These will need to be identified before progressing through the implementation of the development plan; input from others may be crucial at this point if the self-improvement attempts are to be successful. As stated previously, self-analysis can often provide a skewed or biased opinion of oneself, and constructive criticism from colleagues is of far greater importance in determining our abilities and shortfalls.

The actions needed to be undertaken will depend on the work activity or performance area that the dental nurse wishes to improve upon, as follows:

- More experience – the dental nurse has received the necessary theory and underpinning knowledge to perform a task, but has had little opportunity to "put it into practice" yet (such as aspirating effectively for a certain procedure)
- More knowledge – the dental nurse has received some basic information about the topic but requires more depth of knowledge to perform the task adequately (such as knowing what affects the consistency of a dental material during its mixing, so that every mix is satisfactory)
- More training – there is a gap in knowledge and/or skills that will require further training to fulfil the dental nurses' needs (such as taking a post-registration qualification or updating current knowledge with new information)
- More support – the dental nurse has the knowledge and skills required but needs support to recognise their abilities and achieve success

Prioritising

Dental nurses may **desire** to improve their performance for personal reasons, because they are particularly interested in a certain area of dental nursing or because they simply have a thirst for knowledge. Alternatively, they may **require** improvement in their performance to enhance their career prospects, or they may need to update their knowledge to meet their registration requirements with the GDC. Required improvements must take precedence over desirable ones – there is little point in gaining a desired post-registration qualification if the core CPD subjects have not been updated as required by the GDC, as the nurse will then be unable to work anyway.

Similarly, if the area requiring a performance improvement is fundamental to the dental nurse role, such as the ability to aspirate effectively during a chairside procedure, then this skill requires enhancement as a matter of urgency. The alternative is that dental nurse will be unable to carry out their full range of work activities – this may even compromise their employment.

Input from other colleagues will be invaluable at this stage to help the prioritisation process. Indeed, a staff appraisal may have highlighted an issue in the first instance and then the subsequent action plan may well have indicated the way forward. It will also have identified any necessary help and support that the workplace can provide, such as providing funding or study leave and accessing training courses or local CPD events.

Dental nurses can also use available resources to obtain this information for themselves, such as:

- Flyers to the workplace advertising relevant events
- Adverts in dental journals
- Information on the postgraduate deanery website
- Information from the local commissioning body
- Flyers from the local training establishment advertising new courses and updates
- Information on C&G or NEBDN websites

SMART objectives

Using the available resources, dental nurses can then develop their SMART objectives to assist in the formulation of the development plan. SMART is an acronym used in business and education which helps users to focus their efforts when considering their career development pathway and how to achieve their desired/required goals – it makes their personal development plan "do-able". It is similar to but not the same as setting goals for oneself; setting objectives is more specific and should outline how the goal achievement will be measured. So a goal statement could be the broad phrase "improve my dental nursing skills", while the objectives to support this goal will detail the specific actions to be taken to achieve it (such as by attending a specific training event), determine the set timeline over which it is to be achieved (such as over two attendances), and indicate how the successful outcome will be measured (such as by gaining a certificate of competence in the specific area of training).

When used correctly, SMART objectives should help to identify the specific targets dental nurses are aiming at, and therefore also to identify the training and development opportunities that are available to achieve their aims. These objectives are used as follows:

- **Specific** – the objectives stated must be clear and well defined, and in a manner that is understood by the dental nurse's colleagues and employer
- **Measurable** – there must be a method available to measure the outcome of the activity, so that it is known when the objectives have been achieved; for example by the passing of an assessment test, or the gaining of a proficiency certificate
- **Attainable** – there must be a realistic pathway to achieving the objectives, so the end goal must be within reach of the dental nurse
- **Realistic** – achieving the objectives must be possible with the use of any available resources, within the knowledge levels of the dental nurse, and achievable within the time available
- **Time-based** – there must be a realistic time frame within which the objectives should be achieved; this must be neither too short nor too long, and must be agreed with the employer if it is likely to affect the work performance of the dental nurse

The SMART objectives can then be included in the PDP and the appraisal document, and are discussed with the employer, mentor or a senior colleague for input before the performance plan is implemented. They will then also provide a documented record of the outcomes to be achieved, which is accessible to both the dental nurse and to the person responsible for evaluating the nurse's performance and achievements.

Development opportunities

Depending on the area of performance to be improved upon and the actions needed, the dental nurse must determine what resources are available that can be accessed and utilised as development opportunities. These may range from a simple mentoring or coaching agreement with a work colleague or other professional, to attendance at a CPD event or a formal educational programme of study.

A mentor is usually a more experienced work colleague who is able to instruct, advise and support junior staff members as they develop their professional skills within the workplace. A coach is one term given to a fellow professional who is able to instruct or train dental nurses in a specific topic, and this may be someone outside the workplace. A coach may also be referred to as a tutor.

The majority of suitable development opportunities for the dental nurse are likely to be provided as CPD events or as formal educational programmes and training courses.

Continuing professional development

The professional standards, guidelines and legislation that were in place at the beginning of a dental nurse's training and initial qualification are open to improvement and change with time, as in any other job role. To maintain an acceptable level of competence in their profession, all GDC registrants must undergo update training on a regular basis as a condition of their continued registration, with the aim of retaining knowledge and improving skills, as well as being made aware of new information since qualification. To avoid team members having to constantly resit examinations to achieve this, the GDC introduced a system of CPD for all registrants. Certain CPD subjects are compulsory over a 5-year cycle and are referred to as core subjects. For the dental nurse they are as follows:

- Medical emergencies
- Disinfection and decontamination
- Radiological protection
- Legal and ethical issues
- Complaints handling

Lack of up-to-date knowledge by dental nurses in any of these areas could result in patients or colleagues being harmed or worse, or they may be found guilty of negligence or professional misconduct – that is why they are compulsory (core) topics of development. By undergoing CPD in accordance with GDC requirements, registrants will then achieve lifelong learning – every time they attend a CPD event, they will learn new information or skills throughout their professional career.

In addition, dental professionals must also undertake general CPD in topics of their own choice, so, for example, those who work in mainly orthodontic workplaces are likely to attend orthodontic events, while those who work with special needs patients are likely to attend events relevant to that speciality, and so on.

Continuing professional development is categorised as either verifiable or non-verifiable and all of the core topics must be delivered as verifiable CPD.

Verifiable CPD is that offered formally, with written specific aims and learning outcomes given by the organiser/presenter. Certificates of attendance and participation in verifiable CPD activities will be issued and must be kept as evidence of complying with the GDC's hourly requirements for CPD events (Figure 2.3). The certificates may even have to be produced as evidence of verifiable CPD activity, when requested by the GDC at the end of each 5-year cycle (that for dental nurses ends in 2013). Random checks of CPD records allow the GDC to ensure that professional obligations are being met by its registrants, while taking a step back and allowing the profession to regulate itself.

Examples of verifiable CPD events are as follows:

- Attendance on postgraduate courses
- Attendance at local meetings organised by postgraduate tutors, or deaneries

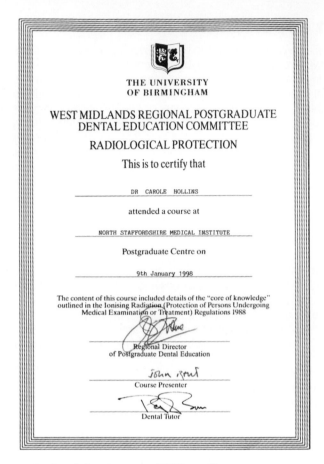

THE UNIVERSITY
OF BIRMINGHAM

WEST MIDLANDS REGIONAL POSTGRADUATE
DENTAL EDUCATION COMMITTEE

RADIOLOGICAL PROTECTION

This is to certify that

DR CAROLE HOLLINS

attended a course at

NORTH STAFFORDSHIRE MEDICAL INSTITUTE

Postgraduate Centre on

9th January 1998

The content of this course included details of the "core of knowledge"
outlined in the Ionising Radiation (Protection of Persons Undergoing
Medical Examination or Treatment) Regulations 1988

Regional Director
of Postgraduate Dental Education

Course Presenter

Dental Tutor

Figure 2.3 Continuing professional development (CPD) certificate.

- Distance-learning programmes with learning outcomes
- Computer-aided learning (CAL) programmes
- Attendance at conferences with stated learning outcomes
- Studying and taking formal examinations in dentally related subjects
- Taking post-registration qualifications
- Attending training events in other than the CPD core subjects

Non-verifiable CPD is that done on an informal basis, often purely on a personal interest basis. Although new information may well be learned during these activities, it cannot be tested or proved that specific learning outcomes have been achieved. Examples include all of those in the following list, although some can also count as verifiable CPD when assessments are set (e.g. in journals) that are scored on completion and records kept. The greater variety will provide the better learning and development opportunities for the dental nurse:

- Reading relevant articles in work-related journals – with or without assessments
- Reading new textbook publications
- Exploring relevant websites on the internet – with or without assessments
- Diversifying skill base by training in new areas of dental nursing
- Attending seminars, conferences and other work-related events

RECORD OF CPD – 2010

DATE	TITLE OF EVENT / ACTIVITY	VENUE	PROVIDER	VERIF.	NON VERIF.	HOURS	COMMENTS
19th Jan	Basic life support and CPR	Medical Institute	West Midlands Deanery	X		4	Hard work!
4th Feb	Journal reading	Home			X	2.5	BDJ articles on perio.
23rd March	Conscious sedation update	Aintree Hospital	Mersey Deanery	X		7	Excellent
11th May	Ethics and legislation update	Medical Institute	West Midlands Deanery	X		3	
10th June	LDC meeting re; CQC	Medical Institute			X	2	
29th June	Oral health workshop	Health Centre	PCT	X		3	Send in travel claim
4th Sept	Dental radiography – core subjects update	M'chester PGC	School of Radiography	X		5	
25th Oct	Communication skills	Leighton Hospital	Mersey Deanery	X		4	
2nd Nov	Journal reading and assessment test	Practice	Dental Update Journal	X		1	Record Keeping update
15th Nov	Medical emergencies drill and update	Practice	St. John	X		2	
8th Dec	Orthodontics update – fixed and functional	B'ham Dental School	West Midlands Deanery	X		5	

Figure 2.4   An example of a continuing professional development (CPD) record sheet.

- Taking an active part in workplace events;
  - Staff meetings
  - Running of quality assurance systems
  - Risk assessment analyses

Written records must be kept by dental nurses of all CPD activities, and it is advisable to complete a simple table of the necessary information on a monthly basis so that events and activities are not forgotten. All completed sheets for a stated year are then kept together with any certificates issued at verifiable events, and are then easily reproducible when requested – an example layout is shown in Figure 2.4.

The types of knowledge gained from all of these example sources will fall into one of the three broad knowledge categories recognised by the profession, and a suitable combination of the three is essential to good dental nursing skills:

- **Scientific knowledge** – models and theories that can be scientifically tested against data gathered and which are therefore verifiable – they can be written down and learned by others
- **Experiential knowledge** – that gained over time by intuition and repetitive practice, including reflection and self-evaluation
- **Ethical knowledge** – that considered to be morally correct, although it is based on beliefs and values rather than facts (see later)

When carried out correctly, then, organised CPD events covering the mandatory areas of dental practice as well as a wider range of subjects relevant to the role of the dental nurse are of great benefit to the registrant. The CPD process should enable recognition of areas that are of interest as well as areas where more knowledge is required, as dentistry and dental nursing are ever-changing disciplines where new materials and techniques are developed regularly.

Completion of CPD should produce some of the following for all dental nurses:

- Increased job satisfaction
- Identification of problem areas
- Improved communication with colleagues
- Improved efficiency
- Improved career prospects
- Greater commitment to the workplace

The planning and undertaking of CPD should be given careful thought by dental nurses to ensure not only that the mandatory requirements of the GDC are met, but also that any other CPD undertaken is of use to their lifelong learning. While the temptation exists to attend only courses of personal interest, a broader coverage of subjects is more desirable and useful to the development of the dental nurse. The following points should also be taken into consideration when planning a CPD activity:

- It can be time-consuming
- It may involve personal expense, as the completion of CPD requirements is the responsibility of dental nurses, not of their employers
- It requires self-discipline to carry out and complete
- It must be structured and organised to be of any real value
- There must be a real educational benefit to undertaking it
- Appropriate courses may not be available locally
- Courses may run during work time, so employers must be amenable to participation
- Courses may also run outside work time, so personal leisure time will be affected

Post-registration qualifications

Once qualified (by whichever training route) and registered with the GDC, dental nurses can access various post-registration qualifications run by the NEBDN, in a variety of specialised areas of dental nursing. These educational programmes and qualifications provide further development opportunities for dental nurses, as well as providing huge job satisfaction when the new skills learned are able to be used regularly in the workplace.

Currently, these higher level qualifications cover the following areas:

- Dental sedation nursing – for those students working in hospitals, clinics and practices where conscious sedation techniques are used (intravenous and inhalation)
- Oral health education – for those students wishing to take responsibility for advising and instructing patients on improving their oral health
- Special care dental nursing – for those students working with patients having special needs
- Dental radiography – for those students involved in all aspects of dental radiographic techniques, including positioning and exposing patients
- Orthodontic dental nursing – for those students working in hospitals, clinics and practices where orthodontic treatment is carried out
- Dental implant nursing – for those students working in hospitals, clinics and practices where dental implants are placed; this qualification is currently work in progress

Other specialised areas of dental nursing are being considered for future post-registration qualifications, including mentoring in the dental workplace and endodontic dental nursing.

Further details of any of these courses, including a list of accredited training providers for each qualification, are available from admin@nebdn.org.

Extended duties

Since dental nurses have become GDC registrants, their roles and those of other dental team members has been assessed to determine if any additional duties could be safely carried out once additional training has been given in the workplace, but without having to sit an examination first. Various duties fall into this category, and are collectively known as "extended duties". They do not include the specialised area of study and examination required for a dental nurse to position and expose a patient to ionising radiation. This skill can only be achieved by acquiring the dental radiography post-registration qualification.

In allowing dental nurses to acquire these extended duties, the GDC released their publication *Scope of Practice* to give guidance on how they can be achieved, without dental nurses working beyond their level of skill.

Obviously, those skills that are specifically provided to other dental team members as part of their registerable qualification training are excluded as skills available to the dental nurse, without undertaking that additional, formal training and qualification.

In all areas of extended duties possible, the GDC publication states that "The scope of your practice is a way of describing what you are trained and competent to do". The key words in this statement are "trained" and "competent". To achieve both in an extended duty, a senior work colleague must provide supervised guidance and training in the chosen topic, produce a written record of the training given, and sign to say that in their opinion the dental nurse is competent to carry out the duty.

Examples of extended duties available to the dental nurse include the following:

● Impression taking (alginate)
● Shade taking
● Suture removal
● Casting of study models from alginate impressions
● Construction of tooth whitening trays
● Pressing the X-ray machine exposure button under the direct supervision of the operator
● Intra-oral photography

Direct access

In April 2013 the GDC announced that it is removing barriers to direct access for some dental care professionals, in particular dental therapists and dental hygienists. Those barriers were removed in May 2013, and the result represents a significant change in how some members of the dental team can now work, as well as how patients and members of the public can access dentistry in the UK.

The decision to allow direct access was the culmination of a review into the current use in particular of dental therapists and hygienists in the dental workplace, and specifically focused on issues of patient safety when patients were seen by dental care professionals. The main results were as follows:

● There was no evidence of significant issues of patient safety resulting from the current clinical activity of dental care professionals
● There was evidence that access to dental care improved as a result of direct access arrangements, of cost benefits to patients and of high levels of patient satisfaction
● There was some evidence that dental care professionals may over-refer patients to dentists, which may ensure patient safety but lead to wasteful use of resources and a high level of "no shows" on referral

However, registrants treating patients direct must only do so if they are appropriately trained, competent and indemnified. They should also ensure that there are adequate onward referral arrangements in place and they must make clear to the patient the extent of their scope of practice and not work beyond it. Also, this decision does not make direct access mandatory and no dental care professional has to offer it to a patient.

The outcome for dental nurses is that they can see patients direct (rather than under supervision) if they are taking part in structured programmes which provide dental public health interventions, such as fluoride application. The outcome for dental therapists and hygienists is far greater, but is not relevant here.

Further information and advice is available from the GDC website at www.gdc-uk.org.

Evaluate the effectiveness of the plan

Once the development plan has been running for a while, its effectiveness at improving the performance of the dental nurse must be evaluated to determine if it is successful or not; if not, then it should be determined what else can be instigated to improve matters where necessary.

The evaluation process can be carried out by the dental nurse alone, but will be more effective if others are involved too, such as a mentor, line manager, practice manager or employer. They will all be able to give an impersonal evaluation and opinion on the performance of the dental nurse, as well as probably being in a better position to action any changes required.

To evaluate the effectiveness of the development plan, the following points must be considered:

- Reflect on the performance of the dental nurse since implementation of the plan
- Demonstrate an improvement in performance
- Regularly review the impact of the plan on the nurse's work
- Implement identified development opportunities

The reflection process is as described previously for reflection on action events, with consideration given to the performance of the dental nurse during certain work activities when looked back on at a later date. Was an improvement in performance seen, and can that be demonstrated as having occurred?

So, for example, can the dental nurse:

- Assist during various procedures now without having to be supervised?
- Carry out new skills correctly and unaided?
- Perform new duties that have been taught in the workplace?

These examples identify ways in which the knowledge-based and skill-based requirements of professional dental nurses have been addressed and improved upon where necessary, but their attitudes and behaviour also form key elements of these professional requirements too.

To implement performance improvements in their ethical knowledge, dental nurses must demonstrate that they follow the principles of "best practice" at all times, irrespective of their own personal values and beliefs. They must therefore strive towards achieving the following:

- Promote equality, diversity, and anti-discriminatory practice at all times
- Respect the patient's rights at all times
- Promote, develop and maintain effective working relationships with other team members
- Never stray outside the legal limits of their own qualifications
- Take an active part in CPD
- Ensure that all changes to effective dental nursing are known and acted upon, so that the concept of "best practice" is always attained

During the reflective process, dental nurses will also consider whether the previously identified priority issues have been addressed. If not, then their actioning must become a matter of urgency, using a new set of SMART objectives to ensure that the issues are definitely addressed in this second round of reflective practice and performance review. Dental nurses will need to consider the reasons why the priority issues were not achieved the first time round, and help or support may be required from the employer if they are to be successful in the future. In particular, previously identified development opportunities (see earlier) may now require implementation.

Compliance with registration requirements

Throughout the working life of the dental nurse, the GDC (as the regulator of all dental professionals) states that it expects the following actions from all its registrants:

- Develop and update your knowledge and skills throughout your working life
- Reflect on your knowledge and skills, and identify both your strengths and weaknesses
- Provide a good standard of care based on up-to-date evidence and guidance
- Follow all the laws and regulations that affect your work

The importance of lifelong learning and participation in CPD activities becomes clear, as these are the methods used to ensure that updated information on relevant topics is made available to dental professionals.

At all times when dental nurses are acting in their capacity as a dental care professional and as a member of the dental team, they must always work in accordance with the standard operating procedures of their workplace. These are the procedures usually followed when carrying out the normal work activities of their particular workplace, which are therefore not able to be varied in a random way.

They will be set out initially as various **policy** documents, which will describe the courses of action that have been adopted by the workplace. A policy may vary from workplace to workplace; one suitable for a hospital department will not be suitable for a small practice, for example. When the policy has been decided and then put into writing as the required course of action to be followed, it will be signed by all employees to show their agreement with its terms; it will then become a **protocol**. So a protocol is a written draft of terms agreed to and signed by all parties as a code of conduct within the workplace – all the protocols together are the standard operating procedures.

In addition, and to ensure patient safety, the dental nurse must also always comply with all legislation and regulations relevant to any dental workplace, and work within the guidelines that are in effect in their own particular workplace. These various issues are discussed in detail in Chapters 1, 4, 7, 12, 13 and 14.

The professional codes of practice and the ethical standards that dental nurses must also follow are contained in the GDC's *Standards for the Dental Team* documentation, which has recently been updated and extended from six key principles with accompanying guidance booklets into nine core ethical principles of practice, with guidance provided within just the one document (Figure 2.5).

The GDC Standards documentation can be downloaded directly from the GDC website at www. gdc-uk.org. The nine core ethical principles of practice are:

1. **Put patients' interests first**
2. **Communicate effectively with patients**
3. **Obtain valid consent**
4. **Maintain and protect patients' information**
5. **Have a clear and effective complaints procedure**
6. **Work with colleagues in a way that is in patients' best interests**
7. **Maintain, develop and work within your professional knowledge and skills**
8. **Raise concerns if patients are at risk**
9. **Make sure your personal behaviour maintains patients' confidence in you and the dental profession**

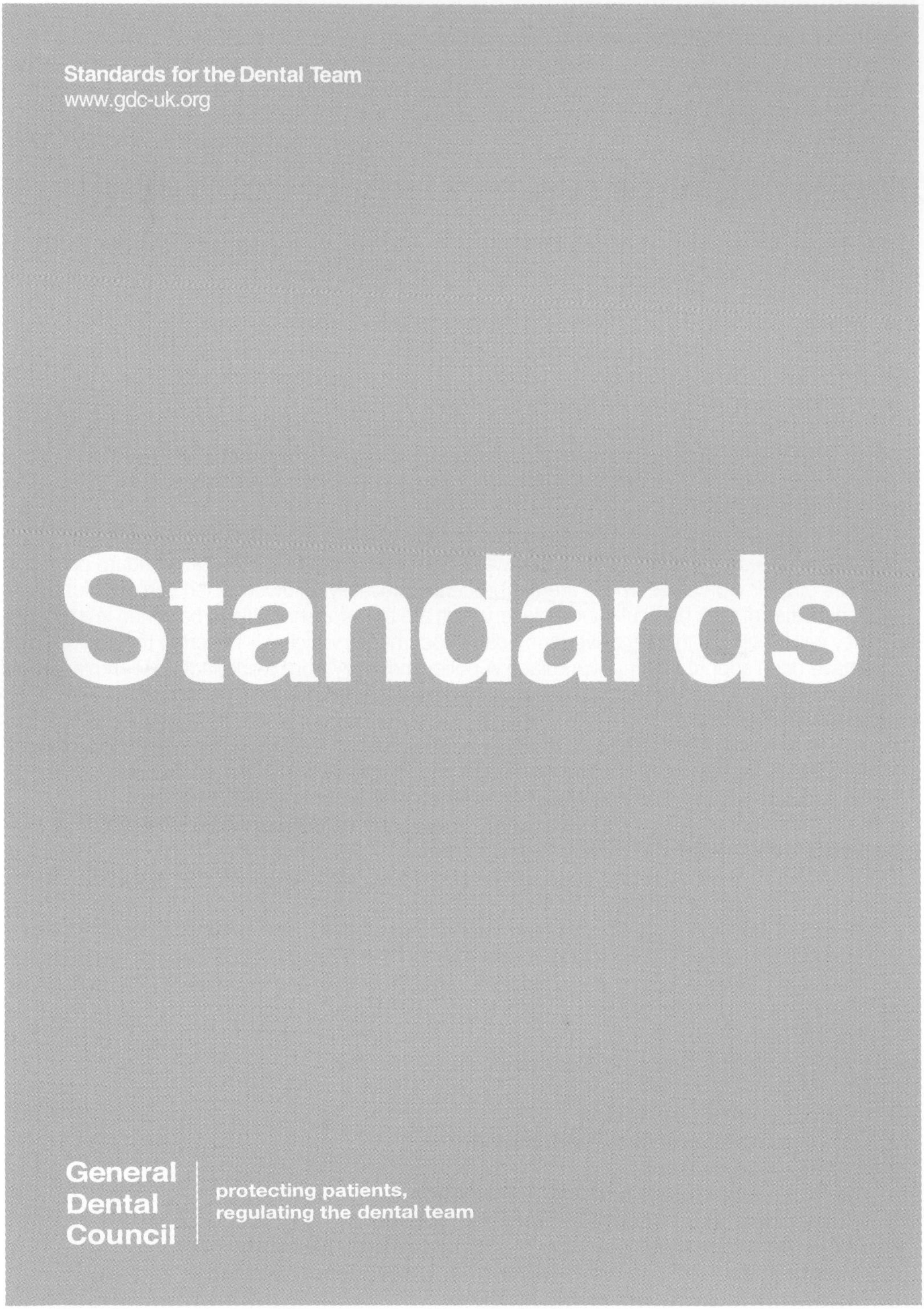

Figure 2.5 General Dental Council's *Standards for the Dental Team* document. Source: General Dental Council.

Each principle has a set of standards attached that must be followed and met by every GDC registrant. Failure to meet the standards is likely to result in their professional registration with the GDC being put at risk of suspension or even erasure. The standards to be followed by members of the dental team are based on the reasonable patient expectations of the dental professionals they come into contact with during their treatment.

The booklet now contains considerable guidance to enable registrants to meet the standards, or to be able to use their own judgment and insight when necessary to justify any variation from the guidance. However, it clearly states that when the word "**must**" is used, the duty is compulsory and is therefore not open to interpretation or variation. Only where the word "**should**" is used will it be accepted that the duty may not apply in all situations and that alternative action may be appropriate.

The nine principles and their guidance information are set out in detail in the following sections, so that all readers can familiarise themselves with their content and apply the relevant ones to their own working environment while studying for their registerable qualification. The document is one publication for all dental professionals, and some of the standards cover areas that are more applicable to team leaders or to those team members who actually provide "hands on" treatment to the patients – dentists, therapists, hygienists and clinical dental technicians.

1   Put patients' interests first

This is the overall principle that all dental professionals must aspire to, and be seen to do so, at all times. All team members have a duty of care towards their patients to ensure that their best interests are at the forefront of all decisions made about them – their treatment and all aspects of its safe delivery, their rights as individuals, their expectations with regard to correctly priced and painless treatment, and their right to redress if they suffer harm during the delivery of that treatment.

In particular, patients have a right to expect that the team will always put their best interests before those of financial gain and business need.

1.1   Listen to your patients

1.1.1   Treatment options must be discussed in a way that the patient can understand, and they must have the opportunity to ask questions and discuss their own expectations and concerns.

1.2   Treat every patient with dignity and respect at all times

1.2.1   You should be aware of how your tone of voice and body language might be perceived – so develop good communication skills and use them throughout your working life (see Chapters 5 and 13).

1.2.2   You should take patients' preferences into account and be sensitive to their individual needs and values – irrespective of whether you agree with them or not.

1.2.3   You must treat patients with kindness and compassion – few patients attend the dental workplace without some level of anxiety, and all staff should show empathy towards them.

1.2.4   You should manage patients' dental pain and anxiety appropriately – there is nothing more belittling or frightening to a fearful patient than to be ridiculed by a blasé member of staff.

1.3   Be honest and act with integrity

1.3.1   You must justify the trust that patients, the public and your colleagues place in you by always acting honestly and fairly in your dealings with them – this applies to business and educational activities, as well as professionally.

1.3.2   You must make sure you do not bring the profession into disrepute – further information about fitness-to-practise issues is available by following the links at www.gdc-uk.org.

1.3.3   You must ensure that any advertising, promotional material or other information that you produce is accurate and not misleading, and complies with the GDC's guidance on ethical advertising – in particular, the words "specialists in" or "experts in" should be avoided, as they tend to imply a higher level of expertise than is often the case.

1.4 Take a holistic and preventative approach to patient care which is appropriate to the individual patient

1.4.1   A holistic approach means you must take account of patients' overall health, their psychological and social needs, their long-term oral health needs and their desired outcomes.

1.4.2   You must provide patients with treatment that is in their best interests, providing appropriate oral health advice and following clinical guidelines relevant to their situation – you may need to balance their oral health needs with their desired outcomes, while accepting that their desired outcomes may not always be achievable or in their best interests. In these instances, the risks, benefits and likely outcomes must be explained fully to help the patient reach a decision.

1.5 Treat patients in a hygienic and safe environment

1.5.1   You must find out about the laws and regulations that apply to your work role – further relevant detail is given in Chapters 1, 4, 7, 12 and 14.

1.5.2   You must make sure that you have all necessary vaccinations and follow guidance relating to blood-borne viruses – this is to prevent cross-infection from patients to staff and from staff to patients.

1.5.3   You must follow the guidance on medical emergencies and training updates issued by the Resuscitation Council (UK) – further relevant detail is given in Chapters 3 and 13.

1.5.4   You must record all patient safety incidents and report them promptly to the appropriate national body – further detail is given in Chapter 1.

1.6 Treat patients fairly, as individuals and without discrimination

1.6.1   You must not discriminate against patients on any grounds – irrespective of your own personal beliefs and values.

1.6.2   You must be aware of and adhere to all your responsibilities as set out in relevant equalities legislation.

1.6.3   You must consider patients' disabilities and make reasonable adjustments to allow them to receive care which meets their needs – in some instances, this may require the patient to be referred to a colleague or to the community services for treatment.

1.6.4   You must not express your personal beliefs (political, religious or moral) to patients in any way that exploits their vulnerability or could cause them distress.

1.7 Put patients' interests before your own or those of any colleague, business or organisation

1.7.1   You must always put your patients' interests before any financial, personal or other gain.

1.7.2   Patients must be clearly informed of those treatments they may receive via the NHS (or other equivalent health service) and those which are only available on a private basis – this is relevant in a mixed practice, where treatment is available by either route.

1.7.3   You must not mislead patients into believing that treatments available via the NHS are only available privately – if the practice only provides private treatment, the patient must be made aware of this before they attend.

1.7.4   Patients must not be pressurised into having treatment privately if it is also available on the NHS.

1.7.5   You must refuse any gifts, payment or hospitality if accepting them could affect (or appear to affect) your professional judgment.

1.7.6 Referrals to another team member must be in the best interests of the patient only, not in yours or another colleagues interests.

1.7.7 If you believe that patients might be at risk because of someone's health, behaviour or performance, you must take prompt and appropriate action.

1.7.8 If a professional relationship with a patient has to be ended, it must not be solely due to a complaint against you, and steps should be taken to make arrangements for the continuation of the patient's treatment elsewhere.

1.8 Have appropriate arrangements in place for patients to seek compensation if they have suffered harm

1.8.1 You must have appropriate insurance or indemnity in place, relevant to your duties – this is a requirement for all registered members of the dental team, and further advice is available from dental companies offering indemnity insurance or from www.gdc-uk.org.

1.8.2 You should ensure you follow the terms and conditions of your personal indemnity insurance at all times, and contact your insurer as soon as possible when a claim is made.

1.9 Find out about laws and regulations that affect your work and follow them

1.9.1 Further detail is given in Chapters 1, 5, 6 and 13.

2 Communicate effectively with patients

This principle covers the necessity for good communication skills by all members of the dental team. If these skills are so poor that the patient cannot understand what is being said to them, for whatever reason (use of jargon, language barrier, no information given, no opportunity to ask for clarification, and so on) then the patient cannot be said to have given consent for the proposed treatment.

2.1 Listen to them and give them time to consider information, taking their views and individual needs into consideration

2.1.1 You must treat patients as individuals and respect any cultural values and differences. You must be sufficiently fluent in written and spoken English to communicate effectively with patients, their relatives, the dental team and other healthcare professionals in the UK.

2.2 Recognise and promote patients' rights and responsibilities for making decisions about their health priorities and care

2.2.1 You must listen to patients and communicate effectively with them at a level they can understand, including explaining treatment options, risks, benefits and costs.

2.2.2 You should encourage patients to ask questions about their options and treatment.

2.2.3 You must give full and honest answers to any questions asked – especially to avoid influencing patients in their choices.

2.3 Give patients the information they need, in a way they can understand, so that they can make informed decisions

2.3.1 You must introduce yourself to patients and explain your role so that they know how you will be involved in their care – some dental workplaces expect more formality with names than others.

2.3.2 Involve any colleagues or patient carers in discussion with patients where appropriate – this must be in line with patient confidentiality requirements.

2.3.3   You should recognise patients' communication difficulties and try to meet their needs – for example, by using an interpreter or avoiding professional jargon.

2.3.4   You should ensure that patients have understood the information given, by asking questions and summarising the main points.

2.3.5   You should make sure that patients have enough information and enough time to ask questions and make a decision.

2.3.6   You must give patients a written treatment plan(s) before their treatment starts, and retain a signed copy in their notes.

2.3.7   The plan must include the proposed treatment, a cost indication, and whether the treatment is via NHS or private services where necessary – where both services are relevant, the plan should indicate which is which for each item.

2.3.8   The plan and costs should be reviewed during treatment and the patient should be informed if any changes occur – a written, updated plan should then be provided.

2.3.9   You must provide patients with clear information about emergency and out-of-hours arrangements.

2.3.10 You should make sure patients have the necessary details to contact you.

2.3.11 You should provide patients with clear information about referral arrangements.

2.4   Give patients clear information about costs

2.4.1   You must display a simple price list where patients can see it.

2.4.2   This information must also be available in practice literature and on websites.

2.4.3   You should inform patients of your rules on guaranteed work – this should include any circumstances leading to exclusions, such as a lack of care on their part.

3   Obtain valid consent

This principle simply covers the patients' right to expect to be asked if they wish to proceed with the treatment they require, before it begins and throughout the course of the treatment. To provide any treatment to a patient without their consent is actually deemed to be assault. The principle therefore explains why the treatment proposed must be fully explained in a manner that the individual patient (or their carer) can understand, before they are able to agree to it or to decline it. A dental professional can advise the patient (or their carer) what they consider to be their best treatment option, but it is entirely up to the patient to decide whether they wish to proceed or not, irrespective of the professional advice given – that is the patient's right. They must never be bullied or coerced into accepting treatment which they do not really want, nor must they be misled or deceived into choosing one option of treatment over another.

3.1   Obtain valid consent before starting treatment, explaining all the relevant options and the possible costs

3.1.1   You must make sure you have valid consent before starting treatment, and do not assume that someone else has obtained the patient's consent beforehand – see Chapter 13 for further detail.

3.1.2   You should document the discussions you have with patients in the process of gaining consent, as well as gaining a signature.

3.1.3   You should find out what your patients want to know as well as what you think they need to know.

3.1.4   You must check and document that patients have understood the information you have given.

3.1.5   You must acknowledge the patients' right to refuse treatment, withdraw their consent, or request that treatment is stopped after it has started, and follow their wishes – possible consequences should be explained and any discussions must be recorded in the notes.

3.1.6   You must obtain written consent where treatment involves conscious sedation or general anaesthesia.

3.2   Make sure that patients (or their representatives) understand the decisions they are being asked to make

3.2.1   You must provide patients with sufficient information and give them a reasonable amount of time to consider that information in order to make a decision – they must not be hurried or coerced into making a decision about their treatment.

3.2.2   You must tailor the way you obtain consent to each patient's needs, by giving them information in a format they can easily understand.

3.2.3   You should encourage patients with communication difficulties to have a trusted person present when gaining consent, so that relevant questions can be asked and your answers explained.

3.2.4   You must always consider whether patients are able to make decisions about their care themselves, rather than assume so – see Chapters 5 and 13 for further detail .

3.2.5   You must check and document that patients have understood the information you have given them – the easiest method is to ask them to repeat back to you what their understanding of your discussions have been.

3.3   Make sure that the patient's consent remains valid at each stage of investigation or treatment

3.3.1   Gaining consent is an ongoing process of communication between patients and all members of the dental team involved in their care.

3.3.2   You must make sure you have specific consent for the treatment to be carried out at each appointment.

3.3.3   You must tailor the way you confirm ongoing consent to each patient's needs, and check that they have understood the information you have given them.

3.3.4   All ongoing consent discussions must be documented.

3.3.5   If the treatment or costs are likely to differ from the originals, you must gain consent for the changes from the patient and document that you have done so.

4   Maintain and protect patients' information

This principle covers patients' expectations with regard to the personal and clinical information that the workplace holds for them. They do not expect any third party to be able to gain access to their personal information without their knowledge or agreement (although legal precedents do exist), but they do expect to be able to access their own information if necessary – clinical records should not be kept secret from the patient themselves. With this in mind, it is therefore obvious why the accuracy of the records is of paramount importance to the dental team, and that no defamatory or derogatory comments are ever included – this is grossly unprofessional.

4.1   Make and keep contemporaneous, complete and accurate patient records

4.1.1   You must make complete and accurate patient records, including an up-to-date medical history, each time that you treat patients – if the dental nurse is to write up a patient's notes, wherever possible they should be dictated by the clinician.

4.1.2   You should record as much detail as possible about the discussions you have with your patients.

4.1.3   You must follow appropriate national advice on retaining, storing and disposing of patient records – see Chapter 13 for further detail.

4.1.4 You must ensure that all documentation is clear, legible, accurate and can be readily under-stood by others, including the initials of the treating clinician where appropriate – this is only relevant where computer records are not held and handwritten records are made instead.

4.1.5 Any amendments to the records must be clearly marked and dated – again, computer records will record this automatically.

4.1.6 Any referral to another health or dental professional must be accurately recorded in the patient's notes, ideally with a copy of the referral maintained.

4.2 Protect the confidentiality of patients' information and only use it for the purpose for which it was given

4.2.1 You must keep patient information confidential, including all information you have learnt in your professional role – see Chapter 13 for further detail.

4.2.2 You must ensure that all non-registered members of the dental team are aware of the importance of confidentiality, and that they maintain it at all times too.

4.2.3 Professional social media must not be used to discuss cases unless the patient cannot be identified, and social networking or blogging sites should be avoided – visit www.gdc-uk.org for further guidance.

4.2.4 You must not discuss patients or their treatment where you can be overheard by others who should not have access to this information – this is particularly relevant in the reception area.

4.2.5 You must explain to patients the circumstances in which you may need to share information with others involved in their healthcare, and record whether or not they gave their permission.

4.2.6 You should ensure anyone you share information with understands that it is confidential.

4.2.7 If patient information is required by others for teaching or research, the patient must be informed and their consent gained, and wherever possible their details must remain anonymous.

4.2.8 Patient information must remain confidential even after the patient's death.

4.2.9 The duty of confidentiality also applies to patient images and recordings, and these must not be made without the patient's permission.

4.3 Only release a patient's information without their permission in exceptional circumstances

4.3.1 This may be necessary if it is in the best interests of the public or the patient, although recorded attempts should be made to gain their permission anyway – see Chapter 13 for further detail.

4.3.2 You should obtain advice from your defence or professional organisation before releasing information without the patient's permission.

4.3.3 You must inform the appropriate social care agencies or the police if you believe that a patient is or could be at risk of significant harm or abuse – visit any of the following for further guidance and advice: www.nice.org.uk, www.cqc.org.uk, www.gdc-uk.org.

4.3.4 You should only release the minimum amount of information necessary to comply with a court order or statutory duty to do so without a patient's permission.

4.3.5 You must document your reasons for releasing confidential information and be prepared to explain and justify your decisions and actions.

4.4 Ensure that patients can have access to their records

4.4.1 Patients have a right of access to their dental records under Data Protection legislation, and if they request access you must comply promptly and in accordance with the law.

4.4.2 You should request guidance from your national Information Commissioner's Office before charging patients for access to their records.

4.5 Keep patients' information secure at all times, whether your records are held on paper or electronically

4.5.1   You must store all patients' information securely at all times – see Chapter 13 for further detail.

4.5.2   You must use a secure method of sending confidential information, including encryption if the information is stored electronically.

4.5.3   Back-up copies of computerised records should be made, so that the information is not lost on failure of the hardware or software.

5   Have a clear and effective complaints procedure

This principle covers what patients expect if they do ever have a complaint about an issue. They expect their complaint to be taken seriously and investigated thoroughly even if it becomes apparent that the complaint is spurious or even malicious. Genuine complaints are useful learning tools for the dental team to improve their service to their patients, while other complaints that are handled correctly provide unshakable evidence that the team are not at fault and that no further action is necessary. Essentially, it prevents unnecessary and costly legal action proceeding against a blameless dental team, or one of its members, while also giving recourse to patients when appropriate.

5.1 Make sure that there is an effective complaints procedure readily available for patients to use, and follow that procedure at all times

5.1.1   You must deal with complaints properly and professionally, by following the written complaints procedure of the workplace at all times – see Chapter 13 for further detail.

5.1.2   All staff must be trained in handling complaints.

5.1.3   Where NHS or other health service treatment is provided, you should follow the procedure set down by that organisation.

5.1.4   Where private treatment is provided, you should make sure that the provision for handling complaints should set similar standards and time limits to those of the NHS.

5.1.5   See Chapter 13 for the full detail of those requirements.

5.1.6   You should analyse any complaints received to help improve your service where relevant.

5.1.7   You should keep a written record of all complaints together with all responses, and separate from the patient records.

5.2 Respect a patient's right to complain

5.2.1   You should not react defensively to complaints, but listen carefully and discover what outcome the patient wants.

5.3 Give patients who complain a prompt and constructive response

5.3.1   You should give the patient a copy of the complaints procedure so that they understand the stages involved and the timescales.

5.3.2   You should deal with complaints calmly and in line with procedure.

5.3.3   You should aim to resolve complaints as efficiently, effectively, and politely as possible.

5.3.4   You must respond within the time limits.

5.3.5   You should inform the patient if more time is required to investigate.

5.3.6   You should give the patient regular updates on progress when the timescales cannot be followed.

5.3.7   You should deal with all the points raised and offer solutions to each where possible.

5.3.8   You should offer an apology and a practical solution where appropriate – but also make the point that an apology is not an admission of liability where appropriate.

62

5.3.9   You should offer a fair solution when a complaint is justified.

5.3.10 You should respond to the patient in writing, in an accurate and legible manner.

5.3.11 You should inform the patient of how to proceed further if they are not satisfied with your complaint handling and decision taken.

6   Work with colleagues in a way that is in patients' best interests

This principle covers teamwork, and the way that patients expect the dental team to perform when providing their treatment, so that everyone pulls together in the best interests of the patient at all times. Each team member should always work to the best of their abilities but not beyond them – they should be efficient in their actions, support each other during the provision of care to a patient, and only work within the remit of their qualifications and training.

6.1   Work effectively with your colleagues and contribute to good teamwork

6.1.1   You should ensure that any team you are involved in works together to provide appropriate dental care for your patients – this is a basic requirement of professionalism.

6.1.2   You must treat colleagues fairly and with respect – as you would wish to be treated by them.

6.1.3   You must treat colleagues fairly in all financial transactions.

6.1.4   You must value and respect the contribution of all team members.

6.1.5   You must ensure that patients are fully informed of the names and roles of the dental professionals involved in their care – by team member photographs, name badges, or simply by verbal introduction.

6.1.6   You should ensure that all non-registrants that you work with are appropriately trained and competent, as you may be held responsible for their actions.

6.2   Be appropriately supported when treating patients

6.2.1   You must not provide treatment if you feel that the circumstances make it unsafe for patients.

6.2.2   You should work with another appropriately trained member of the dental team at all times when treating patients in a dental setting – exceptions to this are when providing out-of-hours emergency care, during a public health programme, and exceptional (unavoidable, non-routine, and unforeseen) circumstances such as sudden illness.

6.2.3   You must assess the possible risk to the patient of continuing treatment when exceptional circumstances occur.

6.2.4   You should be supported by a GDC registrant (or other healthcare registrant) when working in a hospital setting.

6.2.5   You should be supported by a GDC registrant or an appropriately trained care professional in a domiciliary/care setting.

6.2.6   You must make sure there is at least one other person available within the workplace to deal with medical emergencies when you are treating patients – this may have to be the patient's escort in exceptional circumstances.

6.3   Delegate and refer appropriately and effectively

6.3.1   You can delegate the responsibility for a task but not the accountability, if you delegate to someone who has not been appropriately trained – see the *Scope of Practice* document at www.gdc-uk.org for further detail.

6.3.2   You must not pressurise a colleague into accepting a delegated task if they feel unable to carry it out.

6.3.3 You should refer patients elsewhere if the treatment required is outside of your scope of practice.

6.3.4 You should make any request for treatment on referral or clinical advice from a colleague clear and give them full information.

6.3.5 You must explain the referral process to the patient and record it in their notes.

6.4 Only accept a referral or delegation if you are trained and competent to carry out the treatment and you believe that what you are being asked to do is appropriate for the patient

6.4.1 You must be clear about what you are being asked to do and that you have the knowledge and skills to do it.

6.4.2 You should only proceed with the treatment if you are satisfied that what you are being asked to do is appropriate, following any necessary discussion with the colleague – if not, you should seek advice from your defence organisation.

6.5 Communicate clearly and effectively with other team members and colleagues in the interests of patients

6.5.1 You should document any discussions you have with colleagues about a patient's treatment, in the notes.

6.6 Demonstrate effective management and leadership skills if you manage a team

6.6.1 You should make sure that all team members have:
- Proper induction when they first join the team
- Performance management (such as appraisal)
- Opportunities to learn and develop
- Hygienic and safe working environment
- Non-discriminatory working environment
- Opportunities to provide feedback
- Way to raise concerns

6.6.2 You should ensure that relevant team members are appropriately registered with the GDC (or other regulator), or in training before registration, and indemnified.

6.6.3 You should encourage all team members to follow the guidance in the GDC Standards document.

6.6.4 You should make sure that you communicate regularly with all team members.

6.6.5 You must encourage, support and facilitate the CPD requirements of your team – see earlier in this chapter.

6.6.6 You must ensure that all staff are sufficiently trained and prepared to be involved in managing a medical emergency during a treatment session, and that sufficient staff are present to do so.

6.6.7 You should ensure your team has good leadership, clear aims, and understanding of their roles and responsibilities you must find out about current evidence and best practice roles and responsibilities

6.6.8 Their roles and responsibilities include knowledge of their scope of practice.

6.6.9 You should discuss all new policies and procedures to ensure full staff compliance.

6.6.10 You should display information about team members in a patient area.

6.6.11 You should display your GDC registration and the nine principles of the GDC Standards document in a patient area.

7   Maintain, develop and work within your professional knowledge and skills

This principle lays out dental professionals' duties with regard to ensuring that their knowledge and skills are kept up to date at all times, so that the patients receive the best care possible at all times. Patients have a right to expect that the team members providing their care have reached and maintained the required level of professional competence to deliver their care safely and within their personal limits, and that they will refer them on to others when care is required above and beyond those limits.

7.1   Provide good quality care based on current evidence and authoritative guidance

7.1.1   You must find out about current evidence and best practice which affect your work, premises, equipment and business and follow them.

7.1.2   You should record the reason for any deviation from established practice and guidance, and be able to justify your reasons for doing so.

7.2   Work within your knowledge, skills, professional competence and abilities

7.2.1   You must only carry out a task or a type of treatment if you are appropriately trained, competent, confident and indemnified – this includes for any extended duties that a dental nurse may carry out.

7.2.2   You should only deliver treatment and care if you are confident that you have had the necessary training and are competent to do so.

7.2.3   You must only work within your mental and physical capabilities.

7.3   Update and develop your professional knowledge and skills throughout your working life

7.3.1   You must make sure that you know your CPD requirements to maintain your registration and that you carry it out within the required time.

7.3.2   You should take part in CPD activities that improve your practice – see earlier in this chapter.

8   Raise concerns if patients are at risk

This principle covers the patients' expectations with regard to their likely actions when the welfare of someone is at risk by the acts or omissions of a dental professional – whether that vulnerable person is a child patient, an adult patient or another team member. Patients do not expect professionals to "stick together" and attempt to cover up the failings of one of their colleagues when problems come to light; they quite rightly expect the opposite to occur – an open and robust investigation of what went wrong, how it went wrong, who was involved (or to blame) and how to avoid a recurrence of the event in the future.

8.1   Always put patients' safety first

8.1.1   You must raise any concern that patients might be at risk for any reason, even if you are not in a position to control or influence your working environment, and this duty overrides any personal or professional loyalties you have.

8.1.2   You must not enter into a contract or agreement which contains a "gagging clause" that would prevent you from raising concerns, or restrict what you could say when raising concerns.

8.2   Act promptly if patients or colleagues are at risk and take measures to protect them

8.2.1   You must act on your concerns promptly, and if in doubt you must raise a concern rather than leave the issue.

8.2.2   You should not have to prove your concern for it to be investigated, and if the investigation shows there was no problem, this should not be held against you as long as you were acting in the best interests of the patients at the time.

8.2.3   You should raise your concern initially with your employer or manager, unless they are the source of your concern.

8.2.4   In this case, you must raise the issue with your local health commissioner, defence organisation or with one of the following bodies:
- Care Quality Commission (England)
- Healthcare Inspectorate Wales
- Regulation and Quality Improvement Authority (Northern Ireland)
- Healthcare Improvement Scotland

8.2.5   You must raise your concern with the GDC if you believe the patients or the public need to be protected from a registered dental professional – see earlier in this chapter.

8.2.6   You must refer concerns about other healthcare professionals to the relevant regulator.

8.3   Make sure if you employ, manage or lead a team that you encourage and support a culture where staff can raise concerns openly and without fear of reprisal

8.3.1   You must promote a culture of openness in the workplace so that staff feel able to raise concerns.

8.3.2   You should include this culture in your policies and procedures.

8.3.3   You should encourage all staff to raise concerns about the safety of patients.

8.3.4   You must not offer staff a contract that contains a gagging clause.

8.4   Make sure if you employ, manage or lead a team, that there is an effective procedure in place for raising concerns, that the procedure is readily available to all staff and that it is followed at all times

8.4.1   You must make sure that there are written procedures in place to enable staff members to raise concerns.

8.4.2   When a concern is raised it must be taken seriously, investigated promptly and in an unbiased manner.

8.5   Take appropriate action if you have concerns about the possible abuse of children or vulnerable adults (including the elderly)

8.5.1   You must know who to contact for further advice in these situations, and how to refer your concerns to an appropriate authority such as your local social services department.

8.5.2   You must be aware of the local procedures available for the protection of children and vulnerable adults, and follow them if it becomes necessary to raise a concern.

9   Make sure your personal behaviour maintains patients' confidence in you and the dental profession

This principle covers what patients have a right to expect from people they look up to as "professionals". It sets out the behaviour that they consider appropriate for a professional member of the team both during work time and at all other times. It is not considered appropriate to behave in a less than exemplary manner when away from the workplace or outside of normal working hours – patients expect professional standards to be maintained at all times.

In particular, team members should be very careful of their use of social networking sites – the medium is called "social" because it is accessible to many, including patients, colleagues and the GDC. The medium is monitored, and those team members making inappropriate or derogatory comments are quite likely to find themselves at a fitness-to-practise hearing with the GDC.

9.1   Ensure that your conduct, both at work and in your personal life, justifies patients' trust in you and the public's trust in the dental profession

9.1.1   You must treat all team members, colleagues and members of the public fairly, with dignity, and in line with the law – put simply, as you would wish to be treated by others yourself.

9.1.2   You must not make disparaging remarks about another member of the dental team in front of patients, but use the proper channels to raise any concerns where necessary.

9.1.3   You should not publish anything that could affect patients' and the public's confidence in you or the dental profession, in any public media – this includes social networking sites, blogs and other forms of social media – visit www.gdc-uk.org for further guidance.

9.1.4   You must maintain appropriate boundaries in the relationships you have with patients, and not take advantage of your position as a dental professional in these circumstances – in particular, intimate relationships with a patient should not be entered into.

9.2   Protect patients and colleagues from risks posed by your health, conduct or performance

9.2.1   You must consult a suitably qualified colleague immediately if you believe you may be putting people at risk, and follow the advice given.

9.2.2   You must not rely on your own assessment of the risk you pose to patients, but seek occupational health advice as soon as possible.

9.3   Inform the GDC if you are subject to criminal proceedings or a regulatory finding is made against you, anywhere in the world

9.3.1   Criminal proceedings brought against you anywhere in the world may bring your professionalism into question, and as a registered professional with the GDC you have a duty to inform them so that if found guilty, your continuing registration may be reconsidered if appropriate.

9.3.2   You must inform the GDC immediately if you are subject to the fitness-to-practise procedures of another healthcare regulator, either in the UK or abroad, for the same reason as stated in 9.3.1.

9.3.3   Similarly, you must inform the GDC immediately if a finding has been made against your registration by another healthcare regulator, either in the UK or abroad.

9.3.4   You must inform the GDC immediately if you are placed on a barred list held by either the Disclosure and Barring Service (DBS – formerly known as the Criminal Records Bureau) or Disclosure Scotland.

9.4 Co-operate with any relevant formal or informal inquiry and give full and truthful information

9.4.1   You must respond fully and in a timely manner if you receive contact from the GDC in connection with concerns about your fitness to practise, and take advice from your defence organisation over the matter.

9.4.2   You must co-operate with any legally appointed organisation or body during an inquiry, including healthcare regulators, Coroners (or the Procurator Fiscal in Scotland), lawyers or commissioners of health.

Ultimately, along with all other dental professionals (and all other healthcare workers), dental nurses have a "duty of care" to the patients that attend their workplace to follow these nine principles at all times to ensure that their recognition as a member of their profession is always justified.

3

Unit 268: First Aid Essentials

Learning outcomes

1. Be able to understand the role and responsibilities of an emergency first aider
2. Know how to assess an incident
3. Be able to manage an unresponsive casualty who is breathing normally
4. Be able to manage an unresponsive casualty who is not breathing normally
5. Be able to recognise and assist a casualty who is choking
6. Be able to manage a casualty who is wounded and bleeding
7. Be able to manage a casualty who is in shock
8. Understand how to manage a casualty with a minor injury

Outcome 1 assessment criteria

The learner can:
- Identify the role and responsibilities of an emergency first aider
- Describe how to minimise the risk of infection to self and others
- Describe how to complete an incident report form
- Identify the first aid equipment available and describe how it can be used safely

Outcome 2 assessment criteria

The learner can:
- Describe how to conduct a scene survey
- Describe how to make a primary survey of a casualty
- Identify when and how to call for help

Outcome 3 assessment criteria

The learner can:
- Demonstrate how to assess a casualty's level of consciousness
- Demonstrate how to open a casualty's airway and check breathing

Diploma in Dental Nursing, Level 3, Third Edition. Carole Hollins.
© 2014 John Wiley & Sons, Ltd. Published 2014 by John Wiley & Sons, Ltd.
Companion website: www.wiley.com/go/hollins/dentalnursinglevel3

- Demonstrate how to place an unconscious casualty into the recovery position that maintains an open airway, and explain why it is important
- Describe how to treat a casualty who is in seizure

Outcome 4 assessment criteria
The learner can:
- Demonstrate how to administer effective cardiopulmonary resuscitation using a manikin

Outcome 5 assessment criteria
The learner can:
- Describe how to identify a casualty with a partially and completely blocked airway obstruction
- Demonstrate how to treat a casualty who is choking

Outcome 6 assessment criteria
The learner can:
- Demonstrate how to control severe external bleeding

Outcome 7 assessment criteria
The learner can:
- Describe signs and symptoms of shock
- Demonstrate how to manage a casualty who is in shock

Outcome 8 assessment criteria
The learner can:
- Describe how to manage a casualty with:
  - Small cuts, grazes, and bruises
  - Minor burns and scalds
  - Small splinters

This unit must be assessed in line with the document 'Skills for Health First Aid Assessment Principles'.

Details of various elements of theory and underpinning knowledge are included in Chapter 13, and these are also assessed within the written paper.

The theory and underpinning knowledge required to know about and understand the medical emergencies that may occur in the dental workplace, and the emergency treatment required to preserve life in each situation, are discussed in detail in Chapter 13. This chapter explains the dental nurse's roles and responsibilities in relation to emergency first aid skills – those required to provide immediate assistance and emergency medical care to a casualty before professional medical help arrives.

The skills required and able to be demonstrated by the dental nurse include the following:

- Limits of the roles and responsibilities of the first aider
- Incident assessment
- Management of an unresponsive casualty
- Management of an unresponsive casualty with breathing problems
- Management of a choking casualty
- Management of a wounded and bleeding casualty
- Management of a casualty in shock
- Management of minor injuries

The provision of immediate and appropriate emergency first aid to a casualty could be the difference between life and death, and as healthcare workers, dental nurses (and all other members of the dental team) should have these skills at their fingertips in the event of an emergency situation. Any individual can train to become a first aider, but healthcare workers are also trained and knowledgeable in other areas of medicine as part of their job role, and therefore they are obvious individuals to be trained as first aiders. Their skills are not confined to the dental workplace or learned once in a one-off training session – they should be able to be adapted to any emergency situation and should undergo constant update training on a regular basis.

Basic life support (BLS) and resuscitation skills are among the core topics of verifiable continuing professional development (CPD) that must be undertaken by all members of the dental team, throughout their period of registration with the General Dental Council (GDC).

Roles and responsibilities of the first aider

The skills required to be an effective first aider are not simply to have the knowledge of how to deal with specific medical emergency situations; the dental nurse must also be able to risk assess an emergency situation, be able to communicate effectively with the casualty (when conscious) and other individuals, and be able to ensure the casualty receives timely and appropriate first aid assistance until paramedics arrive. The roles and responsibilities can be summarised as follows:

- Health and safety requirements of the workplace
- Infection control and minimising cross-infection
- Correct reporting of Incidents
- Knowledge and use of emergency equipment
- Communication and care of the casualty

Health and safety requirements

In the dental workplace, a health and safety policy should already be available and will have been developed after a risk assessment has been carried out for the premises, usually by the employer. The dental nurse must follow this policy when on the premises at all times, as should all other personnel. This topic is discussed further in Chapters 1 and 12.

Specifically, dental nurses must ensure that they are not responsible for any acts or omissions in relation to the health and safety policy that would put themselves, their colleagues or any other individuals in the workplace at risk of harm, at any time. Obvious examples of poor practice would be failure to follow ionising radiation regulations, failure to wash their hands and wear personal protective equipment (PPE) when dealing with patients, and failure to take adequate precautions when using cleaning chemicals.

Dental nurses must therefore ensure that they are familiar with the following:

- Where the health and safety policy is kept
- Its contents
- The details of any updates or amendments to the policy
- The changes required in their actions following the updates or amendments

When dental nurses are called upon to act as an emergency first aider away from the dental workplace (such as coming upon the scene of a car crash), the knowledge and skills they have in relation to health and safety must be adapted accordingly. They must use their common sense in the emergency situation to ensure that no one else is put at risk while attempting to help any casualties.

Infection control and minimising cross-infection

The control of infection and the avoidance of cross-infection is a hugely important subject to all healthcare workers, including the dental nurse. Exposure to body fluids during the treatment of patients, as well as the close proximity of the working environment, puts all dental staff at risk of cross-infection throughout a normal working day. All are familiar with working while wearing suitable items of PPE, and of the necessity for the thorough decontamination of any items that are to be reused on other patients. Just as important is to ensure that single-use items are treated as such and never reused between patients. Infection control is discussed in detail in Chapter 12.

When the dental nurse is called upon to act as an emergency first aider away from the dental workplace, the same cross-infection risks apply and the same precautions should be taken. All first aiders are advised to carry a set of non-latex clinical gloves with them at all times, as well as a personal face shield device so that they can wear suitable PPE and protect themselves when offering first aid at the scene of an accident. The dental nurse has easy access to these gloves, and the face shields are available through organisations such as St John Ambulance. Further information is available at www.sja.org.uk.

Correct reporting of incidents

All dental nurses should be familiar with the correct procedures to be followed in the event of an accident or a significant event in the dental workplace. Accidents that occur in the workplace fall into one of two categories:

- **Minor accidents** – these result in no serious injury to persons or the premises, and are dealt with "in house" and recorded in the **accident book**
  - A written record of the minor accident must be made and kept by the workplace in the accident book, under the Notification of Accidents and Dangerous Occurrences Regulations (see Figure 1.15)
  - Examples of minor accidents include a trip or fall resulting in no serious injury, a clean (non-infectious) needlestick injury, or a minor mercury spillage that can be safely dealt with using the spillage kit
- **Major accidents** – these result in a serious injury to a person, or severe damage to the premises
  - They are classed as "significant events" and are therefore notifiable incidents that must be reported to the Health and Safety Executive under the Reporting of Injuries, Diseases and Dangerous Occurrences Regulations (RIDDOR)

The reporting of accidents and notifiable incidents are discussed in detail in Chapters 1 and 12.

When the dental nurse acts as an emergency first aider away from the dental workplace, or when handing over to medical professionals following a notifiable incident within the workplace, certain information will be required by the specialists immediately if advanced medical care for the casualty is to be successful. The likely first responders to an emergency call will be paramedics, complete with specialised equipment and drugs to take over the advanced life support of the individual.

They will require an accurate report of the emergency from all rescuers present to determine how best to proceed. The following points, in particular, will require verification:

- **What happened?** Did anyone witness the actual emergency event (trip and fall, road traffic accident, convulsion, heart attack, choking, etc.)?
- **What time?** How long ago did the event occur, and how quickly were rescuers on the scene?
- **Condition?** Was AVPU (alert, verbal, painful, unresponsive – see later) gone through by the rescuers, and if so, what was the casualty's initial level of responsiveness?
- **Basic life support?** Was BLS required, how long was it carried out for, were there any problems in maintaining life before the specialists arrived?
- **Use of the automatic external defibrillator (AED)?** Was the AED administered to the casualty, and if so how many times?
- **Background knowledge?** Are any relatives or friends present with further information on the casualty (including their name), and are any Medic Alert identifiers present?

- **Personal items?** Hand over all of the casualty's personal items to the specialists; they will be able to check identity and medical status, which is especially important in terms of discovering whether any medications are taken, such as an asthma inhaler
- **Remain at the scene** – do not leave until the specialists are happy that they have all the information they require, including your personal and contact details in case the casualty dies, as a statement to the police may be required

In an emergency situation, it is very important that the emergency first aider remains calm throughout, that they can think and act logically, and that they can recall the information given above accurately – the best method to ensure this is to write notes as soon as possible ready for the handover to the paramedics.

Knowledge and use of emergency equipment

All dental workplaces should have first aid provision available for their employees, in the form of a first aid box (see Figure 1.8) which is in an easily accessible position and highlighted with a typical poster showing a white cross on a green background (see Figure 1.9).

In a workplace of five or more employees, at least one person should be trained as an emergency first aider, although as many trained staff as possible would be ideal, so that holidays periods and sick leave are covered too. The contents of the first aid box will have been chosen in light of the risk assessment carried out on the premises, and should include all of the following items in the dental workplace as a minimum:

- Emergency first aid booklet – as a quick reference guide
- Assorted waterproof plasters
- Eye pads
- Assorted medium and large dressings, with scissors
- Triangular bandage and safety pins to secure once applied
- Sealed cleansing wipe packets
- Face shield for non-contact mouth-to-mouth resuscitation
- Burn shield
- Finger dressings
- Space blanket to maintain body temperature
- "Micropore" tape
- Non-latex clinical gloves

Suitable first aid training will cover the use of each item. When the dental nurse has received training it would be advisable to maintain a similar first aid box for personal use away from the dental workplace too – stored in the car, for example. Some of the items will have "use by" dates attached, and there must be a simple process in place to ensure that they are checked on a regular basis so that items can be replaced as necessary. This should be a duty of the first aider and must be delegated within the workplace accordingly.

In addition to the first aid kit, the dental workplace must also have certain specialist resuscitation equipment available on the premises and in good working order, and all personnel must be regularly trained in its use. The management of medical emergencies is a verifiable CPD requirement for all staff in the dental workplace.

The equipment is as follows:

- Emergency drugs box (see later)
- Portable suction unit to clear the airway, in the event of loss of power to the chairside aspirator
- Oxygen cylinder, tubing and face mask
- Positive ventilation bag and reservoir, with tubing

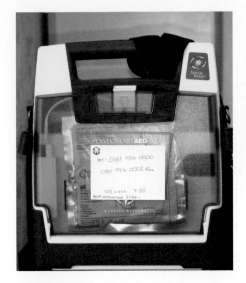

Figure 3.1 An automatic external defibrillator.

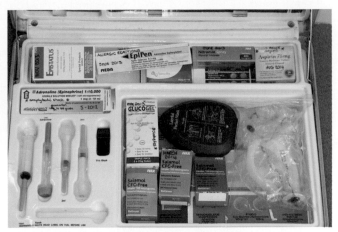

Figure 3.2 An emergency drugs kit.

All dental workplaces must have an external automatic defibrillator (AED) on site too (Figure 3.1). This specialist device is used when a casualty is suspected of having suffered a heart attack and attempts are being made to re-start the heart. Their correct use in an emergency situation can make a significant difference to the likelihood of survival of the casualty, but they must only ever be used by an individual who has received the necessary training and has been certificated as being competent to use the machine.

Emergency equipment/drugs

It has been accepted for many years now that individuals working in a healthcare setting should have a greater level of knowledge and understanding of medical emergencies and emergency first aid than the average lay person, by virtue of the training they have undergone in their chosen profession. Dental personnel are no exception, and workplaces must hold an emergency drugs kit (Figure 3.2) as well as the first aid kit, so that a casualty may receive advanced support from the team in the event of a sudden collapse while in the dental workplace. These emergencies are discussed in detail in Chapter 12, and they are listed as follows:

- Asthma attack
- Anaphylaxis
- Epileptic seizure
- Diabetic hypoglycaemia or coma
- Angina attack that may lead to myocardial infarction

The drugs that should be available in the kit for use with any of these emergency events are shown in the following table. The various causes of the collapse of a casualty must be known and understood by the dental nurse, so that they can assist usefully in the emergency treatment of these individuals should the need arise. While knowing and understanding the functions of the emergency equipment that all dental surgeries must hold, the dental nurse would not be expected to administer any of the drugs available, except as a last resort where they are the only rescuer and the casualty is likely to die otherwise, before specialist help arrives.

Emergency	Drug and dose	Route given
Asthma attack	Salbutamol metered dose 0.1 mg Oxygen	Inhaler Face mask
Anaphylaxis	Adrenaline 1:1000 Oxygen Hydrocortisone 100 mg Chlorphenamine 10 mg/mL	IM injection Face mask IM injection IM injection
Epileptic fit	Oxygen if possible Midazolam buccal gel if fit is prolonged	Face mask Oral
Hypoglycaemia	Conscious – glucogel Unconscious – glucagon 1 mg	Oral IM injection
Angina	GTN metered dose 0.4 mg Oxygen	Sublingual Face mask
Myocardial infarction	Aspirin 300 mg Oxygen	Oral Face mask

IM, intramuscular; GTN, glyceryl trinitrate.

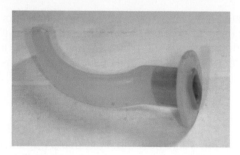

Figure 3.3　A Geudel airway.

In addition, certain equipment is also required to administer these drugs, so the kit must also contain a suitable range of sterile syringes and needles, and a selection of sizes of airways for insertion in the casualty's mouth so that the airway is maintained while the person is unconscious. The usual example is a Geudel airway (Figure 3.3), and while their use in an emergency situation goes a long way towards the survival of the casualty, they must only be administered by trained personnel. As with the first aid kit, the contents of the emergency drugs kit will have "use by" dates which require regular checking and then items replacing as necessary. It is particularly important that out-of-date drugs are not used on a casualty, as they are unlikely to produce the required response and are very likely to harm the person.

Members of the dental team should familiarise themselves with the emergency equipment and practise using it on a regular basis. In particular, they should practise:

- The use of the resuscitation masks and positive ventilation bag
- The use of the portable suction unit for clearing the airway
- The use of artificial airways and their correct insertion technique
- Switching on the oxygen supply, and connecting the tubing and masks correctly
- Opening drug phials and correctly drawing up their contents (out-of-date drugs can be kept on the premises for this purpose, but they must be removed from the emergency kit itself)

When the dental nurse is involved in an emergency incident away from the workplace, there will be no access to these drugs and additional equipment, and the emergency care provided will be that of first aid only to maintain life until the arrival of the paramedics.

Communication and care of the casualty

During an emergency situation, it is likely that the casualty, their companions and other onlookers present will be in a state of shock and distress and unable to think and act logically in an effort to assist the casualty. The first aider must remain calm and decisive throughout, and be able to take command of the situation so that everyone possible is directed to assisting in the emergency.

In the dental workplace, the emergency first aid drill should be practised on a regular basis, with the protocol to be followed having been established so that all members of the dental team are aware of what is required of each of the people involved. In particular, the following points must be addressed:

- Designation of the team leader (usually the senior dentist)
- All staff must stop work and be available to assist with the emergency immediately
- The location of the emergency drugs kit, the AED and the oxygen cylinders and tubing must be known by all staff
- Duties will be delegated by the team leader and must be carried out correctly by those involved – in particular, duties to collect the emergency drugs box, the oxygen, to call 999, to clear other patients away, and to direct the specialist emergency personnel to the casualty
- No duties should be undertaken that staff have not been specifically trained for
- All staff must be competent in BLS techniques and be able to assist as necessary
- Commands from the team leader must be followed immediately and accurately
- Duty of care to the casualty must be upheld at all times

When away from the workplace, the dental nurse may be the most trained and knowledgeable person present, and will therefore have to take on the role of team leader and delegate the relevant duties to other persons present.

Dental nurses must use their verbal and non-verbal communication skills to best effect during the emergency, remaining calm and friendly but maintaining authority so that requests are followed by others. Communication with the casualty may be impossible if the person is unconscious, or difficult if it is an infant or young child, or if the person speaks little or no English. In these examples, the dental nurse must also manage a parent, other family member or a friend of the casualty in an effort to calm them enough to assist in useful communications.

Casualties who are conscious often feel embarrassed at their situation, and dental nurses should do everything possible to help maintain the person's dignity, just as they would with a patient in the workplace. Anyone present who is not immediately involved in assisting with the care of the casualty should be politely but firmly ordered to move away from the immediate vicinity. If casualties are exposed in any way, they should be covered with coats, blankets or anything else to hand without impeding the first aid treatment, but only after they have been assessed for the full extent of any injuries.

Their personal possessions may also be strewn around the accident site, and these need collecting and keeping safe so that they can be handed over to the paramedics on their arrival. If the casualty has been found collapsed with no clue to their identity or the cause of their collapse, it is reasonable for the first aider to search their possessions for identification or items such as a Medic Alert card – but this search should be carried out in front of witnesses wherever possible.

If clothing or other items require to be removed, the casualty should be asked for permission to do so if possible and should be shielded from onlookers, hot sunshine and rain throughout. These duties can be delegated to a responsible person where necessary, so that the first aider can concentrate efforts on directly assisting the casualty.

Incident assessment

When individuals come across an accident or emergency situation, it is natural to want to race in and attend to casualties immediately, but in some instances this may endanger the lives of the first aider themselves. A casualty may have been electrocuted, or overcome by toxic fumes, and these dangers may still be present at the scene when the first aider arrives. Consequently, a few seconds taken to carry out an incident assessment in a logical manner may well prevent others from becoming casualties too, and provides the best chance of survival for the original casualty – first aiders cannot carry out BLS if they have been electrocuted too.

An incident assessment should therefore follow an established pattern, so that nothing is forgotten or missed by the first aider, as follows:

- **Assess the situation** – before approaching the casualty assess:
  ○ Safety – check for dangers to ensure it is safe to attend to the casualty
  ○ Scene – is there more than one casualty requiring help?
  ○ Situation – what has happened to cause the incident; are any witnesses available?
- **Primary survey of the casualty** – better known as "DRSABC" (see the next section)
- **Secondary survey of the casualty** – once emergency treatment has been given, any information about the incident can be determined from the casualty or any witnesses, and then a "head-to-toe" survey is carried out to determine if the casualty has any less obvious injuries present

When carrying out the situation assessment, if it becomes apparent that the area is not safe to approach or that there is more than one seriously injured casualty to attend to, the emergency services must be contacted immediately. The first aider must never approach any casualty until the area is made safe, and if there is more than one casualty then the most seriously injured (those with life threatening injuries) must be attended to first.

Primary survey

The aim of the primary survey is to determine if any life-threatening injuries or conditions are present, and then to manage them until medical help arrives. The five points that must be considered at the scene of any emergency situation (whether in the dental workplace or not) are referred to as **DRSABC** (referred to as "doctors – a – b – c"):

- **D** for **Danger** – checking for dangers within the immediate vicinity of the casualty
- **R** for **Response** – checking for the level of responsiveness of the casualty: the less responsive, the more serious the incident
- **S** for **Shout for help** – when and how to call for emergency assistance
- **A** for **Airway** – checking, clearing and opening the airway
- **B** for **Breathing** – providing effective rescue breaths
- **C** for **Circulation** – carrying out effective chest compressions to circulate the blood

These BLS techniques are discussed in detail later in the chapter.

The correct recognition of the cause of any emergency is vital if casualties are to be correctly treated and their life supported until the emergency services can attend. This is done by being able to recognise the "**signs**" and "**symptoms**" of an emergency.

The signs are what the first aider can see with regard to the casualty, such as:

- Skin colour – is it pink, grey, red, pale?
- Breathlessness – are they gasping, breathing quickly, struggling to inhale or exhale?
- Suddenness of any collapse – did the casualty fall straight to the ground, or did they slowly slump down?

- Actions before collapse, such as clutching the chest
- Condition of the pulse – is it fast, slow, weak, absent?

At the same time, the casualty will feel symptoms which the first aider will ask about if the person is conscious, such as:

- Any pain – is it sharp, dull, throbbing, made worse by anything?
- Location of pain – where is it felt exactly?
- Nausea – does the casualty feel sick, or have they vomited?
- Drowsiness – do they feel sleepy, are they struggling to respond to verbal commands?
- Difficulty breathing – are they struggling to breathe in or out, or both?
- Dizziness – does the casualty feel like they will fall over; is the room spinning?

By assessing the casualty and noting the signs and symptoms exhibited, the dental nurse can determine the next course of action, and often this will be to reassure the conscious casualty and to summon more experienced help.

However, there are two signs that should prompt any first aider to begin BLS immediately:

- **Unconsciousness**
- **Abnormal breathing**

These two signs indicate that the casualty's life is at risk, as sudden unconsciousness may indicate that the heart has stopped beating (**asystole**) or is beating ineffectively (**fibrillating**), and abnormal breathing indicates a compromised airway and possible lack of oxygen to the brain (**hypoxia**). The presence of any of these signs may result in the death of the casualty if not dealt with quickly by the first aider.

The aim of BLS is to maintain a flow of oxygenated blood to the casualty until one of the following happens:

- The casualty recovers and begin to circulate oxygenated blood by breathing unassisted
- The casualty's life support is handed over to specialists, usually paramedics
- The rescuer is too physically exhausted to continue
- The casualty's death is confirmed by an authorised practitioner, such as a doctor at the scene

Whenever possible, first aiders should remain with the casualty and begin cardiopulmonary resuscitation or other emergency first aid (as necessary) while a second person is sent to summon emergency help. If alone with the casualty, the first aider must shout loudly for help or use the emergency system available in the workplace (alarm bell, etc.); if no help is forthcoming the first aider may have to leave the casualty to go and summon help.

This may involve locating a phone and calling "999" or "112" and requesting paramedics, or flagging down a passing vehicle and asking them to raise the alarm, or just finding other people and asking them to raise the alarm while the first aider returns to the casualty and begins BLS.

Secondary survey

A secondary survey should only be carried out by a first aider who has received adequate training to do so; otherwise injuries may be made worse and the risk of cross-infection increased to both the casualty and the first aider. If the casualty is conscious, the dental nurse will inform the person that they are about to be checked from head to toe for other injuries, before beginning the secondary survey. The casualty should be asked if there is any pain or numbness on one side as the survey is carried out, with the first aider using both hands to assess the casualty and compare any differences between the right and left sides. Suitable PPE should be worn if bleeding is present, and any wounds found should not be touched but covered with dressings if possible.

Management of an unresponsive casualty who is breathing normally

When a casualty is first discovered, the primary survey will soon determine whether or not they are unconscious and breathing normally. The first aid treatment that must be carried out is quite different in each circumstance, as an unconscious casualty who is breathing normally will obviously not require cardiopulmonary resuscitation to be carried out, but must have the airway maintained until emergency help arrives.

The "DRSABC" relevant in this situation is described here.

Danger

As with the incident assessment protocol, before approaching the casualty, the immediate area must be checked for possible dangers, such as electric wires running through pooled water, punctured gas canisters, spilt chemicals giving off strong fumes. If hazardous chemicals are suspected of being involved in the emergency situation, the workplace Control of Substances Hazardous to Health (COSHH) file must be consulted at some point for information on first aid actions that may be necessary. This action is best delegated to a spare rescuer, while BLS is being carried out by others.

If possible, any dangers should be made safe by rescuers before approaching the casualty, but not at the risk of endangering themselves in the process. Ideally, this should not involve moving the individual, except in extreme circumstances, such as rising water levels that may cause drowning. This is to prevent any further injury being caused.

Response

The level of responsiveness will determine whether or not the casualty is unconscious. Call loudly to the person, asking if they can hear you or if they are alright, while gently tapping their shoulders. Their responsiveness can quickly be assessed and determined by a system referred to as the "AVPU" code:

- **Alert** – the casualty is fully conscious and able to communicate fully and spontaneously
- **Verbal** – the casualty is not fully conscious, but is able to respond to verbal commands and prompts
- **Painful** – the casualty is semi-conscious at best, but able to respond to painful stimuli such as a gentle pinch
- **Unresponsive** – the casualty shows no response to verbal prompts nor painful stimuli, is unconscious and unable to be roused

If casualties show no response whatsoever, then they are in need of urgent help. Wherever possible, the level of responsiveness should be determined without moving individuals from the position in which they were found, to avoid any further injury.

Shout

If the casualty is unresponsive and therefore unconscious, the rescuer will need help with any attempt at BLS if it is required, as well as to summon specialist help if necessary. If only one rescuer remains to aid the individual while help is being sought, that rescuer may need to continue BLS for a prolonged period of time, and ultimately this may result in their physical exhaustion. If attempts at BLS have to then be abandoned before specialist help arrives, the casualty is likely to die.

Shout very loudly to alert anyone else in the vicinity that an emergency situation has arisen. In the workplace, there may be internal communication systems in place for just such an event, such as intercoms, alarm bells or coded calls, and these must be known about and used appropriately by the dental nurse. Training will have been provided by the employer in the correct protocol to follow.

Airway

The airway needs to be checked for any obstruction, such as vomit or debris or the tongue itself, which may have fallen back and blocked it. Any loose obstruction should be removed by rolling the casualty's head to the side to encourage it to drop out of the mouth. In the dental workplace there will also be electrically operated suction equipment available at the chairside, or a manually operated suction device within the emergency kit that all dental workplaces have to have on the premises (Figure 3.4). However, these must only be used by those staff members who have been trained in their correct use, as they can push debris further down the airway or cause soft tissue injury if not used correctly.

The casualty's airway can then be opened to allow breathing to occur. This can be achieved by tilting the head back by placing the palm of one hand on the casualty's forehead and lifting the chin with the fingers of the other hand at the same time (Figure 3.5).

However, this technique must never be used when an individual has a suspected neck or spinal injury, as to do so would almost certainly cause further damage to the spinal cord. This could result in permanent paralysis of the individual. In these cases the airway can be opened by thrusting the lower jaw forward with both hands, without any head tilting occurring (Figure 3.6). This should avoid any further neck or spinal injury.

Breathing

With the airway open, breathing is assessed quickly over a 10-second period. The rescuer needs to determine if any spontaneous breathing attempts are being made, and their quality, by checking for the following (Figure 3.7):

- **Look** to see if the chest is rising and falling
- **Listen** to any breathing sounds
  - Are they regular or infrequent?
  - Are they quiet or noisy?
  - Are they normal or gasping in nature?
- **Feel** for air flow by placing the cheek close to the casualty's mouth

If it is determined that the casualty is breathing normally at this point, but remains unconscious, then the person's airway must be maintained until the emergency services arrive. The casualty needs to be placed in a position where the airway is not likely to become blocked by their tongue, or by vomit, and this is especially important if the first aider has to leave the casualty to go to summon help.

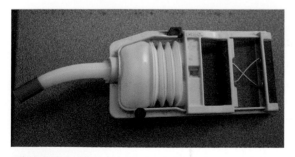

Figure 3.4   A manual suction device.

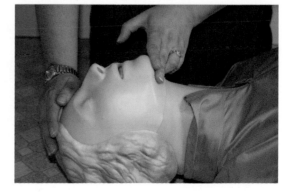

Figure 3.5   Head tilt to open airway.

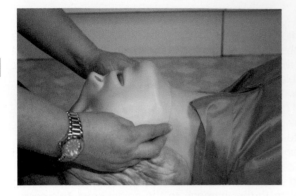

Figure 3.6   Jaw thrust to open airway.

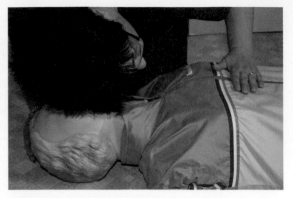

Figure 3.7   Look, listen and feel for signs of breathing.

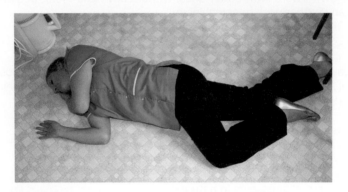

Figure 3.8   The recovery position.

Recovery position

The recovery position involves rolling casualties onto their side and bending their limbs so that they are supported in that position, with the airway open and unobstructed (Figure 3.8). This can only be fully performed when they have no potential injuries to their spine or limbs, otherwise a modified position must be used (see next section).

For casualties lying on their back and breathing, with no injuries, the recovery position is achieved as follows:

- Kneel at one side of the casualty
- Straighten out their arms and legs
- Move their nearest arm out at a right angle and bend it up at the elbow
- Gently pull their other arm and furthest leg towards you, so that the casualty begins to roll towards you
- Place the furthest hand against the side of their face
- Continue to roll them towards you by pulling the furthest leg, until their knee touches the ground
- Keep their hand against the face so that their head rolls onto it
- Once the roll is completed, ensure the airway is open by tilting the head back as necessary
- Adjust the bent leg to stabilise the casualty in this recovery position

The dental nurse will be required to demonstrate putting a casualty into the recovery position to an assessor, as part of the completion of their workplace portfolio. The technique is the same for all age groups except babies. Babies will be unstable if placed in the conventional recovery position, and it is much easier to place them in a safe position while holding them.

If breathing but unconscious, babies should be picked up and held on their side, towards the first aider, with one hand under the head and the other under their side and bottom. They should be tilted down slightly so that the head is lower than their body, allowing the tongue and any fluids to fall forwards away from the airway.

Modified recovery position

If a spinal injury is suspected, such as if the casualty has fallen onto their back from a height, performing the full recovery position manoeuvre may well cause permanent spinal injury and should not be attempted.

Ideally, casualties should be left in the position in which they were found until specialist help arrives, but this may not be advisable if there is a possibility that the airway could become obstructed. In this situation, they must be rolled onto their side and supported in that position using anything available, such as rolled-up coats or other people. While rolling them, their head and spine must be kept in alignment at all times (the "log roll"), so the manoeuvre can only be carried out when more than one individual is present. Similarly, if any limb injuries are suspected, casualties must be rolled without pulling on their limbs, and supported by coats, etc., rather than by bending the limbs to achieve stability.

The most important point is that the airway is opened and remains unobstructed, so that life is preserved. The first aider will need to monitor the breathing and ensure that it continues to be unobstructed until specialist help arrives.

Casualty having a seizure

One cause of a casualty collapsing and becoming unconscious without suffering from breathing problems is an epileptic seizure.

Epilepsy is a pre-diagnosed condition, where there is a brief disruption of the normal electrical activity within the brain, causing a fit, or seizure. The fits can occur mildly (petit mal) and the casualty may appear to be daydreaming, or they may occur in a major form (grand mal). The casualty will lose consciousness with a grand mal seizure.

Signs – sudden loss of consciousness with the casualty falling to the floor, followed by "tonic–clonic" seizure, and possible incontinence. In the tonic phase, the casualty becomes rigid; in the clonic phase, the casualty convulses.

Symptoms – Casualties may experience an altered mood (aura) just before the fit begins, they are dazed on recovery and have no memory of the fit.

Treatment:

- Protect the casualty from injury by moving objects away from them
- Do not attempt to move the casualty yourself
- Remove onlookers from the area and maintain the casualty's dignity
- The tonic–clonic episode usually lasts just a few minutes at the longest
- Allow the casualty to recover, then ensure they are escorted home if they are a known epileptic
- The emergency services must be called if the casualty:
  - Has no previous history of seizures
  - Is in seizure for more than 5 minutes
  - Has continuous seizures
  - Remains unconscious for more than 10 minutes
  - Is injured during the seizure
- If the seizure occurs in the dental workplace, a trained first aider can administer midazolam buccal gel from the emergency drug box

Management of an unresponsive casualty with breathing problems

During the primary survey (DRSABC) the first aider will check whether the casualty is breathing spontaneously or not, and also for the quality of the respiratory efforts. With the airway open, breathing is assessed quickly over a 10-second period as follows:

- **Look** to see if the chest is rising and falling
- **Listen** to any breathing sounds
  - Are they regular or infrequent?
  - Are they quiet or noisy?
  - Are they normal or gasping in nature?
- **Feel** for air flow by placing the cheek close to the casualty's mouth

If the casualty's breathing efforts are absent or abnormal, the emergency services must be called as specialist help is required. Ideally a second person can be sent to do this, but if necessary the lone first aider must leave the casualty and go to call for emergency help. If the emergency has occurred in the dental workplace, the AED must also be brought to the scene at this point.

The first aider must now give early BLS by carrying out cardiopulmonary resuscitation (CPR) to maintain the casualty until the emergency services arrive. This may require moving the casualty to a position where this can be carried out effectively. This is usually achieved by very carefully rolling the individual onto their back with a firm surface underneath, in a safe area and with enough room to manoeuvre as necessary, as BLS may need to be carried out correctly for a prolonged period until specialist help arrives.

Circulation

The final stage of the primary survey is to maintain a circulation to the casualty's organs and body tissues. Any residual oxygenated blood within the casualty needs to be quickly pumped around their body to the brain, which is achieved by the first aider carrying out chest compressions on the casualty. These will only be effective if the heart is adequately compressed between the breastbone (sternum) and the spine, on a firm surface, and at a sufficient rate to actually cause the blood to flow through the circulatory system as required, rather than just swishing backwards and forwards (Figure 3.9).

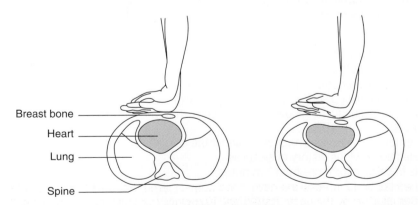

Breast bone
Heart
Lung
Spine

Figure 3.9   Carrying out external cardiac compressions. Source: *Levison's Textbook for Dental Nurses*, 11th edition (Hollins), 2013. Reproduced with permission of Wiley-Blackwell.

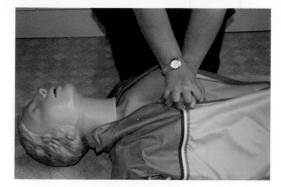

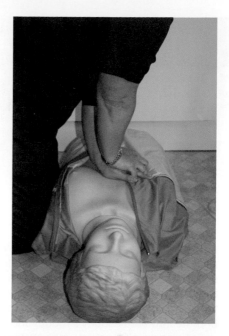

Figure 3.10 Hand lock for chest compressions. **Figure 3.11** Arm lock for chest compressions.

If any spinal or neck injuries are suspected, it would be ideal not to move the casualty from the position in which they were found, to avoid further injury. However, this may not always be possible, especially if the casualty's position prevents successful BLS from being carried out. Ideally, several helpers should be used to very carefully roll the casualty onto their back on a hard surface, keeping the head in line with the spine at all times – this is the "log roll" technique.

In the dental workplace, dental chairs are designed to be firm enough to carry out chest compressions without having to move the casualty onto the floor.

The correct point to apply the compressions is the centre of the chest, which can be quickly located as follows:

- Kneel at the side of the casualty, or stand if the person is still on the dental chair
- Run a finger along the lower border of the individual's ribcage, towards the midline
- Once in the midline, the breastbone will be felt with the finger
- Place the heel of the other hand adjacent to the finger, towards the head of the individual
- Interlock the fingers of both hands over this compression point (Figure 3.10)
- Lean over the individual, keeping the arms straight and the elbows locked (Figure 3.11)

Thirty compressions can now be given at a rate of 100/minute, by compressing the chest by up to a third and then releasing to allow the heart to expand and refill with blood. Once the initial 30 compressions have been administered, two rescue breaths can be given by the lone first aider, or ideally by a second individual.

Rescue breathing

Once the first 30 compressions have been administered, any residual oxygen in the blood will have been used up by the body tissues, and especially the brain. To maintain life, the oxygen now has to be regularly replaced before being distributed around the body again by the chest compressions, and this is achieved by artificial ventilation or rescue breathing.

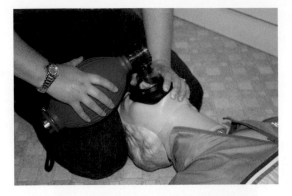

Figure 3.12   Use of the ventilation bag.

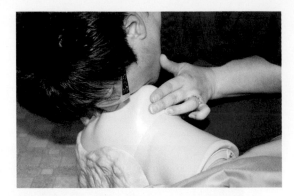

Figure 3.13   Rescue breathing mouth to mouth.

The atmosphere contains about 21% oxygen, but that expired (breathed out) only contains 16%, as our body tissues use up the 5% difference to produce energy for the cells to work. In an emergency situation, rescue breaths are usually given by breathing expired air into the casualty in a mouth-to-mouth technique. If there are facial injuries affecting the mouth, it may be necessary to use a mouth-to-nose technique instead, and with small children or babies the rescuer will breathe into the casualty's mouth and nose together.

The use of emergency oxygen supplies, such as that held by all dental workplaces, will increase the amount of available oxygen for rescue breathing when given using a pocket mask or an Ambu-bag, but the technique can only be successfully used by those trained to do so (Figure 3.12).

The airway will already have been cleared of obstructions during the DRSABC procedure, but will need to be held open now to administer rescue breaths, again using the head tilt/chin lift or jaw thrust technique. Two rescue breaths are then given as follows:

- Maintain the head tilt to keep the airway open
- Place the face shield from the first aid kit over the mouth and nose of the casualty
- Pinch the nostrils closed with the fingers of the hand being used to press onto the forehead
- Support the chin with the other hand while holding the mouth open
- Take a deep breath, then seal the mouth over that of the casualty to ensure no air escapes (Figure 3.13)
- Breathe with normal force into the casualty's open mouth for about 2 seconds, watching from the corner of the eye to ensure that the chest rises
- With the airway still held open, move away from the mouth and watch the chest fall as the air comes out
- Repeat the rescue breath
- If given successfully, follow with another 30 chest compressions as a CPR cycle

Sometimes problems will be experienced while attempting rescue breathing, the commonest one being that the chest does not rise. In the absence of an airway obstruction, this is usually due to the airway not being fully opened, and the head tilt procedure should be repeated until successful. Otherwise, ensure that the nostrils are fully closed and that a good mouth-to-mouth seal is being achieved.

If the abdomen is seen to rise while the breath is being given, it means air is being blown into the stomach, rather than the lungs, by being too forceful or too prolonged. The rescue breath should stop once the chest stops rising, usually after just 2 seconds at a normal breath force.

Dental nurses will be required to demonstrate successful CPR techniques using a manikin to an assessor, as part of the completion of their workplace portfolio.

Cardiopulmonary modifications

The CPR protocols described are to be used for adults and children over the age of 8 years. Babies and young children require less force to be used while carrying out both chest compressions and rescue breathing, to avoid injuring their bodies.

The weight of the foetus in a pregnant woman will also hinder CPR attempts if she is lying on her back, and the usual technique has to be modified for these groups of casualties.

Babies and young children

Anatomically these age groups are different from adults in the following ways:

- They have narrower air passages in the respiratory system
- These air passages are more prone to blockages
- The trachea is more flexible, and so it is easily blocked if airway opening attempts are too severe
- Their tongues are relatively larger than those of adults, which is more likely to obstruct the airway when the baby or young child is unconscious

Cardiac arrest in these younger casualties is rarely due to heart problems, as it is in an adult, but is far more likely to be caused by lack of oxygen to the brain due to airway obstruction.

As the primary survey is being followed, it will soon become apparent if the young casualty is unresponsive and having breathing difficulties or not breathing at all, and it is imperative that rescue breathing is commenced **BEFORE** starting chest compressions. This is because the likely cause of their collapse will be a shortage of oxygen to their vital organs, and any reserves will have been quickly used up by their young bodies and must be replenished as soon as possible.

So the full modified CPR sequence of events in cases involving a baby or a young child is as follows:

- **Danger** – check for dangers as usual
- **Response** – less reliable in younger casualties, so merely determine whether they are unresponsive only
- **Shout** – summon help from anyone in the vicinity, without leaving the casualty
- **Airway** – check the airway for obstruction, especially the tongue, then carefully open the airway, taking care not to overextend the head tilt and so block the trachea
- **Breathing** – look, listen and feel for signs of spontaneous breathing for 10 seconds, and if they are absent **GIVE FIVE RESCUE BREATHS USING THE MOUTH TO MOUTH-AND-NOSE TECHNIQUE**
- **Circulation** – give 30 chest compressions, using two fingers for a baby or one hand for a young child, aiming to compress the chest by one-third of its depth at a rate of 100/minute
- The lone first aider must continue CPR for a full minute before going for specialist help

Pregnant women

Any premenopausal woman who collapses and requires CPR could potentially be pregnant. In some cases, it will be known or obvious that they are pregnant, but otherwise it should always be considered a possibility, especially if resuscitation attempts are failing for no other obvious reason.

In a heavily pregnant woman lying on her back, the uterus (womb) tends to lie over the major blood vessels that return blood from the lower body to the right side of the heart (the inferior venae cavae). If this casualty collapses and requires CPR, the rescuer has the added difficulty of forcing blood through these squashed blood vessels during chest compressions, and the rescue attempt is likely to fail.

Instead, then, the pregnant casualty should be laid slightly on the left side with some form of support under the right buttock so that these major blood vessels are not squashed by the uterus. CPR can then be carried out in the normal way, while maintaining this angled position of the woman throughout.

Monitoring and evaluating CPR

Once the primary survey has been gone through correctly, the need for early BLS established, and CPR attempts are under way, the situation and condition of the casualty must be carefully monitored by the first aider to determine if rescue efforts should continue or be stopped.

There are four instances where CPR attempts should be stopped:

- The casualty recovers and is able to circulate oxygenated blood and breathe without assistance
- Their life support is handed over to specialists (paramedics)
- The rescuer is too physically exhausted to continue resuscitation efforts
- The death of the casualty is confirmed by an authorised practitioner (a doctor at the scene)

Management of a choking casualty

Like the simple faint, choking is an emergency that may well occur in the dental workplace from time to time, due to the nature of dental treatment – patients lying on their back (supine), the use of small instruments during dental treatment, and the presence of tooth debris and fluids in the mouth. However, unlike the simple faint, choking is a very serious situation that could result in death if not dealt with promptly. It can occur in both the conscious or unconscious casualty, by the partial or full blockage of the respiratory tract causing lack of blood oxygenation. The body tissues will become hypoxic, and this can be catastrophic when the brain or heart is affected.

Signs – sudden coughing or wheezing, laboured or noisy breathing, inability to speak, blue lips, clutching at the throat.

Symptoms – aware of respiratory obstruction, breathing difficulties, dizziness as oxygen levels to the brain are reduced.

Treatment:

- Calm and reassure the casualty
- Support the casualty in leaning forward and encourage coughing
- Give five back slaps between the shoulder blades to dislodge the obstruction (Figure 3.14)
- Begin abdominal thrusts (Heimlich manoeuvre) to cause artificial coughing if the obstruction is still present (Figure 3.15)
- If the casualty becomes unconscious, clear and open the airway as described in the primary survey
- Call 999 or 112 if this is unsuccessful

The technique of giving abdominal thrusts is as follows:

- Stand behind the casualty
- Wrap your arms around the casualty, just below the person's ribcage
- Form a fist with one hand and, grasped by the other, position both in the upper abdomen
- Pull both hands in sharply, to cause an artificial cough
- Air will whoosh out at each thrust, hopefully dislodging the obstruction

Dental nurses will be required to demonstrate how to treat a casualty who is choking to their assessor, as part of the completion of their workplace portfolio.

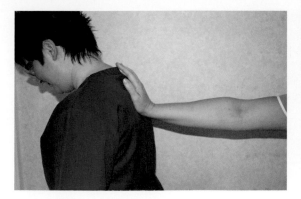

Figure 3.14   Back slaps between shoulder blades.

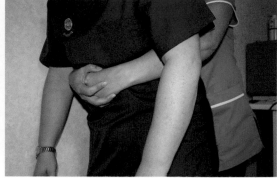

Figure 3.15   Abdominal thrusts.

Choking in young children

The signs and symptoms of choking in a young child will be as for an adult casualty, but they are more likely to experience this emergency due to their lack of awareness of danger and their tendency to put objects into their mouths without realising the consequences.

The procedure to follow is very similar to that for an adult but with less force, and depends on whether the young child is conscious or not. The important point is that rescue breathing should only be carried out on unconscious children, as their airway often becomes clear as their muscles relax during loss of consciousness, and rescue breaths may not be necessary.

The procedure in a choking conscious child is as follows:

- Keep calm and keep the casualty (and any attending parent) calm
- Get the child to cough to try and expel the obstruction
- If unsuccessful, give five back slaps and recheck the mouth
- If unsuccessful, give five chest thrusts from behind against the breastbone, then recheck the mouth
- If unsuccessful, send for help then repeat the back slaps and recheck the mouth
- If unsuccessful, give up to five abdominal thrusts but with less force than that used for an adult, then recheck the mouth
- Continue alternating all three techniques until the obstruction is cleared, the child loses consciousness or specialist help arrives
- If successful, have the child medically checked for any signs of respiratory system damage

If the choking episode is severe and prolonged, or the obstruction is complete, the child will collapse and become unconscious. The rescue procedure is as follows:

- Check the mouth for any obstruction and remove, then open the airway
- Try five times to give two rescue breaths – if the chest rises successfully then carry out chest compressions to circulate the oxygen around the body
- If the chest fails to rise, give five back slaps followed by five chest compressions if the child is still choking
- Recheck the mouth and open the airway, then give another five rescue breaths
- If unsuccessful give another five back slaps followed by five abdominal thrusts
- Continue the cycle until specialist help arrives or the obstruction is removed

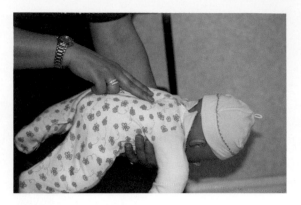

Figure 3.16 Baby back slaps using fingers.

Choking in babies

Babies are easier for the rescuer to handle during a choking episode, as they can be held face down for back slaps and carried towards help while still being aided, rather than having to be left. Obviously, the force used to attempt to dislodge an obstruction must be significantly less than that used for a young child. Also, under no circumstances should abdominal thrusts be attempted on a baby, as the internal organs would be easily damaged by this technique.

Again, as with a young child, rescue breathing should not be attempted unless the baby is unconscious.

If the baby is conscious and choking, the procedure is as follows:

- Check the mouth for any obvious obstruction and remove it
- With the baby held face down along the rescuer's arm, give five back slaps using fingers only (Figure 3.16)
- Turn the baby face up and remove any obstruction
- If unsuccessful, give five sharp chest compressions (as for CPR)
- If unsuccessful, call for specialist help and continue the cycle until the obstruction is removed or the baby becomes unconscious

If the baby becomes unconscious:

- Recheck the mouth and open the airway
- Try five times to give two rescue breaths
- If the chest rises, continue chest compressions to circulate the oxygen
- If not, give five back slaps followed by five chest compressions
- Recheck the mouth for any obstruction and open the airway, then repeat the cycle until specialist help arrives

Management of a wounded and bleeding casualty

A casualty may fall and injure themselves at any time, whether in the dental workplace or not. This may result in an open wound, where the skin is broken and there may be significant bleeding, or a closed wound where the skin is not broken but bruising at the site will indicate that there is bleeding into the tissues around the wound site. If the injury causing the closed wound is severe enough, the casualty may suffer from internal bleeding into the body cavities (the chest or abdomen).

Minor wounds are discussed later.

When casualties are wounded and bleeding either internally or externally, they will require emergency treatment so that their blood loss is controlled and they do not go into shock. Shock occurs when the blood volume within the body falls due to uncontrolled bleeding, and the body organs begin to become damaged due to their resultant lack of blood supply.

When a casualty is wounded and bleeding externally, the first aider must act quickly to control the bleeding while awaiting the arrival of the emergency services. The first aider can do little to help when internal bleeding occurs.

In the dental workplace, it is a requirement to wear PPE when dealing with body fluids or handling instruments contaminated with body fluids, especially blood, and the same is true when dealing with a wounded and bleeding casualty. Cross-infection of the wound and the first aider must be avoided at all times, so non-latex gloves must always be worn when dealing with a bleeding casualty or an open wound.

The aims of emergency first aid treatment with a wounded and bleeding casualty are to:

- Control the bleeding
- Prevent shock occurring
- Get specialist help for the casualty

When the first aider is without assistance, the bleeding must be controlled and the casualty positioned to prevent shock before they are left alone, while the first aider seeks specialist help. If the bleeding is left to continue while help is sought, the casualty is far more likely to go into shock and may even die before the emergency services arrive.

The bleeding is controlled and shock prevented by carrying out the following actions;

- Apply direct pressure to the wound site, with gloved hands
- If a limb is bleeding, it should be elevated above heart level to slow the flow
- If small foreign objects are visible in the wound and they can be removed by quickly flushing the area, do so to reduce the risk of infection
- If a large foreign object is present in the wound (such as a shard of glass), this should not be removed, as its removal is likely to cause further tissue damage
- The first aider must then work around the object to control the bleeding, and without pushing the object further into the wound
- Apply a dressing from the first aid kit to the wound site, fastening it firmly but not so tightly that the circulation is restricted – a tourniquet must not be used
- If blood seeps through the dressing, a second one should be applied over the top
- If blood continues to seep through the dressings, they should be removed, direct pressure applied again, and then new dressings applied
- The casualty should be laid down with the feet raised, in a similar position to that used for a fainting casualty (Figure 3.17)

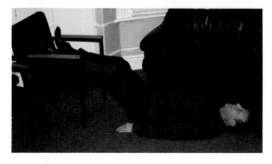

Figure 3.17   Faint recovery position.

- An injured limb should continue to be supported in an elevated position
- Ideally the casualty should be laid on coats, blankets, or the space blanket from the first aid kit to insulate them from the cold ground
- This should help to prevent them going into shock
- The emergency services can now be called

Dental nurses will be required to demonstrate how to control severe external bleeding to their assessor, as part of the completion of their workplace portfolio.

Management of a casualty in shock

Shock usually occurs when a casualty suffers severe blood loss, and the blood volume becomes so reduced the heart cannot pump it to the brain effectively. It may also occur following serious burns, due to the extensive loss of tissue fluid and plasma from the burnt area of skin. The body will begin to shut down other organs in an attempt to pump the reduced blood volume to the brain only, and if prolonged enough this will cause organ failure in the casualty. The blood loss may occur internally and so it will not be evident to the first aider initially. However, internal bleeding should always be suspected if the casualty displays the signs of shock without suffering any obvious fluid loss from an external bleed.

Shock is a life-threatening occurrence in casualties, and they will require urgent emergency treatment to prevent their death. The first aider must be able to recognise the signs of shock developing and take swift action to summon emergency help and prevent the casualty from deteriorating further before that help arrives, by improving the blood supply to the brain.

The signs are:

- Typical signs seen in a fainting casualty initially:
  - Pale complexion, cold and clammy skin
  - Rapid pulse
  - Sweating
- Development of cyanosis as oxygen levels fall
- Pulse becomes weaker
- Rapid but shallow breathing
- Yawning or actual gasping
- May become restless and aggressive before becoming unconscious

The casualty will feel weak, dizzy and nauseous, and complain of feeling thirsty. They may actually vomit. Shock is more likely to develop in an injured casualty who is frightened or in intense pain, so the first aider must do everything possible to calm and reassure the person, while managing the situation.

The treatment is as follows:

- Calm and reassure the casualty
- Treat any external bleeding, as described earlier
- Put the casualty into the faint recovery position, to improve the blood flow to the brain (see Figure 3.17)
- Keep the casualty warm by laying them on a blanket or by wrapping them in the space blanket
- The casualty's reduced blood flow should not be restricted, so loosen all tight clothing if possible
- Do not allow the casualty to drink anything to quench their thirst, but their lips can be moistened if any water is to hand

- Send for the emergency services
- Be prepared to carry out CPR if the casualty deteriorates

Dental nurses will be required to demonstrate how to manage a casualty who is in shock to their assessor, as part of the completion of their workplace portfolio.

Management of minor injuries

The types of minor injuries that the dental nurse may have to manage both in the dental workplace and away from it are as follows:

- Small cuts, grazes and bruises
- Minor burns and scalds
- Small splinters

Small cuts, grazes, and bruises

Cuts and grazes are open wounds and will require cleaning to reduce the risk of infection. They can occur as inoculation or other sharps injuries in the dental workplace, and their specific treatment is described in detail in Chapters 4 and 12.

For simple minor injuries, the treatment is as follows:

- Clean the wound with a sterile cleansing wipe from the first aid kit
- Pat (rather than rub) the wound dry with a sterile gauze pad
- Cover the wound with a sterile dressing and seal it in place with an adhesive dressing
- If the wound was dirty initially, or there is a risk of tetanus, advise the casualty to see their doctor

A small bruise is a closed wound where bleeding has occurred into the surrounding tissues. When no serious injury (such as a fracture) is likely, the bruised area can simply be treated with a cold compress for up to 30 minutes. If the bruising is on a limb, it can be raised to reduce the amount of bleeding into the tissues, and therefore reduce the extent of the bruising.

Minor burns and scalds

A burn is an injury caused by dry heat, corrosive chemicals or irradiation, while a scald is a wet burn caused by steam or hot liquids. Possible causes of burns in the dental workplace include touching hot equipment or instruments, touching naked flames, various chemicals (etching gel, bleach products, other cleaning agents), and uncontrolled exposure to X-rays. Possible causes of scalds in the dental workplace include exposure to steam from the autoclave or washer-disinfector, as well as the use of very hot water.

The damaged area will appear red and possibly swollen and blistered, and the casualty will be in pain. The first aid treatment is to cool the area and prevent infection of the underlying tissues, as follows:

- Remove the casualty from the source of heat
- Wear gloves to reduce the risk of cross-infection
- Immerse the burned area under cold running water for at least 10 minutes, without touching the raw area
- This will cool the burned area and reduce blistering
- Remove any jewellery if possible, but leave any clothing that is stuck to the burned skin in place
- Blisters should be left intact
- The wound may have a non-adhesive sterile dressing applied carefully

Small splinters

A splinter is usually a thin length of wood or glass which has broken away from an object and become embedded in the skin, usually a finger. If it is still projecting from the skin it can be removed with a pair of tweezers by the first aider. The wound should then be washed and dried, and covered with a small adhesive dressing.

If the splinter is too deep or not projecting from the skin, the casualty should be advised to immerse the area in warm soapy water, to clean the area and to soften the skin so that the splinter can be worked loose by gentle pressure. Once the splinter is removed, the wound should be covered with a small adhesive dressing.

4

Unit 304: Prepare and Maintain Environment, Instruments and Equipment for Clinical Dental Procedures

Learning outcomes

1. Be able to apply standard precautions of infection control for all treatments
2. Be able to apply health and safety measures for all treatments
3. Be able to apply methods of sterilisation for dental instruments and equipment
4. Be able to safely dispose of hazardous waste and non-hazardous waste

Outcome 1 assessment criteria
The learner can:
- Wear personal protective equipment for all treatments
- Maintain a clean and tidy environment for all treatments
- Use cleaning equipment and materials in a safe manner
- Adjust environmental factors to meet the needs of the patient and the procedure
- Explain which decontaminants are effective against the different types of microorganisms
- Explain the purpose of adjusting environmental factors

Outcome 2 assessment criteria
The learner can:
- Maintain personal hygiene
- Demonstrate that equipment is functioning prior to use
- Check equipment and materials are safe and secure, and leave them at the correct level of cleanliness, and in the correct location, on the completion of procedures

Diploma in Dental Nursing, Level 3, Third Edition. Carole Hollins.
© 2014 John Wiley & Sons, Ltd. Published 2014 by John Wiley & Sons, Ltd.
Companion website: www.wiley.com/go/hollins/dentalnursinglevel3

- Demonstrate methods of hand cleansing
- Explain what actions to take in the event of equipment failure
- Explain what actions to take in the event of a spillage occurring
- Explain the reporting procedures for hazards and why they should be reported
- Explain the reasons why records must be kept in relation to the servicing of equipment

Outcome 3 assessment criteria
The learner can:
- Prepare instruments and hand pieces for sterilisation
- Carry out sterilisation procedures
- Store sterilised instruments and hand pieces according to practice policy
- Maintain accurate and legible records of sterilisation procedures
- Explain the reason for pre-cleaning instruments prior to sterilisation
- Explain the methods available for testing autoclaves are functioning correctly
- Explain the importance of placing equipment and instruments in the correct location relevant to the different stages of sterilisation
- Explain the potential risks of not decontaminating equipment and instruments
- Explain the potential long-term effects of using damaged or pre-used sterile goods

Outcome 4 assessment criteria
The learner can:
- List the different types of waste
- Dispose of hazardous waste in a safe manner according to practice guidelines
- Explain the dangers of not disposing of waste correctly and promptly

This unit is assessed by:
- observation in the workplace, with examples included in the learner's portfolio
- an appropriate alternative method

Details of various elements of theory and underpinning knowledge are included in Chapter 12, and these are assessed within the written paper.

The theory and underpinning knowledge required to understand the principles involved in the control of infection in the dental workplace are fully discussed in Chapter 12. This chapter explains the dental nurse's role and responsibilities in relation to the following actions:

- Application of standard precautions of infection control for all dental procedures
- Application of health and safety measures for all dental procedures
- Application of suitable sterilisation methods for dental instruments and equipment
- Safe disposal of hazardous and non-hazardous waste

Application of standard precautions of infection control

For any clinical dental procedure to be carried out safely and effectively, the environment, instruments and equipment must all be properly prepared and maintained before, during and after each procedure. These preparation and maintenance tasks are two of the main duties of a dental nurse working at the chairside.

The aim of the preparation procedure is to ensure that all of the instruments and equipment to be used are clean and free of all contamination by microorganisms from a previous patient or from dental staff. They can then be safely used in the prepared environment (the dental surgery) without the risk of passing on, or cross-infecting, the next patient or member of staff.

Similarly, the aim of the maintenance procedure is to ensure that all the instruments and equipment used are then disposed of safely or cleaned to a high enough standard that they can be reused without the risk of cross-infecting the next patient, and so on. Likewise, the environment must also be cleaned thoroughly so that it is safe to be reused.

The risk that the microorganisms pose is that they can spread disease and infection from one person to another, either directly from person to person or indirectly via contaminated instruments or equipment. Those microorganisms that are capable of causing disease are referred to as pathogenic microorganisms, while those unable to cause disease are called non-pathogenic microorganisms.

The required underpinning knowledge involving the basics of microbiology and pathology, the actions of the microorganisms and the way in which they cause disease, and the body's defence mechanisms against them is discussed in detail in Chapter 12.

Standard precautions

These were previously referred to as "universal precautions" and have been adopted in healthcare work in an effort to protect staff from inoculation and contamination risks, and to protect patients from being exposed to the risk of cross-infection, from both dental staff and from other patients.

The basic principle is to assume that any patient may be infected with any microorganism at any time, and as such pose an infection risk to all dental staff and to other patients. A detailed medical history questionnaire, completed at the patient's initial attendance and updated at every appointment thereafter, will identify the majority of problems.

However, patients may be infected with a microorganism without showing any signs of disease, and may therefore be unaware of the risk they pose to others – these patients are called carriers. Also, patients may choose not to disclose their full medical history to the dental staff and would then be assumed to be "safe" to treat.

So, if all patients are considered to be a possible source of infection and are treated as such, the infection control techniques used in the dental environment will be good enough to reduce all cross-infection risks to a minimum, by maintaining an acceptable level of cleanliness at all times.

The terms "cleaning" and "cleanliness" in a clinical context are quite different from a layperson's concept of them, and definitions of the relevant terms used here are as follows:

- Social cleanliness – clean to a socially acceptable standard, but not disinfected nor sterilised
- Disinfection – the destruction of bacteria and fungi, but not spores or some viruses (the technique usually involves the use of chemicals)
- Sterilisation – the process of killing all microorganisms and spores to produce asepsis (the technique usually involves the use of special equipment that operates under high temperatures and pressure)
- Asepsis – the absence of all living pathogenic microorganisms
- Decontamination – the process used to remove contamination from reusable items, so that they are safe for further use on patients and safe for staff to handle. It may also be referred to as "reprocessing" and involves the following four stages:
  - Cleaning
  - Disinfection
  - Inspection
  - Sterilisation

The standard precautions to be applied for all dental procedures are the following:

- Correct use of personal protective equipment (PPE)
- Maintenance of a clean and tidy working environment

- Correct use of cleaning equipment
- Correct use of decontaminants against the different types of microorganisms
- Maintenance of suitable environmental factors

Personal protective equipment

These items are worn to form a barrier between the dental nurse, and other dental personnel, and any microorganism contamination. This contamination may be from direct sources, such as body fluids, body tissues and airborne particles or from indirect sources, such as contaminated instruments, equipment and aerosol spray. It is a legal requirement for dental employers to provide the following protective equipment for their staff (Figure 4.1):

- Gloves of varying quality, to prevent skin contact with contaminants:
  - Household gloves for handling chemicals and while scrubbing instruments
  - Clinical (non-sterile) gloves for non-surgical dental procedures
  - Surgical (sterile) gloves for surgical procedures
- Eye protection to prevent contaminant material entry or eye injury:
  - Safety glasses
  - Safety goggles (with wrap around side arms)
  - Visor
- Face masks of surgical quality should be worn whenever dental handpieces or ultrasonic equipment are in use, to prevent the inhalation of aerosol contamination and pieces of flying debris
- High-temperature-wash uniform, to be worn in the work area only
- Plastic apron to be worn over the uniform when soiling may occur during surgical procedures or while cleaning the surgery

In normal use then, dental staff working in the surgery environment should be kitted out as shown in Figure 4.2.

The gloves, in particular, must be removed and changed whenever moving from a contaminated (dirty) area to a clean area or when first handling clean items after assisting at the chairside. Appropriate examples are:

- During a chairside procedure, when:
  - Going into drawers or cupboards to locate additional items
  - About to ready materials for mixing
  - The gloves are damaged and their effectiveness is compromised

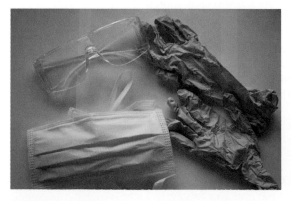

Figure 4.1   Items of personal protective equipment.

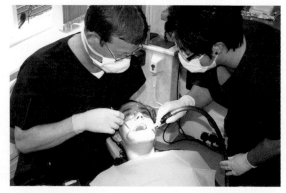

Figure 4.2   Personal protective equipment items in use.

- When finishing a chairside procedure, and before:
  - Touching the patient records or computer keyboard
  - Escorting the patient out of the surgery area
  - Beginning to clean the surgery area

Maintenance of a clean and tidy work environment

The whole of the dental workplace should be cleaned to a socially acceptable standard on a daily basis, and this is usually carried out by a domestic cleaner. In clinical areas, however, a far higher standard of cleaning is necessary because these are the areas where contamination of the environment by microorganisms and body fluids is greatest, and where the highest chance of cross-infection is likely to occur.

The standard to be achieved in the clinical environment is that of disinfection. This involves the use of various chemicals to inhibit the growth of or ideally kill, bacteria, viruses and fungi. However, most are not effective against bacterial spores and some of the harder-to-kill viruses.

Those products that kill bacteria, viruses or fungi are referred to as bactericidal, viricidal or fungicidal, respectively. Those that just inhibit the growth of microorganisms such as bacteria, without killing them, are referred to as bacteriostatic.

Products in common use in the dental workplace include the following (see Figure 1.21):

- **Bleach-based cleaners** – containing sodium hypochlorite and used to disinfect all non-metallic and non-textile surfaces, and to soak laboratory items
- **Aldehyde-based cleaners** – can be used on metallic surfaces and to soak laboratory items
- **Isopropyl alcohol wipes** – to disinfect items such as exposed X-ray film packets for safe handling during processing
- **Chlorhexidene gluconate** – as an irrigating disinfectant during root canal treatments, and as a skin cleanser

Before any session of dental procedures commences, the dental nurse will have cleaned and set up the surgery area ready for the first patient. This is achieved as follows:

- The electric and water supplies should be switched on to all static equipment (dental chair, suction unit, etc.) if not already done
- Any portable items not likely to be required for the first procedure should be placed in cupboards or drawers or removed from the surgery, so that the work surfaces are clear of any clutter
- The work surfaces are wiped down using the disinfectant solution or disinfectant wipes supplied in the workplace
- The controls of any large equipment items that are likely to be contaminated during the procedure must be protected by a barrier technique, including:
  - Dental chair controls, if not foot-operated
  - Dental light controls and handles
  - Computer keyboard, if various screens are in use
  - Bracket table handles and controls
- In some surgery settings, the aspirator pipes and handpiece tubing may also require barrier protection if they are of a design which is difficult to wipe down thoroughly (such as corrugated piping)
- Once connected correctly, the handpieces and scaler unit are run for approximately 30–60 seconds into the spittoon, to ensure that they are working correctly and their water supply is effective
- Any items that do not function correctly must be disconnected from the electrical supply and the matter reported to the correct person – e.g. the operator, a senior colleague, a line manager
- The correct instruments are laid out for the procedure, in easy reach of the operator and the dental nurse, and covered with a disposable bib until the patient is seated
- Those items which are supplied in lidded trays can remain covered, while those in pouches can remain sealed until they are about to be used

After each procedure, and before the start of the next one, the following actions will be taken by the dental nurse while wearing appropriate PPE:

- All sharps are carefully disposed of in the sharps box
- Barrier covers are removed and disposed of as hazardous waste
- All other hazardous waste items are correctly segregated and disposed of in the correct containers/sacks
- All static items of equipment are wiped down using the correct disinfectant
- All autoclavable items are transferred safely to the decontamination room for processing
- All surfaces are wiped down and disinfected using the correct solution
- PPE is discarded and new protective items are applied
- The surgery area is set up for the next procedure, as detailed earlier

Correct use of cleaning equipment

Cleaning equipment in this context is all of those items used for general cleaning as well as for sterilisation purposes. General cleaning items include all of the following, and must be used in strict accordance with the infection control policy of the dental workplace:

- Disinfectant solutions and wipes
- Cleaning cloths (microfibre or disposable) and floor mops – these may be used as coloured sets for use in clinical or non-clinical areas only, rather than one set for all areas
- Vacuum cleaners, floor polishers and steam cleaners – these tend to be used by domestic cleaners rather than chairside staff
- Specific disinfectant solutions for aspirators

Sterilisation equipment includes those items specifically for use on reusable surgery items, which require specialist decontamination and sterilisation before they can be used again safely. They are used by dental staff rather than by domestic cleaners, and include the following:

- Instrument brushes and water bowls
- Ultrasonic bath
- Washer-disinfector
- Autoclave

The correct solutions and items must be used at all times by the dental nurse, and only after receiving suitable training in their correct usage. So, if an item must undergo sterilisation in an autoclave before re-use, it must never be cleaned in any other way. If an item is disposable, it must never be re-used. If a certain disinfectant is to be used on a blood spillage, no other solution must be used instead, and so on.

The types of decontaminants available are shown above, and the infection control policy of the workplace must be consulted to ensure that the correct products are used under the various circumstances and by the correct method shown. The dental nurse should also be aware of the Control of Substances Hazardous to Health (COSHH) advice in relation to these products and how to avoid their misuse and the occurrence of accidents.

Maintenance of suitable environmental factors

The environmental factors to be considered are heating, lighting, ventilation, and humidity.

In a hospital or clinic environment, these factors are likely to be under the control of a maintenance department and therefore not as easily adjusted as they may be in smaller dental workplaces. However, the immediate surgery environment can be altered by local actions, as follows:

- Radiators can be turned up, down or off
- Overhead lights can be turned on or off, as can additional lighting provided at the chairside from the dental unit
- Windows can be opened to improve ventilation and decrease humidity, although care should be taken when carrying out surgical procedures, as increased air flow may spread aerosol and airborne contamination more easily
- Fans can provide an increased air flow too, but should be used with caution as indicated earlier

In particular, the following points will need specific consideration in the dental workplace:

- Higher temperatures will:
  - increase the risk of patients and staff feeling unwell and fainting
  - reduce the setting time of many dental materials
  - increase the levels of mercury vapour in the surgery environment, where amalgam is used and waste amalgam collected
  - make patient haemorrhage more likely during surgical procedures
- Cooler temperatures will:
  - be uncomfortable to work in for prolonged periods
  - increase the setting time of many dental materials
- Poor lighting will compromise the operator while providing dental treatment and may result in injury to the patient or staff
- Excessively bright lighting may result in eye strain for the operator and the dental nurse
- Poor ventilation will:
  - result in a stuffy working atmosphere which will make staff feel tired, listless or sleepy, and their concentration may lapse – this may result in accidents or an injury to the patient
  - allow vapours and fumes to gather more easily and more potently
- Increased air flow may spread aerosols and airborne contamination more easily
- High humidity:
  - may affect the mixing and setting of some dental materials
  - will result in the patient and staff feeling uncomfortable, hot and sweaty

Although there is no legally set temperature limit above which work should be abandoned, the lower limit is 16 °C and this should be adhered to by all dental workplaces, for the comfort of patients and staff alike.

Application of health and safety measures

During the delivery of dental care and the carrying out of any dental procedures, all dental personnel must follow the relevant health and safety legislation and regulations to ensure that patients, staff and visitors to the premises come to no harm. The health and safety legislation seeks to protect staff and patients while on the premises by making the staff aware of any potential hazards at work and encouraging them to find the best ways of making their particular premises safer for all concerned. In legal terms, the employer has a statutory duty to ensure that, as far as is reasonably practicable, the health, safety and welfare at work of all employees and all visitors (including patients) are protected at all times.

The specific actions that dental nurses must take to ensure that they are not personally responsible for causing harm to others or contributing to their harm when health and safety issues arise, involve the following areas:

- Personal hygiene and effective hand washing
- Knowledge of the correct functioning of equipment, the actions to take when equipment fails, and the reasons why maintenance records must be kept

- Knowledge of the correct storage of equipment and materials
- Actions to take in the event of a spillage
- Reporting procedures for hazardous occurrences

Personal hygiene and hand washing

Cross-infection is a very real occupational hazard to those who work in the healthcare sector, but it is a two-way risk as contamination can pass both from patients to staff, and from staff to patients. All staff members therefore have a professional duty of care to patients to ensure that their level of personal hygiene is exemplary at all times when in the dental workplace and this includes the following:

- **Hair** – any style that is longer than shoulder length must be tied back when working in the surgery area and clips must be used to prevent strands from falling across the face. When left loose, dental nurses will be continually pushing the hair out of their face during treatment sessions, while wearing contaminated gloves for each patient, so that saliva (and worse) is easily transferred to their hair and then to the next patient.
- **Nails** – although gloves must be worn whenever dental nurses are working in the surgery, they are more easily punctured if the nails are long or not well maintained and ragged. False nails and nail varnish may harbour unseen contamination beneath their surface and should not be worn when working at the chairside.
- **Jewellery** – finger rings may pierce gloves if they are of any design other than a plain band, and should be removed when working at the chairside. No pieces of jewellery should be worn on the wrists (including a watch) as they will be open to contamination from splatter during treatment sessions and are impossible to clean effectively. Necklaces and earrings should not dangle when the dental nurse is leaning over the patient and must be removed if they do so. Facial piercings may require removal in some workplaces if they are considered to pose a threat to the patient's health and safety when working at the chairside. Some employers may consider that having numerous or obvious facial piercings is less than professional for health-care staff who work in close proximity to patients.
- **Footwear** – this must fully enclose the foot to protect it from damage by dropped instruments or chemicals and must be flat-heeled so that the likelihood of tripping and falling is reduced.
- **Uniform** – this should be provided by the employer and must be worn at all times while in the workplace, to protect the patients and other staff from contamination brought in on their own clothes. The uniform must be removed before leaving the workplace, so that work contamination is not transferred to the general public. Uniform items must be kept clean (by washing at high temperature) and in a good state of repair – any torn or stained items must be discarded.
- **Hand washing** – the hands are the biggest source of potential cross-infection in any health-care workplace and they must be suitably cleaned whenever necessary throughout each working day. Details are given in the following section.

Hand washing techniques

Hand hygiene covers the topics of the different methods of hand washing as well as the recommended use of hand gels for disinfection purposes, as an alternative or in addition to washing, depending on the circumstances. Hand hygiene should be a required topic of coverage in staff induction training in all dental workplaces.

Dedicated hand washing sinks must be available in the dental workplace, and marked as such. They should be located in each surgery area and in the decontamination room, and have taps that can be operated either by the elbow or by foot to avoid contamination from dirty hands. Dispensers of antibacterial liquid soap, disinfectant gel (sanitiser), and moisturiser should be available at each sink (Figure 4.3).

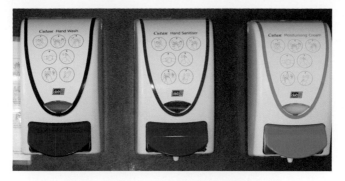

Figure 4.3   Sink-side dispensers.

The three levels of hand hygiene recognised are as follows:

- **Social** – to become physically clean from socially acquired microorganisms, using general-purpose liquid soap
- **Hygienic (clinical)** – to destroy microorganisms, maintain cleanliness and avoid direct cross-infection, using an approved antibacterial hand cleanser
- **Surgical** – to significantly reduce the numbers of normally resident microorganisms on the hands before an invasive surgical procedure is carried out, using an approved antibacterial hand cleanser

Social hand washing is that of a general level of cleanliness and should be carried out at the start and end of each session, before preparing food or eating, and especially after using the toilet facilities. It follows a similar technique to that used for hygienic hand cleansing (see later), but should take just 10–15 seconds as it need not include the wrists or forearms.

Hygienic hand washing should be performed whenever dental nurses are working in the surgery environment, before putting on the first pair of gloves for a chairside treatment session. It may need to be repeated several times throughout the day, depending on the volume and types of treatments carried out. This hand washing method should also be used before donning gloves to carry out instrument decontamination duties.

The correct procedure for hygienic hand washing should be displayed in poster form at each dedicated sink, and the instructions are as follows (see Figure 1.3):

- Turn on the tap using the foot or elbow control to prevent contamination of the tap itself (Figure 4.4)
- Wet both hands under running water of a suitable temperature
- Apply a suitable antibacterial liquid soap from the specially operated dispenser and wash all areas of both hands and wrists thoroughly – this should take up to 30 seconds to carry out correctly
- Nail brushes are not advised unless they are autoclavable, as they can become contaminated with repeated use
- Rinse both hands under running water, holding them up so that the water does not flow back over the fingers
- Dry the hands thoroughly, using single-use disposable paper towels
- Heavy-duty gloves must be worn whenever the cleaning of dirty instruments is being carried out
- Clinical gloves must be worn whenever patients are being treated and discarded between patients – these should be non-powdered and of a non-latex material, such as nitrile or vinyl, to avoid the development of skin sensitisation conditions

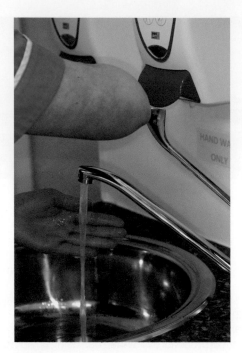

Figure 4.4   Elbow-operated tap in use.

Whenever an invasive surgical procedure is to be carried out (oral, periodontal or implant surgery), this hand washing procedure should be extended to include the forearms too and should be carried out for a minimum of 2 minutes to be completed effectively. Special surgical-grade hand wash should be used, with a sterile, single-use scrubbing brush.

At the end of the cleaning, the hands should be held up during rinsing to allow the water to drain off the elbows, and then the hands and forearms should be dried with sterile paper towels. Sterile gloves should then be placed on both hands. This "scrubbing-up" procedure is known as the surgical (aseptic) technique of hand washing.

Equipment maintenance

As detailed earlier, when setting up the surgery for a treatment session, all the equipment must be checked for its correct functioning before the first patient arrives. For the equipment items within the surgery itself, the following checks are made once the electrical and water supplies have been switched on:

- Dental chair – operate the controls to ensure that the chair body moves up and down, and the chair back reclines and returns to an upright position. Any unexpected noises, peculiar smells or false actions should be reported to a more senior colleague immediately. The electrical supply should be disconnected in the meantime, and a "DO NOT USE" sign placed on the chair until it has been attended to by an engineer
- Aspirator – all of the high- and slow-speed aspirator pipes should be activated and the suction strength checked by placing a hand over each pipe end. Poor suction indicates a blocked pipe and this will need clearing before the aspirator can be used safely, otherwise the electrical motor may overheat. Loss of suction completely indicates that the reservoir is full and this will need emptying and cleaning before use, although the task should have been carried out at the

end of the last treatment session. Any unexpected noises, peculiar smells or false actions should be reported to a more senior colleague immediately. The electrical supply should be disconnected in the meantime, and a "DO NOT USE" sign placed on the aspirator until it has been attended to by an engineer

- Hand pieces and ultrasonic scaler – these should be connected correctly to their relevant compressed air supplies on the bracket table, and then each one should be run into the spittoon for 30–60 seconds to ensure that they are working and have a functioning water supply. If the air or water supply is not functioning, check beneath the bracket table that all of the supply switches are on, that the compressor valve is open and that the water bottle is full. If any hand piece or scaler fails to work, it should be replaced so that treatment can commence. The faulty equipment can be handed to a senior colleague to arrange for repair
- X-ray machine – this should be switched on so that the illuminated settings dial is lit (Figure 4.5). The isolator switch is activated to ensure that the machine supply is overridden and becomes inactivated, and then the machine is switched off. No further tests must be carried out by the dental nurse alone, as an ionising radiation exposure may occur. Any alarms, peculiar smells or false actions should be reported to a more senior colleague immediately. The electrical supply should be disconnected in the meantime and a "DO NOT USE" sign placed on the X-ray machine until it has been attended to by an engineer

For the equipment items away from the surgery, the following checks are made once the electrical and water supplies have been switched on:

- Automatic processing machine – when first switched on, the various temperature and fluid level warning lights may be illuminated until the machine readies itself for use (Figure 4.6). If they

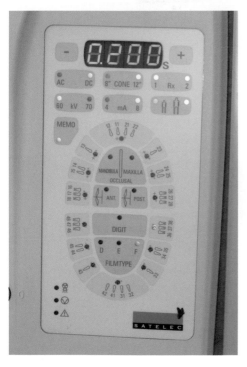

Figure 4.5 Illuminated X-ray machine controls.

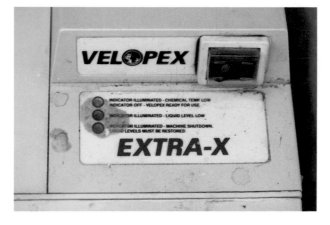

Figure 4.6 Velopex machine warning lights.

104

remain lit after a few minutes, the fluid levels can be checked manually within the machine and topped up as necessary, and in particular the tank drain plugs can be checked for their tightness. If the temperature light remains lit, the heating unit is not operating correctly and the machine cannot be used. Once the machine indicates it is ready for use, a test film can be processed. Any unexpected noises, peculiar smells or false actions should be reported to a more senior colleague immediately. The electrical supply should be disconnected in the meantime and a "DO NOT USE" sign placed on the processor until it has been attended to by an engineer

- Autoclave – the reservoir should be filled with reverse osmosis or purified water, and the working parameters of the first cycle must be checked and recorded as evidence that sterilisation has occurred. This can be done manually or automatically using "TST" strips (Figure 4.7) or similar resources. Printouts (Figure 4.8) must be retained and stored as evidence of correct working, and vacuum autoclaves should also undergo a Helix (Figure 4.9) or Bowie-Dick test to ensure that sealed items are being sterilised. Any unexpected noises, peculiar smells or false

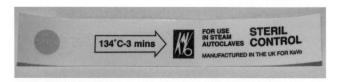

Figure 4.7   "TST" strip for checking autoclave function.

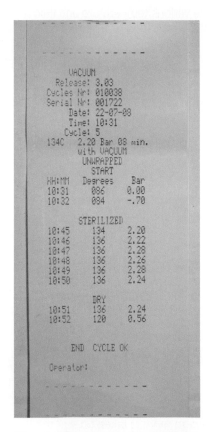

Figure 4.8   An autoclave log printout.

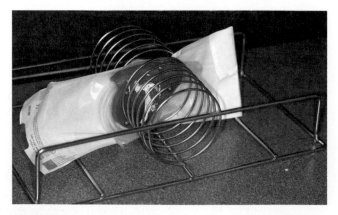

Figure 4.9   Helix device for checking vacuum autoclave function.

actions should be reported to a more senior colleague immediately. The electrical supply should be disconnected in the meantime and a "DO NOT USE" sign placed on the autoclave until it has been attended to by an engineer

- Washer-disinfector – some designs have automatic data-logging devices incorporated into their design that produce printouts of their operational parameters for each cycle (in a similar way to those produced by some autoclaves). These should be retained and stored as evidence of the machine's correct functioning. The water reservoir must be filled with reverse osmosis or purified water, and the detergent reservoir should be checked and topped up as necessary. A manual check of the decontaminated items can be made to ensure that the machine is functioning correctly. Any unexpected noises, peculiar smells or false actions should be reported to a more senior colleague immediately. The electrical supply should be disconnected in the meantime and a "DO NOT USE" sign placed on the washer-disinfector until it has been attended to by an engineer

- Ultrasonic bath – this should be filled with a solution of the special detergent and reverse osmosis or purified water, ready for use. The lid of the bath must be present and down when the machine is in use, to prevent fluid splatter and aerosol contamination of the surrounding area. The vibratory action of the bath can be checked before use by switching the timer on for a brief spell. Any unexpected noises, peculiar smells or false actions should be reported to a more senior colleague immediately. The electrical supply should be disconnected in the meantime and a "DO NOT USE" sign placed on the ultrasonic bath until it has been attended to by an engineer

Full details of the maintenance of decontamination and sterilisation equipment are given in Chapter 12.

When faults do occur with any item of equipment, a recorded maintenance log can be consulted to see if similar problems have occurred previously with the same machine. When evidence exists that routine servicing and maintenance checks have been carried out according to manufacturer's instructions, and the device has failed again, it may indicate an inherent problem that will require the replacement of the equipment item under warranty, and therefore at no cost to the workplace. Obviously, if no servicing and maintenance records are kept then a new machine will have to be purchased instead.

Servicing records can also be used to make retrospective checks on equipment that may have been used during the treatment of a patient who subsequently becomes ill, e.g. from cross-infection or ionising radiation exposure. The records can be used to determine timescales of faulty operation and therefore track other patients who may have been exposed to the same health risk. Failure to keep the required records may put the workplace at risk of prosecution by the Health and Safety Executive (HSE), and at risk of a misconduct hearing by the General Dental Council. All staff members must therefore follow the health and safety policy of the workplace at all times.

Storage of equipment and materials

After use, all equipment that had protective barriers in place should be stripped down and wiped with a suitable disinfectant – each workplace will have its own regime, which the dental nurse must be familiar with, trained in, and follow explicitly. As a general rule, bleach-based solutions must not be used on metallic items as they will corrode the metal. Some equipment items have heavy-duty plastic covers available, and these should be put into place where relevant.

When items of portable equipment are not in use they should be disconnected from the electric supply and stored in cupboards or drawers, with any cables and tubing neatly rolled up so that they do not become entangled. Larger equipment items may have to remain standing in their place (such as the dental chair), but should also be disconnected and stored neatly. Chairs should be raised up bodily, with the backrest upright so that the minimum room is taken up and the floor space around them can be cleaned efficiently.

X-ray machines are usually fastened to the surgery wall and should be folded against it to take up the minimum space and to avoid someone banging into the machine while in the surgery. Other equipment items should be electrically isolated and stored in a similar fashion.

Any equipment that has wheels to allow easier manoeuvring should have them locked once the item is in its storage place, so that it is secure and safe. Heavy items must be stored so that they will not topple over and cause an injury and all items must be moved so that they do not block doorways while in storage. No items should be left outside locked rooms, such as in corridors, as they are not secure from being tampered with.

Materials must also be kept in locked rooms, cupboards or drawers – the potential for accidents and injury if they are accessible to the public is huge. All lids should be securely in place so that leaks and spillages do not occur. Large containers and heavy items should not require lifting or moving, wherever possible, to avoid personal injury to staff members or others.

When materials were in use during dental procedures, they should have been handled with clean hands and gloves, but it does no harm to wipe down the sealed containers at the end of the session with a disinfectant wipe too. All items should be returned to their usual place of storage so that they can be found and used again at a later date. In multi-surgery workplaces, the main surgery is often used as the storage area for expensive equipment and materials, and they are "borrowed and returned" as necessary by the other surgeries.

Actions to take in the event of a spillage

Spillages can and do occur in the dental workplace and they are a hazard to anyone in the area because of the risks they pose, as follows:

- Wet spillages can cause falls and injuries
- Chemical spillages can give off noxious fumes and vapours or damage the surface they contaminate
- Body fluid spillages can cause cross-infection to others

Water spillages

These can occur when an equipment item fails, causing a water leakage. Potential items include:

- Bracket table and all hand pieces or scaler, due to a pipe becoming disconnected or the water bottle leaking
- Aspirator unit reservoir, due to a pipe becoming disconnected or the reservoir overflowing
- Sinks, due to a drain blockage, a burst pipe or being over filled
- Sterilisation and decontamination equipment, due to a pipe becoming disconnected, the reservoir being overfilled or the failure of a door seal

If the item is connected to the mains water supply, this should be turned off as soon as possible at the stopcock, to stop further water leakage. If any electrical items are standing in the water, the electricity must be switched off too, to prevent possible electrocution. Only then should the area be approached.

A hazard sign must be set up to highlight the danger to everyone (see Figure 1.2) and reduce the risk of anyone slipping on the wet surface. The water must then be soaked up using paper towels and a mop so that the floor surface is dry again. If there is any risk of the water leaking under cupboards, rolled-up towels must be placed around the spillage so that it is contained.

Final drying may require additional ventilation, and the hazard sign must not be removed until the area is fully dry. If the spillage is due to a faulty piece of equipment, this must remain out of use until it has been repaired or has been replaced.

Chemical spillages

The chemicals used in the dental workplace will have undergone a risk assessment to determine the risks they pose, how to minimise the risks, and whether they can be replaced by an alternative chemical where the risk is considered too great. This is a specific COSHH assessment and is a legal requirement in all dental workplaces. The dental nurse should be aware of the COSHH file and the information it contains, so that it can be referred to if and when an accident occurs.

Depending on the chemical involved, these types of spillage may also be wet and require the actions described in the previous section. In addition, some chemical spillages are dangerous to health, such as:

- Liquid mercury – used for amalgam fillings, this is toxic whether inhaled, absorbed through the skin or mucous membranes or ingested
- Processing chemicals – used to process X-ray films, both the fixer and the developer give off noxious fumes
- Disinfectants – used for infection control purposes, bleach-based products, in particular, give off noxious chlorine fumes

Although it is called liquid mercury, it actually falls as globules of metal rather than as a "wet" liquid (see Figure 1.16) and it will roll easily into any available nooks and crannies in the area. As its toxic fumes can be given off for years after the accident, large spillages must be handled by the Environmental Protection Agency to ensure the long-term safety of all staff. When just a few globules have been released and are contained, they can be collected in a disposable syringe and placed in the waste amalgam tub.

Small spillages can be handled "in house" using the mercury spillage kit (see Figure 1.19), as follows:

- Stop work and report the incident to the dentist immediately
- Put on full PPE
- Globules of mercury or particles of amalgam must be smeared with a mercury-absorbent paste from the mercury spillage kit – this consists of equal parts of calcium hydroxide and flours of sulphur mixed into a paste with water
- It should be left to dry and then removed with a wet disposable towel and placed in the waste amalgam storage container (see Figure 1.13)
- The area should be well ventilated throughout
- Risk-assess the incident to determine if protocols require amendment and change

Processing chemical spillages should be handled as a wet spillage, with the following inclusions:

- Ventilate the area throughout the clean-up procedure
- Wear PPE, especially a face mask and eye protection
- The wet chemicals should be poured into the relevant waste storage drums used for spent processing chemicals
- Once the wet chemicals have been mopped up, clean the contaminated surface with the usual floor cleaning solution or with a detergent-based solution if the work surfaces were involved

Disinfectant spillages should be handled as a wet spillage, with the following inclusions:

- Ventilate the area throughout the clean-up procedure, especially when bleach-based products have been spilled
- Wear full PPE
- Thick bleach tends to have a greasy, slippery surface and is best cleaned over with the usual water-based floor cleaning solution, so that a slippery surface does not remain as the spillage dries

Any disposable products used to clean chemical spillages (other than mercury) can be disposed of as non-infectious hazardous waste.

Body fluid spillages

These are usually of blood, although occasionally vomit or urine may also be involved. The risk posed by these spillages is one of cross-infection to all other persons in the area, especially with blood. The actions to take after a spillage are as follows:

- Isolate the area from all other personnel and patients
- Wear full PPE
- Contain the spillage using paper towels and remove as much as possible once the towels are soaked
- Place the towels in the infectious hazardous waste sack
- Cover the remaining spillage with a fresh 1% solution of sodium hypochlorite (bleach) and wipe it up, disposing of all contaminated towels as earlier
- Once all traces of the body fluids have been removed, clean the area with the usual floor or work surface cleaning solution and allow to dry thoroughly
- Ventilate the area to assist drying and remove any unpleasant odours

All spillages should be recorded in the accident book or to the HSE when serious spillages occur, under the Reporting of Injuries, Diseases, and Dangerous Occurrences Regulations (RIDDOR – see the following section).

Reporting of hazards

Any hazard that occurs in the dental workplace could potentially result in someone being injured (or killed) either at the time or at a later date, especially if an incident occurs that could be prevented in future but no remedial action has been taken. In other words, lessons have not been learned from the first incident.

Within each workplace, "in house" reporting procedures will be in place which the dental nurse must be aware of and which must be followed at all times. The procedures should have been identified during the induction training of all new staff.

Accidents that occur in the workplace fall into one of two categories:

- **Minor accidents** – these result in no serious injury to persons or the premises and are dealt with "in house" and recorded in the accident book
  - ○ A written record of the minor accident must be made and kept by the workplace in the accident book, under the Notification of Accidents and Dangerous Occurrences Regulations (see Figure 1.15)
  - ○ Examples of minor accidents include a trip or fall resulting in no serious injury, a clean (non-infectious) needlestick injury or a minor mercury spillage that can be safely dealt with using the spillage kit
- **Major accidents** – these result in a serious injury to a person or severe damage to the premises
  - ○ They are classed as "significant events" and are therefore notifiable incidents that must be reported to the HSE under RIDDOR

Notifiable incidents do not include those occurring to a patient while undergoing dental treatment, but do cover all persons on the premises otherwise.

Once notified, the HSE will carry out an investigation into how the incident occurred, to determine whether it was purely an accident or whether the practice or a staff member was at fault. Advice will then be given on how to avoid similar incidents in future, but in serious cases, prosecution may follow. Where necessary, the Environmental Protection Agency will also be notified so that the necessary clean-up operation can be carried out.

The significant events covered by the regulations fall into one of three categories – injuries, diseases or dangerous occurrences. Further information is available at www.hse.gov.uk/riddor.

As with any other workplace, the occurrence of an accidental injury while on the premises is a rare event in the dental world – but nevertheless they can, and do, happen. Minor injuries, as discussed earlier, are handled "in house" as they result in no serious harm to anyone.

However, major injuries do result in causing serious harm or even death to the casualty.

The **injuries that must be reported under RIDDOR** are as follows:

- Fracture of the skull, spine or pelvis
- Fracture of the long bone of an arm or leg
- Amputation of a hand or foot
- Loss of sight in one eye
- Hypoxia (oxygen deprivation to the brain) severe enough to produce unconsciousness
- Any other injury requiring 24-hour hospital admission for treatment

Members of the dental team may be exposed to common diseases in the workplace on a daily basis from patients (such as simple colds or chest infections) or they may be exposed away from the workplace – in this case they are at risk of transmitting the infection to others in the workplace themselves. Dental personnel are also at risk of exposure to more serious pathogens by direct contact with infected blood and saliva from patients, and particularly by receiving an inoculation injury (see later).

The risk of infection by airborne diseases is increased significantly when the workplace is inadequately ventilated or poorly temperature-controlled, and by cross-infection when the workplace is inadequately cleaned.

The **diseases that must be reported under RIDDOR** are any that cause acute ill health by infection with dangerous pathogens or infectious materials, such as:

- Legionella – causing Legionnaires' disease
- Hepatitis B or hepatitis C infection – both linked to the development of liver cancer
- Human immunodeficiency virus (HIV) – causing acquired immunodeficiency syndrome (AIDS)

In the hospital environment or in those with poor personal hygiene, dental personnel may also be exposed to or even transmit, other dangerous pathogens; such as Methicillin-resistant *Staphylococcus aureus* (MRSA – referred to as one of the "superbugs" by the lay public) or *Clostridium difficile* (an intestinal microorganism associated with diarrhoea and tetanus).

A dangerous occurrence is a significant event that could result in a serious injury or death to anyone on the premises at the time that it happens. It would result in the attendance of the emergency services (ambulance, fire, and/or police) as well as specialists in service provision, depending on the cause (gas, electric, service engineer, environmental health officer, etc.)

The **dangerous occurrences that must be reported under RIDDOR** are as follows:

- Explosion, collapse or burst of a pressure vessel (an autoclave or compressor)
- Electrical short circuit or overload that causes more than a 24-hour stoppage of business
- Explosion or fire due to gases or inflammable products that causes more than a 24-hour stoppage of business
- Uncontrolled release or escape of mercury vapour due to a major mercury spillage
- Any accident involving the inhalation, ingestion or absorption of a hazardous substance which results in hypoxia that is severe enough to require medical treatment

Most of the dangerous occurrences listed involve a catastrophic failing of an electrically operated equipment item, resulting in a fire or an explosion. Fire is a daily hazard that can occur in any workplace and as discussed previously, a risk assessment of the dental workplace will identify several specific fire hazards.

In addition to the fire potential from chemicals and gases, all dental equipment is electrically operated and may short circuit, malfunction or spark and cause a fire at any time, especially if not serviced and maintained correctly. Larger electrical items of dental equipment, such as the dental chair and inspection light or autoclaves, have to be serviced and maintained by trained personnel on a regular basis.

Inoculation injury

Nearly all dental procedures involve the use of sharp items; these include local anaesthetic needles, sharp instruments or scalpel blades. All must be handled with great care by staff to avoid an inoculation injury.

Every dental workplace must have a policy in place to avoid a sharps injury and it should ideally include all of the following points:

- The dentist using a local anaesthetic needle should be the person responsible for its re-sheathing and safe placement in a sharps bin, so that injury to others does not occur as there is no transference of the sharp item from one person to another
- Needle guards should be used when re-sheathing needles, so that they can be placed within their plastic sheath without being held in the fingers
- Heavy-duty rubber gloves and full PPE should be worn by any staff responsible for instrument cleaning and debridement before sterilisation

Although a sharps injury from a sterile, unused instrument may be momentarily painful, it is of no consequence save to reconsider the level of care taken by the staff member involved. However, if a contaminated inoculation injury occurs, the following actions must be carried out:

- Stop all treatment immediately and attend to the wound
- Squeeze the wound to encourage bleeding, but do not suck the wound
- Wash the area with soap and running water, then dry and cover the wound with a waterproof dressing
- Note the name, address and contact details of the source patient if a contaminated item is involved, so that the person's medical history can be checked immediately
- Complete the accident book if the patient is a low risk
- Report to the HSE if the patient is a known or suspected high risk
- Report the incident to the senior dentist/line manager
- The consultant microbiologist at the local hospital must be contacted immediately if the source patient is a known or suspected HIV or hepatitis C carrier, as emergency antiviral treatment must commence within 1 hour of the injury

The contact details for the consultant microbiologist should be readily available within the infection control policy documentation, and updated whenever necessary.

Application of suitable sterilisation methods

The theory and underpinning knowledge required to understand the purpose of correct decontamination and sterilisation methods are discussed in detail in Chapter 12.

The various methods used that must be carried out on a day-to-day basis by the dental nurse are given here, and cover the following areas:

- Transportation of items to the decontamination room
- The decontamination room layout
- Preparation of items for sterilisation, by decontamination
- Sterilisation procedures
- Storage of sterilised items

Transportation to the decontamination room

In large dental workplaces, especially hospitals and clinics, the patient treatment areas may be located some way from the decontamination room. In some environments, a central sterilisation facility may be in use, which is off-site from the treatment areas.

Wherever the decontamination of instruments and handpieces is carried out, their transportation to that area must be carried out safely, so that there is no possibility of contaminated debris or fluids falling from the items and cross-infecting the route as they are transported. A simple system that can be followed is for all of the reusable items from a dental procedure to be loaded into a portable plastic container, sealed with a clip-on lid and then carried directly to the decontamination room by the dental nurse.

Each workplace will have its own procedure in place which should be equally as effective, and the method should be correctly followed by all staff members, at all times. In the hospital environment, there are often dedicated staff members charged with the task of safely collecting and transporting the items to a central decontamination area, rather than having everyone involved in the process.

Decontamination room layout

The need for a separate area to process reusable items away from the clinical area is an obvious one, and many dental workplaces have operated with separate facilities for some time, although it is likely to become a requirement in some countries of the UK under the latest Department of Health guidelines.

The process of decontaminating, sterilising, and reusing instruments in the surgery is often referred to as "reprocessing". Ideally, all reprocessing activities should be carried out in a designated decontamination room that is physically separated from the clinical area. To achieve maximum efficiency of preventing the occurrence of cross-infection of instruments from one patient to another, the area needs to operate in a strict (but logical) order, as follows:

- The separate areas within the room should be set out in the following order:
  - Set-down area for dirty items
  - Hand washing sink
  - Instrument washing sink
  - Ultrasonic bath (if required)
  - Rinsing sink or bowl
  - Washer-disinfector
  - Illuminated magnifier for inspection
  - Autoclave
  - Packaging and storage
- When followed strictly, the dirtiest items are received in an area furthest away from where the items are at their cleanest, after reprocessing – so they are physically separated from each other as far as possible
- The decontamination stages they are taken through become more and more precise in their effectiveness as they are followed – so gross debris is removed initially, then visible debris, and then microscopic debris during the sterilisation stage
- Dental nurses will clean or change their gloves before handling the items at each stage, to avoid recontaminating the instruments as they become cleaner
- The requirement of a clean to dirty air flow system within the room also ensures that any aerosol or airborne contamination is physically drawn away from the clean zone
- A single worktop area should run the length of the room, with enough length to allow the autoclave to be well away from the cleaning/decontamination area
- The worktop should be sealed along its length and should be made of an easily cleanable surface (so smooth rather than indented)
- The dirty and clean zones should be clearly labelled as such, to avoid cross-contamination of the two areas

Preparation of items for sterilisation

From the description in the previous section, it can be seen that the preparation stages can involve some or all of the following techniques:

- Manual cleaning
- Debridement with ultrasonic bath
- Decontamination with washer-disinfector

Full details of the merits of each are discussed in Chapter 12, and the dental nurse may be required to carry out any of them in the dental workplace.

Handpieces

Various different makes of air turbine and slow-speed handpiece are available nowadays, and the manufacturer's instructions should always be followed in relation to their cleaning, lubrication and sterilisation to prolong the life of the item. Currently, it is accepted that full sterility of the handpiece is unlikely with any type of autoclave available at the moment, so the emphasis is more on reducing the risk of cross-infection rather than completely eliminating it.

However, all hand pieces should be able to undergo the following:

- External cleaning using a suitable cleaning agent
- Lubrication of bearings before and/or after cleaning and sterilisation, according to the manu-facturers' instructions
- Sterilisation in an autoclave

Handpieces should never be immersed and decontaminated in an ultrasonic bath (the bearings that drive the bur rotation will be irreparably damaged), but some are suitable for decontamination in washer-disinfectors where indicated by the manufacturer. The point at which bur removal should occur may also vary between makes and, once again, the manufacturers' instructions should be consulted for the correct procedure to be followed.

Dental instruments

Dental hand instruments that are used to assess patients and provide dental treatment itself tend to be made of high-quality metals – especially stainless steel. Some are also available with ceramic coatings, for use with composite restorative materials. Their metallic content reduces the likelihood of surface corrosion, so wire brushes should not be used to remove hardened debris as this scratches the surface and allows corrosion to occur. Microscopically, the scratches and corroded areas will harbour microorganisms very easily.

The basic procedure to manually clean items safely and effectively is as follows:

- Wear suitable PPE – to avoid inoculation injury, thick household gloves should be worn when-ever any items are cleaned manually, as well as face and eye protection
- Always clean the items as soon as possible after use, to avoid contaminants drying onto their surfaces – this is far more difficult to remove than wet contamination
- Use cold water and a suitable detergent in a dedicated instrument cleaning sink/bowl – hot water "fixes" contaminants such as blood on to the item surface and makes it far more difficult to remove
- Use nylon-bristled, autoclavable scrubbing brushes to remove difficult contaminants, as wire bristles will scratch the metal surfaces and allow corrosion and rusting to occur
- The items should be scrubbed while under the water surface, to avoid spraying contaminants into the immediate vicinity

112

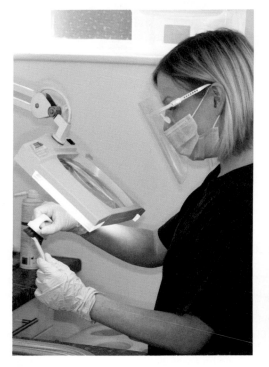

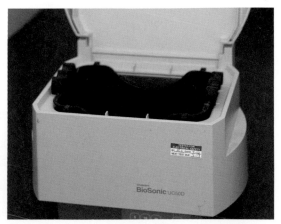

Figure 4.10 Use of the illuminated magnifier for instrument inspection.

Figure 4.11 An ultrasonic bath.

- A separate sink/bowl of distilled or reverse osmosis water should be used to rinse the items after cleaning, to remove any detergent and loose contamination
- Tap water must not be used as it will contain unwanted chemicals, and its level of "cleanliness" is dependent on the water utility provider rather than the workplace
- The items should be visibly inspected (ideally using an illuminated magnifier – Figure 4.10) to ensure that all contamination has been removed; if any is found the item should be re-cleaned and rinsed again
- The items should then be autoclaved as soon as possible before they can dry in the air – this can result in corrosion or recontamination otherwise
- Those that are to be bagged before vacuum sterilisation should be dried thoroughly first

The basic procedure to decontaminate items using the ultrasonic bath (Figure 4.11) is as follows:

- Heavy soiling with blood and other visible contaminants should be reduced by briefly soaking the items in cold detergent solution beforehand and then rinsing
- Hinged items (such as extraction forceps) should be opened, and assembled items (such as amalgam carriers) should be disassembled
- All items should be placed on the bath tray and be fully immersed beneath the solution, to allow debridement to occur effectively
- The bath should not be overloaded with items, as debridement will not be effective
- The timer should be set according to the manufacturer's instructions, the lid closed on the machine, and the programme started – the lid must be closed to prevent aerosol contamination of the vicinity
- When the timer ends, the basket and its contents should be lifted and allowed to drain, then the items should be rinsed in a dedicated sink / bowl of distilled or reverse osmosis water

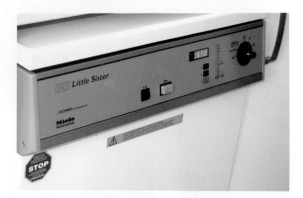

Figure 4.12   A washer-disinfector machine.

- The items should be visibly inspected to ensure debridement has occurred, and put through the process again if debris remains
- The ultrasonic bath cannot be used to debride handpieces
- Items should be sterilised as soon as possible after being decontaminated, as for manually cleaned items

The washer-disinfector machine (Figure 4.12) operates in a similar fashion to a specialist dishwasher machine, and some makes are suitable for the safe disinfection of dental handpieces, as well as other dental items and instruments. They should be carefully loaded in a similar fashion to a dishwasher, with no items lying over each other, and with all items placed upright in the special baskets provided so that they receive the full effects of the washing and disinfection cycle.

Each typical machine cycle goes through five stages during the cleaning and disinfection process and the cycle cannot be stopped before completion or altered so that any stages are missed. The stages are as follows:

- Flush
- Wash
- Rinse
- Thermal disinfection
- Drying

The duties of the dental nurse are to ensure the water and detergent reservoirs are full and to load the instruments correctly in the machine before starting the cycle.

Sterilisation procedures

Once the reusable items have been decontaminated by either manual or automated means, they are ready to be rendered safe for reuse on another patient by undergoing sterilisation. The machines used in the dental workplace to achieve sterilisation are called autoclaves, and there are two basic types – "N" type and "B" type. A third specialised type ("S" type) is available for use, but is more frequently seen in the hospital environment.

Full details of the "N" and "B" types are discussed in Chapter 12, but the basic difference is that "N" types sterilise by the downward displacement of high-temperature steam under pressure (Figure 4.13), while the "B" types sterilise by producing a vacuum within the chamber (Figure 4.14). Vacuum autoclaves are therefore recommended for use with all items that have a narrow lumen, such as metal triple syringe tips, and items can be sealed within sterilisation pouches before they are placed in the autoclave, rather than after completing the cycle.

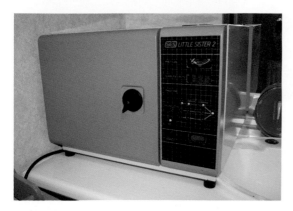

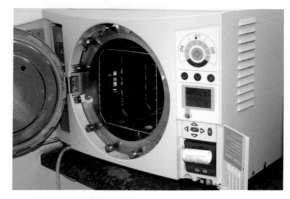

Figure 4.13   Downward displacement autoclave.   **Figure 4.14**   A vacuum autoclave.

The duties of the dental nurse are to ensure the water reservoir is full, and to correctly load the items onto the perforated trays (bagged or not) in a single layer before sealing the door and starting the cycle. Once the cycle is under way, the autoclave cannot be opened again until the sterilisation process has been completed.

Manual and automated test records must be kept for each autoclave in a legible manner, as discussed in Chapter 12.

Storage of sterilised items

The correct handling and storage of items once they leave the autoclave is imperative in ensuring that their sterility is maintained until they are required for use again. The obvious ways of achieving this are:

- Remove from the autoclave and handle while wearing clean PPE
- Dry using a single-use cloth or towel
- Place within a device to act as a barrier between the items and the general atmosphere to avoid aerosol and microorganism recontamination, such as:
  - Sealed view pouch
  - Lidded tray
  - Sterilisation bag (for use with vacuum autoclave only)

With all autoclaves, the sterilised items must be dry before any further packaging occurs, before storage. Residual moisture allows recontamination of the items with microorganisms, a more likely scenario, so it must be removed by using the "drying cycle" of the autoclave or by manually drying the items as soon as they are removed from the autoclave. Similarly, a damp cloth or towel that is repeatedly used to dry the items is also more likely to become contaminated with time, so single-use towels must be available.

For downward displacement autoclaves, all items must be sterilised unwrapped and then dried and wrapped after removal from the machine. As they must therefore be handled to do so, it is currently recommended that the storage packages are date-stamped so that the items are used or re-sterilised within a year (Figure 4.15). Until recently, this timeline had been set at just 21 days for downward displacement autoclaves, and 60 days for vacuum autoclaves. If the items are to be used again during that session, they can be covered only, rather than fully wrapped.

With vacuum autoclaves, items can complete the sterilisation cycle while enclosed in pouches and lidded trays on a drying cycle, and then further packaged at the end of the cycle. The outer packaging is then date-stamped for 1 year.

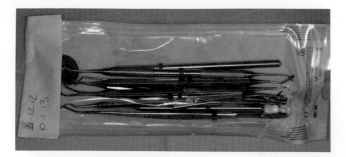

Figure 4.15   A date-stamped sterilisation pouch.

Once all items have been dried and packaged, they should be stored in their designated place within the dental workplace. While it is currently still acceptable to store packaged items in the clinical area for ease of access, they must be kept within drawers or cupboards until immediately before use and as far away from the chairside as possible. However, in the clinical area, the potential for recontamination is greater than in other areas of the workplace due to the aerosol scatter created during dental treatment, as well as due to the throughput of the patients.

The least contaminated area of the workplace should be the "clean zone" of the actual decontamination area itself, where the sterilised items are produced and where the public have no access. For this reason, best-practice guidelines recommend that all sterilised items are stored within the clean zone of the decontamination room, collected from there by staff when their use is imminent and taken to the clinical area as required for use.

Safe disposal of hazardous and non-hazardous waste

The current classification of waste produced in the dental workplace has four broad types requiring segregation and storage on the premises:

- Offensive waste
- Trade waste
- Hazardous waste:
  - Infectious (clinical)
    - Sharps
    - Soft
  - Non-infectious (chemical)
- Non-hazardous waste

Offensive waste is defined as "wastes which are non-infectious, do not require specialist treatment or disposal but may cause offence to those coming into contact with it". In the dental workplace this will include any PPE, cleaning towels, X-ray films and other similar items that have not been contaminated with body fluids, medicines, chemicals or amalgam, as well as toilet hygiene waste.

Trade waste includes items such as dental equipment (dental chairs, curing lights, portable suction units, etc.), as well as commercial electronic waste like computer screens, televisions, fluorescent lighting tubes and batteries.

Dental workplaces produce a wide range of both hazardous and non-hazardous wastes, and in order to segregate the waste correctly, it must first be identified and then classified in line with the current regulatory guidance. All waste should only be handled while wearing suitable PPE, otherwise staff members risk exposing themselves to cross-infection.

For quick and easy identification of each category of waste produced in the dental workplace, various colour-coded containers are used to help segregate the various items. In addition, on all documentation, the European Waste Catalogue (EWC) codes should be used – however, details of these codes are not relevant to the student dental nurse.

Details of the storage containers to be used are detailed below:

- Offensive waste – yellow sack with black stripe, tied at the neck
- Non-hazardous medicines and out of date stock – blue-lidded yellow rigid container (see Figure 1.24)
- Soft infectious (clinical) hazardous waste – orange sack, no more than three-quarters full and tied at the neck (see Figure 1.25)
- Sharps infectious (clinical) hazardous waste – all-yellow rigid container, no more than two-thirds full (see Figure 1.26)
- Non-infectious (chemical) hazardous waste:
  - Processing chemicals – separate securely lidded, rigid containers (see Figure 1.27)
  - Waste amalgam/mercury – white, securely lidded container with a mercury vapour suppressant sponge insert (see Figure 1.13)
  - Amalgam-containing teeth and spent capsules – white, securely lidded containers with a mercury vapour suppressant sponge insert (Figure 4.16)

There may be occasional national variations to some of the hazardous waste containers used, and dental nurses must ensure that they are aware of these in their local dental workplace.

When full, all waste containers must be securely stored on the premises until they are collected by an authorised waste handler. There should be no public access to the storage area, and the

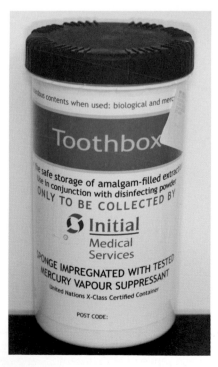

Figure 4.16   A waste 'tooth pot'.

yellow and orange sacks should be further placed in waterproof bins (dustbins are ideal) so that any fluid leakage that may occur is safely contained within the bin.

Most waste collectors operate on a monthly collection cycle, although dental workplaces that produce large quantities of waste may require a more frequent delivery schedule.

Waste handling training

All dental personnel who are likely to be involved in handling any healthcare waste must be correctly trained to do so. The training should cover all of the following points:

- Risks associated with each category of waste (such as sharps injury, exposure to toxic vapours, cross-infection, etc.)
- Correct classification, segregation and storage procedures, in line with the healthcare waste policy of the workplace
- COSHH information on all non-infectious hazardous waste chemicals used on the premises
- Safe handling, including the use of appropriate PPE and moving techniques
- Correct procedures in the event of spillages or accidents
- Correct completion of relevant documentation – transfer notes and consignment notes

If waste is not handled, segregated, stored and disposed of correctly, any of the following may happen:

- Cross-infection to staff member, patient, waste collector or member of the public
- Sharps injury to the same
- Environmental contamination with chemicals
- Poisoning of staff member, patient, waste collector or member of the public

5

Unit 305: Offer Information and Support to Individuals on the Protection of Their Oral Health

Learning outcomes

1. Be able to communicate with individuals
2. Be able to provide oral hygiene advice to suit the individual

Outcome 1 assessment criteria:
The learner can:
- Check the individual's identity and gain valid consent
- Give individuals the opportunity to discuss and seek clarification
- Provide information to individuals ensuring that it is accurate and consistent with organisational guidelines
- Answer any questions clearly and in a manner that minimises fear and anxiety
- Refer questions beyond their role to an identified member of the team
- Explain the methods and importance of effective communication, taking into account personal beliefs and preferences
- Explain the system for internal referrals to other team members

Outcome 2 assessment criteria:
The learner can:
- Provide individuals with oral health information
- Prepare and use oral health education aids
- Advise individuals on suitable oral hygiene techniques

Diploma in Dental Nursing, Level 3, Third Edition. Carole Hollins.
© 2014 John Wiley & Sons, Ltd. Published 2014 by John Wiley & Sons, Ltd.
Companion website: www.wiley.com/go/hollins/dentalnursinglevel3

- Demonstrate methods of caring for dentures
- Give advice on maintaining orthodontic appliances

This unit is assessed by:
- observation in the workplace, with examples included in the learner's portfolio
- an appropriate alternative method

Details of various elements of theory and underpinning knowledge are included in Chapter 15, and these are assessed within the written paper.

The theory and underpinning knowledge required to understand the scientific principles involved in the management of oral diseases and dental procedures, including the information and oral hygiene techniques required to protect an individual's oral health, are fully discussed in Chapter 15. This chapter explains the dental nurse's role and responsibilities in relation to disseminating this oral health information and advice to the individual. The individual may be the patient, a guardian, another healthcare worker, a family member or a carer.

The dental nurse will require suitable skills in the following areas, to be able to give the oral health information correctly and support the individual adequately:

- Communication skills
- Ability to recognise when to refer to colleagues for advice
- Provide appropriate oral health information
- Demonstrate and advise on appropriate oral hygiene techniques

Initially, individuals who are to receive the information and advice will require to be identified correctly, as well as clarifying the reason for their attendance, before valid consent can be gained. When they are not patients, they may have no records at the workplace, so detailed notes of the session must be kept by the dental nurse and stored in line with the correct policy of the dental workplace. Where an individual is attending on behalf of a patient (whether the patient is present or not), the notes can be kept within that patient's records.

Correct identification of the patient

The day list will refer to each patient attending that day by name, and/or date of birth, and/or address, and/ or some kind of patient identification marker – such as a unique computer number or the patient's NHS number for example.

Whatever the system in place, the dental nurse should be familiar with it and be able to access the patient's records so that a cross-reference check can be made with the notes present and the expected procedure to be carried out. So if the previous notes refer to the patient requiring specific oral hygiene advice but the day list indicates that they are attending for a dental procedure, one of the following scenarios has occurred which must be checked with the operator and the patient before proceeding any further:

- The records and the day list entry are for two different patients
- The records are incomplete and a change in treatment has been decided without being recorded
- The records are correct and the day list entry is incorrect
- The records are incorrect and the day list entry is correct

Any of these scenarios could quite easily have occurred and the matter should be referred to a more senior colleague (ideally the operator concerned) so that the dental nurse can assist in determining the way forward – to identify the correct patient and the correct procedure to be carried out that day.

The records required may be hard copies in full (i.e. a "pack" of handwritten patient notes, with paper copies of the medical history, previous treatment plans, consent forms and so on) or they may be fully computerised and only accessible "on screen", or they may be a combination of the two. Whatever their presentation, they should be collected by the dental nurse and presented in the preventive dental unit so that the operator can access them and check their content too.

In large dental workplaces, such as dental schools and hospitals, dental nurses can check the patient identity by asking patients to confirm their name, date of birth and address and that they have knowledge of the reason for their attendance on the day. The final decision to confirm the patient's identity is the duty of the operator.

In smaller workplaces, many of the patients are recognisable to the staff by sight – some may even be known by their first names – but identity and procedure checks should still always be carried out to avoid any mishaps.

Gaining valid consent

The issue of consent is discussed in detail in Chapter 13.
Valid consent is that which achieves all of the following:

- Informed – the individual has been given full information about the information and advice to be offered and so is able to make an informed decision as to whether to proceed or not
- Specific – the consent has been gained expressly for the delivery of oral health advice and oral hygiene instruction
- Relevant – the consent has been given by the individual who is to receive the information or advice, whether it is for themselves or for another individual

Thus the individual will be told what will be involved in the session, why it is necessary and what the consequences will be of not receiving the information and advice. The information must be given in a way that the patient understands – this may involve the use of visual aids, an interpreter or sign language. Individuals must have all of their questions answered in a way that is understandable, without the use of dental terminology if it is not appropriate, and where the dental nurse is unable to answer any of their questions, the necessary information must be gained from another team member. That team member may be another dental care professional or the dentist.

Communication skills

Good communication between members of the dental team and their patients and other individuals is crucial if they are to take an active role in managing their own oral health or are responsible for the management of another person's oral health. Not only is it a necessity if any consent given for treatment is to be valid (see preceding section), but it will also lead to greater understanding between all parties, especially if individuals are unsure about treatment options or are making choices that may damage their own or another person's oral health.

Communicating means "to give or exchange information" and this can be done both verbally and non-verbally using the following methods:

- **Talking** – either face to face with the individual or by telephone
- **Written explanations** – which reiterate any verbal information given
- **Information leaflets or posters** – which can be read and then discussed verbally as necessary
- **Other visual aids** – demonstration models, oral health product samples, disclosing tablets
- **Body language** – which can be open and friendly or defensive and "stand-offish"
- **Eye contact** – maintaining eye contact shows attentiveness, whereas breaking eye contact indicates that the individual is being dismissed by the listener
- **Facial expressions** – again, these can be friendly or not (smile, frown, querying, laughing, etc.)

- **Body position** – sitting to listen to the individual is more attentive than standing, especially if the body position of the listener is turned away from the speaker too
- **Touching** – this is sometimes used to reinforce points, although it is not acceptable in some situations and with some individuals and should only be used where there is a friendly and well-established rapport between them and the dental nurse concerned

When good communication is required between the dental nurse and an individual to get a specific message across that is in the best interests of a patient, there may be complicating factors that must be taken into account. For example, the method of delivery of suitable oral health messages will be different for each of the following groups:

- Adults
- Children and young people
- Older people (with or without complications such as deafness, poor vision, etc.)
- Individuals with special needs (physical or mental)

In addition, the dental nurse must also take into account the individual's social and ethnic background and the issues that these factors may raise. The individual's personal beliefs and preferences may be wholly different from those of the dental nurse – the standard of their oral health may be of far less importance to them than it is to a dental nurse working in a healthcare environment, who sees the ravages that poor oral health can cause on a daily basis. Nevertheless, their communication skills must be adapted to suit the situation in an effort to get important health messages across.

The dental nurse's efforts may be compounded further when the individual's first language is not English – in these situations a family member or friend should be available to act as an interpreter on behalf of the individual who requires the oral health information and advice. The NHS provides oral health leaflets in a variety of languages, as well as in large print for those with impaired vision, and these resources should be available in the workplace and used wherever necessary.

The differing risk factors associated with good oral health that occurs between age groups, social groups and ethnic groups are discussed in detail in Chapter 15.

In some circumstances, then, it may be more appropriate to disseminate the oral health information and advice to someone other than the actual patient, as follows:

- A parent or guardian of a young child
- A carer and/or family member who looks after an elderly person – the carer will be aware of any particular issues or difficulties the patient may have in relation to carrying out good oral hygiene
- A carer and/or family member who cares for a patient with special needs – good communication with some patients in this group is often difficult for the dental team, but the carer will be very skilled in doing so. Carers will also be able to advise the dental nurse on any particular issues the patient may have in relation to carrying out good oral hygiene
- A family member or friend acting as an interpreter
- An individual responsible for the oral care of a group of vulnerable adults, such as those in a nursing home

The decision as to who will attend the oral health session and receive the information and advice may be made at the oral health assessment appointment, by the dentist or another dental care professional. Otherwise, the matter should be discussed at the time with the individual and referred for a decision to a more senior colleague, as necessary. In some cases it may be more appropriate for the patient in question to be seen by another member of the dental team, especially when problems have been identified which are preventing the person from achieving good oral health:

- The presence of calculus, which will require professional removal by the hygienist, therapist or dentist
- The presence of caries, which will require assessment by the dentist

- The presence of poorly fitting dentures, which will require assessment by the dentist
- The presence of a broken orthodontic appliance, which will require repair by the orthodontic therapist or the dentist

Each dental workplace will have its own system of internal referral to another team member in these situations and the dental nurse must be aware of it and follow the specific protocol that is relevant.

In summary, then, valid consent must be gained from the appropriate individual for the oral health session to go ahead and the individuals who are to attend must be decided upon so that the session can be booked. A dedicated room within the workplace is an ideal setting for the session to take place – often referred to as a preventive dental unit or an oral health room – and it should be sited away from the usual noise and bustle of the workplace so that the session can proceed without interruption. The dental nurse should take time to plan the session beforehand, to ensure that all the necessary information will be delivered. Any visual aids that may be useful should be made available, including any particularly relevant oral health leaflets for individuals to take away and refer to again at a later date.

It may also be useful for the dental nurse to run through the aims and objectives of the planned session with an appropriate team member, to ensure that the relevant points will be covered and that the information and advice to be given is consistent with the ethos of the dental workplace.

The specific communication methods that tend to be suitable for each age group are summarised here:

Adults:

- The use of specific oral health leaflets from dental suppliers – e.g. relevant to periodontal disease or smoking and oral health
- The opportunity to discuss particular points and seek clarification, perhaps about information given previously or about advertised oral health products
- One-to-one discussions of relevant oral health issues with the dental nurse in a non-patronising manner
- The non-use of dental jargon unless it is appropriate, but without condescension
- The adoption of an attentive manner, so that the patient's own difficulties and problems relating to oral health maintenance are listened to and understood
- Any queries raised need answering at a level that the patient will understand and may require referral to another member of the dental team if this is beyond the role of the dental nurse
- Eye contact should be maintained with the patient during the discussions to ensure the correct level of attention is given
- Reflective replies to the patient's queries and concerns should be given, which relate to the person's individual experiences

Young people:

- The use of relevant leaflets and dental literature, many of which are specifically aimed at this age group
- Definitely a one-to-one approach to give oral health messages for members of this age group who are easily embarrassed
- Some will tend to react better in small groups, especially with similarly aged siblings or friends
- Careful consideration of the language and terminology used throughout the session – some may be too embarrassed to ask for explanations when they do not understand
- Use of visual aids when appropriate, to maintain their attention and have them involved in the session rather than just listening to lots of advice
- Reference to suitable celebrities as examples of the points being made, if possible – this age group, in particular, are open to this kind of influence

- Authority and control of the situation need to be maintained by the dental nurse throughout the session, but in a friendly manner
- The dental nurse should never lose patience with these individuals, no matter how obstreperous they become – some will simply not be interested in the information and advice being given, others may show embarrassment by making a joke out of the situation, for example
- Good patient management by the dental team at this age should produce attentive and responsible adults in the future

Children:

- Respond best to a group approach when learning new information, wherever possible
- Often have a short attention span and their interest in a subject can soon be lost or they can be easily distracted
- Short and interactive sessions are best, with plenty of opportunities for individual involvement by the child
- The use of disclosing tablets to show the presence and position of bacterial plaque
- Supervise individual attempts at tooth brushing, to determine how to improve plaque removal
- Develop relevant games to play, especially any involving current TV or film characters
- Encourage parental involvement in the oral health sessions wherever possible, as the parents need to maintain and promote the oral health messages discussed at home

Provide appropriate oral health information

Good oral health is present when a patient has no oral disease present or has received successful dental intervention to stop existing oral disease and repair or control any damage it has caused. The oral diseases involved are:

- Dental caries
- Non-carious tooth surface loss due to poor technique or diet:
    - Abrasion
    - Erosion
- Gingivitis and periodontal disease

All of these diseases can be prevented or controlled by providing individuals with the particular information they require to understand the cause of the problem and to educate them in how their own actions can reduce the risks of experiencing the disease that is relevant to them.

The theory and underpinning knowledge of oral diseases are discussed in detail in Chapter 15.

Dental caries

Dental caries occurs due to a combination of certain types of bacteria being present within dental plaque that use non-milk extrinsic (NME) sugars to produce acids that cause enamel demineralisation. There are therefore three main areas of caries prevention available to the patient and the dental team:

- Control the build-up of bacterial plaque – to practise its regular removal by using good oral hygiene techniques (see later)
- Increase the tooth resistance to acid attack – by incorporating fluoride into the enamel structure (see Chapter 8)
- Modification of the diet – to include fewer cariogenic foods and drinks and to reduce their frequency of intake

Non-carious tooth surface loss

The two examples included here have similar causative factors as other oral diseases and are controllable by the patient:

- Abrasion is caused by incorrect tooth brushing action
- Erosion is caused by excessive dietary intake of acidic drinks and foods

Gingivitis and periodontal disease

The main cause of gingivitis and periodontal disease is consistently poor oral hygiene, along with contributory factors such as smoking and, in some cases, an unfortunate genetic predisposition to periodontal problems. So, the prevention of these diseases can be achieved in most patients, whereas it can only be controlled in others:

- Control the build-up of bacterial plaque – to practise its regular removal by using good oral hygiene techniques (see later)
- Modify the contributory factors – e.g. by giving advice on smoking cessation
- Control the host response – in patients predisposed to periodontal problems, by more frequent dental attendance for monitoring and evaluation, and intervention where necessary (see Chapter 8)

Educating individuals in how to remove bacterial plaque successfully, on a daily basis and for the rest of their lives, is the most important aim for the dental team to achieve in helping them to maintain a good standard of oral health. Oral hygiene techniques are discussed in detail in the next main section.

Individuals' knowledge and skills in relation to their own oral health are evaluated by adequate communication with them. The aim of good communication is to identify their level of motivation and, if poor, what the specific problems are for them – what is preventing them from achieving and then maintaining a good standard of oral health? The oral health information that is offered can thus be adapted to suit their particular circumstances.

During consideration of the issues, all of the following points will be looked at and taken into account by the dental nurse and the senior team member involved in the individual's oral health assessment:

- Do they just need direct advice, help and support to adequately achieve good oral health, such as one-to-one oral hygiene instruction with a member of the dental team?
- Are factors involved that prevent them from achieving good oral health, such as a disability or a habit-related problem, like smoking?
- Is the cause of their poor oral health a dietary issue, such as high sugar or acid intake?
- Are they simply disinterested in their oral health or are they unaware that they have a problem?
- Are general health factors involved that either exacerbate or actually cause the oral health problem?
- Is a serious general health problem present which overrides their oral health problems?
- Are there barriers to good communication with certain groups or do specific communication skills need to be applied?

The oral health information given here is that which the dental nurse may give to the individual and will focus on diet and specific issues such as smoking, before moving on to advice about plaque control.

Diet

The most important modifications to the diet that are required to reduce the incidence of dental caries is the reduction (or ideally the elimination) of NME sugars and the reduction of dietary acids by patients from their daily food and drink intake.

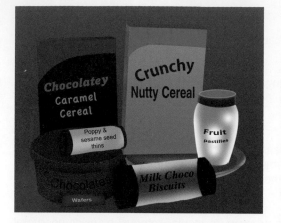

Figure 5.1 Collection of unhealthy snacks. Source: *Levison's Textbook for Dental Nurses*, 11th edition (Hollins), 2013. Reproduced with permission of Wiley-Blackwell.

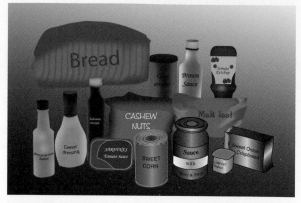

Figure 5.2 Collection of "hidden sugar" products. Source: *Levison's Textbook for Dental Nurses*, 11th edition (Hollins), 2013. Reproduced with permission of Wiley-Blackwell.

The dental nurse will offer information and advice on the following:

- Identify the sources of these products in available foodstuffs and separate them as bad foods and hidden sugars
- Identify the sources of these products in the individual's diet – possibly with the use of a diet sheet
- Advise the individual on the importance of the frequency of sugar/acid intake
- Make suggestions about changes that can be made to the diet that may help the individual

A visual resource of unhealthy foods and drinks that are readily available to the individual can be shown (Figure 5.1) to emphasise the number of products that should be reduced or avoided. The resource may be a poster or leaflet or dental nurses can collect food and drink wrappers and make their own poster – this is often more effective as it can be personalised and altered as required for different groups of individuals. The products linked to caries that are consumed by children are likely to be different from those consumed by and causing caries in adults.

Products that may be included are:

- Sweets and other confectionery
- Biscuits and cakes
- Carbonated drinks
- Pure citrus fruit juices – care should be advised with excessive intake of citrus fruits such as oranges, lemons, grapefruits and limes between meals
- Tea and coffee with sugar

Hidden sugar foods will be introduced as those where NME sugars have been artificially added during the manufacturing and processing of foods for taste and preservation purposes, very often in foods that individuals would not expect to be harmful to their teeth. This is especially the case with "low fat" products.

A visual resource of "hidden sugar" products can be produced in a similar fashion (Figure 5.2) and will often make the oral health points more clearly still, as individuals realise that there are some "healthy foods" on the poster. Products that may be included are:

- Cooking sauces, especially those with a tomato base
- Table sauces, including ketchup
- Flavoured crisps
- Fruits tinned in syrup
- Some tinned vegetables, including baked beans and sweet corn
- Some breakfast cereals
- Jams, marmalades and chutneys
- Some low-fat products, as sugar is often artificially added to improve their taste
- Tinned fish and meat in tomato sauce
- Soups
- Savoury crackers and biscuits
- Some processed ready meals
- Energy drinks

The individual's own diet can then be analysed to determine how many of these foods and drinks are consumed daily and, in particular, at what time during the day they are most likely to be consumed – at mealtimes, between meals, after breakfast, at supper time, before or after brushing the teeth and so on. The timing of the food intake will have a huge impact on the individual's risk of developing caries.

The information required may be quite detailed and individuals are more likely to be accurate in their account if they have completed a diet sheet before the oral health session which can be brought along and referred to by the dental nurse. This can be designed by the dental nurse and needs to be straightforward and easy for individuals to complete. It should ideally be completed over at least one weekday and a Saturday or Sunday, as there are likely to be differences in their activities during the week. Twenty-four-hour time slots can be included if patients take food and/or drinks overnight.

A simple example is shown here.

Tuesday	Food or drink	Oral hygiene
6 am	Cereal with sugar, orange juice	
7 am		Tooth brushing
8 am		
9 am		
10 am	Biscuit, coffee with two sugars	
11 am		
12 pm	Pizza, chocolate muffin, diet coke	
1 pm		Chewing gum, not sugar-free
2 pm		
3 pm	Diet coke	
4 pm		
5 pm	Salt and vinegar crisps	
6 pm		

127

Tuesday	Food or drink	Oral hygiene
7 pm	Chicken salad and chips, glass of wine	
8 pm	Glass of wine	
9 pm	Glass of wine	Tooth brushing and mouthwash
10 pm		
11 pm	Glass of diet lemonade	
12 am		

In the example shown, the individual has a 14-hour period where NME sugars and acidic drinks are consumed regularly during a typical weekday, but no oral hygiene is carried out. The frequency of the food and drink intake is enough to counteract the protective saliva buffering that occurs after meals and is likely to result in caries eventually. In addition, after the bedtime tooth-brushing session the individual consumes an acidic drink which will cause enamel erosion.

The dental nurse can use the diet sheet to recommend which foods should be reduced or avoided, when it is safer to consume them otherwise, at what times oral hygiene techniques should be carried out and if any specific products will be helpful, such as sugar-free chewing gum, enamel protect mouthwash and so on.

For some individuals diet sheets may need to be completed by a parent, family member or carer – as long as the information is accurate this is of no consequence.

Dental nurses will also specifically recommend other food products in the diet as "detergent foods" to be taken after a meal when tooth brushing is not possible or as a healthy snack alternative. Detergent foods are raw, firm, fibrous fruits or vegetables, such as apples, pears, carrots and celery. By virtue of their tough fibrous consistency, they require much chewing and stimulate salivary flow, thereby helping to scour the teeth clean of food remnants. Although plaque is unaffected by detergent foods, they can remove some of the food debris which nourishes all plaque bacteria and enables some of them to produce acid. Although cheese at the end of a meal has no direct detergent effect, it stimulates salivary flow, neutralises acid and enhances remineralisation of enamel, due to its calcium content. Hard cheeses are more beneficial than soft cheeses.

Loose food debris can also be removed by using sugar-free chewing gum, although its excessive use should be discouraged in all patients where evidence of attrition or bruxing appears. Chewing gum should be confined to immediately after a meal – it should not be continually chewed throughout the day.

Specific issues

For general health reasons as well as for good oral health, all individuals who smoke should be advised of the long-term effects of the habit on their bodies and in particular on the risks they will have of developing oral cancer or periodontal disease. Smokers who express an interest in trying to quit should be referred to the dentist or a suitable dental care professional for advice on how to access the NHS "quit smoking" schemes in their area. Information leaflets should be available at the dental workplace and these can be handed out as necessary (Figure 5.3).

Other visual aid resources that can be used to make the point are photographs of cancers and extensive periodontal disease, and these products may also be available from dental suppliers as posters or leaflets. Models of dental arches showing periodontal disease are also available as useful resources, some of the better ones having "loose teeth" which can actually be pulled out of the model.

When giving specific oral health information which is targeted at harmful habits such as smoking, the dental nurse must always respect individuals' personal choices and accept the decision they make

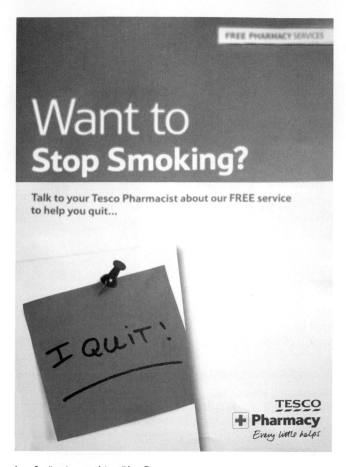

Figure 5.3   An example of a "quit smoking" leaflet.

about their own bodies. They must not be preached at or judged in a discriminatory way because of their lifestyle choices – the appropriate oral health information must be delivered accurately and in a friendly manner and then the individual must decide whether to act or not.

Some individuals may be identified as having a special need that causes specific issues, such as a lifetime of taking sugared medication or an inability to adequately open the mouth for effective oral hygiene procedures to be carried out. Dental nurses may have to refer to other team members for help in these cases.

Demonstrate and advise on appropriate oral hygiene techniques

The aim of all oral hygiene techniques is to:

- Remove bacterial plaque from tooth surfaces to reduce the risk of caries
- Remove bacterial plaque from the gingival crevice to reduce the risk of gingivitis and the development of periodontal disease
- Remove bacterial plaque from dentures and orthodontic appliances
- Use oral health products that are specifically suited to the individual

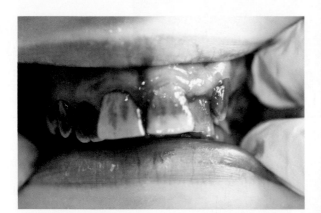

Figure 5.4   Plaque visible on teeth after using
a disclosing liquid. Source: *Levison's Textbook for
Dental Nurses*, 11th edition (Hollins), 2013.
Reproduced with permission of Wiley-Blackwell.

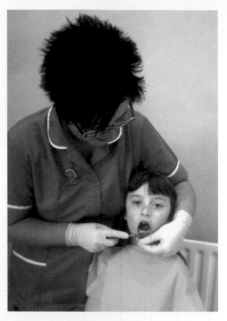

Figure 5.5   Supervised child tooth brushing.

Controlling bacterial plaque on a daily basis is the main method available to individuals to assist them in the protection of their oral health. It is the role of the dental team to ensure that they are taught the oral hygiene methods that are most suitable to them and that these are performed on a frequent enough basis to avoid damage to their oral health.

As fresh plaque is a creamy white colour, its presence is not obviously apparent to the individual and the dental nurse may consider the use of disclosing agents so it becomes clearly visible during the oral hygiene session. This technique is particularly useful with children and young people and should be carried out as follows:

- Explain to the individual (and their parent or guardian) the purpose of the procedure
- Apply a waterproof bib to the individual, to protect their clothing
- Have the person standing or sitting by a sink and facing a large mirror
- Use a disclosing liquid to paint the tooth surfaces to highlight the plaque
- Alternatively, ask the individual to chew a disclosing tablet for 1 minute, to swish the chewed mixture around the mouth and then spit it out into the sink
- Wipe the person's lips but do not allow them to rinse
- The plaque will be visible as a coloured stain on the teeth (Figure 5.4)

Once visible, the individual can be instructed in how to remove the plaque by fully removing the stain present. Areas of the dental arch where particularly heavy accumulations are visible can be pointed out by the dental nurse for special attention – these are likely to be around crowded teeth, on the left side of the mouth for left-handed individuals and on the right side of the mouth for right-handed individuals.

Where a parent or guardian will be responsible for the individual's plaque removal, dental nurses will demonstrate the correct position to be taken (Figure 5.5) and then allow the parent to carry out the disclosing stain removal.

Plaque can be easily and regularly removed by the individual at home by carrying out a regular combination of the following oral hygiene techniques on a daily basis:

- Tooth brushing, using a toothpaste recommended by the dentist, therapist or hygienist
- Interdental cleaning
- Using suitable mouthwashes

Tooth brushing demonstration and advice

Tooth brushing removes the bacterial plaque from the flat surfaces of the teeth – labial, buccal, lingual, palatal and the occlusal surfaces of the posterior teeth. The demonstration should be carried out on a suitably large model initially, so that individuals can see exactly what the dental nurse is doing with the toothbrush, as the nurse talks through the technique. They can then perform the brushing on themselves, using a suitable toothbrush and watching themselves in the mirror.

The dental nurse will have asked individuals to bring their own brush to this session, so its suitability can be assessed and advice given on a better product where necessary:

- Toothbrushes with a small head and multi-tufted medium nylon bristles are probably the most effective for the vast majority of individuals
- Good-quality, rechargeable electric toothbrushes avoid the need for consistently good manual techniques and are more likely to achieve prolonged high standards of oral hygiene (Figure 5.6). These are particularly useful when individuals are dependent on a carer for their oral hygiene, as the plaque removal achieved is better
- The brush is rinsed to wet the bristles and a portion of the recommended toothpaste added
- Each dental arch is divided into three sections: left and right sides and front
- Side sections are subdivided into buccal, lingual and occlusal surfaces; front sections are divided into labial and lingual
- When instructing individuals, these areas should be referred to in terms they can understand, such as "cheek side", "tongue side", "lip side" and so on
- This amounts to eight groups of surfaces in each jaw and at least 5 seconds should be spent on each group
- The use of egg timers or similar devices can be suggested so that individuals obtain an idea of how long the recommended "2 minute" brushing cycle actually is; some electric brushes have a timer incorporated into their design to ensure the brushing cycle is long enough
- Individuals should be encouraged to develop their own start and end point within the oral cavity and then follow it systematically at each brushing session so that a methodical routine is developed – so, for example, lower left side (all surfaces) followed by lower front (all surfaces) and then lower right side (all surfaces), before moving to the upper arch
- The most effective technique of brushing will vary between individuals, but for gingival crevice plaque removal they should be advised to have the brush head angled towards the gum as they brush from side to side (Figure 5.7)
- A forceful "sawing" action of brushing must be discouraged, as this produces tooth abrasion (Figure 5.8)
- Each area is brushed in turn and the mouth is then cleared by spitting out the toothpaste and oral debris
- The individual should be instructed not to rinse the mouth out, as this removes the residual toothpaste and prevents its chemical constituents from continuing to act in the mouth – this

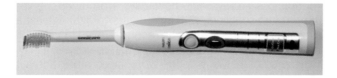

Figure 5.6   A Sonicare electric toothbrush.

132

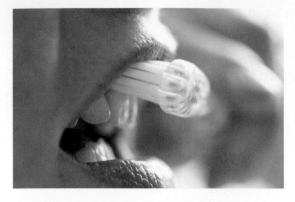

Figure 5.7   Gingival crevice brushing.

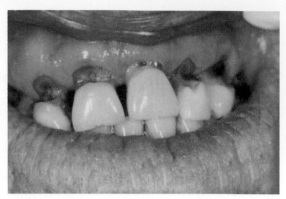

Figure 5.8   Extensive abrasion cavities.

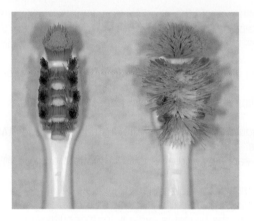

Figure 5.9   New and worn toothbrushes.

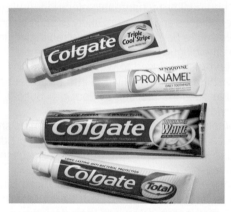

Figure 5.10   Examples of different toothpastes.

is particularly important when fluoridated toothpastes are used, as their topical fluoride effect is important in protecting the enamel
- Parents will need to perform effective tooth brushing on children up to the age of around 8 years, to ensure that all plaque is removed and to teach the child how to brush correctly
- Brushes should be rinsed afterwards and allowed to dry – they only have a limited life and need to be replaced every few months as the bristles curl down and render the brush ineffective (Figure 5.9)

Toothpastes

A huge variety of toothpastes are available nowadays, from shops' own brands to specialised ones from oral health product suppliers, with ingredients to fight against all aspects of common oral disease. Examples of all products likely to be recommended to individuals should be available in the preventive dental unit, so that the dental nurse can refer specifically to those that are suitable at each oral hygiene session. Many dental workplaces stock and sell various oral hygiene products to ensure that individuals are using those that have been recommended. Various types of toothpaste are shown in Figure 5.10.

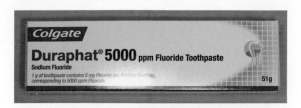

Figure 5.11   High-concentration fluoride toothpaste.

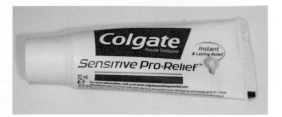

Figure 5.12   Desensitising toothpaste.

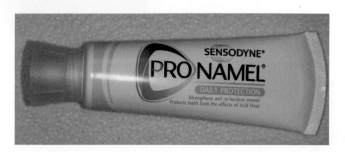

Figure 5.13   Enamel repair toothpaste.

The particular features of some of the targeted products that may be recommended are as follows:

- High-concentration fluoride toothpaste (Figure 5.11) to give additional protection when high caries rates are evident
- Plaque suppressant toothpastes to limit the amount of plaque that is able to form
- Calculus suppressant toothpastes for those individuals who build calculus easily
- Desensitising toothpaste (Figure 5.12) to reduce the painful effects of tooth sensitivity
- Whitening toothpastes, but only good-quality, non-abrasive types should be recommended
- Enamel repair toothpastes (Figure 5.13) for individuals with erosion damage

Interdental cleaning

However good the tooth-brushing technique, it is still impossible to clean interdental spaces perfectly with a toothbrush alone, unless a specialist electric brush is used. Consequently, these mesial and distal contact areas between adjoining teeth are more prone to developing caries and periodontal disease. To clean the interdental areas adequately, several oral health aids are available to assist patients to remove plaque that has formed here, as follows:

- **Dental floss** and **dental tape** are thread-like aids that are widely used to achieve interdental plaque removal; however, correct usage depends to some extent on the patient's manual dexterity and on receiving sound oral health instruction (Figure 5.14)
- "**Flossette-style**" handles hold the length of floss in place so that individuals can floss with one hand, therefore making the procedure less cumbersome, especially for posterior teeth where access is difficult for most people (Figure 5.15). They are also very useful when one person is responsible for the interdental cleaning of another
- **Interdental brushes** are a typical "bottle-brush" design (Figure 5.16) and are able to clean in spaced interdental areas (Figure 5.17), as well as around the individual brackets of fixed orthodontic appliances

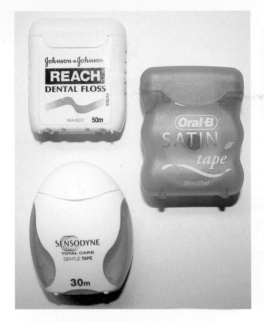

Figure 5.14   Dental flosses and tapes.

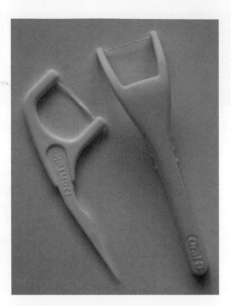

Figure 5.15   Interdental flossettes.

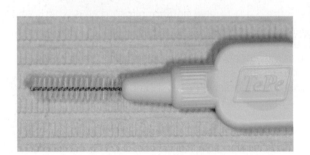

Figure 5.16   Interdental brush detail.

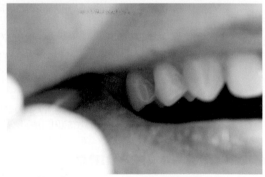

Figure 5.17   Use of an interdental brush for posterior cleaning.

- **Woodsticks** (although they may also be plastic!) are also available to dislodge solid pieces of food debris from interproximal areas, as well as to massage the gingivae here; however, their use should be restricted to competent adults whenever possible, as they can easily be stuck into the gum and cause problems if used incorrectly or by an inexperienced patient

The correct flossing demonstration and instructions that the dental nurse will give to those individuals who have adequate dexterity for the technique are as follows:

- Use a suitable demonstration model so that the individual can clearly see the actions as they are carried out
- Break off a sufficient length of the floss to wrap the ends several times around the index fingers and leave a 2-inch length between the hands
- Alternatively, tie the length into a loop and stretch it between the index fingers

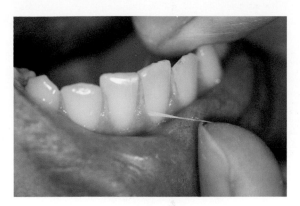

Figure 5.18   Flossing technique.

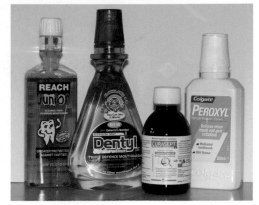

Figure 5.19   Types of mouthwash.

- With the fingers holding the length in place, use the thumbs to control the 2-inch piece and guide it into an interdental area
- The floss is then wrapped around the mesial or distal surface of one of the teeth (Figure 5.18) and "sawed" across the tooth surface, from the gingival area first
- This scrapes off the plaque and carries it towards the oral cavity, away from the gingiva
- Remove any debris from the floss
- Repeat the action in the same interdental area, wrapping it around the other tooth surface
- Repeat the action in the next interdental area
- If a flossette device is used, the head is pushed or pulled to wrap the floss piece around one tooth surface or the other once it is in the interdental area
- The floss or flossette should be discarded as soon as any shredding is evident
- Ideally, fluoridated products should be used whenever possible for maximum benefit to the teeth

With interdental brushes, the dental nurse will recommend the correct size for the individual – the wider the interdental space present, the larger the brush size possible so the bristles make contact with the tooth surfaces. The heads of some can also be angled and bent to make interdental access easier, especially when cleaning posterior teeth.

Use of mouthwashes

A wide range of mouthwashes are currently available, ranging from shops' own brands to specialised products from dedicated oral health product suppliers (Figure 5.19). Widely available types are as follows and individuals should have specific products recommended for use by the dental team, once their particular oral health needs have been assessed:

- General-use mouthwashes containing various ingredients to promote good oral hygiene
- Desensitising mouthwashes for use with generalised tooth sensitivity (Figure 5.20)
- Some are used specifically in the presence of oral soft tissue inflammation as a first aid measure or after oral surgery and contain hydrogen peroxide, which helps to eliminate anaerobic bacteria (Figure 5.21)
- Specialised mouthwashes are also available for patients suffering from both acute and chronic periodontal infections – they contain chlorhexidine, which is an antiseptic plaque suppressant (Figure 5.22)
- High-concentration fluoride mouthwashes for individuals at high risk of caries and orthodontic patients (Figure 5.23)

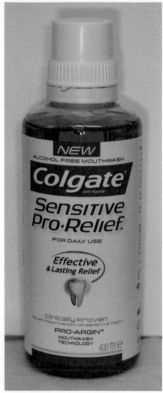

Figure 5.20   A desensitising mouthwash.

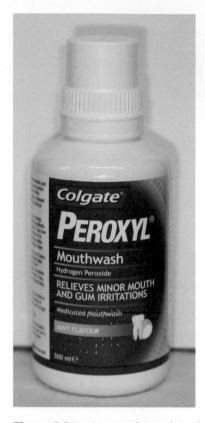

Figure 5.21   A peroxyl mouthwash.

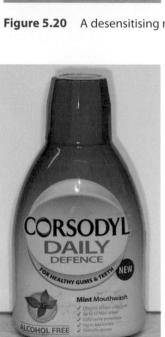

Figure 5.22   A corsodyl daily mouthwash.

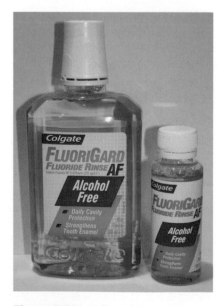

Figure 5.23   A fluoride mouthwash.

The dental nurse will advise the individual to use a recommended mouthwash in addition to a good tooth brushing regime and not instead of it. Mouthwashes are best used before bedtime so that their particular formulation is not washed off the teeth by food or drink. Some mouthwashes may be used several times a day and for young orthodontic patients they may take a small bottle to school for use after lunch.

Oral hygiene advice for denture wearers

Dentures provide additional areas for bacterial plaque to accumulate, besides that which develops on the teeth and in the gingival crevices. Individuals who wear dentures must be specifically instructed in the correct cleaning of the prostheses to avoid an increased risk of oral disease. This includes edentulous individuals who may develop a fungal infection called denture stomatitis if they fail to remove and clean their prostheses. Some individuals who receive the oral hygiene advice will be carers who attend to the oral health duties of others in nursing and residential homes and it is important that they are encouraged to develop a system of correct cleaning techniques without mixing up several sets of dentures at a time. If this is allowed to happen, individuals will be exposed to cross-infection and will potentially develop oral problems from wearing ill-fitting dentures.

The dental nurse will give the following instructions to individuals on the wear, care and cleaning of the new dentures, as follows:

- A demonstration of how to insert and remove the dentures is given if the denture wearer is actually present, with individuals then practising the techniques in front of the mirror
- They should be advised to avoid wearing dentures overnight, if possible, to avoid the development of oral fungal infections (thrush)
- The dentures should be stored overnight in a denture pot containing water, or ideally in a soaking agent such as Steradent (for all-acrylic dentures) or Dentural (for metal dentures)
- The dentures should be cleaned after each meal if possible, using a denture brush and denture toothpaste – some ordinary toothpastes may be too abrasive for use on the acrylic teeth
- The dental nurse can demonstrate the technique of cleaning all of the denture surfaces, especially those that fit against the dental ridges
- The dentures must be cleaned over a bowl of water, to avoid damage if they are dropped
- The individual should be advised to avoid soaking the dentures in bleach-based cleansers if any metal components are included in the design
- The denture wearer must eat soft foods initially, while the oral soft tissues acclimatise to the prostheses
- Denture wearers will have to take time to chew foods thoroughly, to avoid causing indigestion by swallowing large food particles
- Individuals can help to harden the oral soft tissues by carrying out hot salt water mouthwashes initially; otherwise the new dentures are likely to rub the soft tissues and make them sore
- The dental nurse must advise denture wearers to return to the surgery if any ulceration occurs beneath the dentures, as further adjustments are likely to be required to remove high spots and deep flange edges

Oral hygiene advice for orthodontic patients

Fixed appliances

Every tooth is incorporated into a fixed orthodontic appliance, so there are a lot of stagnation areas and the potential for oral damage to occur is huge. Routine twice-daily tooth brushing alone is insufficient to maintain adequate standards of good oral hygiene and special instructions and techniques are recommended for individuals undergoing fixed orthodontic therapy. The dental nurse should give the following advice to patients and their parent or guardian at the same time, as they will be responsible for supervising the oral hygiene techniques and the necessary diet controls between appointments.

The dental nurse can demonstrate the cleaning techniques on a model set up with a fixed appliance and then allow patients to follow the actions in their mouth:

- Careful manual tooth brushing should be carried out after each meal
- This should not be a vigorous scrubbing style of brushing, as it is likely to dislodge parts of the appliance
- Good-quality electric toothbrushes, such as Sonicare and Oral B, may be safely used instead
- Fluoridated toothpaste must always be used
- Daily use of interdental brushes to clean around each bracket individually
- Avoidance of cariogenic and acidic food and drinks, for the full period of treatment
- Avoidance of sticky foods, for the full period of treatment
- Use of fluoride mouthwash daily, to minimise the risk of decalcification
- Regular use of disclosing tablets, to highlight problematic areas where plaque is being retained and thus to minimise the risk of decalcification

Removable appliances

As with removable prostheses, orthodontic appliances are capable of acting as stagnation areas and holding food debris and plaque against the teeth and gingivae, unless a good standard of oral hygiene is maintained.

Although some dentists prefer patients to wear appliances during meals, it is possible that more acrylic breakages will occur in this case. The instructions for patients wearing removable appliances are as follows:

- Wear as directed by the dentist
- Clean the appliance and teeth after each meal, using a toothbrush and toothpaste
- The appliance should be removed from the mouth for cleaning
- The dental nurse will demonstrate the cleaning technique required to show that all surfaces must be cleaned and the care that must be taken when cleaning around springs and other components
- The cleaning must be carried out over a bowl of water to avoid breakages if it is dropped
- Avoid cariogenic and acidic foods and drinks, as advised
- If the appliance is to be removed for meals, ensure it is placed safely in a rigid container to avoid breakages during mealtimes

The same oral hygiene advice is relevant to those patients fitted with a functional appliance, except that they must always remove their appliance before eating a meal.

6

Unit 306: Provide Chairside Support during the Assessment of Patients' Oral Health

Learning outcomes

1. Be able to prepare the dental environment for an oral health assessment
2. Be able to record a range of oral health assessments

Outcome 1 assessment criteria

The learner can:

- Identify the different types and functions of dental records and charts
- Record assessments spoken by other team members using the correct notation on the correct dental charts
- Record the medical conditions that can affect an individual's dental treatment
- Provide examples of the terminologies and charting notations/symbols used in dental assessment
- Provide examples of dental charting using manual and computerised systems

Outcome 2 assessment criteria

The learner can:

- Retrieve and make available the correct patient's charts, records and images which are necessary for the assessment to be undertaken
- Select and arrange the equipment, instruments, materials and medicaments that are required for a full clinical assessment of the mouth
- Process and store dental charts, records and images in a manner that maintains their confidentiality

Diploma in Dental Nursing, Level 3, Third Edition. Carole Hollins.
© 2014 John Wiley & Sons, Ltd. Published 2014 by John Wiley & Sons, Ltd.
Companion website: www.wiley.com/go/hollins/dentalnursinglevel3

This unit is assessed by:
- observation in the workplace, with examples included in the learner's portfolio
- an appropriate alternative method

Details of various elements of theory and underpinning knowledge are included in Chapter 13, and these are assessed within the written paper.

The theory and underpinning knowledge required to understand the principles involved in the assessment of a patient's oral health are fully discussed in Chapter 13. This chapter explains the dental nurse's role and responsibilities in relation to preparing for and the recording of information for the following assessments:

- Soft tissues
- Hard tissues
- Charting
- Orthodontic assessment

Those responsibilities are to the operator (the person carrying out the procedure – usually the dentist, but in some cases it may be the orthodontic therapist as they can carry out Index of Orthodontic Treatment Need (IOTN) assessments following the General Dental Council's review into direct access issues) and also to the patient who is undergoing the assessment, and the patient's guardian where relevant.

The roles and responsibilities of the dental nurse involve the following actions:

- Identifying the various types of patient records
- Retrieving the correct patient records
- Setting up the correct items for the particular assessment
- Correctly recording the verbal assessment information given by the operator
- Correctly recording any relevant medical conditions
- Processing and storing the assessment information while maintaining confidentiality

Oral health assessments are carried out every day in the dental workplace as the starting point of a patient's diagnosis and treatment planning journey with various members of the dental team. Recording of the assessment results is invariably carried out by the dental nurse, and inaccurate recording of any of the information can lead to incorrect or no treatment being received by the patient. This will compromise the oral health of that patient at some point, so a full understanding of assessment methods and the knowledge to record the information accurately are essential skills required by dental nurses.

Types of patient records

The records that are made during an oral health assessment will vary between patients and depend on the purpose of the assessment and the likely treatment to be offered. Some patients will attend for a recall appointment, where their current level of oral health is assessed and any restorative treatment identified. Other patients will attend with specific problems such as a fractured tooth or bleeding gums, while others will be assessed for specific treatment needs, such as orthodontics.

The full range of dental records and charts that may be required are discussed in the following sections.

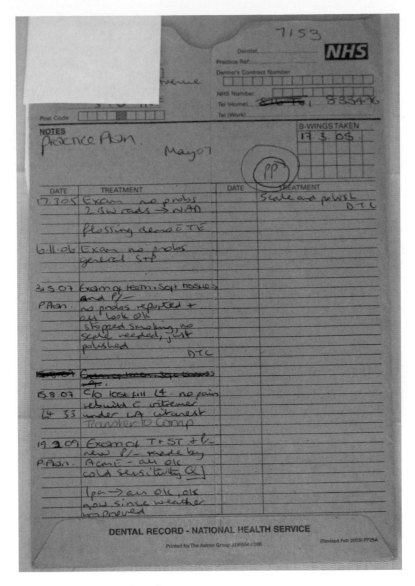

Figure 6.1   A typical NHS FP25 record card.

Personal details

The personal details identify the correct patient who requires the assessment. These are either provided as a hard copy on a written record card, or as information stored on a computer in a patient file. The record should contain the following information, to allow patient identification and to provide contact details: title, full name, address, date of birth, home and work telephone numbers.

In dental hospitals and clinics, these records may be in a similar format to those used in medical hospital wards – an A4 booklet with various page inserts – but in smaller dental workplaces they are more likely to be the typical NHS FP25 style record card (Figure 6.1).

Medical history

During an oral assessment, some patients may present with a lesion affecting their oral mucosa that indicates they are suffering from a disease, or they may have a medical condition or be taking prescribed medication which affects the oral tissues in some way. The natural process of ageing also has an effect on the normal appearance of the oral soft tissues. The changes to the oral tissues that may be seen are discussed in detail in Chapter 13.

All patients will have a full medical history taken when they initially attend the workplace, and this is then updated at each assessment appointment thereafter. Full details of any past and present illnesses and other medical issues must be regularly updated on the medical history form, and signed and dated as being updated at that time. A verbal confirmation of no changes at each treatment appointment is then satisfactory. The assessment of any updated entries or declarations is solely the responsibility of the dentist, although the information can be collected by the dental nurse.

Dental charts

These are available in standard formats so that they can be accurately read and understood across many potential language barriers between members of dental teams in different countries. Tooth charts, in particular, record the necessary information using internationally recognised symbols and notations, which are discussed in detail in Chapter 13 – a completed example is shown in Figure 6.2.

Besides tooth charts which can record both the primary and secondary dentition, there are also two periodontal charts in common use:

- Basic periodontal examination (BPE) chart – used as a quick reference guide for recording the overall periodontal status of a patient and identifying areas where a more detailed assessment is required (Figure 6.3)
- Full periodontal assessment sheet (Figure 6.4) – various formats are available which give detailed information on the periodontal status of individual teeth throughout both arches, recording pocket depths, tooth mobility, bleeding points, presence of plaque, and so on

Some operators also use a pre-illustrated soft tissue assessment sheet (Figure 6.5) to record any identified soft tissue lesions that are present during an oral health assessment. Unlike tooth and BPE charts, the soft tissue assessment sheets are only used when a lesion is found, rather than as a screening tool to be completed at every assessment.

Radiographs

Dental images are taken of oral structure for many reasons, and provide an insight into areas of the teeth and jaw bones that would otherwise be inaccessible to the dentist. They can assist in diagnosis and treatment planning as follows:

- Hard tissue pathology:
  - Teeth
  - Jaw bones
  - Facial bones
- Soft tissue pathology:
  - Abscesses
  - Cysts
  - Tumours
- Presence or absence of unerupted teeth
- Skeletal classification for orthodontic assessment and treatment planning
- Iatrogenic problems:
  - Overhanging restorations
  - Residual caries
  - Perforated root canals

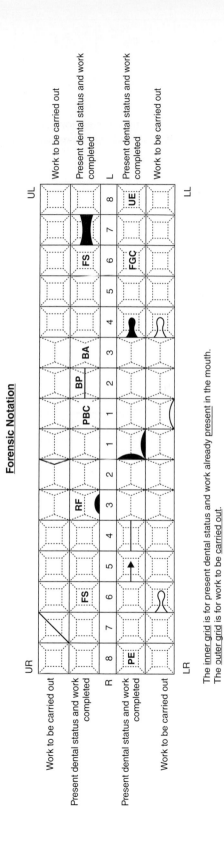

Figure 6.2 An example of completed charting grid. Source: *Levison's Textbook for Dental Nurses*, 11th edition (Hollins), 2013. Reproduced with permission of Wiley-Blackwell.

2	0	4
2	1	3

Figure 6.3 Example of a completed basic periodontal examination (BPE) chart. Source: *Levison's Textbook for Dental Nurses*, 11th edition (Hollins), 2013. Reproduced with permission of Wiley-Blackwell.

144

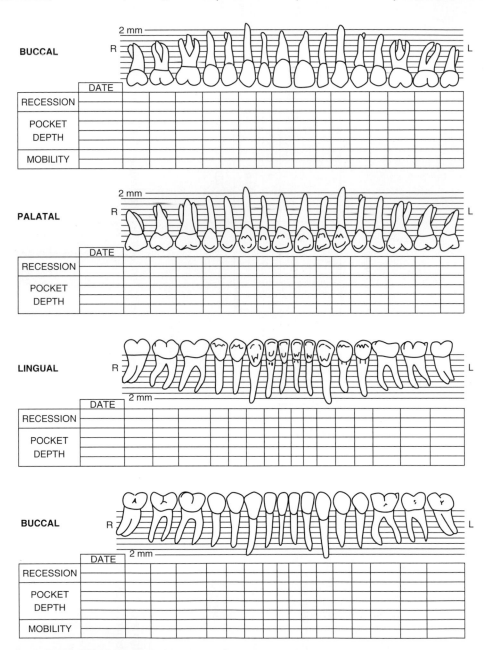

Figure 6.4 A detailed periodontal assessment sheet. Source: *Levison's Textbook for Dental Nurses*, 11th edition (Hollins), 2013. Reproduced with permission of Wiley-Blackwell.

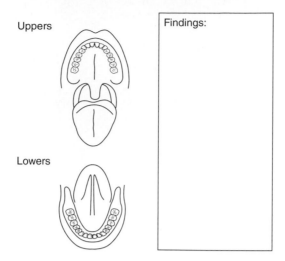

Uppers

Findings:

Lowers

Figure 6.5   A soft tissue assessment sheet. Source: *Levison's Textbook for Dental Nurses*, 11th edition (Hollins), 2013. Reproduced with permission of Wiley-Blackwell.

(a)   (b)

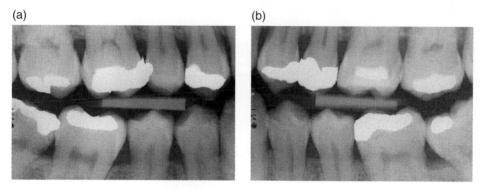

Figure 6.6   A horizontal bitewing radiograph. Source: *Basic Guide to Dental Procedures* (Hollins), 2008. Reproduced with permission of Wiley-Blackwell.

Radiographs are produced either digitally or as hard copies – the details of their production and processing are discussed in Chapter 14.

The dental image required for a particular assessment will vary as follows:

- Intra-oral views:
  - Horizontal bitewing for routine assessment of posterior teeth (Figure 6.6)
  - Vertical bitewing for assessment of posterior bone levels
  - Periapical for assessment of individual teeth (Figure 6.7)
  - Anterior occlusal for assessment of the anterior areas of the maxilla or mandible
- Extra-oral views:
  - Dental pantomograph (Figure 6.8) for:
    - Third molar assessment
    - Orthodontic assessment
    - Periodontal assessment
    - Jaw pathology
  - Lateral skull view (Figure 6.9) for orthodontic assessment and jaw measurement
  - Lateral oblique for lower third molar assessment

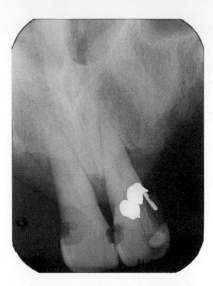

Figure 6.7 A periapical radiograph. Source: *Levison's Textbook for Dental Nurses*, 11th edition (Hollins), 2013. Reproduced with permission of Wiley-Blackwell.

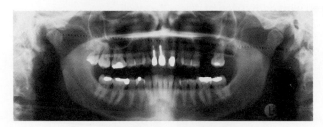

Figure 6.8 A dental pantomograph.

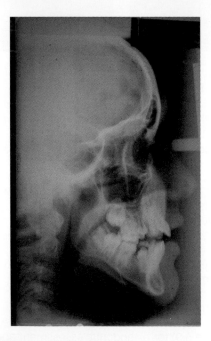

Figure 6.9 A lateral skull view.

Photographs

These can be taken to record various aspects of the dentition or soft tissues for future reference. They can be produced using conventional cameras (especially "Instamatic" types), digital cameras with "macro" lenses for close-up shots, or specialist intra-oral digital cameras. Specialised computers and equipment are required for this last technique.

Photographs are used during oral health assessments for the following purposes:

- To record soft tissue lesions to aid diagnosis
- To record the extent of injury following trauma
- To record the teeth and occlusion in a pre-treatment state, to assist particularly in orthodontic treatment planning
- To record potentially sinister lesions that can be emailed to specialists immediately, to aid a speedy diagnosis

Study models

It is sometimes necessary for the dentist to consider the patient's occlusion at the assessment appointment before being able to decide on any treatment necessary, e.g. when providing partial dentures or orthodontic treatment. Impressions are taken of both dental arches and then cast up to produce a set of study models (Figure 6.10).

Study models are used during oral health assessments for the following purposes:

- Occlusal analysis in complicated crown or bridge cases
- Orthodontic cases, to determine if extractions are required and which type of appliance is necessary
- Occlusal analysis where full mouth treatment may be necessary, to determine the functioning of the dentition
- Where tooth surface loss is evident, either by erosion from acidic foods and drinks or by attrition due to tooth grinding, so that the progression of the tooth wear can be monitored and treatment determined

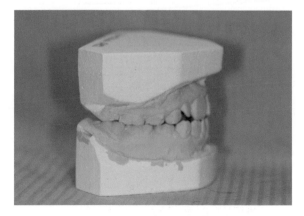

Figure 6.10   A set of study models.

Orthodontic measurements

An orthodontic assessment will be carried out when a patient is being considered for orthodontic treatment, and is not routinely performed otherwise. The assessment can be carried out by a dentist or an orthodontic therapist and involves viewing, taking and recording measurements of various aspects of the patient's occlusion, so that the severity of the malocclusion can be scored. An example of an orthodontic assessment sheet is shown in Figure 6.11. The scoring system is referred to as the Index of Orthodontic Treatment Need (IOTN) and is used to determine if patients are eligible to receive orthodontic treatment via the NHS or whether they need to seek treatment privately.

The usual records and measurements taken during an orthodontic assessment are:

- Classification of occlusion
- Overjet and overbite measurements
- Presence and location of crowding in each dental arch
- Presence of any retained deciduous teeth
- Note of any peculiarities, such as tooth rotations, arch spacing, unerupted permanent teeth, and so on
- IOTN score

ORTHODONTIC ASSESSMENT

NAME: *Jeremy Bloggs*

DOB: *12.12.1999*

DATE: *1ˢᵗ April 2013*

CLASSIFICATION	I	II div 1	II div 2	III
		X		
OVERJET	*11ᴍᴍ*	Reverse	Edge to edge	
OVERBITE	*50%*	Increased	Reduced	AOB
RETAINED DECIDUOUS TEETH	*E* _____ *I* ___ *E* _____ / *I*			
UPPER ARCH CROWDING *None*	Mild	Moderate	Severe
	Labial	And/or	Buccal
LOWER ARCH CROWDING	Mild X	Moderate	Severe
	Labial X	And/or	Buccal
ROTATIONS	*LL4 erupted DB rotated, taking excess arch space*		
ADDITIONAL NOTES	*Need to start functional appliance to reduce overjet asap but OH needs improving first – plaque present generally at gingival margins* *Needs 1 to 1 with OH educator and disclosing*		
IOTN SCORE	*5a*		

Figure 6.11   An orthodontic assessment sheet.

Retrieve and make available the patient records

The records required may be hard copies in full (so a "pack" of hand written patient notes, with paper copies of their medical history, previous treatment plans and consent forms, and so on), or they may be fully computerised and only accessible "on screen", or they may be a combination of the two. Whatever their presentation, they should be collected by the dental nurse and presented in the assessment area so that the operator can access them and check their content too.

In large dental workplaces, such as dental schools and hospitals, the dental nurse can check the correct patient identity by asking them to confirm their name, date of birth, and address, and that they know the reason for their attendance on the day. The final decision to confirm the patient's identity is the duty of the operator.

In smaller workplaces, many of the patients are recognisable to the staff by sight – some may even be known by their first names – but identity and procedure checks should still always be carried out, to avoid any mishaps. Once the patient has been correctly identified, the records and assessment area can be prepared.

The records to be set out will include the following:

- Notes written at the previous appointments
- Medical history form, to be checked to highlight any potential concerns – for example, does the patient gag while having impressions taken, or have an allergy to latex?
- The medical history can be checked by the dental nurse and any recognised potential issues pointed out to the operator
- Relevant radiographs that have been taken previously
- The radiographs must be correctly orientated and displayed, either as digital images on the computer or as hard copies on film
- Hard copies must be correctly mounted on the viewing screen:
  - Intra-oral views with the pimple facing out (to indicate left from right), and upper teeth with their roots above the crown and lower teeth with their roots below the crown
  - Bitewing radiographs with the pimple facing out and the molar teeth on the outer edges of each view (to indicate left and right quadrants, as well as distinguish upper from lower teeth)
  - Extra-oral views with the "L" marker in the bottom right-hand corner of the radiograph as it is positioned on the viewing screen, to indicate the patient's left side
- With hard copy records, dental and periodontal chartings may be stored as separate paper inserts in the patient's record folder – these should be laid out for the operator to view
- Computerised records may store this information as drop-down files within each patient's computer folder – these will require opening so that the operator can flick from one set of information to another easily
- Similarly, previous orthodontic assessments and photographs may be stored as separate hard copy inserts or as a drop-down file in the computerised records, and should be accessed accordingly
- Previous study models may be stored in a specific location in the workplace, usually in a box system with the patient's details written on both the box and the models
- If required, these should be retrieved and set out for the operator in the assessment area

Setting up for the assessment

Various items besides the patient's written or computerised records will be set up at the full clinical assessment appointment by the dental nurse, depending on the particular stage of the assessment to be carried out. The operator will require routine items of personal protective equipment (PPE) to be available, as they will be inspecting the oral cavity of the patient and are likely to be in contact with saliva. The routine PPE items are gloves, face mask or visor, and safety glasses if a face mask is worn.

Observing hard and soft tissues

The items that are likely to be required for this stage of a full clinical assessment are as follows:

- Mouth mirror – used to reflect light on to the hard and soft tissue surfaces, to retract the soft tissues to provide clear vision, and to protect the soft tissues during the assessment
- Angled probe – used to detect soft tooth surfaces and margins on existing restorations
- Tweezers (Figure 6.12) – used to hold cotton wool pledgets to wipe tooth surfaces dry or to place cotton wool rolls
- Moisture control items – cotton wool rolls and cotton wool pledgets (Figure 6.13)
- Briault probe – two-ended probe specially designed to detect interproximal caries, either mesially or distally (Figure 6.14)
- Soft tissue assessment sheet (see Figure 6.5) – to record any soft tissue findings

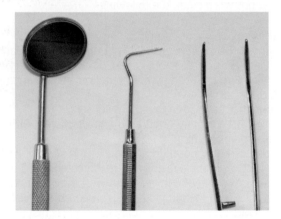

Figure 6.12 Mouth mirror, angled probe and tweezers. Source: *Levison's Textbook for Dental Nurses*, 11th edition (Hollins), 2013. Reproduced with permission of Wiley-Blackwell.

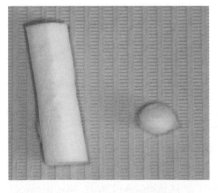

Figure 6.13 Cotton wool roll and cotton wool pledget.

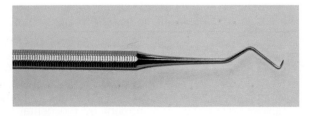

Figure 6.14 Briault probe.

Measuring and making records

This stage of the assessment involves the accurate recording of the verbally reported tooth and periodontal findings of the operator by the dental nurse into the notes or onto specially designed charts and assessment sheets, and therefore requires knowledge of the anatomical structure of the oral cavity. The basic structure and function of oral and dental anatomy are discussed in detail in Chapter 13, and charting techniques are summarised in the next section.

To record the tooth and gingival findings accurately, the following items are likely to be required, in addition to those listed in the preceding section:

- Dental charting sheet – to record any necessary information on the state of the teeth; this may be an extension of an existing charting record, or a new chart altogether (see Figure 6.2)
- BPE record sheet – to record the overall state of the periodontal tissues (see Figure 6.3)
- Periodontal record sheet – to record the detailed state of the periodontal tissues in patients with some degree of periodontal disease (see Figure 6.4)
- BPE or other periodontal probe – to take the periodontal tissue measurements (Figure 6.15)
- Film packet/cassette and relevant holder – to take any necessary dental images, as listed earlier
- Viewing screen – to view any hard copy dental radiographs if a digital system is not in use

Orthodontic assessment

This assessment is usually (but not always) carried out on child patients to determine any malocclusion and whether orthodontic treatment (or referral) is required. Patients may attend specifically for an orthodontic assessment or it may be carried out as part of their routine oral health assessment:

- Orthodontic assessment sheet – to accurately record the assessment findings (see Figure 6.11)
- Mouth mirror – to view the teeth
- Measuring ruler – to record the overjet and help to record the overbite (Figure 6.16)
- Alginate impression material items – to take impressions for study models (material, water at room temperature, mixing bowl and spatula, stock impression trays; Figure 6.17)
- Sheet of pink wax – to record the current occlusal bite so that the study models can be trimmed and set up correctly
- Film packet/cassette and relevant holder – to take any necessary dental images, as listed above
- Viewing screen – to view any hard copy dental radiographs if a digital system is not in use

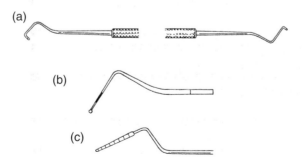

Figure 6.15   Periodontal probes. (a) Calculus probe, (b) BPE/CPITN probe and (c) pocket measuring probe. Source: *Levison's Textbook for Dental Nurses*, 11th edition (Hollins), 2013. Reproduced with permission of Wiley-Blackwell.

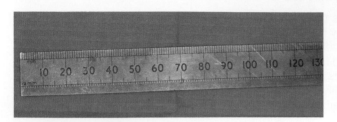

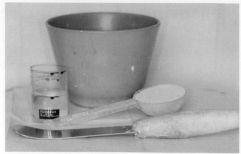

152

Figure 6.16   A measuring ruler to record the overjet and help record the overbite.

Figure 6.17   Alginate mixing equipment.

Recording the verbal assessment information

During the oral health assessment, operators will make a verbal report of their findings which the dental nurse must record accurately onto the relevant assessment sheet or computer screen. Many operators have a set routine for their assessment procedure, and the dental nurse will need to be familiar with each one. For example, some will carry out a full clinical assessment in the following order, on all patients:

Observation of hard and soft tissues → tooth charting → BPE charting → full periodontal charting → taking of necessary radiographs

Although this is a logical order of assessment, other operators will have their own style. An orthodontic assessment may be carried out at any point, or after all of these procedures have been completed. Similarly, many operators follow a set order of assessing the dentition and the periodontium, such as:

Upper right → upper left → lower left → lower right

During each stage of the assessment, the dental nurse will be writing down the information or entering it into the computer, and must do so accurately. If the operator speaks too quickly or too softly, the dental nurse must make them aware of any difficulty in recording the necessary information, and not be afraid to ask for points to be repeated as required. An incomplete or inaccurate assessment record is of no value to either the operator or the patient.

Observation of hard and soft tissues

Soft tissue assessment is carried out at each dental examination and in a systematic manner, otherwise there is a risk that areas will be missed out and lesions present remain uninvestigated. Unless an abnormality or lesion is discovered during the assessment, it is normal procedure to state "nothing abnormal diagnosed" (NAD) as the only required entry in the patient's records. If something does require recording, a soft tissue assessment sheet (see Figure 6.5) will need to be completed with the relevant details entered. The oral areas to be checked are as follows:

- Labial, buccal and sulcus mucosa – checked for their colour and texture, the presence of any white or red patches, and a note taken of the moisture level
- Palatal mucosa – both the hard and soft palates, the oropharynx and the tonsils (if present)
- Tongue – checked for colour and texture, symmetry of shape and movement, the level of mobility; all surfaces are checked, especially beneath the tongue, as this is one of the commonest sites for oral carcinoma to develop

- Floor of mouth – checked for colour and texture, the presence of any white or red patches, and the presence of any swellings

The presence of a lesion will be marked on the sheet (e.g. with a star or a circle) and any relevant measurements taken will be noted. Additional information, such as the colour of the lesion or the lack of moisture, will be recorded in the notes section of the sheet too.

Tooth charting

With tooth charting, a two-grid system is used (forensic notation) which separates the current dental status from any treatment required. Each anterior tooth charted diagrammatically is shown with four surfaces and an incisal edge or canine cusp, and each posterior tooth with five surfaces as shown in Figure 6.18.

The teeth are recorded from the centreline backwards for both the deciduous and the permanent dentition, and the charting grid is arranged as follows:

- Inner grid – shows current dental status and dental treatment already present in the mouth
- Outer grid – records all dental treatment that needs to be carried out

For the purpose of tooth charting, current dental status refers to the following notations only:

- The presence or absence of a tooth
- The presence of a root
- The notation of any tooth that is stated as unerupted, and charted as "UE"
- The notation of any tooth that is stated as partially erupted, and charted as "PE"
- The position of a tooth in relation to the normal dental arch, and may be stated as "instanding" or "buccal to the arch", for example

The condition of the teeth and the presence of any restorations can then be charted in a code form on the inner grid, and work to be carried out is recorded in the outer grid. The notable exception to the usual rules of inner grid versus outer grid is the charting of a fracture to a tooth. A fracture can range from a minimal incisal edge chip to a tooth, which requires no treatment (and is therefore charted on the inner grid as it represents "current dental status"), to a full fracture of the crown of the tooth from its root at gingival level (and is therefore charted on the outer grid, as it represents "dental treatment that needs to be carried out").

The charting symbol in both these instances of a fracture is "#", so the dental nurse must be careful to determine if an indication is made as to whether the tooth is to be restored or not, as this will determine which grid should be used for the notation.

Palmer notation

This is based on the division of the dentition into four quadrants when looking at the patient from the front: upper right and left, and lower left and right. Using either the letters representing the deciduous dentition or the numbers representing the permanent dentition, each tooth can then be written and identified individually. With the increased use of computers to record patients' dental records, including tooth chartings, the use of the quadrant symbol has been superseded by the use of the following:

- UR for upper right
- UL for upper left
- LL for lower left
- LR for lower right

So, individual teeth are charted as, for example, UR4 (upper right first premolar) and LLD (lower left first deciduous molar), and so on.

154

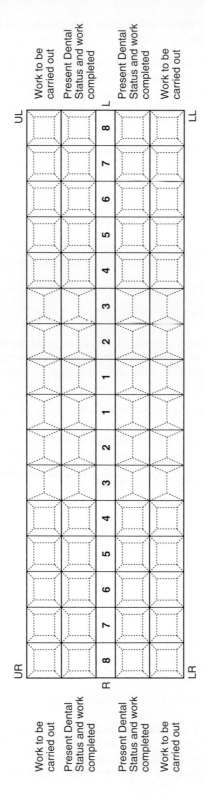

Figure 6.18 A manual charting grid. Source: *Levison's Textbook for Dental Nurses*, 11th edition (Hollins), 2013. Reproduced with permission of Wiley-Blackwell.

The Palmer system relies on the use of the English language for its correct interpretation, and a more international system of tooth charting is also available that is not language dependent, but is based on numbers only.

Two-digit FDI World Dental Federation notation

This international system was designed by the World Dental Federation and replaces the quadrant symbol or use of UR, UL, etc. with a quadrant number as well as a tooth number, as follows:

- Upper right – permanent quadrant 1, deciduous quadrant 5
- Upper left – permanent quadrant 2, deciduous quadrant 6
- Lower left – permanent quadrant 3, deciduous quadrant 7
- Lower right – permanent quadrant 4, deciduous quadrant 8

The quadrant number forms the first digit while the second identifies an individual tooth as 1 to 8 in the same way as the Palmer system. Reading clockwise from the upper right third molar, all 32 permanent teeth and 20 deciduous teeth have their own two-digit number indicating their quadrant (first digit) and identity (second digit) as shown:

18 17 16 15 14 13 12 11	21 22 23 24 25 26 27 28
48 47 46 45 44 43 42 41	31 32 33 34 35 36 37 38

And for deciduous teeth:

55 54 53 52 51	61 62 63 64 65
85 84 83 82 81	71 72 73 74 75

The lower left second premolar, for example, is written as 35 and pronounced "three-five", not "thirty-five", and the upper right deciduous first molar would be written as 54 and pronounced "five-four", and so on.

To enable the dental team to describe and discuss individual teeth and the treatment they may require, each surface of every tooth has its own name in relation to the midline of each jaw, and the anatomical structures that they sit against. It is this tooth surface nomenclature that allows the charting of every patient to be recorded accurately.

The general terminology in use for describing the tooth surfaces is summarised here:

- Labial – surface adjacent to the lips, applies in both arches and relates to incisor and canine teeth
- Buccal – surface adjacent to the buccinator muscle of the cheeks, applies in both arches and relates to premolars and molars
- Palatal – surface adjacent to the palate, applies to all maxillary teeth (Figure 6.19)
- Lingual – surface adjacent to the tongue, applies to all mandibular teeth
- Occlusal – biting surface of posterior teeth, applies to both arches and relates to premolars and molars
- The sharply raised points of these surfaces are called cusps, and the crevices between them are the fissures
- Incisal – biting edge of anterior teeth, applies to both arches and relates to incisors (canines have a cusp rather than an edge)
- Mesial – interdental surface of all teeth closest to the midline of each arch, so the front interdental surface
- Distal – interdental surface of all teeth furthest from the midline of each arch
- Contact point – the point where the mesial and distal surfaces of adjacent teeth are in contact with each other (Figure 6.20)
- Cervical – the neck region of any tooth, on the buccal, labial, palatal, or lingual surface

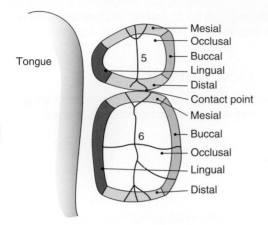

Figure 6.19 Surfaces of the teeth – mesial aspect. Source: *Levison's Textbook for Dental Nurses*, 11th edition (Hollins), 2013. Reproduced with permission of Wiley-Blackwell.

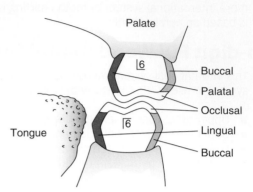

Figure 6.20 Surfaces of the teeth – occlusal aspect. Source: *Levison's Textbook for Dental Nurses*, 11th edition (Hollins), 2013. Reproduced with permission of Wiley-Blackwell.

BPE and periodontal charting

As with tooth charting, a system has been developed whereby the presence of periodontal disease can be quickly recorded during routine oral assessment, by dividing the mouth into sextants and recording the presence and depth of any unnatural spaces down the side of the teeth – these are called periodontal pockets. This recording technique is called a BPE assessment and is noted as shown in Figure 6.3.

Healthy periodontal tissues appear pink, firmly attached to the necks of the teeth with a gingival crevice no deeper than 3mm and do not bleed when touched. Teeth are firmly held in their sockets by the periodontal supporting tissues, and no plaque is present on the tooth surfaces.

Specially designed periodontal probes (such as a BPE probe – Figure 6.21) are used to record the presence and depth of any periodontal pockets discovered in each sextant of the dental arches; the coding system used is as follows:

- Code 0 – healthy gingival tissues with no bleeding on probing
- Code 1 – pocket no more than 3.5mm, bleeding on probing, no calculus nor other plaque retention factor present
- Code 2 – pocket no more than 3.5mm but plaque retention factor detected
- Code 3 – pocket present up to 5.5mm deep
- Code 4 – pocket present deeper than 5.5mm
- Code * – gingival recession or furcation involvement present

Higher codes therefore indicate a more serious periodontal problem. Where codes greater than 3 are recorded, a full periodontal assessment will be carried out to record the pocket depths of each tooth in that sextant, so that specific problem areas can be identified and intensive periodontal treatment can be initiated. In addition, the presence of any bleeding and plaque found will be recorded, as well as the mobility of any tooth. Tooth mobility is graded as follows:

- Grade I – side-to-side tooth movement less than 2mm
- Grade II – side-to-side tooth movement more than 2mm
- Grade III – vertical movement present

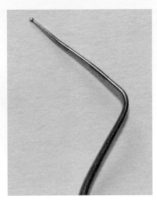

Figure 6.21   Basic periodontal examination (BPE) probe.

All of these assessments can be recorded manually, either on the patient's record card or on specific pre-printed charts (see Figure 6.4), or directly into the relevant files of computerised record systems.

Dental nurses will be required to provide anonymised examples of the following records within their workplace portfolio for inspection by their assessor:

- Examples of manual dental charting records
- Examples of computerised dental charting records
- Examples of the terminologies and charting symbols/notations used during the assessment

Orthodontic assessment

The terminology used to record an orthodontic assessment is quite specific and is recorded either directly into the patient's records or onto a designated assessment sheet.

When normal occlusion is not present, the patient is described as having a type of malocclusion which is recorded as an orthodontic classification, as follows:

- Class I – ideal occlusion generally (Figure 6.22), although it is possible for the molar teeth to be correct but there still to be crowding present anteriorly
- Class II division 1 – the lower jaw is behind the correct position and the anterior teeth are proclined (Figure 6.23)
- Class II division 2 – the lower jaw is behind the correct position and the anterior teeth are upright or retroclined (Figure 6.24)
- Class III – the lower jaw is in front of the correct position and the anterior teeth bite edge to edge or with the lowers in front of the upper incisors (Figure 6.25)

Normally, the upper incisors slightly overlap the lower ones vertically and horizontally and special names are given to this overlap; vertical overlap is called the overbite (measured as a percentage of lower tooth coverage) and horizontal overlap is called the overjet (measured in mm), as shown in Figure 6.26.

Other information to be recorded will vary between patients and be individual to them, such as the location in either arch of crowding (labial, or left or right buccal), and the presence of any retained deciduous teeth, and so on. When recording information about individual teeth, such as a rotation or a buccal displacement from the arch, the dental nurse will refer

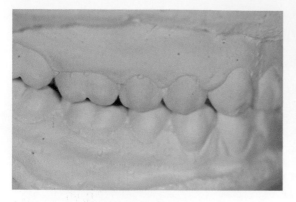

Figure 6.22   Class I occlusion.

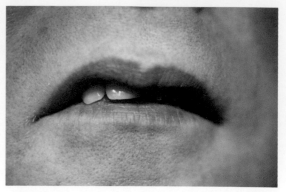

Figure 6.23   Class II division 1 malocclusion with lip trap.

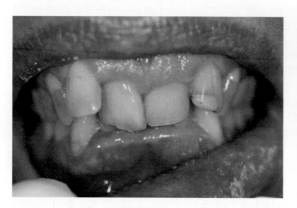

Figure 6.24   Class II division 2 malocclusion with increased overbite.

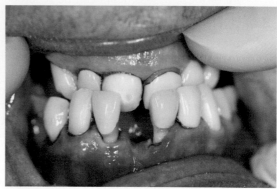

Figure 6.25   Class III malocclusion with reverse overjet.

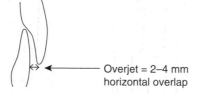

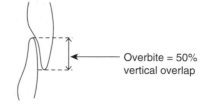

Figure 6.26   Overjet and overbite. Source: *Levison's Textbook for Dental Nurses*, 11th edition (Hollins), 2013. Reproduced with permission of Wiley-Blackwell.

to the tooth in the usual charting notation used in the workplace, i.e. as the UR3 or as 13, for example.

The final information to be recorded will be the IOTN score, which will be determined by the operator and then recorded by the dental nurse. IOTN scores are always recorded as a number from 1 to 5, indicating the degree of severity of the case in ascending order, followed by a coded letter that will indicate the worst feature of the case. So, for example, IOTN 4d indicates a tooth displacement from the arch that will require orthodontic realignment, and IOTN 5a indicates a large overjet that will require orthodontic reduction. Dental nurses are not required to know the various IOTN codes, only how they should be correctly recorded during the assessment.

During the orthodontic assessment, it may be decided that a set of study models and a wax bite record are required to permanently record the malocclusion as it presents on that day. The dental nurse will assist during the taking of the alginate impressions and the wax bite as follows:

- Apply PPE to the patient
- Mix the alginate to the correct consistency
- Load the impression trays
- Monitor and support the patient during the impression-taking procedure
- Warm the wax sheet in warm water
- Assist the patient with rinsing and cleaning up as necessary
- Disinfect the impressions and the wax bite
- Correctly package and label the items ready for removal to the laboratory

Recording relevant medical conditions

The importance of having an accurate medical history for every patient is discussed in detail in Chapter 13.

The medical history can be recorded on a written sheet (Figure 6.27) or entered in a computer file in the correct patient's computer records, and once the initial information has been recorded, the questionnaire will require updating at every assessment appointment thereafter. The dental nurse will complete the form with the patient and accurately record all the information that is given. So in the example form shown, any questions that have a tick in the "yes" column should then have further information added in the notes section, or on a separate sheet if necessary. The spelling of prescribed medications can be checked in the *British National Formulary* and the dosage of each item should be recorded as well.

The medical history should be taken in an area of the workplace that guarantees patient privacy so that they will divulge all relevant information willingly – very often this is the assessment area itself, which will be at a remove from other persons. In particular, information about the patients' alcohol and tobacco usage will be required, as these habits can have a significant effect on their overall general and oral health. Various medical conditions and medications can also affect a patient's dental treatment, and particular reference should therefore be made to the following:

- Smoking history – for its relationship to the incidence of oral cancer
- Alcohol consumption – for its relationship to the incidence of oral cancer
- History of herpes infection – especially a history of a primary herpes infection or of a "cold sore", as these patients may be infectious to the dental team when lesions are present
- History of HIV infection – these patients will be infectious and therefore are hazardous to all dental personnel
- History of hepatitis – although dental staff must be vaccinated against hepatitis B, other forms of hepatitis occur that are equally as infectious and therefore hazardous to all dental personnel
- Diabetes – whether a patient has type 1 or type 2 diabetes, they will be prone to xerostomia, oral infection and poor wound healing
- Epilepsy – a side-effect of some medications used for this condition allows gingival hyperplasia to develop which will affect the patient's ability to clean the teeth effectively

CONFIDENTIAL MEDICAL HISTORY
To provide the best and safest treatment, your dentist needs to know of any problems that
may affect your treatment.

NAME _____

SEX: MALE/FEMALE _____

ADDRESS _____

_____

TEL NO: HOME _____ WORK _____

DATE OF BIRTH _____ OCCUPATION _____

WHEN DID YOU LAST RECEIVE DENTAL TREATMENT? _____

DOCTOR'S NAME AND ADDRESS _____

_____

	YES	NO	IF YES, PLEASE GIVE DETAILS
Are you attending or receiving treatment from a doctor, clinic, hospital or specialist?			
Are you taking any medicines, tablets, drugs or injections or using any creams or ointments?			
Are you taking or have taken any steroids in the last 2 years?			
Are you allergic to Penicillin?			
Are you allergic to any medicines, foods or materials?			
Are you pregnant or a nursing mother?			
Are you HIV positive?			
Have you had Rheumatic Fever or chorea?			
Have you had jaundice, liver, kidney disease or hepatitis?			
Have you been hospitalised for any reason?			
Have you ever had your blood refused by the blood transfusion service?			

Figure 6.27 An example of a medical history form.

	YES	NO	IF YES, PLEASE GIVE DETAILS
Have you ever been told you have a heart murmur, heart problem, angina or high blood pressure?			
Have you ever had a bad reaction to a local or general anaesthetic?			
Have you had a joint replacement or other implant?			
Do you have arthritis?			
Do you have a pacemaker or have you had heart surgery?			
Do you suffer from hay fever, eczema or any other allergy?			
Do you suffer from bronchitis, asthma or other chest condition?			
Do you have fainting attacks, giddiness, blackouts or epilepsy?			
Do you or anyone in your family have diabetes?			
Do you bruise or bleed easily following a tooth extraction or injury?			
Do you carry a warning card?			
Do you think there are any other aspects concerning your health that your dentist should know about?			
Are your a smoker/drinker? If so, how many of the following do you consume per day?	Cigarettes		Alcoholic units

SIGNED   DATE

Figure 6.27   *(Continued)*

- Hypertension and heart disease – similarly, some prescribed medications for these conditions allow gingival hyperplasia to develop
- History of stroke – these patients are likely to be taking an anticoagulant, such as aspirin or warfarin, and great care will be needed if they are to undergo extractions or minor oral surgery procedures

- Eating disorders – the self-induced vomiting associated with conditions such as bulimia will result in enamel erosion and soft tissue burns
- Digestive disorders – disorders such as Crohn's disease and ulcerative colitis often manifest as oral ulceration in the patient

It is the responsibility of the operator to check the medical history form and question the patient further to clarify any medical issues that have been highlighted in its initial completion or update.

Maintaining confidentiality of the information

Once the oral health assessment has been completed and all the relevant information acquired, the patient's dental charts, records and images must be stored in accordance with the information governance requirements of the workplace, to ensure that they remain confidential. These requirements may vary between workplaces, and dental nurses will be required to show evidence of knowledge of those relevant to themselves in their particular workplace.

In particular, the information governance policy will give an overview of how information should be handled in the workplace, including the following specific areas:

- Storage of data – there should be a secure area of the premises which has no public access that is used for the storage of hard copies of patient records. Within that area the records should also be held in a locked file system, so that they are further secured. Computer records should be protected by the use of password access, and this should be known by staff members only
- Consent to view data – normally, all patient records are accessible to every staff member, except perhaps the most junior of dental team members, but otherwise there must be strict protocols in place with regard to access to patient records by anyone else. The exceptions that do exist, including patients' right to access their own records, are discussed in Chapter 13
- Maintenance of patient confidentiality – patient details and the contents of their records must not be disclosed to other patients, even amongst families, unless someone is acting as a guardian for another. Patient details must not be left in public areas of the workplace where they may be viewed by others, especially not in a surgery area or at the reception desk in full view of the next patient. If the records cannot be filed in a secure area immediately after the assessment, they should be stored in a locked cupboard in the surgery area until they have been written up and checked by the operator. Computer records must be saved in the file before the screen is changed, otherwise they will be lost, and a daily backup system must be used (with secure storage off-site) to ensure the records are correctly retained
- Situations where information disclosure may be required – these are discussed in Chapter 13

Dental workplaces will vary with regard to their particular storage systems in use – some may store all hard copies of information together (i.e. written records with dental images together) while others may have separate storage systems for each. Dental nurses must always follow the policies and protocols of their own particular workplace, and ensure that they are never personally responsible for any breaches of patient confidentiality.

7

Unit 307: Contribute to the Production of Dental Images

Learning outcomes

1. Be able to provide the support and resources necessary for the taking of dental images
2. Be able to process dental films
3. Be able to contribute to the quality assurance process of dental images

Outcome 1 assessment criteria

The learner can:
- Maintain health and safety throughout imaging procedures
- Provide the correct resources for the taking of dental images
- Identify different intra-oral and extra-oral radiographs and ask patients to remove any items that may interfere with the radiographic image
- Offer patients support during the taking of a radiographic image
- Refer any questions that are beyond their role to an appropriate member of the team

Outcome 2 assessment criteria

The learner can:
- Process dental films using the correct resources for the imaging equipment used
- Ensure that the quality of the image is maintained during processing
- List the chemicals used in dental processing and their purposes

Diploma in Dental Nursing, Level 3, Third Edition. Carole Hollins.
© 2014 John Wiley & Sons, Ltd. Published 2014 by John Wiley & Sons, Ltd.
Companion website: www.wiley.com/go/hollins/dentalnursinglevel3

Outcome 3 assessment criteria
The learner can:
- Store or save images produced according to the organisation's established procedure
- Keep accurate records of quality assurance checks
- List methods of mounting radiographs

This unit is assessed by:
- observation in the workplace, with examples included in the learner's portfolio
- an appropriate alternative method

Details of various elements of theory and underpinning knowledge are included in Chapter 14, and these are assessed within the written paper.

The theory and underpinning knowledge required to understand the scientific principles involved in the safe use of ionising radiation in dentistry are fully discussed in Chapter 14. This chapter explains the role and responsibilities of dental nurses in relation to their required contribution to the production of dental images, and includes the following:

- Maintain the health and safety of all persons throughout any imaging procedures
- Set up for the taking of dental images
- Process the dental films and mount them correctly
- Store or save the dental images correctly
- Contribute to quality assurance checks

Their responsibilities are to the operator (the person carrying out the procedure – usually the dentist, but in some cases it may be a suitably qualified dental care professional) and also to the patient who is undergoing the imaging procedure, and the patient's guardian where relevant.

Maintain the health and safety of all persons

This requires an understanding of the hazardous nature of ionising radiation which is discussed in detail in Chapter 14. There is no "safe" level of use of ionising radiation – every X-ray exposure can cause some amount of tissue damage in the patient, or in anyone else in the imaging area who is exposed to the X-ray beam. An overdose can cause serious health effects, ranging from a mild burn to leukaemia and, ultimately, death.

For this reason, specific legislation is in place to ensure full compliance with the health and safety aspects of ionising radiation by all dental workplaces, under the following regulations:

- Ionising Radiation Regulations 1999 (IRR99)
- Ionising Radiation (Medical Exposure) Regulations 2000 (IR(ME)R2000)

While IRR99 is concerned with the protection of staff and IR(ME)R with the protection of patients, the aim of both sets of regulations is to keep the number of X-ray exposures, and their dose levels, to the absolute minimum required for clinical necessity at all times. In relation to these regulations, dental nurses must be fully knowledgeable of the following:

- The actions they can take in relation to imaging procedures
- The actions they cannot take in relation to imaging procedures
- How to protect patients and others from unwanted ionising radiation exposure

The following table details the duties that can and cannot be carried out by dental nurses in relation to the various stages involved in the production of dental images.

Duty	Radiography qualified dental nurse	NEBDN qualified dental nurse	NVQ qualified dental nurse	Trainee dental nurse
Patient ID	X	X	X	X
Positioning	X	NO	NO	NO
Setting exposure	X	NO	NO	NO
Pressing exposure button	X	X In the presence of the "set up" operator	X In the presence of the "set up" operator	X In the presence of the "set up" operator
Processing	X	X	X	X
Quality audit	X	X	X	X
QA test exposures	X	X In the presence of the "set up" operator	X In the presence of the "set up" operator	X In the presence of the "set up" operator
QA programmes	X	X	X	X

NEBDN, National Examining Board for Dental Nurses; NVQ, National Vocational Qualification.

Only those persons (including suitably post-registration qualified dental nurses) who have received formal training and assessment in the setting up of an imaging machine and the choice of the exposure level can legally expose any person to ionising radiation. To undertake these actions safely requires detailed knowledge and understanding of the physics involved in the use of ionising radiation, and this is well beyond the level of knowledge achieved at register-able qualification.

Similarly, the dental nurse may be required to press the exposure button of the machine, either when irradiating a patient or when carrying out a test exposure, but only on the instruction of the operator, as only they have the knowledge to set the machine correctly and to decide when it is safe to press the button.

One area where the dental nurse can help to avoid unnecessary exposures and therefore help to contribute to the health and safety aspects of the procedure is patient identification.

Correct identification of the patient

The day list will refer to each patient attending that day by name, and/or date of birth, and/or address, and/ or some kind of patient identification marker – such as a unique computer number, or the patient's NHS number.

Whatever the system in place, the dental nurse should be familiar with it and be able to access the patient's records so that a cross-reference check can be made between the notes present and the expected exposure procedure to be carried out. So if the previous notes refer to the patient requiring a set of bitewing radiographs, but the day list indicates that the patient is attending for a dental pantomograph exposure, one of the following scenarios has occurred which must be checked with the operator and the patient before the ionising radiation procedure is carried out:

- The records and the day list entry are for two different patients
- The records are incomplete, and a change in the dental image required has been decided without being recorded
- The records are correct and the day list entry is incorrect
- The records are incorrect and the day list entry is correct

Any of these scenarios could quite easily have occurred and the matter should be referred to a more senior colleague (ideally the operator concerned) so that the dental nurse can assist in determining the way forward – to identify the correct patient and the correct exposure procedure to be carried out that day.

In large dental workplaces, such as dental schools and hospitals, the dental nurse can check the correct patient identity by asking them to confirm their name, date of birth and address, and that they know the reason for their attendance on the day. The final decision to confirm the patient's identity is the duty of the operator.

In smaller workplaces, many of the patients are recognisable to the staff by sight – some may even be known by their first names – but identity and procedure checks should still always be carried out to avoid any mishaps. Once the patient has been correctly identified, the correct resources for the exposure can be prepared by the dental nurse.

Other health and safety actions

In relation to IRR99 the dental nurse must have received documented training and then comply with the following:

- Local rules in association with each X-ray machine in the dental workplace, in particular:
  - The location of the 1.5-metre controlled area and the 2-metre safety zone (see Figure 1.28)
  - The location of the isolator switch in case of malfunction
  - The contingency plan in case of malfunction
  - The name of the workplace's Radiation Protection Supervisor (RPS), as the person to contact in case of malfunction
  - The methods in place to ensure that no person but the patient can enter the controlled area during exposure, and to follow them at all times
- Comply with the dental workplace requirements with regard to the use of monitoring badges
- Comply with the General Dental Council's continuing professional development requirements with regard to ionising radiation updates, which is a core topic

In relation to IR(ME)R 2000, the dental nurse must have received documented training and then comply with the following:

- Only carry out those duties that they are legally able to, specifically:
  - Patient identification
  - Setting up the resources to enable exposure to occur
  - Pressing the exposure button, but only when requested by the "set up" operator
  - Processing and mounting of radiographs
  - Contribute to quality assurance programmes
- Correctly store dental films so that they do not become damaged before use
- Maintain processing equipment correctly, so that retakes are not necessary

- Use processing chemicals correctly to avoid accidents, and be aware of Control of Substances Hazardous to Health (COSHH) guidelines in relation to any accident and follow them accordingly
- Maintain the security of controlled areas at all times in accordance with the workplace policies, to avoid the possibility of accidental exposures

The principles of justification and optimisation of dental images are the responsibility of the IR(ME) R practitioner alone and are not relevant to dental nurses:

- **Justification** – the decision that the dental image is required to enable diagnosis and treatment to proceed, and that the benefits to the patient will outweigh the risks of being exposed to ionising radiation
- **Optimisation** – the principle of ALARA/P (as low as reasonably achievable/possible), so that the minimum dose of radiation is given for the minimum exposure time to produce a viable dental image

Set up for the taking of dental images

The resources required to be made ready will depend on the dental image that is to be taken, and this will be indicated in the patient records. There are various types of film used but all are either those taken within the oral cavity (intra-oral films) or those taken outside the oral cavity (extra-oral films).

Intra-oral films are supplied in child- and adult-size packets (Figure 7.1), and are used to produce the following views:

- **Horizontal bitewing** (see Figure 6.6) – shows the posterior teeth in occlusion, and is taken to view:
  - Interproximal areas and diagnose caries in these regions
  - Restoration overhangs in these areas
  - Recurrent caries beneath existing restorations
  - Occlusal caries
- **Vertical bitewing** (Figure 7.2) – shows an extended view of the posterior teeth, from mid-root of the uppers to mid-root of the lowers as a minimum, and is taken to view:
  - Periodontal bone levels of the posterior teeth
  - True periodontal pockets
- **Periapical** (see Figure 6.7) – shows one or two teeth in full length with their surrounding bone, and is taken to view the area and the teeth in close detail

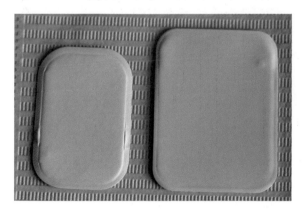

Figure 7.1   Intra-oral films: (a) child size; (b) adult size.

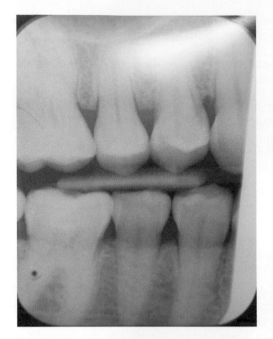

Figure 7.2   A vertical bitewing radiograph.

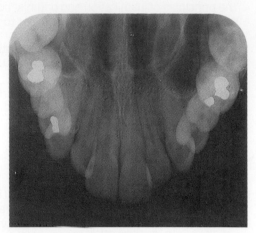

Figure 7.3   Maxillary anterior occlusal.

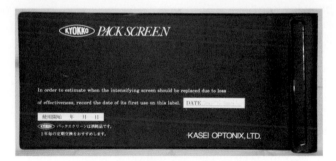

Figure 7.4   Extra-oral dental panoramic tomograph (DPT) cassette.

- **Anterior occlusal** (Figure 7.3) – shows a plane view of the anterior section of either the mandible or the maxilla, and is used especially to view the area for unerupted teeth, supernumerary teeth and cysts

The intra-oral film packets are supplied ready-loaded by the manufacturers, but require one of a variety of holders to allow correct patient and film positioning to be achieved before exposure.

Extra-oral films are used to produce much larger images showing many structures, and are supplied in cassettes (Figure 7.4) to produce the following views:

- **Dental panoramic tomograph (DPT)** (see Figure 6.8) – shows both jaws in full and their surrounding bony anatomy, and is taken for orthodontic and wisdom tooth assessments, as well as to help diagnose pathology and jaw fractures
- **Lateral oblique** – shows the posterior portion of one side of the mandible, including the ramus and angle and the lower molar teeth, and is an alternative to a DPT to view the position of

unerupted third molar teeth (these are used infrequently now, as the image produced on a well-aligned DPT is far superior)
- **Lateral skull radiograph** (see Figure 6.9) – this is a view of the side of the head, taken in a specialised machine called a **cephalostat** (which may be present as an attachment to a DPT machine, or as a "standalone" device); it is used to monitor jaw growth and determine orthognathic surgery techniques in complicated cases of malocclusion

Extra-oral cassettes are expensive items and, as they do not become contaminated by the patient, they can be re-used. The cassette must be reloaded with a new film after each use, as the previously exposed film is removed from the cassette to be processed and produce the radiograph.

169

Knowledge of the correct setting up of the area for the procedure

In some dental workplaces, the intra-oral X-ray machine is in the surgery area, so that images can be taken during treatment with the patient sitting in the chair. If the surgery area is already in use then only the specific resources required for the imaging procedure need to be set out, but otherwise the correct setting up procedure must be followed.

As this is not a clinical procedure, social hand washing only is sufficient before resources are handled.

Once the hands are clean and any wounds covered with a waterproof plaster, the area can be prepared as follows:

- The electricity supply to the dental chair, the X-ray machine and the computer (where relevant) is switched on
- The patient records are accessed on the computer, or the paper copies are laid out on the work surface in easy reach of the operator
- Relevant previous radiographs are correctly mounted on the viewing screen, in easy reach of the operator
- Wearing clean gloves, the correct resources are laid out for the images to be taken (see later)
- Mouth rinse, cup and tissues are made ready for the patient if intra-oral views are to be taken

When an intra-oral view is to be taken, the following must be set out:

- Choice of child- and adult-size intra-oral film packet (adult patients with a small mouth may not tolerate adult-size films)
- Sensor plate and cable if digital images are used (Figure 7.5)
- Manual film holder, depending on which view or views are to be taken:
  - Horizontal bitewing (Figure 7.6)
  - Vertical bitewing (Figure 7.6)
  - Anterior periapical (Figure 7.7)
  - Posterior periapical (Figure 7.7)
- Disinfectant wipes – to clean and handle the exposed film packet on its removal from the patient's mouth
- Alternatively, a plastic disposable barrier pocket for the digital sensor plate
- Container for the patient to deposit any removable prosthesis before exposure

Extra-oral imaging machines are usually located in a separate room away from the surgery area, so that they can be used by various operators while others are seeing patients in the surgery. The setting up of the area is the same as for the intra-oral machine, detailed earlier.

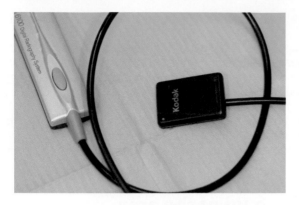

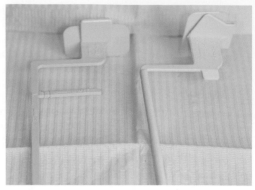

Figure 7.5   Digital sensor plate and cable.

Figure 7.6   Bitewing holders: horizontal (left) and vertical (right).

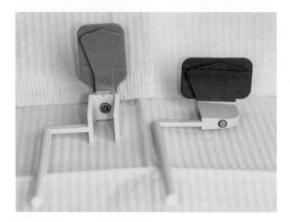

Figure 7.7   Periapical holders: anterior (left) and posterior (right).

When an extra-oral view is to be taken, the following must be set out:

- Loaded film cassette (see Figure 7.4) – this must be checked as loaded either in the darkroom or in the front chamber of the automatic processor, to avoid exposing the film to daylight
- Incisal wedge when a dental pantomograph is to be taken, to ensure the teeth are opened from normal occlusion during exposure so that they are not superimposed over each other – a cotton wool roll is often used by operators for this purpose
- Container for the patient to deposit any removable prosthesis or jewellery (e.g. earrings, tongue stud, necklace) before exposure

When instructed to do so by the operator, the patient can be brought into the imaging area. Parents and guardians should not be allowed into the area, so they are not exposed to the ionising radiation. However, younger patients and some with special needs may be uncooperative unless a parent or guardian is present – the operator will decide if this is acceptable or not. The dental nurse must ask the patient to remove any item that may interfere with the image – this includes removable prostheses, all items of jewellery within the jaw area (e.g. earrings, tongue studs, lip rings), and any hair clips worn in the same region.

While the patient is made ready for the exposure by the operator, the dental nurse may be required to load the film packet into the holder. This must be done carefully to ensure that the

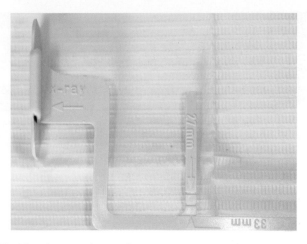

Figure 7.8   Close-up of holder showing beam direction arrow.

packet is positioned the correct way round, so that the front of the film receives the ionising radi-ation beam. The majority of holders are marked in some way to aid with this orientation, e.g. with arrows indicating the direction of the beam (Figure 7.8).

The dental nurse should encourage the patient to be cooperative while the film and holder are positioned, and while the machine collimator is lined up by the operator. Above all, the patient must be told to keep still during the exposure. The dental nurse must step out of the 2-metre safety zone before the exposure is made, along with all other personnel.

When instructed to do so by the operator (and not before), the dental nurse may press and hold the exposure button until the audible buzzer ceases – the exposure is then complete.

The exposed film and its holder are removed by the operator and received by the dental nurse, wearing gloves and with a disinfectant wipe in hand to remove any saliva contamination. The holder will be decontaminated and sterilised for reuse. When a digital image has been taken, the protective sheath will be disposed of as hazardous waste. When an extra-oral view has been taken, the dental nurse will receive the cassette from the operator and take it to the processing area. It must not be opened until safely in the darkroom or the front chamber of the automatic processor.

Process the dental films and mount them correctly

Digital images will be produced on the computer screen immediately, via the cable connecting the sensor to the computer, and do not require processing.

All other films must be put through the correct series of chemicals to produce a permanent image on the film – this is called processing and can be carried out in an automatic processor or manually (in a darkroom).

Automatic processing

The machine used (such as a Velopex machine) consists of a base containing the chemical and water tanks, with conveyor belt-style rollers that carry the film through the machine during processing (Figure 7.9). These are all beneath a removable, light-tight lid which has hand entry ports so that the film packet or cassette can be put into the light-tight chamber before being opened. If the film is exposed to visible light before being processed, the image will be permanently lost.

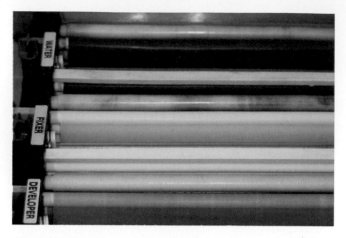

Figure 7.9 Velopex processing machine – internal detail.

The automatic processing procedure is as follows:

- Observe the warning light system to check that the chemical and water levels are adequate, and that the temperature is correct for processing (see Figure 4.6)
- When the temperature is correct, the warning light will go out and the machine is ready for use
- Intra-oral film packets are taken into the machine through the hand ports, while wearing clean gloves
- Extra-oral cassettes are placed into this section by lifting and replacing the lid, and then they can be opened and handled via the hand ports
- The rollers become operational once the processing start button within this first chamber is pressed
- The film packet is carefully opened and the plastic envelope, black paper and lead foil are all dropped to the base of the tank, for removal later
- The film is then held by its sides only, as finger marks on the surface will damage the image
- The film is carefully inserted into the entrance to the rollers, and it will be gently tugged into the machine to be processed
- Once the film has passed through the machine, and been processed and dried, it will reappear at the delivery port at the back and can be safely handled and viewed

Manual processing

Manual processing follows the same procedure as that occurring in an automatic processor, but is carried out by hand and in a darkroom – this is a light-tight, lockable room containing the processing chemicals and water tanks that are heated and maintained in the temperature range 18–22 °C, and illuminated by a red or orange "safe light".

Four tanks will be present, as follows (Figure 7.10):

- Lidded developing tank – containing the alkaline developing fluid that produces the initial latent image; the lid is only removed during developing as the solution will deteriorate in air
- The image is still unstable in visible light at this point
- First water tank – to wash off the developing solution after the correct developing time, using tap water

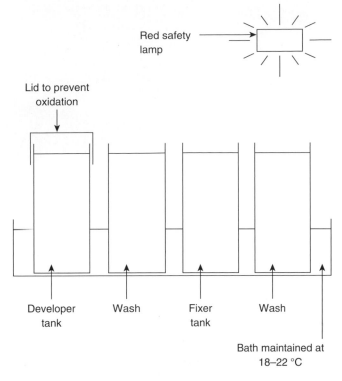

Figure 7.10 Darkroom layout.

- Fixing tank – containing the acid fixing solution which permanently fixes the image onto the celluloid film, so that it can be viewed in visible light
- Second water tank – to wash off the fixing solution after the suitable fixing time, again using tap water

It must be possible to see to some degree inside the darkroom rather than it being completely dark, so an orange or red safe light will be present under which the processing can be carried out without exposing the film to actual visible light, and thereby ruining the image. The room must be lockable from within so that the door cannot be opened by anyone else during the processing procedure, as this would result in the accidental exposure of the film to light and the destruction of the image before it has been fully processed.

The manual processing procedure is as follows:

- Check that the chemical and water levels are adequate
- Check the temperature of the solutions and determine the developing and fixing times required from the chemical manufacturer's guidelines provided
- Check that a timing clock and suitable film hangers are available in the room
- Wipe surfaces dry of any previously spilt chemicals or water, if necessary
- Lock the door and switch off all lights except the safe light
- Open the film packet or cassette, locate the film and clip it to one of the hangers available, carefully handling the film by its edges only, to avoid spoiling it with fingerprints
- Remove the developer lid, immerse the hanger in the solution so that the film is completely covered by the solution and start the timer

174

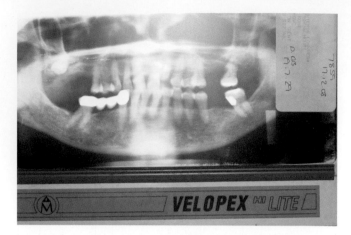

Figure 7.11   Viewing screen.

- When the timer sounds, remove the hanger and film and immerse in the first water tank, agitating the hanger to ensure thorough washing occurs
- Shake off excess water, then fully immerse the hanger and film in the fixer solution, and start the timer
- Replace the developer lid to prevent the solution being weakened by exposure to air, which would allow oxidation to occur otherwise
- When the timer sounds, remove the hanger and film and immerse in the second water tank, agitating the hanger to ensure thorough washing occurs
- Switch on the ordinary light
- Shake off excess water and dry the film – a slow-running hairdryer is suitable for this, as the radiograph must not be dried too quickly

To mount and view the radiographs they must be correctly orientated on the viewing screen (Figure 7.11). This is a light box which illuminates the film from behind so that the image is visible, and there is often a magnifying glass present so that the radiograph can be viewed in greater detail by the operator. The screen and magnifying glass can be wiped with a disinfectant wipe if necessary to remove any water marks or fingerprints before the radiographs are positioned.

It is imperative that the radiographs are mounted and positioned correctly, otherwise the left teeth will be viewed as the right, the uppers as lowers, and vice versa.

Various plastic envelope designs are available to mount all types of intra-oral films nowadays, but they must be loaded correctly by the dental nurse first. All intra-oral films have a raised pimple in one corner which must be facing out to view the film correctly, and not back to front. It is irrelevant which corner of the film the pimple is in, but it must face out towards the person viewing the radiograph.

Extra-oral cassettes are marked with an "L" to indicate the patient's left side, and unless the cassette has been placed upside down in the machine, the film is easily orientated on the viewer so that it is viewed as if looking at the patient from the front (see Figure 6.8).

Dental nurses should also use their knowledge of oral anatomy to check for themselves – molar teeth are posterior to all other teeth, so correct mounting of bitewing films, for instance, should result in the molar teeth appearing on the outer side of both films, with their pimples palpable in one corner (see Figure 6.6). Upper periapical films should be mounted with the roots above the crowns of the teeth, as they are in the patient's maxilla (Figure 7.12), and lowers with their roots below the crowns (Figure 7.13), and so on.

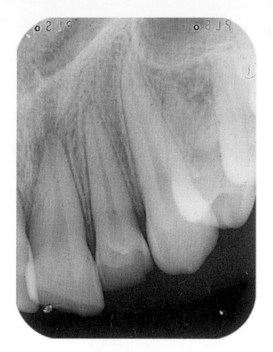

Figure 7.12 Correctly mounted upper periapical radiograph.

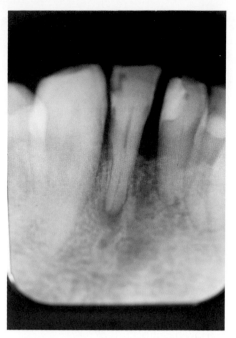

Figure 7.13 Correctly mounted lower periapical radiograph.

Store or save the images correctly

Once the operator has viewed the images, made a diagnosis and formulated a treatment plan, they must be stored or saved in the patient's records so that they can be viewed again and referred back to in future, as necessary.

Digital images must be locked into the computer records, under the correct patient's details, in the same way that all other information is saved on the hard drive. Each software program will have its own system and dental nurses must be familiar with that used in their own dental workplace. If for any reason they have not received suitable instruction in this procedure, they must never attempt to try and save the images anyway – one incorrect command to the computer can delete any amount of information, and in the case of deleted dental images this will result in the patient having to undergo repeat exposures and risking the possibility that one of the those exposures will cause tissue damage resulting in serious health problems in the future.

Hard copies of intra-oral films are usually stored in the patient's record card or in a manual filing system of radiographs alone, and in the correct orientation for viewing. Whichever technique is used, the radiograph must be marked with the patient's identifying details and the date of the exposure so that it can always be found, viewed and re-filed correctly.

Various types of plastic wallet are available from suppliers to do this, for bitewing and periapical views, or a combination of the two. Indelible ink pens must be used to write the identification details so that they do not wear off over time. With larger radiographs such as anterior occlusal views and dental pantomographs, a sticky label can be written on and used to record the required information, ensuring that it is stuck onto the film without obscuring any part of the image.

Dental nurses must use whichever system is followed in their dental workplace. If no training has been received in this area, a senior colleague (dentist, line manager, or similar) must be informed and handed the radiographs so that they are not lost.

Contribute to quality assurance checks

Quality assurance (QA) checks are carried out to determine if procedures are being correctly followed by all staff and to identify when problems have occurred so that they can be rectified and not repeated in the future. The overall aim is to ensure patient safety at all times when they undergo exposure to ionising radiation.

A QA system is run in all dental workplaces with regard to the analysis of dental images – this is a requirement under both IR(ME)R and clinical governance. In addition, similar systems can be run in the workplace to monitor other areas of dental radiography, such as equipment, working procedures or staff training, and so on.

With suitable training, the running of the QA system of radiograph analysis can easily be carried out by the dental nurse – the aim being to reduce all exposure, handling and processing faults to a minimum or to eliminate them completely.

To protect both patients and the dental team from unnecessary ionising radiation exposure, it is the duty of all concerned to ensure that the occurrence of these faults are kept to a minimum or eliminated completely. To do this involves assessing the quality of the films processed to determine the following:

- How readable is the film?
- Is a fault present?
- What is the fault?
- How has it occurred?
- How can it be prevented from recurring?
- Is re-exposure of the patient necessary?

When run correctly, the QA system should achieve the following:

- Involve a simple-to-use scoring system that is understood and followed by all staff
- Easily identify any areas of concern
- Develop solutions to the problems identified
- Limit the number of patient exposures to the minimum required for clinical necessity
- And, therefore, achieve ALARA/P

A simple-to-use scoring system set out in clinical governance guidelines is as follows:

- **Score 1 – excellent** quality radiograph with no errors present (Figure 7.14)
- **Score 2 – diagnostically acceptable** quality, minimal errors present that do not prevent the radiograph from being used for diagnosis (Figure 7.15)
- **Score 3 – unacceptable quality**, where errors prevent the radiograph from being used for diagnosis, and will therefore involve a retake (Figure 7.16)

Examples of score 2 are the following:

- Where mild angulation faults by the operator have produced foreshortened or elongated images, but the whole tooth is still visible and disease can be diagnosed
- Where coning has occurred but the area under investigation is still fully visible on the radiograph
- Where handling faults have scratched the film, but not in the area under investigation
- Reversed radiograph, where the packet has been exposed back to front in the patient's mouth but is still readable on the viewing screen
- Where the processing chemicals are becoming spent so that the image is not as dark as usual, but the radiograph is still readable on the viewing screen

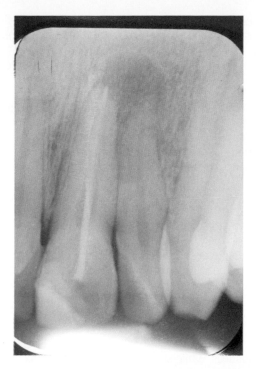

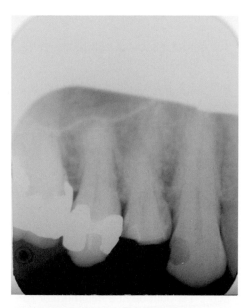

Figure 7.14   Radiograph scoring 1 on the quality assurance (QA) scale, showing a periapical abscess.

Figure 7.15   Radiograph of UR5 scoring 2 on the quality assurance (QA) scale.

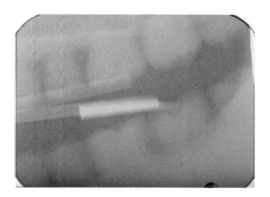

Figure 7.16   Radiograph scoring 3 on the quality assurance (QA) scale.

Examples of score 3 are the following:

- Where severe angulation faults by the operator have produced foreshortened images that are unreadable
- Where severe angulation faults by the operator have produced elongated images which run off the radiograph, so part of the tooth is missing
- Where coning has occurred and the tooth under investigation has been missed off the radiograph
- Where handling faults have scratched the film in the area under investigation, so that diagnosis cannot be achieved

- Where processing chemicals are too weak or cold to produce an image
- Where processing chemicals are too concentrated or too warm, so that the film is over-processed and no image is visible
- Where a malfunction of the processor causes loss of the film or its exposure to daylight before processing while it is being located

The dental nurse can contribute to the quality assurance checks by assisting in (or carrying out) their analysis as follows:

- Determine which radiographs are to be viewed – so a retrospective analysis can be run by viewing the previous 100 exposures recorded, irrespective of the operator or the type of view taken
- Count and total the number of each type of view – e.g. four dental pantomographs, 70 bitewing radiographs (35 pairs), and 26 periapicals
- Total the number of score 1 for each type of view – this will have been recorded at the time of processing
- Of the remaining radiographs which are therefore all scores 2 and 3, total the score 2 and score 3 and note the reason for that score – this will have been recorded at the time of processing
- An analysis can then be made of any patterns of score 2 or score 3 – is the same operator involved each time; is the same X-ray machine used each time; is the same fault produced each time?
- The findings must be recorded and passed onto the RPS in the workplace, so that errors can be investigated and resolved

Score 1 should be at a minimum of 70% of all exposures, while score 3 should be at a maximum of 10%. The results need to be easily recorded after every exposure so that they can be analysed on a regular basis and any problems identified. A typical recording system used at the time of processing, and which therefore produces the information for the QA check to be run, is shown here.

Date	Operator	Patient ID	Radiograph	QA score	Details
4.4.12	DTH	4173	L/R BWs	1 and 1	N/A
4.4.12	JM	854	PA UL6,7	2	Coned, unable to use holder
5.4.12	TNL	1559	DPT	1	N/A
5.4.12	DTH	6212	PA UR2	1	N/A
5.4.12	CSH	377	AO-maxilla	2	Elongated but canines visible
6.4.12	JM	5458	L/R BWs	1 and 2	R BW coned
6.4.12	TNL	905	PA UL4	3	Missed apex for endo - retake
6.4.12	TNL	905	PA UL4	1	N/A

Details of the view taken are shown in the fourth column, with the QA score of 1, 2 or 3 in the fifth column. When 2 or 3 is scored, a note on the fault found must be made in the final column to show that analysis has taken place. Obviously, all films with score 1 require no further detail to be added.

All columns require completion for every radiograph analysis, otherwise patterns of faults between operators and views cannot be determined. For example, one operator may not routinely use film holders when taking periapicals, so a pattern of scores 2 and 3 may emerge for these views and for this operator only. Analysis will conclude that the operator has no faults with other views, so it is safe to assume that the fault lies with attempting to align the periapicals without a holder and that a holder must therefore be used routinely in future.

As stated earlier, the same information can be used, for example, to analyse the functioning of X-ray and processing machines or the chemical top-up and renew protocols followed by the workplace. The information gathered and analysed during these QA checks can then be used to identify machine faults, operator errors or changes in protocols that may be required.

As always, the dental nurse must receive suitable, recorded training in the required QA techniques before being considered competent to run them unsupervised. The training information should be recorded in the "radiation file" (see Chapter 14).

8

Unit 308: Provide Chairside Support during the Prevention and Control of Periodontal Disease and Caries, and the Restoration of Cavities

Learning outcomes

1. Be able to recognise the nature of oral diseases and their prevention
2. Be able to provide support to the individual and operator before, during and after treatment

Outcome 1 assessment criteria

The learner can:

- Identify methods of controlling plaque
- List the treatments available for controlling caries
- List the treatments available for controlling periodontal disease
- Identify the different methods and uses of fluoride

Outcome 2 assessment criteria

The learner can:

- Retrieve and make available the correct patient's charts, records and images, and identify the planned treatment correctly

Diploma in Dental Nursing, Level 3, Third Edition. Carole Hollins.
© 2014 John Wiley & Sons, Ltd. Published 2014 by John Wiley & Sons, Ltd.
Companion website: www.wiley.com/go/hollins/dentalnursinglevel3

- Select the equipment, instruments, materials and medicaments for:
  - Prevention and control of dental caries
  - Prevention and control of periodontal disease
  - Provision of amalgam restorations
  - Provision of composite restorations
  - Provision of glass ionomer restorations
- Aspirate the treatment area and maintain a clear field of operation
- Protect soft tissues using instruments and materials appropriately
- Select and offer the operator:
  - A suitable matrix system to aid the placement of restorations
  - The correct quantity of the appropriately mixed restorative material
  - Any materials or equipment required for finishing the restoration
- Demonstrate the safe handling and disposal of amalgam

This unit is assessed by:
- observation in the workplace, with examples included in the learner's portfolio
- an appropriate alternative method

Details of various elements of theory and underpinning knowledge are included in Chapter 15, and these are assessed within the written paper.

181

The theory and underpinning knowledge required to understand the scientific principles involved in the management of oral diseases and dental procedures, including the prevention and control of disease and the restoration of cavities, are fully discussed in Chapter 15. This chapter explains the dental nurse's role and responsibilities in relation to the following procedures before, during and after they are carried out:

- Prevention and control of periodontal disease by:
  - Scaling and polishing
  - Debridement
- Prevention and control of caries using:
  - Fissure sealants
  - Fluoride treatments
- Restoration of cavities using:
  - Temporary restorations
  - Amalgam restorations
  - Composite restorations
  - Glass ionomer restorations

These responsibilities are to the operator (the person carrying out the procedure – usually the dentist, but in some cases it may be the therapist or the hygienist) and also to the patient who is undergoing the procedure, and the patient's guardian where relevant.

The techniques and procedures used in the prevention and control of periodontal disease and dental caries form the bulk of the day-to-day work of the dental team, and as the work becomes a matter of routine it is easy to forget that some patients will be fearful at the prospect of this treatment. A huge part of the dental nurse's day-to-day role is to be calming, friendly and supportive and to anticipate the concerns and needs of the patient throughout these procedures.

Before the procedure

The vast majority of dental workplaces operate on one appointments system or another, so that the working day can be correctly planned and all of the necessary instruments, materials and equipment are known to be available as required. There would be little point in a patient attending for a cavity restoration procedure, for example, if the workplace had run out of amalgam or composite material. Forward planning is therefore a key element in the successful completion of a busy working day and, along with the skills in the following list, is among the abilities required by a competent dental nurse to provide successful chairside support for disease prevention and control procedures, and for the restoration of cavities:

- Correct identification of the patient
- Correct identification of the procedure
- Knowledge of the records and images required by the operator for the procedure
- Knowledge of the correct setting up of the area for the procedure
- Knowledge of the instruments, materials and equipment that may be required for the procedure
- Knowledge of the actions to take if the dental nurse is unable to fully prepare for the procedure

Correct identification of the patient

The day list will refer to each patient attending that day by name and/or date of birth and/or address and/ or some kind of patient identification marker – such as a unique computer number or the patient's NHS number.

Whatever the system in place, the dental nurse should be familiar with it and be able to access the patient's records so that a cross-reference check can be made between the notes present and the expected procedure to be carried out. So if the previous notes refer to a tooth to be filled using amalgam, but the day list indicates that the patient is attending for a first-stage endodontic procedure that day, one of the following scenarios has occurred which must be checked with the operator and the patient before the procedure begins:

- The records and the day list entry are for two different patients
- The records are incomplete and a change in treatment has been decided without being recorded
- The records are correct and the day list entry is incorrect
- The records are incorrect and the day list entry is correct

Any of these scenarios could quite easily have occurred, and the matter should be referred to a more senior colleague (ideally the operator concerned) so that the dental nurse can assist them in determining the way forward – to identify the correct patient and the correct procedure to be carried out that day.

The records required may be hard copies in full (so a "pack" of handwritten patient notes, with paper copies of the patient's medical history, previous treatment plans and consent forms, and so on), or they may be fully computerised and only accessible "on screen", or they may be a combination of the two. Whatever their presentation, they should be collected by the dental nurse and presented in the treatment area so that the operator can access them and check their content too.

In large dental workplaces, such as dental schools and hospitals, the dental nurse can check the correct patient identity by asking patients to confirm their name, date of birth and address, and that they know the reason for their attendance on the day. The final decision to confirm the patient's identity is the duty of the operator.

In smaller workplaces, many of the patients are recognisable to the staff by sight – some may even be known by their first names – but identity and procedure checks should still always be carried out to avoid any mishaps. Once the patient has been correctly identified, the records and treatment area can be prepared.

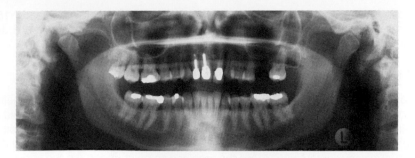

Figure 8.1   Correctly mounted dental pantomograph.

The records to be set out will include the following:

- Notes written at the previous appointment or when the decision was made to carry out the particular procedure – these will remind the operator of the reasons for the treatment decisions taken
- Medical history form, to be checked to highlight any potential concerns – for example, is a certain local anaesthetic required, or does the patient have an allergy to latex?
- Consent form, indicating that the patient has given valid consent to the procedure (see Chapter 13)
- Radiographs of the relevant tooth – these will allow the operator to plan the procedure and the technique used, and show any potential difficulties such as a deep cavity or curved roots on the tooth involved

The dental nurse can also access the records for the following purposes:

- The notes may refer to the patient's level of anxiety, so the dental nurse is aware of the heightened need to be supportive and helpful to the patient throughout the procedure – the issue should also be pointed out to the operator
- The medical history can be checked and any recognised potential issues pointed out to the operator
- Patients can also be asked to confirm if there have been any changes to their medical history since they were last seen, and these are then recorded appropriately and pointed out to the operator
- The consent form can be checked to ensure it covers the planned procedure and that it has been signed and dated by the patient, or that it requires to be signed and dated by the patient today – any discrepancies can be pointed out to the operator
- The radiographs must be correctly displayed to show the tooth under treatment, either as digital images on the computer or as hard copies on film
- Hard copies must be correctly mounted on the viewing screen:
  - Intra-oral views with the pimple facing out (to indicate left from right), and upper teeth with their roots above the crown and lower teeth with their roots below the crown (see Figure 7.13)
  - Bitewing radiographs with the pimple facing out and the molar teeth on the outer edges of each view (to indicate left and right quadrants, as well as to distinguish upper from lower teeth – see Figure 6.6)
  - Extra-oral views with the "L" marker in the bottom right-hand corner of the radiograph as it is positioned on the viewing screen, to indicate the patient's left side (Figure 8.1)

Correct identification of the procedure

The patient is attending for one of the procedures listed, and the actual one should be referred to in the notes and on the day list (although some computer software systems are not programmed to allow individual procedures to be booked – they just record a time slot as a "filling" without specifying the material to be used).

The reasons for carrying out each procedure are discussed in detail in Chapter 15. The records and images required by the operator in order to carry out the procedure are detailed in the preceding section.

Knowledge of the correct setting up of the area

As with all dental procedures, the treatment area (surgery) must be clean before being set up for a prevention and restoration session, and left in a similar condition afterwards, to avoid any possibility of cross-infection occurring. The principles of infection control are discussed in detail in Chapter 12.

Before the surgery is prepared for use, the dental nurse must ensure that they do not inadvertently introduce any contamination into the area and so must undertake the correct hand washing technique before applying the correct personal protective equipment (PPE). As a clinical procedure is to be carried out, the appropriate hand washing technique is as follows:

- Turn on the tap using the foot or elbow control, to prevent contaminating the tap (see Figure 4.4)
- Wet both hands under running water of a suitable temperature
- Apply a suitable antibacterial liquid soap from the dispenser (Figure 8.2) and wash all areas of both hands and wrists thoroughly – this should take at least 30 seconds to carry out thoroughly, and the correct routine is illustrated on the poster that is present at each hand washing station (see Figure 1.3)
- Nail brushes are not advised unless they are autoclavable, as they can become contaminated with repeated use
- Rinse both hands under running water, holding them so that the water does not flow back over the fingers
- Dry the hands thoroughly, using disposable paper towels for single use

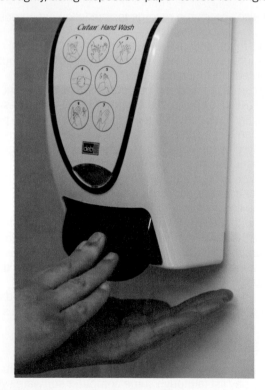

Figure 8.2   Use of a soap dispenser.

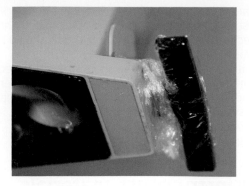

Figure 8.3 Barrier protection on handles.

The equipment and instruments can now be handled safely, unless the dental nurse has any cuts or abrasions on the hands, in which case the lesion should be covered with a waterproof dressing and a pair of clinical gloves must be worn before any items are handled.

The surgery itself is then made ready as follows:

- The electric and water supplies should be switched on to all static equipment (dental chair, suction unit, etc.) if this has not already been done
- Any portable items not likely to be required for the procedure should be placed in cupboards or drawers, or removed from the surgery, so that the work surfaces are clear of any clutter
- The controls of any large equipment items that are likely to be contaminated during the procedure must be protected by a barrier technique, including:
  - Dental chair controls, if not foot-operated
  - Dental light controls and handles (Figure 8.3)
  - Computer keyboard, if various screens are in use
  - Bracket table handles and controls
- In some surgery settings, the aspirator pipes and handpiece tubing may also require barrier protection if they are of a design that makes them difficult to wipe down thoroughly (such as corrugated piping)
- The patient records are accessed on the computer, or the paper copies are laid out on an area of the work surface away from the surgical field (to minimise their contamination)
- Relevant radiographs are correctly mounted on the viewing screen, in easy reach of the operator
- PPE is laid out ready for the patient, the operator and the dental nurse:
  - Protective glasses, disposable bib, tissues – for the patient
  - Protective glasses or visor, face mask, gloves – for the operator and dental nurse
- Mouth rinse and cup are made ready for the patient
- Suitable aspirator tips are connected to the suction unit, both wide-bore and a finer surgical tip should be available
- The correct local anaesthetic equipment and materials are laid out for use, in easy reach of the operator and dental nurse, and covered with a disposable bib until the patient is seated:
  - Topical anaesthetic and cotton wool rolls (where relevant)
  - Syringe (aspirating type if a nerve block is likely)
  - Short or long needle (depending which tooth is involved)
  - Local anaesthetic cartridges
  - Resheathing device
- The local anaesthetic solution should be checked by the operator for suitability before use

- The correct instruments are laid out for the procedure (see later), in easy reach of the operator and the dental nurse, and covered with a disposable bib until the patient is seated:
  - If they are stored in an enclosed tray system, the lid should be replaced once the tray has been checked for all items present
  - If they are within sterile pouches, these should remain sealed until just before their use
- Single-use items, materials and medicaments should be gathered together, made ready for use and covered with a disposable bib until the patient is seated:
  - Suitable matrix system
  - Restorative materials
  - Mixing pad/block and spatula

186

Knowledge of the instruments, materials and equipment required

Plaque is a thin transparent layer of saliva, oral debris and normal mouth bacteria which sticks to the tooth surface and can only be removed by cleaning. It is then replaced within a few hours by a new deposit of plaque, and its presence in the mouth may be regarded as a natural occurrence. The harm it causes comes from food debris which sticks to the plaque during meals and snacks and provides a plentiful supply of nourishment for its bacteria and other microorganisms. They accordingly flourish, the plaque grows thicker, and caries and periodontal disease begin.

If the plaque is in contact with a tooth surface, it will result in caries developing there unless the plaque is removed. If the plaque is in contact with the gingiva, it will result in gingivitis and then periodontitis developing unless the plaque is removed.

All methods involved in the prevention and control of caries and periodontal disease are therefore related to the control of bacterial plaque, by:

- Removing it from tooth surfaces and gingival crevices – by adequate **oral hygiene techniques** by the patient, and **scaling and debridement** by the dental team
- Preventing it from damaging the teeth when it is present – by increasing tooth resistance by the use of **fluorides**:
  - **Topical fluorides** – applied externally to the tooth
    - Fluoride gel and varnish applied by the dental team
    - Oral hygiene products applied by the patient (toothpaste, mouthwash, etc.)
  - **Systemic fluorides** – ingested and incorporated into the tooth from within
    - Fluoridated public water supply at one part per million
    - Fluoride drops and tablets
- Removing stagnation areas – by **fissure sealing** and **good restorative dentistry**

Prevention and control of periodontal disease by scaling and debridement

Accessible plaque is removed by tooth brushing and interdental cleaning, the oral hygiene techniques which are carried out by the patient on a daily basis. Subgingival plaque and calculus are inaccessible to patients and are removed by members of the dental team during scaling and debridement. Supragingival calculus will also require professional intervention, as it cannot be dislodged by tooth brushing alone. Surface stains are then removed and a smooth tooth surface produced by polishing after the plaque and calculus have been removed.

The equipment, instruments and materials that will be required for the procedures, with their functions listed, are shown in the following table.

Item	Function
Ultrasonic scaler (Figure 8.4)	Powered scaler run on compressed air which vibrates ultrasonically to dislodge calculus from the tooth and root surfaces Can be used supragingivally or subgingivally
Supragingival scalers: sickle, push, Jaquette	Short shanked hand instruments which are designed to be scraped across the tooth surface to dislodge plaque and calculus Cushing push scaler is specifically designed to be pushed though the interproximal areas of anterior teeth to clean these surfaces
Subgingival curettes: Gracey and others (Figure 8.5)	Long shanked hand instruments which are designed to reach into the subgingival areas to be scraped across the root surface and dislodge plaque, calculus and contaminated cementum
Periodontal hoe	Long shanked hand instrument which has a similar function to curettes and has been largely superseded by them
Slow handpiece and polishing cup/brush (Figure 8.6)	Rotary polishing devices which are loaded with prophylactic paste and used in a similar fashion to an electric toothbrush, to remove any residual surface staining and produce a smooth tooth surface
Prophylaxis paste	Various products which contain gritty material such as pumice in a paste, and their abrasiveness helps to remove tooth staining

187

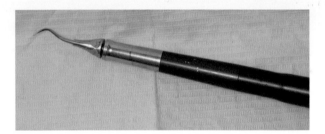

Figure 8.4   An ultrasonic scaler.

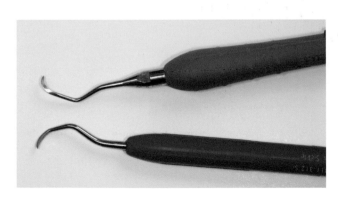

Figure 8.5   Curettes.

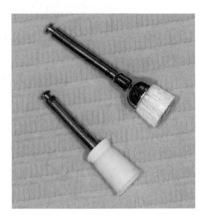

Figure 8.6   Polishing cup and brush.

Prevention and control of caries using fissure sealants

Fissure sealants are materials composed of composite or glass ionomer that are used to seal the naturally occurring stagnation areas of pits and fissures on posterior teeth. These areas are therefore protected from damage by acid attacks and bacterial plaque, and the onset of dental caries is prevented.

The equipment, instruments and materials that will be required for the procedure, with their functions listed, are shown in the following table.

Item	Function
Handpiece and polishing cup or round bur	To clean the surface of the tooth and fissure so that the sealant material is able to adhere effectively. If the fissure is sticky (with demineralisation) it can be run out with the bur first, so that healthy enamel is present
Pumice powder	To be mixed with water as a slurry and used with the polishing cup to clean the tooth surface. Conventional polishing pastes have an oily base which will prevent the sealant from sticking to the tooth
Acid etchant with applicator	Coloured gel or liquid, applied to the tooth surface to chemically roughen the enamel and improve the adhesion of the sealant material
Resin with applicator	Liquid resin applied to the etched tooth surface and minimally light-cured to make it sticky and tacky
Sealant material with applicator	Flowable composite or glass ionomer material which is run into the prepared fissure to seal it, by light-curing. Any air bubbles in the material are "popped" before curing, as they will be weak points that may cause the failure of the sealant

Prevention and control of caries by fluoride application

Fluoride can be applied to all of the teeth in a gel format or to individual susceptible teeth using a varnish application, such as Duraphat varnish (Figure 8.7). These are examples of topical fluoride applications.

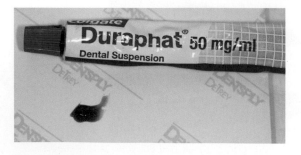

Figure 8.7   Duraphat varnish.

The gel technique requires full mouth coverage using pre-formed applicator trays (similar to rubberised "gum shield" appliances, in a range of small, medium and large sizes), while the varnish technique requires the material and a suitable applicator.

Restoration of cavities

Many operators have personal preferences for the instruments they routinely use during a cavity restoration procedure, and the more usual ones are shown in the following table, with their functions listed. They are often set out in a lidded tray system, referred to as a "conservation tray". These instruments are the same, whatever filling material is to be used.

Item	Function
Mouth mirror	To aid the dentist's vision, to reflect light onto the tooth, to retract and protect the soft tissues
Right-angle probe	To feel the cavity margins, to feel softened dentine within the cavity, to detect overhanging restorations
Excavators	Small and large spoon-shaped, used to scoop out softened dentine
Amalgam plugger	To push filling materials into the cavity and adapt them to the cavity shape, leaving no air spaces and forcing excess mercury to the surface of the filling for removal during carving
Burnisher	Ball-shaped or pear-shaped, to press and adapt the restoration margins fully against the cavity edges so that no leakage occurs under the restoration
Flat plastic	To remove excess filling material and mercury from the restoration surface and create a shaped surface that encourages food particles to flow off naturally, rather than become lodged around the restoration
College tweezers	To pick up, hold and carry various items such as cotton wool pledgets
Gingival margin trimmer	To trim the margin of the cavity to ensure no unsupported enamel or soft dentine remains – their use is becoming obsolete with the wider range of burs available
Enamel chisel	To remove any unsupported enamel from the cavity edges – their use is becoming obsolete with the wider range of burs available

To remove caries and shape the cavity correctly to receive the filling material, the air turbine hand piece and a range of suitable diamond burs, as well as the slow handpiece and a range of suitable stainless steel burs, will also be required (Figure 8.8). The full range of burs is usually stored in a lidded bur block stand which is made available at the start of the procedure so that the operator can choose the particular bur that is required (Figure 8.9).

Material differences

When a temporary restoration is to be placed, one of the materials in the following table will be used. The same materials may also be used as a base beneath a permanent amalgam restoration.

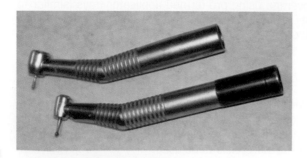

Figure 8.8 Handpieces.

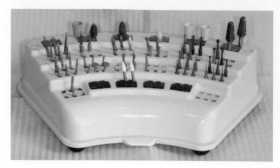

Figure 8.9 A bur block stand.

Material	Mixing	Advantages
Zinc oxide and eugenol cement	Glass slab or waxed pad and spatula – rolls easily into a sausage shape when ready for use	Contains clove oil which acts as a sedative to the pulp tissues
Zinc phosphate cement	Cool glass slab and spatula for slow setting Warm glass slab or waxed pad and spatula for fast setting	Produces a hard restoration when set Can be left as a temporary filling for several months
Zinc polycarboxylate cement	Glass slab or waxed pad and spatula – must be cleaned off before setting as it is very difficult to remove otherwise	Most adhesive material

When a permanent restoration is to be placed, one of the following materials will be used:

- Amalgam
- Composite
- Glass ionomer

The advantages and disadvantages of each material, and their uses are discussed in detail in Chapter 15. Each can be used with a calcium hydroxide liner beneath, and with deep cavities this can be placed beneath a base material too. The additional and specific items and materials required for their use are shown below for each material.

Amalgam

Item	Function
Liner and/or base material	To protect the pulp from thermal shock – there are various available, including calcium hydroxide and the temporary cements, which are all suitable under amalgam restorations
Matrix system	To prevent overspill in cavities of two or more surfaces – usual systems are Siqveland (Figure 8.10) or Tofflemire; the bands are single use

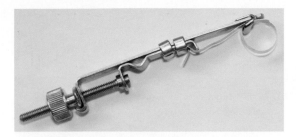

Figure 8.10 The Siqveland matrix system. Source: *Levison's Textbook for Dental Nurses*, 10th edition (Hollins), 2008. Reproduced with permission of Wiley-Blackwell.

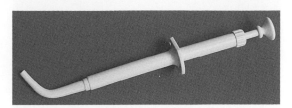

Figure 8.11 A plastic amalgam carrier. Source: *Levison's Textbook for Dental Nurses*, 10th edition (Hollins), 2008. Reproduced with permission of Wiley-Blackwell.

Item	Function
Wedges	Placed interdentally with matrix system, to tightly adapt the band to the tooth. Both wooden wedges and plastic wedges are available
Amalgam carrier (Figure 8.11)	Autoclavable "gun" used to pick up and carry the amalgam to the cavity, where it is squeezed out
Amalgam plugger	Instrument to pack and condense the amalgam into the cavity so that no air spaces remain – usually on the conservation tray
Finishing instruments	To ensure the restoration is adapted to the tooth and is not high in occlusion. Various items are in use – Wards carver, flat plastic instrument, burnisher, greenstone drills, articulating paper; hand instruments are usually on the conservation tray

Composite

Item	Function
Liner or base material	To protect the pulp from chemical shock – calcium hydroxide lining, and glass ionomer base in deep cavities
Matrix system (Figure 8.12)	Transparent matrix strips, to allow curing of the composite through it. Various holder systems are available or they are held in place manually
Plastic instruments	To place the composite and remove excess before curing. Various designs are available, the commonest one being a flat plastic instrument. There are ceramic-tipped instruments that avoid the material sticking to the instrument
Curing light and protective shield (Figure 8.13)	The majority of modern composites available are light-cured to set
Finishing instruments	To ensure no overhangs are left and that the surface of the restoration is smooth and not high in the occlusion. Various items are used – specially shaped plastic instruments, abrasive strips (Figure 8.14), polishing discs, polishing burs of various designs, articulating paper

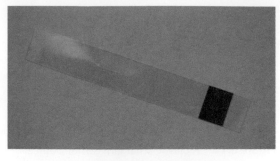

Figure 8.12   A transparent matrix strip.

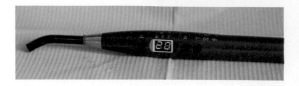

Figure 8.13   A curing light.

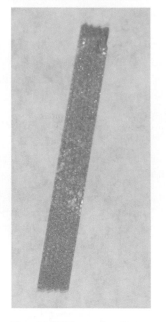

Figure 8.14   A finishing strip.

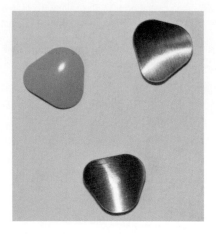

Figure 8.15   A glass ionomer cervical matrix system.

Glass ionomer

Item	Function
Liner	Calcium hydroxide, if any is required, to protect the pulp from the acrylic acid
Plastic instruments	To place the glass ionomer and remove any excess material – usually available on the conservation tray
Cervical matrix (Figure 8.15)	Foil-coated and pre-shaped for use when restoring class V abrasion cavities. Cannot be used if the glass ionomer is a light-cured type of material, as the matrix is opaque
Finishing materials	Varnish or unfilled resin, wiped over the restoration surface to prevent moisture contamination Articulating paper to check the occlusion

Knowledge of the actions to take if preparation cannot be completed

If any instruments, materials or items of equipment are not readily available for use immediately before the procedure is scheduled to start, the dental nurse must report the matter to an appropriate person immediately. This may be the operator, a senior dental nurse (or line manager) or the practice manager.

The final preparation that the dental nurse must carry out is to check with the patient that any prescribed pre-treatment instructions have been followed correctly. In particular, the following points should be clarified:

- Have all routine medications been taken as requested?
- If the procedure is being carried out under any form of conscious sedation technique, have they complied with all of the relevant additional points as requested?
- If the patient is a child or a vulnerable adult, are they in attendance with a suitable adult escort to look after and see them safely home after the procedure?
- If the patient is frail or excessively nervous, are they in attendance with a suitable adult escort for the same purpose?
- Have they (or their guardian) read and understood any pre-treatment information provided – do they have any further questions?
- Have they (or their guardian) been given enough information to provide valid consent for the procedure, and have they given that consent?

When it becomes apparent that one or more of these points have not been followed, the dental nurse must report the matter to the operator immediately, and allow them to discuss the situation further with the patient. It is not the role of dental nurses to act beyond their level of competence by making unilateral decisions about any of these issues – the responsibility lies with the operator.

During the procedure

Usually, the dental nurse will collect patients (and their guardian where relevant) from the reception area and escort them to the surgery, rather than the operator. The dental nurse should be welcoming and friendly towards patients (and their guardian) and use the time to put them at their ease.

With experience, dental nurses will develop their communication skills and their own style of patter that they can use successfully, and patients will respond positively to a good dental nurse with obvious empathy to their situation. Communication skills are discussed in detail in Chapter 5, and the skills of reflection and developing oneself in practice are discussed in Chapter 2.

The abilities required by a competent dental nurse to provide support during the procedure include the following points:

- Preparation of the patient
- Assistance during the administration of local anaesthesia, where necessary
- Identification and correct handling of the instruments, materials and equipment throughout the procedure
- Adequate provision of moisture control and tissue retraction throughout the procedure, where necessary
- Correct mixing of the liner, the base and the restorative material
- Monitoring and support of the patient

Although forward planning of the procedure should avoid the possibility, it may be necessary for the dental nurse to retrieve unprepared instruments and items during the procedure. If so, then gloves must be removed and replaced with a new pair each time that the surgical area is left and re-accessed.

Preparation of the patient

A final check is made by the operator of the patient's identification and that consent has been given to undergo the procedure.

The dental nurse will then assist patients into the dental chair and ready them for the start of treatment as follows:

- Help them to remove their coat if necessary, and hang it up
- Assist them into the dental chair – they may need physical support or the chair may need to raised or lowered, for example
- Apply their required PPE:
  - Safety glasses – these need to be tinted if the curing light is to be used to set materials
  - Protective bib
  - Some patients like to have a tissue in hand too
- Monitor patients for signs of anxiety, and notify the operator as necessary
- Reassure patients in a calm and friendly manner – many appreciate the opportunity of a hand to hold at this point, although this action can be passed to an escort/guardian if appropriate

Assistance during the administration of local anaesthesia

Local anaesthetic will usually be required for cavity restoration procedures and sometimes for scaling and debridement treatment if a patient suffers from sensitive teeth.

The operator and the dental nurse apply their own PPE (safety glasses/visor, face mask, gloves).

The disposable cover used to hide the items while the patient enters and settles in the dental chair is removed from the equipment, and the operator must check that the correct items and local anaesthetic are prepared. The topical anaesthetic is applied to a cotton wool roll and handed to the operator for application in the patient's mouth. While this takes effect, the syringe is loaded ready for use, quietly and out of sight of the patient:

- Noisy clattering of metallic items can be particularly unnerving for patients, so items must be handled proficiently at all times
- The local anaesthetic cartridge is loaded into the syringe correctly, with the cap end at the bottom where the needle will be applied
- If an aspirating technique is to be used, any screw-in plunger is locked into the cartridge bung before the needle is added
- The needle is screwed onto the threaded end of the syringe, with the guard in place
- On removal of the topical anaesthetic, the needle guard is loosened but left over the needle, and the loaded syringe is offered to the operator (Figure 8.16)
- As the operator receives the syringe, the dental nurse keeps hold of the loosened needle guard so that it becomes unsheathed as it is transferred over
- The guard is then placed into the re-sheathing device, ready for the operator when the anaesthetic procedure is completed (see Figure 1.29)
- Successive cartridges are handed to the operator as required during the administration procedure
- When the administration is complete, the equipment is re-sheathed by the operator without being handled by the dental nurse (this avoids increasing the likelihood of an inoculation injury)

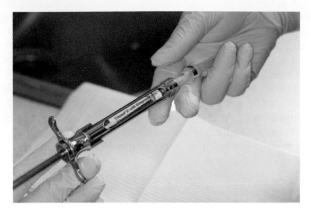

Figure 8.16 Handing over the loaded syringe.

Identification and correct handling of the instruments

Prevention and control of periodontal disease

During a scaling and polishing or debridement procedure, the scalers and/or curettes are laid out on the bracket table for the operator to use as required. The ultrasonic scaler will already be connected to the bracket table, and a polishing cup or brush will be loaded into the slow hand-piece. A reasonable-sized blob of prophylaxis paste will be available in a well or on a disposable sheet, and the operator will dip the cup/brush into this for polishing the teeth, as required.

The dental nurse will be available to aspirate effectively and to carefully retract the soft tissues throughout the procedure. When hand instruments are in use, the dental nurse will carefully remove any oral debris from the instruments with a tissue as the operator works.

Prevention and control of caries

During a fissure sealant procedure, as described earlier, the dental nurse will be available to assist in isolating the tooth by soft tissue retraction so that the etchant material causes no harm. Good aspiration will also be provided as the tooth is washed and dried, and the materials will be passed to the operator in the correct order. While the fissure sealant material is being light-cured to set, the dental nurse may either direct the light or hold the tinted shield in place, or both, or they may be responsible for maintaining aspiration and soft tissue retraction while the operator carries out these tasks.

During a topical fluoride application procedure, dental nurses will aspirate while the teeth are cleaned of any surface debris. They will load the trays with the fluoride gel and hand them to the operator for insertion, or load the varnish on the applicator and hand to the operator for application to the tooth. While the gel trays are in place, dental nurses ensure that moisture control is adequate for the patient, usually with the use of a low-speed aspirator such as a saliva ejector.

Restoration of cavities

Conservation trays are usually kept as pre-set loaded trays, which just require the lids to be removed before use and placed within easy reach of the operator and dental nurse. Items that are stored separately in pouches can be opened and placed on the tray with the other items before treatment begins.

When the operator has finished with an instrument, it is either placed back on the tray or passed safely back to the dental nurse, who receives them and places them on the tray. Routine conservation treatment is not carried out under surgical conditions, so it is acceptable to reuse instruments throughout the procedure.

During the procedure, the dental nurse is likely to also be aspirating and retracting soft tissues, so the receiving and passing of instruments will also require the use of both hands. Experience will improve this ability with time, but all members of the dental team must develop a routine of never passing items across the patient's face while performing instrument transfer – it only takes one dropped item to permanently scar or blind a patient.

When any items are handled that are not disposable or able to be sterilised after the procedure, such as bottles and lids, the dental nurse must remove and replace any contaminated gloves to do so. Similarly, when amalgam capsules are inserted into the amalgamator, the machine must not be handled with contaminated gloves.

The cavity restoration procedure for each of the materials and the role of the dental nurse throughout is as follows:

- Access is made to the carious lesion using the air turbine and suitable diamond burs
- All caries is removed from the cavity using burs and excavators and without breaching the pulp chamber
- The cavity is undercut so that the amalgam restoration does not fall out, but this is not necessary for composite or glass ionomer fillings
- Moisture control techniques are used by the dental nurse so that all fluids and debris are removed from the mouth and so that the cavity remains dry during material placement
- Adequate soft tissue retraction with aspirators or mouth mirrors is done by the dental nurse, without causing trauma to the patient
- A lining or base is placed on the floor of the dry cavity to protect the pulp, if required, or the temporary filling material is mixed (see later)
- A Siqveland or Tofflemire matrix system will be adapted to the tooth to prevent amalgam spillage during placement, whenever a class II cavity is involved
- A transparent strip is similarly used during a class III or class IV composite restoration
- When a class V glass ionomer filling is used, a foil matrix may be required but can only be placed once the material has filled the cavity
- To ensure full adaptation of the metal matrix band to the tooth in the interproximal area, a wedge may be pushed between the tooth and its neighbour to give a tight fit
- The alloy and mercury are mixed in the amalgamator (see Figure 1.18) and the amalgam produced is inserted into the cavity in increments, using the amalgam carrier
- Each incremental load is fully pushed and condensed into the cavity, using the amalgam plugger
- Once filled, any excess amalgam is carved off the tooth and the surface of the restoration is shaped so that food debris is naturally directed away from the interproximal areas, mimicking the normal occlusal fissure pattern of the tooth
- The edges of the amalgam are adapted fully to the tooth surface by use of a burnisher instrument, so that no gaps or ridges remain
- All excess amalgam and mercury are removed from the oral cavity through the high-speed suction
- When a composite material is in use, the tooth is etched, washed and dried, and then resin is tacked into the cavity using minimal exposure of the curing light
- The composite material is then loaded into the cavity, often from a gun-operated compoule tube (Figure 8.17), before curing each increment
- Some glass ionomer materials are also delivered in this way, while others are a powder/liquid system and require hand mixing by the dental nurse before use
- Hand instruments such as a flat plastic are used to adapt the composite or glass ionomer material to the cavity before setting
- The matrix band is removed and the restoration is checked for overhangs
- Any overhangs present with a composite restoration can be removed with finishing strips or burs
- The occlusion is checked with articulating paper and adjusted as necessary
- Glass ionomer fillings are adjusted as little as possible and coated with light cure resin or varnish before the aspirator is removed

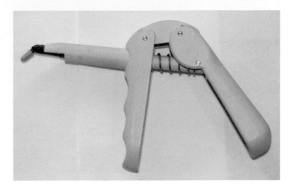

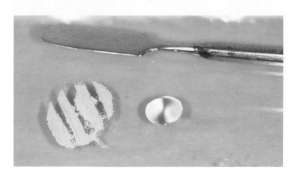

Figure 8.17   Composite compoule in gun device.   **Figure 8.18**   Zinc oxide–eugenol cement – to mix.

Any waste amalgam is retained safely in a pot until after the procedure, so that it can be disposed of correctly.

When a base material or a temporary filling is to be placed, the dental nurse is responsible for mixing it correctly before the material is inserted into the cavity. Each of the three materials available requires mixing to a stiff consistency that is just malleable enough to be manipulated and adapted to the cavity walls before setting occurs. The technique is described here.

Zinc oxide and eugenol

Presented as zinc oxide powder and eugenol liquid ("oil of cloves"), the cement is made by mixing increments of the yellowy powder with a drop of the clear eugenol liquid on a glass slab with a spatula (Figure 8.18). Older varieties of the product can be thickened if necessary by squeezing in a napkin to remove some of the eugenol liquid, otherwise full setting of the cement produced takes a few hours.

When ready for use, the cement should be able to be rolled into a "sausage shape" with the spatula, without sticking to it or smearing across the glass slab.

Zinc phosphate

Presented as zinc oxide powder and phosphoric acid liquid, the cement is prepared by mixing increments of the white powder with the clear liquid on a glass slab with a spatula (Figure 8.19).

Setting of the cement takes a few minutes depending on various factors:

- A warm slab accelerates the setting time
- A cold slab slows down the setting time
- A thick mix sets more quickly than a thin mix
- A dry slab must be used as moisture accelerates setting
- Powder contaminated by moisture in the air will set too quickly for use, so it is most important to screw the cap on tightly, immediately after using the bottle of liquid

These various factors can be used to advantage, depending on the particular use of the cement at the time. If a long setting time is required, such as when cementing a bridge, a cold dry slab can be used to give the maximum setting time possible, so that the cement can be loaded into each retainer and then fully positioning the bridge, before it begins to set.

This ability to control its setting time is the overriding advantage of zinc phosphate cement.

Experience soon teaches a dental nurse how much powder and liquid to set out, but occasionally too little or too much powder will be put on the slab. In the former case more powder

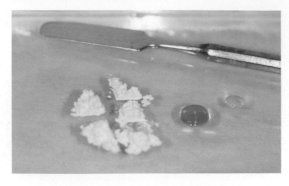

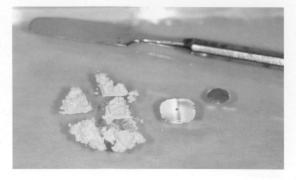

Figure 8.19   Zinc phosphate cement – to mix.   **Figure 8.20**   Zinc polycarboxylate cement – to mix.

can be added from the bottle, but the mixing end of the spatula must not be used for this purpose as it will contaminate and spoil the whole bottle. Excess unused powder may only be returned to the bottle if you are certain that it has not been contaminated by any liquid or mixed cement on the slab.

A cool, thick glass slab should be used for mixing zinc phosphate cement. Thin slabs are warmed by the dental nurse's hand and can make the cement set too quickly.

Zinc polycarboxylate

This is presented as white zinc oxide powder and clear, viscous polyacrylic acid liquid, or as these two components combined in the powder and sterile water as liquid (Figure 8.20). In each case, the cement is prepared by mixing increments of the powder with the liquid or sterile water on either a glass slab or a waxed paper pad with a spatula. A measure is provided by the manufacturer for exact measurement of each increment.

The advantage of using the anhydrous system with sterile water is that only one bottle of material is needed and there is no liquid to deteriorate, or to be used up too soon, or left over when the powder bottle is empty. Furthermore, as the polyacrylic acid liquid is viscous (thick and "gloopy" in consistency), it can be difficult to dispense from the bottle and also difficult to mix. Mixing with water is much easier and quicker.

Excess cement must be wiped off the spatula and instruments, before it fully sets, as it is difficult to remove by manual scrubbing and unlikely to be removed by the action of the ultrasonic bath.

Adequate provision of moisture control and tissue retraction

During the procedure dental nurses will be expected to use the relevant instruments and equipment correctly, to assist the operator in the following techniques:

- **Moisture control** – removal of moisture (saliva, blood, irrigation solution) from the operative area so that adequate vision is possible by the operator and so that the patient is not choking on a mouthful of fluid, using:
  - Wide-bore aspirator for fast fluid removal, as well as some soft tissue retraction
  - Saliva ejector in the floor of the mouth during filling placement (Figure 8.21)
  - Use of cotton wool rolls and pledgets for precise moisture control around and within the tooth (see Figure 6.13)
- **Irrigation** – from the air turbine handpiece during the cavity access and preparation procedure, to avoid heat damage to the tooth

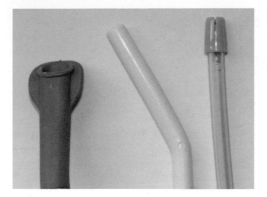

Figure 8.21   Aspirator and ejector tips. Source: *Levison's Textbook for Dental Nurses*, 10th edition (Hollins), 2008. Reproduced with permission of Wiley-Blackwell.

- **Tissue retraction** – to avoid damage to the soft tissues from burs and drills and to provide good vision for the operator, using:
  ○ Flanged wide-bore aspirator tips to retract the cheek, lips or tongue
  ○ Special cheek retractors, although these tend to be reserved for extraction and minor oral surgery procedures
  ○ Mouth mirror to retract the tongue or lips, and to reflect light to illuminate the operative field

Retraction of any soft tissues for any prolonged length of time can be quite tiring for dental nurses, and if they need to stop for a rest or reposition the retractor, operators must be forewarned so that they do not continue drilling or cutting as the soft tissues collapse across the operative field.

Monitoring and support of the patient

Throughout the whole procedure, the patient must be monitored and supported by the dental team, and this duty particularly falls to the dental nurse. The dental nurse must remain calm, friendly and helpful throughout, by taking the following general actions:

- Providing support during mouth rinsing, including helping the patient to avoid spillages once the local anaesthetic has been administered and wiping the mouth as necessary
- Holding the patient's hand if requested to do so, and if it is possible (with particularly fearful patients, especially children, a second person may need to carry out this duty)
- Alerting the operator immediately if it is suspected the patient can actually feel pain
- Constantly reassuring the patient in a calm and even tone, and repeatedly encouraging them by saying phrases such as "You're doing really well"
- Avoiding the use of fearful phrases
- Once the procedure is over, congratulating the patient and reassuring again
- Wiping any blood and debris from the patient's face before they are discharged
- Removing the patient's PPE when it is safe to do so
- Assisting the patient from the surgery area when the operator indicates that it is okay to do so

In particular, the dental nurse must constantly assess and monitor patients in relation to them feeling any pain during the procedure. Signs of pain may be grimacing, wincing or crying and should be pointed out to the operator if they have not noticed – this may be achieved by attracting their attention out of sight of the patient, and quietly indicating the fact by facial expressions such as raising the eyebrows and dropping the eyes to the patient several times.

After the procedure

Once the procedure has been completed, patients will require various checks to be made before being allowed to leave, as follows:

- Check that they have been sufficiently cleaned of materials and waste debris
- Check that they feel well enough to go home
- Give the relevant postoperative instructions if requested to do so, in relation to allowing the local anaesthetic to wear off and avoiding the use of the tooth as necessary
- Check whether the operator requires a further appointment to be made, and organise the making of the appointment – this may involve notifying reception to make the appointment or actually making it while the patient is still present

Immediately after the procedure has been completed, all dirty PPE should be removed and placed in the hazardous waste sack. The dental nurse can then apply clean gloves to assist the patient while they have a mouth rinse or be allowed to spit out, and then while their facial area is cleaned of all debris.

All of the used instruments should be left in situ, either out of the patient's view or covered with disposable bibs until the patient has left the surgery. The dental nurse should escort patients to the reception area if the surgery is not used for making appointments.

The abilities required by a competent dental nurse to provide support after the procedure includes the following points:

- Hand over the patient to reception for discharge
- Complete the patient records
- Correctly handle and dispose of waste amalgam
- Decontaminate the surgery and instruments

Complete the patient records

Some operators prefer to write the patient records themselves, while others will dictate exactly what they want the dental nurse to write. As with all records, they must be accurate, legible, avoid the use of any derogatory or slang terms, and refer only to accepted shorthand phrases that can be easily translated if necessary.

If the dental nurse is required to complete the records alone, these should be made available for the operator to check and then sign to say that they have done so – their accuracy is ultimately the responsibility of the operator. The issues of record-keeping and confidentiality are discussed in detail in Chapter 13.

The points that must be included in the records are:

- Written for the correct patient in their records, either on paper or on computer
- Date of procedure and date of writing (if different) – these will be recorded automatically on computer records
- Ideally completed on the day of the procedure, and as soon after its completion as possible
- Identify the operator and the dental nurse – this may be obvious in a small surgery setting, but less so in hospital departments and clinics
- Identify the procedure undertaken
- The charting must be updated to indicate the completion of a restoration, where necessary (using the relevant charting notations as necessary – see Chapter 13)
- Note the local anaesthetic used and the number of cartridges (batch numbers tend to be recorded centrally rather than in every set of patient notes)
- Give a brief description of the procedure
- Record the procedure carried out, including any restorative materials used

- Record any treatment complications accurately, where relevant – additional LA used, difficulty accessing the full cavity, and so on
- Record when the patient was notified of a problem where relevant, such as any reason why the procedure was not completed, and indicate that the patient was informed of this event
- Record any major complications and their outcome, where relevant
- Record if another appointment was required, and subsequently made
- Signed or initialled by the writer, when completed, and counter-signed by the operator as necessary – computer records can be set to automatically indicate the writer, but rely on pass-words to be accurate

Correct handling and disposal of waste amalgam

201

Despite the many advantages of amalgam over other permanent restorative materials, its one big disadvantage is the fact that it contains mercury, which is known to be toxic. When exposed to excessive amounts over time, members of the dental team are at risk of developing mercury poisoning, which can be fatal, so waste amalgam must be handled very carefully at all times.

Mercury poisoning can occur in the following ways:

- **Inhalation** of the vapours
- **Absorption** through the skin, the nail beds, the eyes and wounds on the hands
- **Ingestion** through swallowing

Precautions to be followed by all staff

The routine use of PPE, such as gloves, mask and safety glasses, or visors worn for protection against cross-infection will provide corresponding protection against mercury hazards.

To avoid absorption of mercury through the skin, the basic rules of cross-infection control should be followed:

- Always wear disposable gloves when handling mercury, mixing amalgam and cleaning amalgam instruments
- Do not wear open-toed shoes in the clinical area, as the floor may be contaminated by spilled mercury or dropped amalgam
- Do not wear jewellery or a wristwatch when working at the chairside as they may harbour particles of amalgam

To avoid pollution of the air by mercury vapour:

- Ideally, a pre-loaded capsule system should be in use (see Figure 1.12), rather than the old-fashioned system of bottled mercury and alloy powder being manually loaded into the amalgamator
- If the latter system is still in use, containers of mercury must be tightly sealed and stored in a cool, well-ventilated place
- When transferring mercury from a stock bottle, great care must be taken not to spill any. It is very difficult to find and recover mercury that has been dropped on the floor or working surface, as it is a liquid metal and rolls away easily
- For removal of old amalgam fillings, the use of a high-speed handpiece with diamond or tungsten carbide burs, water spray and efficient aspiration helps to reduce the aerosol of amalgam dust and mercury vapour, while the use of rubber dam will protect the patient
- Surgery staff must wear full PPE throughout such procedures, as they should for all chairside procedures
- All traces of amalgam must be removed from instruments before autoclaving, otherwise vapour will be released as the autoclave heats up – this is especially pertinent with amalgam carriers

- Keep the surgery well ventilated
- Amalgamators and the capsules therein should be checked after use as cases have been reported of mercury leakage from capsules during mixing
- Amalgamators must be stood on a tray lined with aluminium foil so that any droplets can be easily collected and disposed of as hazardous waste, using a disposable syringe
- The machines must also have a lid over the capsule holder, so that leaking capsules do not throw their dangerous contents into the surgery during mixing
- All premises using amalgam must have a mercury spillage kit so that any accidents can be dealt with swiftly and correctly – dental nurses must be familiar with this kit and how to use it correctly when a mercury spillage occurs

Mercury spillage

Accidental spillage of mercury or waste amalgam must always be reported to the dentist or other senior staff member. If a spillage occurs, globules of mercury can be drawn up into a disposable intravenous syringe (see Figures 1.16 and 1.17) or bulb aspirator and transferred to a mercury container (see Figures 1.13 and 1.14), while small globules can be collected by adherence to the lead foil from X-ray film packets. Waste amalgam can be gathered with a damp paper towel. For larger spillages, the following protocol should be followed:

- Stop work and report the incident to the dentist immediately
- Put on full PPE
- Globules of mercury or particles of amalgam must be smeared with a mercury-absorbent paste from the mercury spillage kit (see Figure 1.19)
- This consists of equal parts of calcium hydroxide and flours of sulphur mixed into a paste with water
- It should be left to dry and then removed with a wet disposable towel and placed in the storage container
- Risk-assess the incident to determine if protocols require amendment and change
- Larger spillages still require the evacuation of the premises, the sealing of the area and the involvement of Environmental Health to remove the contamination as a specialist procedure
- The Health and Safety Executive will be notified under Reporting of Injuries, Diseases and Dangerous Occurrences (RIDDOR) regulations, so that an investigation can be carried out to determine if the practice procedure needs to be changed to prevent a recurrence of the spillage

Decontaminate the surgery and instruments

The aspects of infection control and health and safety that are relevant to surgery and equipment decontamination (especially cleaning methods), infection control and sterilisation are fully discussed in Chapters 4 and 12.

In summary, they are as follows:

- All sharps are carefully disposed of in the sharps box – this includes local anaesthetic needles and used metal matrix bands
- All waste amalgam is placed in the waste amalgam tub, all used capsules are placed in the waste amalgam capsule tub
- All autoclavable items are placed in a washer-disinfector unit or an ultrasonic bath and decontaminated thoroughly before being placed in the autoclave for sterilisation
- All contaminated waste is placed in hazardous waste sacks or sharps bins
- All surfaces are disinfected using the correct solution

9

Unit 309: Provide Chairside Support during the Provision of Fixed and Removable Prostheses

Learning outcomes

1. Be able to support the patient and the operator for fixed and removable prostheses
2. Be able to prepare equipment, instruments and materials for fixed prostheses
3. Be able to select and prepare impression materials for fixed and removable prostheses
4. Be able to prepare equipment, instruments and materials for removable prostheses and orthodontic appliances

Outcome 1 assessment criteria
The learner can:
- Provide the necessary charts and records
- Select the appropriate impression materials
- Provide support and monitor the patients whilst impressions are in the mouth
- Provide the necessary equipment required for the taking of shades, supporting the operator in this procedure
- Provide the necessary equipment and materials for taking occlusal registrations
- List the methods for protecting and retracting the soft tissues during treatment

Outcome 2 assessment criteria
The learner can:
- Prepare and list the equipment, instruments and materials for:
  - Preparation of temporary/permanent crowns and bridges

Diploma in Dental Nursing, Level 3, Third Edition. Carole Hollins.
© 2014 John Wiley & Sons, Ltd. Published 2014 by John Wiley & Sons, Ltd.
Companion website: www.wiley.com/go/hollins/dentalnursinglevel3

    ○ Fitting temporary/permanent crowns and bridges
    ○ Adjustment of temporary/permanent crowns and bridges
- Select the correct type of adhesive material required for the fitting of fixed prostheses
- Provide the instruments required for trimming, cleaning and checking the final adjustment of fixed prostheses

Outcome 3 assessment criteria

The learner can:
- Select the correct type of impression material for taking impressions for fixed prostheses
- Prepare the correct quantity of impression material:
    ○ To the correct consistency
    ○ Within the handling and setting time relative to the material and ambient temperature
    ○ Using the correct technique
- Load impression materials correctly on the impression tray
- Disinfect impressions appropriately on removal from the patient's mouth
- Store the impressions so that their accuracy is maintained
- Complete laboratory tickets with legible and accurate information regarding the stage, shade and requirements, and attach it securely to the packaging

Outcome 4 assessment criteria

The learner can:
- Provide and list the equipment, instruments and materials required for:
    ○ Try-in stage of a removable prosthesis
    ○ Fitting stage of a removable prosthesis
- List the range of orthodontic treatments available
- List the equipment, instruments and materials that are used in the following stages of fixed and removable orthodontic treatments:
    ○ Fitting
    ○ Monitoring
    ○ Adjusting

This unit is assessed by:
- observation in the workplace, with examples included in the learner's portfolio
- an appropriate alternative method

Details of various elements of theory and underpinning knowledge are included in Chapter 15, and these are assessed within the written paper.

The theory and underpinning knowledge required to understand the scientific principles involved in the management of oral diseases and dental procedures, including fixed and removable prostheses, are fully discussed in Chapter 15. This chapter explains the dental nurse's role and responsibilities in relation to these procedures at the following stages:

- Preparation, temporisation and fitting of fixed prostheses
- Construction and fitting of removable prostheses
- Fitting, monitoring and adjusting of fixed and removable orthodontic appliances

Their responsibilities are to the operator (the person carrying out the procedure – usually the dentist, but in some cases it may be the orthodontic therapist) and also to the patient who is undergoing the procedure, and the patient's guardian where relevant.

Fixed prostheses are the tooth restorations or replacements that are cemented within, or onto, a tooth and include the following prostheses:

- Temporary or permanent crown – a cap or shell-like device made to cover three-quarters to the whole surface of a single tooth
- Temporary or permanent bridge – two or more crown-like units joined together as a single device, at least one of which is to replace a missing tooth
- Veneer – a facing made to fully cover the labial surface of a tooth
- Inlay – an insert into a tooth cavity that has been constructed in a laboratory

All are provided for varying reasons but involve the use of similar impression and cementation materials and the use of similar instruments as well.

Removable prostheses are all types of dentures – appliances that are made in the laboratory in various stages to replace missing teeth. They can be removed from the mouth by the patient (e.g. for cleaning) and reinserted again easily, without the use of cements. Generally, removable prostheses are made to replace several missing teeth rather than just one or two, as bridges do, or even to replace all the teeth in some patients.

When there are no teeth left in a jaw, it is said to be edentulous (edentate) and the artificial replacement is called a full or complete denture; if some teeth are still present, the replacement is called a partial denture. The majority of dentures are made entirely of acrylic, although many may also be constructed with a base of chrome-cobalt metal.

All removable prostheses are constructed on models made from impressions taken in the patient's mouth, and these models are also used to construct the interim stages of the appliance. All types of removable prostheses are provided for varying reasons but involve the use of similar impression materials and are constructed through the same stages.

Orthodontic appliances are used to align teeth within each arch and to correct the occlusion between the two jaws. They are either fixed appliances, which are cemented in a similar way to fixed prostheses, or they are removable appliances that are constructed in a similar way to removable prostheses, but do not require the interim construction stages for their completion. However, once fitted, they do require regular monitoring and adjustment as the treatment progresses.

The provision of all three areas of treatment in this unit will involve the taking of impressions at some point, which can be a cause for anxiety amongst some patients, especially children. In addition, the tooth preparation necessary for fixed prosthetic procedures usually involves the use of local anaesthetic, so a huge part of the dental nurse's role at these times is to be calming, friendly and supportive and to anticipate the concerns and needs of the patient throughout the procedure.

Before the procedure

The vast majority of dental workplaces operate on one appointments system or another, so that the working day can be correctly planned and all of the necessary instruments, materials and equipment are known to be available as required. There would be little point in a patient attending for a fixed prosthetic preparation procedure, for example, if the workplace had run out of crown preparation burs or the appropriate impression material. Forward planning is therefore a key element in the successful completion of a busy working day and, along with the skills in the following list, is among the abilities required by a competent dental nurse to provide successful chairside support for fixed and removal prosthetic procedures:

- Correct identification of the patient
- Correct identification of the procedure
- Knowledge of the records and images required by the operator for the procedure
- Knowledge of the correct setting up of the area for the procedure

205

- Knowledge of the instruments, materials and equipment that may be required for the procedure
- Knowledge of the actions to take if the dental nurse is unable to fully prepare for the procedure

Correct identification of the patient

The day list will refer to each patient attending that day by name and/or date of birth and/or address and/ or some kind of patient identification marker – such as a unique computer number or the patient's NHS number.

Whatever the system in place, the dental nurse should be familiar with it and be able to access the patient's records so that a cross-reference check can be made between the notes present and the expected procedure to be carried out. So if the previous notes refer to a tooth to be restored with a filling, but the day list indicates that the patient is attending for a crown prepara-tion, one of the following scenarios has occurred which must be checked with the operator and the patient before the procedure begins:

- The records and the day list entry are for two different patients
- The records are incomplete and a change in treatment has been decided without being recorded
- The records are correct and the day list entry is incorrect
- The records are incorrect and the day list entry is correct

Any of these scenarios could quite easily have occurred and the matter should be referred to a more senior colleague (ideally the operator concerned) so that the dental nurse can assist them in determining the way forward – to identify the correct patient and the correct procedure to be carried out that day.

The records required may be hard copies in full (i.e. a "pack" of handwritten patient notes, with paper copies of their medical history, previous treatment plans and consent forms and so on) or they may be fully computerised and only accessible "on screen", or a combination of the two. Whatever their presentation, they should be collected by the dental nurse and presented in the treatment area so that the operator can access them and check their content.

In large dental workplaces, such as dental schools and hospitals, the dental nurse can check the correct identity by asking patients to confirm their name, date of birth and address, and that they know why they are attending on the day. The final decision to confirm the patient's identity is the duty of the operator.

In smaller workplaces, many of the patients are recognisable to the staff by sight – some may even be known by their first names – but identity and procedure checks should still always be carried out, to avoid any mishaps. Once the patient has been correctly identified, the records and treatment area can be prepared.

The records to be set out will include the following:

- Notes written at the previous appointment or when the decision was made to carry out the particular procedure – these will remind the operator of the reasons for the treatment decisions taken
- Medical history form, to be checked to highlight any potential concerns – for example, is a certain local anaesthetic required, or does the patient have a respiratory problem that may make impression taking more difficult?
- Consent form, indicating that the patient has given valid consent to the procedure (see Chapter 13)
- Radiographs of the relevant tooth or teeth – these will allow operators to remind themselves of any particular concerns, such as a difficult angulation of a tooth requiring a crown
- Study models for orthodontic patients in particular
- Any prosthesis or appliance to be fitted

The dental nurse can also access the records for the following purposes:

- The notes may refer to the patient's level of anxiety if impressions are to be taken, so the dental nurse is aware of the heightened need to be supportive and helpful to the patient throughout the procedure – the issue should also be pointed out to the operator
- The medical history can be checked and any recognised potential issues pointed out to the operator
- Patients can also be asked to confirm if there have been any changes to their medical history since they were last seen, and these are then recorded appropriately and pointed out to the operator
- The consent form can be checked to ensure it covers the planned procedure and that it has been signed and dated by the patient (or their guardian), or that it requires to be signed and dated today – any discrepancies can be pointed out to the operator
- The radiographs must be correctly displayed to show the tooth or teeth under treatment, either as digital images on the computer or as hard copies on film
- Hard copies must be correctly mounted on the viewing screen:
  - Intra-oral views with the pimple facing out (to indicate left from right), and upper teeth with their roots above the crown and lower teeth with their roots below the crown (see Figure 7.13)
  - Extra-oral views with the "L" marker in the bottom right-hand corner of the radiograph as it is positioned on the viewing screen, to indicate the patient's left side (see Figure 8.1)
- Check that any prosthesis or appliance to be fitted is:
  - Present
  - For the actual patient
  - At the correct stage

Correct identification of the procedure

The patient is attending for one of the procedures in the following list, and the actual one should be referred to in the notes and on the day list (although some computer software systems are not programmed to allow individual procedures to be booked – they just record a time slot as "bridge preparation" or "orthodontic view" procedure).

For a fixed prosthesis appointment, the procedure will be one of the following options:

- Crown preparation or crown fitting (temporary or permanent)
- Bridge preparation or bridge fitting (temporary or permanent)
- Veneer preparation or fitting
- Inlay preparation or fitting

For a removable prosthesis appointment, the procedure will be one of the following options:

- First or second impressions, with or without shade taking
- Occlusal registration, with or without shade taking
- Try-in (may just be a chrome base to try first) or re-try
- Fitting

For an orthodontic appliance, the procedure will be one of the following options:

- Working model impressions for removable appliance construction
- Removable appliance fitting
- Fixed appliance bonding
- Fixed or removable appliance monitoring and adjustment

- Fixed appliance debonding and fit retainer
- Removable retainer fit

The records and images required by the operator in order to carry out the procedure are detailed in the preceding section.

Knowledge of the correct setting up of the area

As with all dental procedures, the treatment area (surgery) must be clean before being set up for a fixed or removable prosthetic session, and left in a similar condition afterwards, to avoid any possibility of cross-infection occurring. The principles of infection control are discussed in detail in Chapter 12.

Before the surgery is prepared for use, the dental nurse must ensure that they do not inadvertently introduce any contamination into the area, and so must undertake the correct hand washing technique before applying the correct personal protective equipment (PPE). As a clinical procedure is to be carried out, the appropriate hand washing technique is as follows:

- Turn on the tap using the foot or elbow control, to prevent contaminating the tap (see Figure 4.4)
- Wet both hands under running water of a suitable temperature
- Apply a suitable antibacterial liquid soap from the dispenser (Figure 8.2) and wash all areas of both hands and wrists thoroughly – this should take at least 30 seconds to carry out thoroughly, and the correct routine is illustrated on the poster that is present at each hand washing station (see Figure 1.3)
- Nail brushes are not advised unless they are autoclavable, as they can become contaminated with repeated use
- Rinse both hands under running water, holding them so that the water does not flow back over the fingers
- Dry the hands thoroughly, using disposable paper towels for single use

The equipment and instruments can now be handled safely, unless the dental nurse has any cuts or abrasions on the hands, in which case the lesion should be covered with a waterproof dressing and a pair of clinical gloves must be worn before any items are handled.

The surgery itself is then made ready as follows:

- The electric and water supplies should be switched on to all static equipment (dental chair, suction unit, etc.) if this has not already been done
- Any portable items not likely to be required for the procedure should be placed in cupboards or drawers, or removed from the surgery, so that the work surfaces are clear of any clutter
- The controls of any large equipment items which are likely to be contaminated during the procedure must be protected by a barrier technique, including:
  ○ Dental chair controls, if not foot-operated
  ○ Dental light controls and handles (see Figure 8.3)
  ○ Computer keyboard, if various screens are in use
  ○ Bracket table handles and controls
- In some surgery settings, the aspirator pipes and handpiece tubing may also require barrier protection if they are of a design that makes them difficult to wipe down thoroughly (such as corrugated piping)
- The patient records are accessed on the computer, or the paper copies are laid out on an area of the work surface away from the surgical field (to minimise their contamination)
- Relevant radiographs are correctly mounted on the viewing screen, in easy reach of the operator
- Relevant study models are set out in easy reach of the operator
- PPE equipment is laid out ready for the patient, the operator and the dental nurse:

○ Protective glasses (tinted if the curing light is to be used), disposable bib, tissues – for the patient
○ Protective glasses or visor, face mask, gloves – for the operator and dental nurse
- Mouth rinse and cup are made ready for the patient
- Suitable aspirator tips are connected to the suction unit
- For fixed prostheses, the correct local anaesthetic equipment and materials are laid out for use, in easy reach of the operator and dental nurse, and covered with a disposable bib until the patient is seated:
  ○ Topical anaesthetic and cotton wool rolls (where relevant)
  ○ Syringe (aspirating type if a nerve block is likely)
  ○ Short or long needle (depending on which tooth/teeth is/are involved)
  ○ Local anaesthetic cartridges
  ○ Re-sheathing device
- The local anaesthetic solution should be checked by the operator for suitability, before use

209

Knowledge of the instruments, materials and equipment required
Fixed prosthesis preparation

The instruments, materials and equipment required for a fixed prosthesis preparation procedure are very similar across the categories, from crowns through to inlays. The instruments required, with their functions, are listed in the following table. The preparation procedure itself is discussed in detail in Chapter 15.

Item	Function
Diamond burs (Figure 9.1)	Tapered so that no undercuts are produced on the prepared tooth or teeth, otherwise the fixed prosthesis will not seat fully on to the tooth
Air turbine handpiece	For use with the burs during tooth preparation
Retraction cord (Figure 9.2)	Cord soaked in an astringent solution (adrenaline or alum) that is then packed into the gingival crevice to cause shrinkage of the gingiva away from the prepared tooth – this provides a definitive tooth margin which is reproduced in the impression and also the cast model
Impression trays (Figure 9.3)	Variety of plastic or metal boxed trays, sized to fit fully over the dental arch – upper and lower styles Also triple tray system
Crown-former (Figure 9.4)	Pre-formed plastic or polycarbonate tooth-shaped formers, in a variety of sizes and available for each tooth shape – required when preparing for crowns or bridges
Beebee crown shears (Figure 9.5)	Short beaked shears for cutting and shaping the margins of temporary crowns
Shade guide (Figure 9.6)	Shaded teeth in holder, to determine the required shade of the prosthesis by comparing each example to the adjacent teeth and determining the best match available
Post system (Figure 9.7)	Required if a post crown is being provided

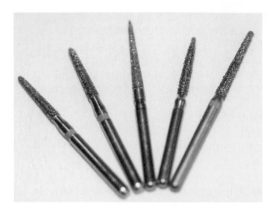

Figure 9.1   Crown preparation diamond burs.

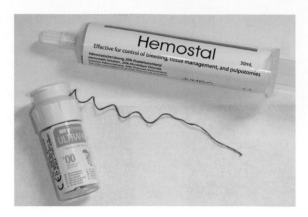

Figure 9.2   Retraction cord and solution.

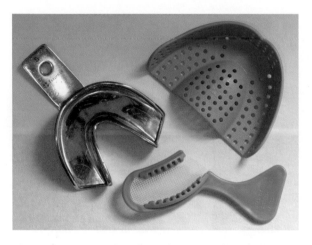

Figure 9.3   Examples of suitable impression trays.

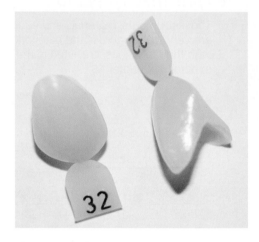

Figure 9.4   A crown former.

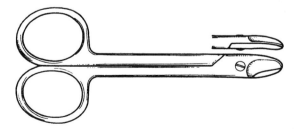

Figure 9.5   Beebee crown shears. Source: *Levison's Textbook for Dental Nurses*, 11th edition (Hollins), 2013. Reproduced with permission of Wiley-Blackwell.

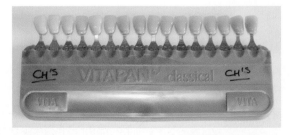

Figure 9.6   A shade guide.

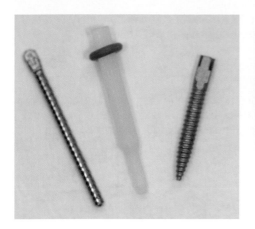

Figure 9.7   Post systems.

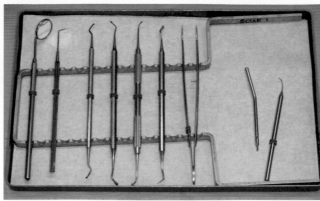

Figure 9.8   A conservation tray.

211

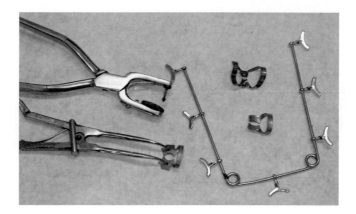

Figure 9.9   Rubber dam equipment.

In addition, a routine conservation tray of instruments will be required, as shown in Figure 9.8, and some operators will also prefer to work under rubber dam, so the instruments shown in Figure 9.9 should also be laid out.

The materials required at this stage will be suitable impression materials for both the working arch (where the tooth preparation has occurred) and the opposing arch (to record the occlusion), and their mixing equipment, as well as the temporary cement, as follows:

- Working arch:
  - ○ Elastomer material with mixing gun, mixing machine or waxed pad and spatula
- Opposing arch:
  - ○ Alginate material with bowl and spatula, or mixing machine
- Temporary cement:
  - ○ Zinc oxide and eugenol-based temporary luting cement (or similar) to hold the temporary crown or bridge in place
  - ○ Glass ionomer-based cement for veneer tooth coverage
  - ○ Temporary filling material for inlay preparation
  - ○ Appropriate mixing pad/glass slab and spatula for each

All these materials are discussed in detail in Chapter 15. The mixing and decontamination techniques to be used for the impression materials are discussed later in this chapter.

Fixed prosthesis fitting

As the name suggests, the fitting appointment is concerned with the permanent cementation of the fixed prosthesis to the tooth/teeth, using one of the available luting cements to do so. Again, local anaesthetic equipment, a routine conservation tray and possibly rubber dam will be required, as well as the items in the following table.

Item	Function
Fine articulating paper	To accurately check the occlusion of the prosthesis when fitted – indicates any high spots (premature contacts) by leaving a coloured mark on it and on the opposing tooth
Miller forceps (Figure 9.10)	Used by some operators to hold the articulating paper in place. Many operators place the articulating paper with their fingers only
Variety of polishing burs (Figure 9.11)	To smooth over any areas of the prosthesis requiring reduction while the occlusion is corrected, so that a smooth, polished surface remains
Patient mirror	To allow patients to view the prosthesis before fitting and ensure they are happy with the shade and alignment

In addition, the operator's choice of one of a range of luting cements and their mixing equipment will be required for the actual cementation of the fixed prosthesis. A wide variety of cements is available, and the preferred choice of the operator will probably be known by the dental nurse due to the familiarity of the dental team. If not, the operator should be asked about this before the procedure begins, so that all of the required items are set up and ready to be used.

The choices available are listed in the following table, and luting cements are discussed in detail in Chapter 15.

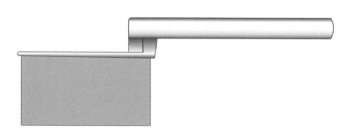

Figure 9.10   Miller forceps and articulating paper.
Source: *Levison's Textbook for Dental Nurses*, 11th edition (Hollins), 2013. Reproduced with permission of Wiley-Blackwell.

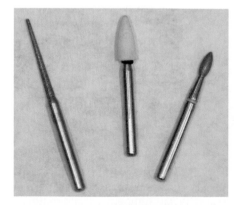

Figure 9.11   Polishing burs.

Type	Action	Mixing
Zinc phosphate	Mechanically adhesive to rough inner surface of prosthesis and surface of tooth	Glass slab and spatula
Zinc polycarboxylate	Chemically adhesive to tooth and inner surface of prosthesis	Glass slab and spatula
Glass ionomer	Chemically adhesive to tooth and inner surface of prosthesis	Waxed pad and spatula
Polyester resin	Chemically adhesive and inert in saliva	Waxed pad and spatula
Self-cure resin	Chemical bonding between tooth and prosthesis	Double syringe mix
Light-cure resin	Light-cure bonding between tooth and prosthesis	Double syringe mix
Dual-cure resin	Combination of self-cure and light-cure bonding between tooth and prosthesis	Double syringe mix

Modern types of cement tend to be provided in double syringe form with no mixing necessary, but older types (such as phosphate, polycarboxylate and glass ionomer cements) require correct proportioning and thorough mixing before use, using the items listed in the third column. The resin-based cements also require etchant or primer materials to ensure a good bond is achieved between the tooth and the inner surface of the fixed prosthesis, and they tend to be available as a mixing kit with all the necessary materials and applicators within.

Removable prosthesis appointment

As indicated earlier, various stages are involved in the construction of a removable prosthesis, and different equipment, instruments and items are required for each stage. Dental nurses will know from the patient records and/or the day list which stage is to be carried out that day and can set up the surgery as necessary. Once completed, each stage must be decontaminated and returned to the laboratory for the technician to make the next stage.

The items for each stage are described in the following sections.

First impressions

These are taken to produce the initial working model for the prosthesis construction and are sent to the laboratory for casting up.

Item	Function
Stock impression trays (Figure 9.12)	To be sized and used to take the initial impressions, so that special trays can be constructed – they may be upper and/or lower, and edentulous or dentate (boxed)
Alginate impression material and room temperature water	To be mixed in a mixing bowl with spatula, loaded into the trays and inserted to produce the initial impressions

Item	Function
Shade and mould guides (Figure 9.13)	To determine the colour and shape of the denture teeth, to be as close in appearance to any remaining teeth as possible – usually a different shade guide than that used for fixed prostheses
Work ticket or docket (Figure 9.14)	To record the patient and dentist details, the denture design and base material to be used, the tooth shade and mould, the type and position of any clasps, and the return date

Second impressions

These are taken to provide more detail and better accuracy of the completed prosthesis, and many operators often incorporate this stage with that of the bite registration.

Item	Function
Study models and special trays (Figure 9.15)	To take the more accurate second impressions where required, in order to produce the working models
Alginate or elastomer impression material	To take the more accurate second impressions of the arch where the prosthesis is to be fitted
Work ticket	To record the next stage request and the return date

Bite registration

This stage records the way that the patient normally bites, so that the prosthesis can be made to accurately fit into that bite, rather than to alter it. With edentulous patients, their occlusal face height has to be measured as a guide for the technician, as the patient has no actual bite to refer to (because they have no teeth).

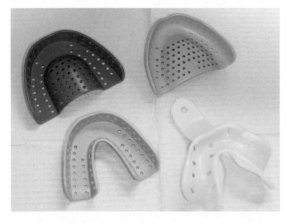

Figure 9.12   Stock impression trays – edentulous and boxed.

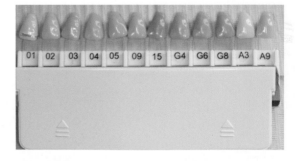

Figure 9.13   A denture shade guide.

ACME DENTAL LABORATORIES LTD. M.H.R.A. REF. CA 008044
136 WATERLOO ROAD, BURSLEM, STOKE-ON-TRENT ST6 3HB
Telephone: 01782 817621 Fax: 01782 824142

DAMAS
Dental Appliance Manufacturers
Audit Scheme

DAMAS
Dental Appliance Manufacturers
Audit Scheme

Dentist _____ Job No. _____

Surgery Address _____

THIS IS A CUSTOM MADE DEVICE FOR THE EXCLUSIVE USE OF

Patient Mr./Mrs. _____

Special U ☐   Acrylic ☐   Shade ☐   Mould ☐   Teeth ☐

Trays L ☐

<u>RETURN DATES</u>   *Please tick box*

Bite _____   Received _____   PVT ☐

Try in _____   Received _____   IND ☐

Retry _____   Received _____   N.H.S ☐

Finish _____   Received _____

<u>DENTURES</u>

Notes   I.D.Names ⬭

NON STERILE DEVICE   LABORATORY FEE _____

STATEMENT.   This device conforms to the relevant requirements set out in

Annex I of the Medical Devices Directive

Inspected and Signed by

Figure 9.14   A work ticket (docket). Source: *Levison's Textbook for Dental Nurses*, 11th edition (Hollins), 2013. Reproduced with permission of Wiley-Blackwell.

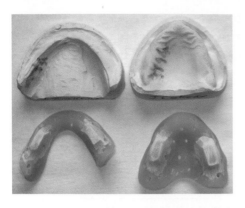

Figure 9.15 Special trays and initial models.

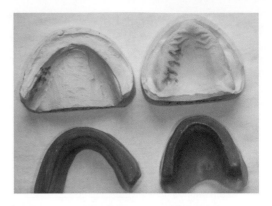

Figure 9.16 Wax bite rims with models.

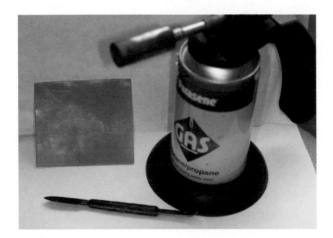

Figure 9.17 Pink wax, wax knife and burner.

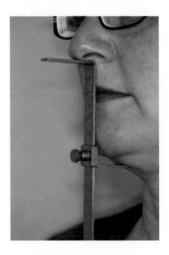

Figure 9.18 Willis bite gauge in position.

Item	Function
Wax bite rims (Figure 9.16)	Adjusted in height so that correct face height of the patient can be recorded
Heat source (Figure 9.17)	To warm the hand instruments and rims for adjustment
Wax knife (Figure 9.17)	To remove or add additional wax to the rims, as necessary
Bite registration paste (optional)	To be mixed and applied to the rims, so that they are held in the correct position once set
Pink sheet wax (Figure 9.17)	For addition to the rims, as necessary
Willis bite gauge (Figure 9.18)	To record the desired occlusal face height in edentulous patients, where no natural teeth remain as a guide
Work ticket	To record the next stage request and return date

Try-in

This stage is a trial insertion of the removable prosthesis before it is sent to the technician for completion. The prosthesis may be a wax base, with or without stainless steel clasps (technicians differ over this point), or it may be a chrome-based design with the teeth held in wax. Final adjustments can be made to the wax, the stainless steel clasps, the teeth and their shade at this point, and minimal adjustments to the chrome base.

Item	Function
Try-in prostheses	To determine if fit, occlusion and aesthetics are correct before finishing the dentures
Heat source	To warm the wax and make adjustments, as necessary
Le Cron carver (Figure 9.19)	To make fine adjustments to the wax area of the try-in, as necessary
Wax knife	To warm and smooth the wax after adjustments, as necessary
Shade and mould guides	To check or alter the shade or mould, as necessary
Pink sheet wax	For addition to the try-in, as necessary
Adam pliers	To adjust stainless steel or chrome clasps
Pink stone with straight handpiece	To make minimal adjustments to the chrome base, as necessary. If the chrome base is inaccurate, it will need remaking at this point
Patient mirror	To allow patients to view the try-ins and decide if they are happy with the appearance before completion of the dentures
Work ticket	To record any changes required for a retry or to record the fit return date

Fitting

The completed removable prosthesis is fitted satisfactorily and given to the patient to wear.

Item	Function
Completed removable prostheses	To fit, to the patient and dentist's satisfaction
Straight handpiece and selection of trimming burs and carborundum polishing stones (Figure 9.20)	To remove any acrylic pearls or occlusal high spots before polishing and smoothing the adjusted area for comfort
Patient mirror	To allow patients to view the completed prostheses
Articulating paper or occlusal indicator wax	To identify occlusal high spots, for adjustment as necessary
Pressure relief paste	To identify high spots on the denture fitting surface, for removal as necessary

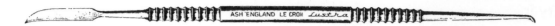

Figure 9.19   Le Cron carver. Source: *Levison's Textbook for Dental Nurses*, 11th edition (Hollins), 2013. Reproduced with permission of Wiley-Blackwell.

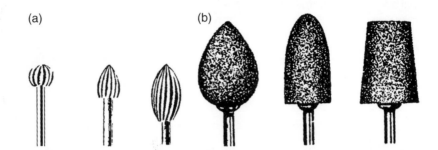

Figure 9.20   Acrylic burs (a) and stones (b).

Orthodontic appliances

A set of pre-treatment study models is always required before any orthodontic treatment is carried out, whether fixed or removable appliances are used, and the equipment and items for this stage are as for any alginate impression technique.

Removable appliance fitting and adjustment

Removable appliances are constructed with an acrylic base and various stainless steel clips and springs incorporated in their design, for retention and tooth movement, respectively. As with other removable prostheses, they are able to be removed for cleaning and so on, so no cements are required for their fitting.

The equipment and items required are as listed in the following table.

Item	Function
Adam universal pliers (Figure 9.21)	To adjust all metal springs and retractors, as necessary
Straight handpiece and acrylic trimming bur (Figure 9.22)	To adjust all acrylic areas of the appliance, as necessary
Measuring ruler	To record any measurable tooth movement, such as the overjet
Expansion screw key, where necessary	To count the number of turns applied to the screw between visits, to ensure compliance by the patient

Fixed appliance bonding and adjustment

Fixed appliances are bonded to most of the teeth in one arch, with some components requiring resin-based cements (as for fixed prostheses) and other components requiring conventional luting cements, such as glass ionomer or zinc polycarboxylate products. The instruments required for these are as for those listed in the earlier section on fixed prostheses.

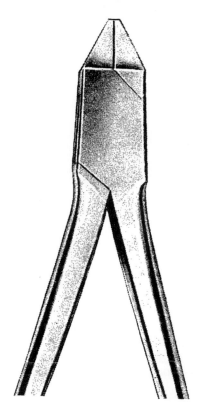

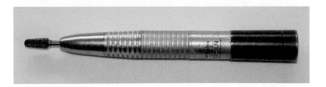

Figure 9.22   Straight handpiece and acrylic trimming bur.

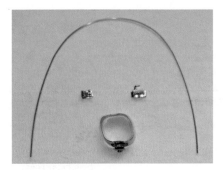

Figure 9.21   Adams universal pliers.
Source: *Levison's Textbook for Dental Nurses*,
11th edition (Hollins), 2013. Reproduced
with permission of Wiley-Blackwell.

Figure 9.23   Archwire, bracket and
molar band with tube.

The specific equipment and instruments required for the bonding and adjustments appointments are listed in the following table.

Item	Function
Archwire (Figure 9.23)	Flexible nickel titanium or stainless steel wires, to fasten into the brackets or bands
End cutters	Right-angled cutters to trim the ends of the archwire after replacement
Alastiks	Rubber bands to hold the archwire into the slots of each bracket
Alastik holders	Ratcheted holders (similar to artery forceps) to apply the alastiks to the brackets
Brackets (Figure 9.23)	Metal or ceramic components to attach to each tooth, if any have been lost since the previous appointment
Bands (Figure 9.23)	Metal rings to attach to molars in particular, although bands are available for all teeth and were the only attachments available before brackets were developed

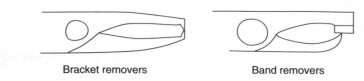

Bracket removers   Band removers

Figure 9.24 Bracket and band removers.

Item	Function
Bracket holders	To hold and position each bracket to the centre of the tooth, if any replacements are required
Bracket and band removers (Figure 9.24)	To remove brackets, bands and any residual bond material before replacing, if necessary
Bonding materials	Acid etch and orthodontic resin bond material – to hold brackets onto the tooth
Band cement	Any luting cement material, to hold bands onto the molar teeth

At the bonding appointment the appliance will be initially bonded to the teeth, to start the tooth movement treatment. At the adjustment appointments, the archwires will be replaced and tied back in again, and sometimes a dislodged bracket or band may require replacement too. Rather than having to select a specific archwire, bracket or band, the dental nurse will be able to lay out an orthodontic kit containing a selection of the components, and the operator will then choose the item required.

Retainer fit

At the end of any orthodontic treatment, the tooth movement will have been completed and the teeth will be held in their new positions by a retainer. Some operators use the actual appliance as a retainer initially, before fitting a specially made one at a later date. A final post-treatment set of study models will also be taken at this appointment as a record of the tooth movement and occlusion achieved. These will be taken with alginate, and the equipment and materials required are as for any alginate impression technique.

Otherwise, the equipment and instruments required at this appointment are listed in the following table.

Item	Function
Bracket and band removers	To remove the various components of the fixed appliance from the teeth, without damaging the teeth or causing pain to the patient
Retainer	A passive removable appliance similar to the removable prosthesis, or a vacuum-formed "gum shield" design, or a passive wire bonded to the palatal or lingual aspect of the teeth when fixed appliances have been used
Scale and polish equipment	To clean the teeth of any plaque or calculus debris once a fixed appliance has been removed
Air turbine and polishing burs	To remove any residual bond material from the teeth after a fixed appliance has been debonded

Knowledge of the actions to take if preparation cannot be completed

If any instruments, materials or items of equipment are not readily available for use immediately before the procedure is scheduled to start, the dental nurse must report the matter to an appropriate person immediately. This may be the operator, a senior dental nurse (or line manager) or the practice manager. In particular, the dental nurse must ensure that any laboratory items required for the appointment have been returned and are ready for use.

The final preparation that the dental nurse must carry out is to check with the patient that any prescribed pre-treatment instructions have been followed correctly. In particular, the following points should be clarified:

- Have all routine medications been taken as requested?
- If impressions are to be taken, has the patient refrained from having a meal in the last hour, to avoid the possibility of vomiting?
- If the procedure is being carried out under any form of conscious sedation technique, has the patient complied with all of the relevant additional points as requested?
- If the patient is a child or a vulnerable adult, are they in attendance with a suitable adult escort, to look after and see them safely home after the procedure?
- If the patient is frail or excessively nervous, are they in attendance with a suitable adult escort for the same purpose?
- Has the patient (or guardian) read and understood any pre-treatment information provided – are there any further questions?
- Has the patient (or guardian) been given enough information to provide valid consent for the procedure, and has that consent been given?

When it becomes apparent that one or more of these points have not been followed, the dental nurse must report the matter to the operator immediately, and allow them to discuss the situation further with the patient. It is not the role of dental nurses to act beyond their level of competence by making unilateral decisions about any of these issues – the responsibility lies with the operator.

During the procedure

Usually, the dental nurse will collect patients (and their guardians, where relevant) from the reception area and escort them to the surgery, rather than the operator. The dental nurse should be welcoming and friendly towards patients (and guardians) and use the time to put them at their ease.

With experience, dental nurses will develop their communication skills and their own style of patter that they can use successfully, and patients will respond positively to a good dental nurse with obvious empathy to their situation. Communication skills are discussed in detail in Chapter 5, and the skills of reflection and developing one's own self in practice are discussed in Chapter 2.

The abilities required by a competent dental nurse to provide support during the procedure include the following:

- Preparation of the patient
- Assistance during the administration of local anaesthesia, where necessary
- Assistance during the placement of rubber dam, where necessary

- Identification and correct handling of the instruments, materials and equipment throughout the procedure
- Adequate provision of moisture control and tissue retraction throughout the procedure, where necessary
- Mixing impression materials and loading trays
- Correct handling of impressions and items to be returned to the laboratory
- Mixing luting cements and temporary cements
- Monitoring and support of the patient

Although forward planning of the procedure should avoid the possibility, it may be necessary for the dental nurse to retrieve unprepared instruments and items during the procedure. If so, then gloves must be removed and replaced with a new pair each time the surgical area is left and re-accessed.

Preparation of the patient

A final check is made by the operator of the patient's identification and consent to undergo the procedure. The dental nurse will then assist patients into the dental chair and ready them for the start of treatment as follows:

- Help them to remove their coat if necessary and hang it up
- Assist them into the dental chair – they may need physical support, for example, or the chair raising or lowering
- Apply their required PPE:
  - Safety glasses – these need to be tinted if the curing light is to be used to set materials
  - Protective bib
  - Some patients like to have a tissue in hand too
- Monitor the patient for signs of anxiety, and notify the operator as necessary
- Reassure the patient in a calm and friendly manner – many appreciate the opportunity of a hand to hold at this point, although this action can be passed to an escort / guardian if appropriate
- When orthodontic appliances are to be fitted to children, it is usual for the guardian to be present in the surgery throughout the procedure, and the dental nurse can direct them to an appropriate seat

Assistance during the administration of local anaesthesia

Local anaesthetic will usually be required for fixed prosthetic procedures only. The operator and the dental nurse apply their own PPE (safety glasses/visor, face mask, gloves).

The disposable cover used to hide the items while patients enter and settle in the dental chair is removed from the equipment, and the operator must check that the correct items and local anaesthetic are prepared. The topical anaesthetic is applied to a cotton wool roll and handed to the operator for application in the patient's mouth. While this takes effect, the syringe is loaded ready for use, quietly and out of sight of the patient:

- Noisy clattering of metallic items can be particularly unnerving for patients, so items must be handled proficiently at all times
- The local anaesthetic cartridge is loaded into the syringe correctly, with the cap end at the bottom where the needle will be applied
- If an aspirating technique is to be used, any screw-in plunger is locked into the cartridge bung before the needle is added
- The needle is screwed on to the threaded end of the syringe, with the guard in place

- On removal of the topical anaesthetic, the needle guard is loosened but left over the needle, and the loaded syringe is offered to the operator (see Figure 8.16)
- As the operator receives the syringe, the dental nurse keeps hold of the loosened needle guard so that it becomes unsheathed as it is transferred over
- The guard is then placed in the re-sheathing device, ready for the operator when the anaesthetic procedure is completed (see Figure 1.29)
- Successive cartridges are handed to the operator as required during the administration procedure
- When the administration is complete, the equipment is re-sheathed by the operator without being handled by the dental nurse (this avoids increasing the likelihood of an inoculation injury)

223

Assistance during the placement of rubber dam

The rubber dam kit is usually kept in a lidded tray, and the items should be separated out so that they can be picked up more easily. Many operators apply rubber dam without any assistance from the dental nurse, while others will require the hole to be punched and perhaps the clamp forceps to be loaded. Once the dam is successfully in place on the tooth, the dental nurse may assist in applying it to the dam frame and passing additional items such as floss to ensure the tooth is fully exposed (Figure 9.25).

Some operators prefer to have a saliva ejector placed in the floor of the patient's mouth once the rubber dam is in place.

Identification and correct handling of the instruments, etc.

Conservation trays are usually kept as pre-set loaded trays, which simply require the lids removing before use and placing within easy reach of the operator and the dental nurse. Items that are stored separately in pouches can be opened and placed on the tray with the other items before treatment begins.

When the operator has finished with an instrument, it is either placed back on the tray or safely passed back to the dental nurse, who receives it and places it on the tray. Routine prosthetic treatment is not carried out under surgical conditions, so it is acceptable to reuse instruments throughout the procedure.

During the procedure, the dental nurse is likely also to be aspirating and retracting soft tissues, so the receiving and passing of instruments will require the use of both hands. Experience will

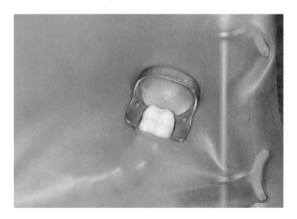

Figure 9.25   Rubber dam in place on lower molar tooth.

improve this ability with time, but all members of the dental team must develop a routine of never passing items across the patient's face while performing instrument transfer – it only takes one dropped item to permanently scar or blind a patient.

Adequate provision of moisture control and tissue retraction

This is required during both fixed prosthetic procedures and fixed orthodontic appliance procedures, but not for removable prostheses. When rubber dam is in place for fixed prosthetic procedures, adequate moisture control and tissue retraction are far easier to achieve for the dental nurse, as the tooth is isolated from the rest of the mouth by the dam.

During the procedure the dental nurse will be expected to use the relevant instruments and equipment correctly, to assist the operator in the following techniques:

- **Moisture control** – removal of moisture (saliva, blood, irrigation solution) from the operative area so that adequate vision is possible by the operator and so that the patient is not choking on a mouthful of fluid, using:
  - ○ Wide-bore aspirator for fast fluid removal, as well as some soft tissue retraction
  - ○ Saliva ejector beneath the rubber dam, which may need repositioning from time to time
- **Irrigation** – from the air turbine handpiece during tooth preparation and adjustments procedures, to avoid heat damage to the tooth
- **Tissue retraction** – to avoid damage to the soft tissues from burs and drills, and to provide good vision for the operator, using:
  - ○ Flanged wide-bore aspirator tips to retract the cheek, lips or tongue
  - ○ Special cheek retractors, although these tend to be reserved for extraction and minor oral surgery procedures
  - ○ Mouth mirror to retract the tongue or lips, and to reflect light and thus illuminate the operative field

Retraction of any soft tissues for any prolonged length of time can be quite tiring for the dental nurse, and if they need to stop for a rest or to reposition the retractor, the operator must be forewarned so that they do not continue drilling or cutting as the soft tissues collapse across the operative field.

Mixing impression materials and loading trays

Various impression materials may be used during fixed and removable prosthetic procedures, and alginate is also used during orthodontic treatment, so dental nurses must be skilled in mixing any material required and loading impression trays adequately for any of these procedures. Details of the impression materials available are discussed in Chapter 15.

Those likely to be used are:

- Alginate
- Elastomer material:
  - ○ Silicone
  - ○ Polyether and similar materials

Alginate impression material

This is the most commonly used impression material in the dental workplace, as it is easy to mix and relatively cheap. It is used for the following:

- Opposing arch models for crown, bridge, inlay and veneer construction
- Models for the construction of full and partial acrylic dentures
- Models for the construction of removable orthodontic appliances

- Study models, before and after orthodontic treatment
- Models for the construction of special trays and orthodontic retainers

The mixing and loading technique is as follows (Figure 9.26):

- Select the correct impression tray(s) with the handle inserted
- Unperforated trays (usually metal) will require an adhesive application, to prevent the alginate lifting off the tray when it is removed from the mouth
- Shake the lidded powder container to evenly distribute the contents
- Measure out the required amount of water (at room temperature) using the water measure provided
- Prepare a levelled scoop of powder using the scoop provided, in a 1:1 ratio of water:powder
- Put the powder in the mixing bowl and add the water into a central well
- Mix the contents by spatulating the wet powder against the side of the bowl, to remove all air bubbles

225

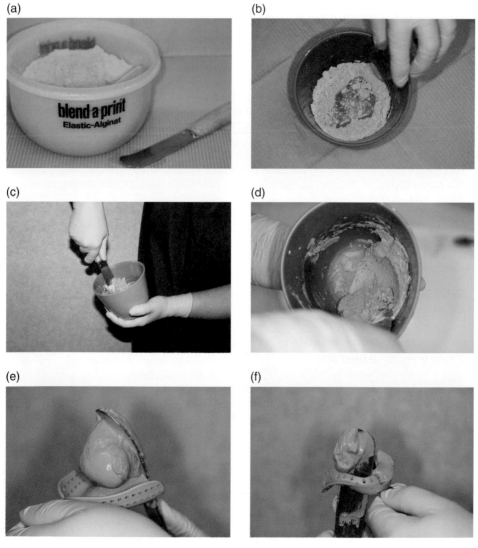

Figure 9.26   Alginate mixing stages (a–d) and tray loading (e, f).

- When a firm and even mix is achieved, load the tray:
  - ○ Upper trays, from the back and spread forwards
  - ○ Lower trays, from the lingual edges and spread out, one side at a time
- Pass the loaded tray to the operator

Silicone impression material

These materials are the more commonly used ones for taking accurate impressions, where alginate is not suitable. They will be used for the following:

- Working models for fixed prostheses – crowns, bridges, and so on
- Working models for chrome cobalt dentures, using a special tray

They have a variety of presentations and their mixing is determined accordingly:

- Tubs of heavy-bodied putty with liquid or paste activator
- Tubes of light-bodied paste with liquid or paste activator
- More recently, preloaded gun syringes that mix the constituents automatically

The various mixing and loading techniques are described in the following:

Putty or paste with activator:

- A measured scoop or length of putty or paste is placed on the supplied waxed pad, which has graduation marks to allow measurement of the liquid or paste activator (Figure 9.27)
- The liquid activator is measured by the number of drops, while the paste activator is measured by length of expressed material
- For putty products, the two constituents are folded into each other with a spatula, then picked up and hand-mixed until an even colour is produced, with no streaks of unmixed material visible
- For paste products, the two constituents are fully spatulated on the mixing pad
- When fully mixed:
  - ○ Load the tray with the putty in a sausage shape to mimic the dental arch
  - ○ Hand the paste to the operator on the pad, so that it can be applied to the prepared tooth
  - ○ Pass the loaded tray to the operator

Preloaded gun syringes:

- Express small blobs of material from the syringes to ensure they are unblocked before applying a new mixing tube (Figure 9.28)

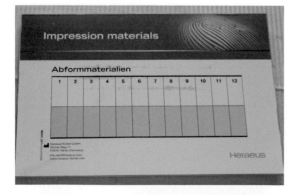

Figure 9.27   A graduated elastomer mixing pad.

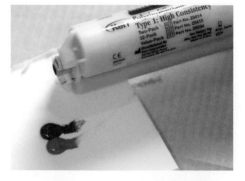

Figure 9.28   Expressed material before applying mixing tube.

- The constituents are automatically mixed as the gun is worked
- Express the putty material in a sausage shape around the tray and hand to the operator
- The operator will have applied the mixed paste to the prepared tooth

When the putty base materials are mixed by hand, it is possible for the mixing and setting times to be affected by some types of rubber PPE gloves used. If mixing is to occur by hand, then, it is advisable that vinyl gloves are worn, as other types could affect the setting of the silicone impression.

The silicones can be used in either a one-stage technique (the most widely available, and using addition cured silicones) or a two-stage technique (using condensation cured silicones).

With the former, both the heavy-bodied putty and the light-bodied paste are mixed at the same time – the dental nurse mixes the putty while the operator mixes the paste. The putty is loaded into the impression tray while the paste is either syringed on to the prepared tooth or placed on it using a flat plastic instrument. Both materials then set and are removed together in the impression tray.

With the latter, the putty is mixed, loaded into the tray, inserted into the mouth and allowed to set first. It is then carefully removed and spaced in the area of the preparation, while the mixed paste is syringed or wiped on to the tooth. The set putty and tray are reinserted and the whole is removed when the paste has set. Again, the dental nurse mixes the putty and the operator will apply the paste to the prepared tooth.

Adhesive is usually supplied by the manufacturer to avoid the impression pulling out of the tray, but perforated trays can also be used. If adhesive is used, the dental nurse will apply this to the tray before mixing begins.

The setting time for the silicones is usually 4 minutes or more, so adequate moisture control by the dental nurse to maintain patient comfort is of great importance during this period. This is usually achieved by supporting a saliva ejector in the floor of the mouth while the impression sets.

Polyether impression material

These elastomer materials are highly accurate alternatives to silicone-based impression materials and have similar uses. Some operators use them as a personal preference for fixed prosthetic work.

They are presented as two pastes, which are usually different colours to ensure that uniform mixing occurs. They are mixed in equal proportions by spatulation on a waxed paper pad and then collected into special syringes for administration to the prepared tooth (Figure 9.29).

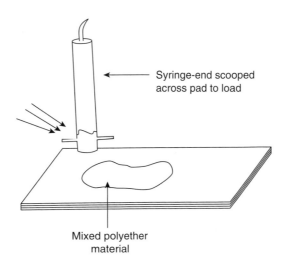

Syringe-end scooped across pad to load

Mixed polyether material

Figure 9.29   Polyether collection technique.

The remaining material is loaded into the impression tray. Again, adhesive is supplied by the manufacturer. They have a similar setting time to silicones but set more stiffly than other elastomers and therefore need to be removed with a sharp displacing action from the mouth, otherwise they can be difficult to remove.

Correct handling of impressions and other items

As all of the impressions taken, as well as the various stages of denture construction, have been inside the patient's mouth, they will obviously be contaminated by saliva and perhaps even blood. To avoid cross-infection from the patient to both staff and the technician, the impressions, bite rims and try-in items must be disinfected immediately after removal from the mouth.

Once set and removed from the mouth by the operator, impressions must be adequately disinfected and then wrapped, ready to be transferred to the laboratory, as follows:

- Rinsed under cold running water to remove any visible debris
- Fully immersed in a disinfectant bath of a recommended impression disinfectant, such as a solution of up to 10% sodium hypochlorite (bleach)
- Immersed for up to 10 minutes
- Rinsed under cold running water again, to remove the disinfectant solution
- Alginate impressions – covered with wet gauze and sealed in an air-tight bag
- Elastomer impressions – blown dry using the triple syringe and sealed in an air-tight bag
- All stored at room temperature or below before transportation to the laboratory
- Work ticket enclosed – detailing dentist, patient name and age, prosthesis to be constructed, material to be used, shade, additional features, date of delivery for fitting, disinfection details

The work ticket details should also be recorded onto the patient's record card or computer notes.

Intermediate stages of denture construction (rims and try-ins) are carefully disinfected in a similar manner, dried and then placed on to the working models and sealed within the air-tight bag. When wax stages of denture items are being handled, they must never be rinsed or immersed in warm water, as they will melt and distort.

Some dental workplaces use a sticky-label system to indicate to the technician that the item has been disinfected. Alternatively, this can just be written on to the work ticket and initialled by the dental nurse.

Mixing luting cements and temporary cements

At a fixed prosthesis fitting appointment, or the bonding of a fixed orthodontic appliance, various luting cements and materials are used which the dental nurse must mix correctly and assist the operator in applying to the teeth during the procedure.

At a fixed prosthesis preparation appointment, once the impressions have been taken, some type of temporary coverage of the prepared tooth or teeth must be placed, for the following reasons:

- To avoid sensitivity problems with the tooth/teeth
- To maintain the space around the prepared tooth/teeth for the fixed prosthesis to fit over accurately
- To maintain the occlusion between the prepared tooth/teeth and the opposing teeth, so that the fixed prosthesis will fit accurately
- For aesthetics

A temporary crown or bridge will require cementing to the teeth, an inlay preparation will require a temporary filling to be placed, and sometimes a veneer preparation will require a labial covering to improve the aesthetics anteriorly. Temporary crowns and bridges may be cemented with the same materials as those used for permanent prostheses and fixed orthodontic bands, or with specific temporary cement products such as Tempbond. This material is supplied as a two-tube paste system, which is simply mixed by spatulation in equal portions on a paper pad to an even colour and then loaded into the temporary prosthesis before applying to the tooth.

Those powder-liquid luting cements that actually require hand-mixing, such as zinc phosphate, must be done in such a way that produces a material of creamy consistency that can be applied to the inner surface of the prosthesis before it is placed on to the tooth, and that is thin enough to allow the full placement of the prosthesis before setting begins.

Zinc phosphate

Presented as zinc oxide powder and phosphoric acid liquid, the cement is prepared by mixing increments of the white powder to the clear liquid on a glass slab with a spatula (see Figure 8.19). Setting of the cement takes a few minutes depending on various factors:

- A warm slab accelerates the setting time
- A cold slab slows down the setting time
- A thick mix sets more quickly than a thin mix
- A dry slab must be used, as moisture accelerates setting
- Powder contaminated by moisture in the air will set too quickly for use, so it is most important to screw the cap on tightly, immediately after using the bottle of liquid

These various factors can be employed to advantage, depending on the particular use of the cement at the time. If a long setting time is required, such as when cementing a bridge, a cold dry slab can be used to give the maximum setting time possible, so that the cement can be loaded into each retainer and allow full positioning of the bridge before it begins to set.

This ability to control its setting time is the overriding advantage of zinc phosphate cement.

Experience soon teaches a dental nurse how much powder and liquid to set out, but occasionally too little or too much powder will be put on the slab. In the former case, more powder can be added from the bottle, but the mixing end of the spatula must not be used for this purpose as it will contaminate and spoil the whole bottle. Excess unused powder may only be returned to the bottle if you are certain that it has not been contaminated by any liquid or mixed cement on the slab.

A cool, thick glass slab should be used for mixing zinc phosphate cement. Thin slabs are warmed by the dental nurse's hand and can make the cement set too quickly.

Zinc polycarboxylate

This is presented as white zinc oxide powder and clear, viscous polyacrylic acid liquid, or as these two components combined in the powder and sterile water as liquid (see Figure 8.20). In each case, the cement is prepared by mixing increments of the powder with the liquid or sterile water on either a glass slab or a waxed paper pad, with a spatula. A measure is provided by the manufacturer for the exact measurement of each increment.

The advantage of using the anhydrous system with sterile water is that only one bottle of material is needed and there is no liquid to deteriorate, or to be used up too soon, or left over when the powder bottle is empty. Furthermore, as the polyacrylic acid liquid is viscous (thick and "gloopy" in consistency), it can be difficult to dispense from the bottle and also difficult to mix. Mixing with water is much easier and quicker.

Excess cement must be wiped off the spatula and instruments, before it fully sets, as it is difficult to remove by manual scrubbing and unlikely to be removed by the action of the ultrasonic bath.

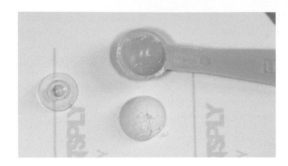

Figure 9.30   Glass ionomer powder, scoop and liquid.

Glass ionomers

These are composed of a powdered glass-like mixture of aluminosilicate particles and polyacrylic acid, which is measured accurately with a scoop and then mixed with water (Figure 9.30). As the material is adhesive to all tooth tissues, it is the preferred choice of hand-mixed luting cement of many operators. Glass ionomers are mixed by the same method as the zinc cements.

Light-cure and dual-cure materials

These luting cements are usually composed of a resin-based material, such as composite, and the prepared tooth must be chemically roughened before they are applied to improve the retention of the prosthesis. They are also used to bond the brackets of a fixed orthodontic appliance to the teeth, in a similar technique. The procedure is as follows:

- Once the prosthesis has been checked for the accuracy of its fit, shade and occlusion, the surface is blown dry with the triple syringe
- The dental nurse can apply a thin layer of primer to the inner surface of the prosthesis, which will then evaporate dry
- Acid etch is handed to the operator either in a gel syringe (see Figure 1.20) or in a well with an applicator, for application to the surface of the tooth
- After the required time, the etchant is washed off the tooth and aspirated away, and the tooth is dried
- Liquid resin is applied to the etched surface and made tacky by exposure to the curing light for about 10 seconds, ensuring that the orange shield is used to prevent eye damage to the operator and the dental nurse
- The luting material is then mixed and loaded into the fixed prosthesis or onto the back of the orthodontic bracket and carefully handed to the operator
- Once applied in the correct position on the tooth, the edges of the prosthesis are cured for the required time (usually around 40 seconds)
- Final checks and adjustments are made on the occlusion of the prosthesis using articulating paper and relevant burs, until the operator is satisfied

Monitoring and support of the patient

Throughout the whole procedure, the patient must be monitored and supported by the dental team, and this duty falls to the dental nurse in particular. Impression taking is a particularly unpleasant experience for many patients, and some may be so fearful that they feel nauseous beforehand. At other times, a wet sloppy mix of material, especially alginate, will drip off the back of the impression tray while in the mouth and actually cause the patient to vomit. Other patients do not find the procedure distressing in any way.

The dental nurse must remain calm, friendly and helpful throughout, by taking the following general actions:

- Providing support during mouth rinsing, including helping patients to avoid spillages once the local anaesthetic has been administered, and wiping their mouth as necessary
- Holding a patient's hand if requested to do so, and if it is possible (with particularly fearful patients, especially children, a second person may need to do this)
- Alerting the operator immediately if they suspect a patient can actually feel pain (see later)
- Constantly reassuring patients in a calm and even tone, and repeatedly encouraging them by saying phrases such as "You're doing really well"
- Avoiding the use of fearful phrases
- If patients feel nauseous, provide a bowl and tissues for them to use if necessary, holding the bowl for them and constantly reassuring them in a calm tone of voice
- It may be necessary to hold their hair out of the way too
- If a patient actually vomits, do not express distaste or annoyance – the patient will feel embarrassed enough without being shamed too
- Once the procedure is over, congratulating the patient and reassuring them again
- Wiping any blood and debris from a patient's face before discharge
- If they have vomited, ensuring that they are fully cleaned and made presentable before they leave the surgery
- Removing their PPE when it is safe to do so
- Assisting them from the surgery area when the operator indicates that they can leave

In particular, the dental nurse must constantly assess and monitor patients for pain during the procedure. Signs of pain could be grimacing, wincing or crying and should be pointed out to the operator if they have not noticed – this may be achieved by attracting the operator's attention out of sight of the patient, and quietly indicating the fact by facial expressions such as raising the eyebrows and dropping the eyes to the patient several times.

After the procedure

Once the procedure has been completed, patients will require various checks to be made before they are allowed to leave, as follows:

- Check that they have been sufficiently cleaned of blood and debris
- Check that they feel well enough to go home, especially if they felt ill during the impression stage
- Give the relevant oral hygiene instructions, especially when a new prosthesis or appliance has been provided
- Check whether the operator requires a further appointment to be made and organise the making of the appointment – this may involve notifying reception to make the appointment or actually making it while the patient is still present

Immediately after the procedure has been completed, all dirty PPE should be removed and placed in the hazardous waste sack. The dental nurse can then apply clean gloves to assist patients while they rinse out their mouths or spit out the contents, and then while their facial area is cleaned of all debris.

All the used instruments should be left in situ, either out of the patient's view or covered with disposable bibs until the patient has left the surgery. The dental nurse should escort patients to the oral health room or to reception, if the surgery is not used for oral health advice and making appointments.

The abilities required by a competent dental nurse to provide support after the procedure include the following:

- Provide oral hygiene instructions
- Hand over the patient to reception for discharge
- Complete the patient records
- Decontaminate the surgery and instruments

Provide oral hygiene instructions

232

Specific oral hygiene instructions must be given to every patient who has a fixed or removable prosthesis fitted, as well as to all orthodontic patients. Their regular, twice-daily manual brushing regime will not be adequate in the majority of cases to remove bacterial plaque and ensure that caries does not develop, especially if the diet is not good either.

Fixed prostheses

No matter how well-fitting the crown or bridge is to the tooth, microscopically the junction between the two is a potential stagnation area for plaque to gather. Thorough brushing at the margins of the crown will ensure that plaque does not accumulate and cause recurrent caries or periodontal problems.

The general oral health messages to be relayed to patients following crown or bridge cementation are as follows:

- Regular and thorough tooth brushing daily
- Use of fluoride toothpaste and a medium textured toothbrush
- Regular flossing to clean crown margins interproximally
- Careful use of floss so as not to dislodge the crown
- Attend for dental examinations so that margins can be checked professionally
- Sensible diet, low in non-milk extrinsic sugars
- Regular use of a good-quality mouthwash to reinforce plaque control

In addition, bridges provide a challenge to the patient with regard to adequate oral hygiene, as they are fixed prostheses producing stagnation areas actually beneath the pontics. As well as the oral hygiene instructions for crowns, patients with bridges need to be instructed in the use of "superfloss" (Figure 9.31). This is a type of dental floss with a stiff end, which can be threaded under the pontic by the patient, and then drawn through to a sponge part which is used to clean beneath the pontic. When used regularly, it keeps this region of the bridge plaque-free and prevents caries undermining the retainers, which would have catastrophic consequences.

More recently, sonic toothbrushes has been shown to provide excellent cleaning in these areas, without dislodging the bridge, and these are being recommended more frequently in these cases.

Removable prostheses

Instructions are given on the wear, care and cleaning of the new dentures, as follows:

- A demonstration of how to insert and remove the dentures is given, with the patient then practising the techniques in front of the mirror and under the operator's supervision
- Avoid wearing them overnight if possible, to avoid the development of oral fungal infections (thrush)
- Store them overnight in a denture pot containing water, or ideally a soaking agent such as Steradent (for all-acrylic dentures) or Dentural (for metal dentures)

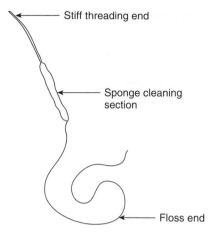

Figure 9.31   Superfloss.

- Clean after each meal if possible, using a denture brush and denture toothpaste – some ordinary toothpastes may be too abrasive for use on the acrylic teeth
- Clean over a bowl of water to avoid damage to the denture if it is dropped
- Avoid soaking in bleach-based cleansers if any metal components are included in the design
- Eat soft foods initially, while the oral soft tissues acclimatise to the prostheses
- Take time to chew foods thoroughly to avoid causing indigestion by swallowing large food particles
- Harden oral soft tissues by carrying out hot salt water mouthwashes initially, otherwise the new dentures are likely to rub the soft tissues and make them sore
- Return to the surgery if any ulceration occurs beneath the dentures, as further adjustments are likely to be required to remove high spots and deep flange edges
- Dentate patients must continue to attend for oral health assessment at their regular recall interval, and edentulous patients are advised to attend at least once every 2 years, but ideally annually

Orthodontic appliances
Patient advice for fixed appliances

Every tooth is incorporated into a fixed appliance, so the number of stagnation areas, and the potential for oral damage to occur, is far greater than for individual fixed prostheses. Routine twice-daily tooth brushing alone is insufficient to maintain adequate standards of good oral hygiene, and special instructions and techniques are recommended for patients undergoing fixed orthodontic therapy:

- Careful manual tooth brushing should be carried out after each meal
- Good quality electric toothbrushes, such as Sonicare and Oral B, may be safely used instead
- Use of fluoridated toothpaste
- Daily use of interdental brushes to clean around each bracket individually
- Avoidance of cariogenic and acidic food and drinks for the full period of treatment
- Avoidance of sticky foods for the full period of treatment
- Use of fluoride mouthwash daily to minimise the risk of decalcification
- Regular use of disclosing tablets to highlight problematic areas where plaque is being retained, in order to minimise the risk of decalcification

Patient advice for removable appliances

As with removable prostheses, orthodontic appliances are capable of acting as stagnation areas and of holding food debris and plaque against the teeth and gingivae, unless a good standard of oral hygiene is maintained.

Although some dentists prefer patients to wear appliances during meals, it is possible that more acrylic breakages will occur if this is the case. The instructions necessary for patients wearing removable appliances are as follows:

- Wear as directed by the dentist
- Clean the appliance and teeth after each meal, using a toothbrush and toothpaste
- Avoid cariogenic and acidic foods and drinks, as advised
- Attend all dental appointments for the necessary adjustments
- Contact the surgery immediately if there are any breakages or the appliance is lost
- Expect the appliance to feel tight initially after each adjustment
- Contact the surgery if any prolonged or excessive symptoms occur
- If the appliance is to be removed for meals, ensure it is placed safely in a rigid container to avoid breakages during mealtimes

The same oral hygiene advice is relevant to those patients fitted with a functional appliance, except that they must always remove their appliance before eating a meal.

Once the relevant oral hygiene advice has been given where necessary, the patient can be escorted to reception and handed over to the administration staff while a further appointment is made (if necessary) and then discharged.

Complete the patient records

Some operators prefer to write the patient records themselves, while others will dictate exactly what to write to the dental nurse. As with all records, they must be accurate, legible, avoid the use of any derogatory or slang terms, and refer only to accepted shorthand phrases that can be easily translated if necessary.

If the dental nurse is required to complete the records alone, they should be made available for the operator to check and then sign to say that this has been done – their accuracy is ultimately the responsibility of the operator. The issues of record-keeping and confidentiality are discussed in detail in Chapter 13.

The points that must be included in the records are:

- Written for the correct patient in the records, either on paper or on computer
- Date of procedure and date of writing (if different) – these will be recorded automatically on computer records
- Ideally completed on the day of the procedure, and as soon after its completion as possible
- Identify the operator and the dental nurse – this may be obvious in a small surgery setting, but less so in hospital departments and clinics
- Identify the procedure undertaken and the shade of any prosthesis to be constructed
- The charting must be updated to indicate the fitting of a permanent prosthesis (using the relevant charting notations as necessary – see Chapter 13)
- Note the local anaesthetic used and the number of cartridges (batch numbers tend to be recorded centrally rather than in every set of patient notes)
- Give a brief description of the procedure
- Record any shade taken, the luting cement used and whether a temporary prosthesis was placed
- Record any treatment complications accurately, where relevant – additional local anaesthetic used, patient ill with impression, and so on

- Record when the patient was notified of a problem, where relevant, such as any reason why a prosthesis was not completed, and indicate that the patient was informed of this event
- Record any major complications and their outcome, where relevant
- Record that oral hygiene instructions were given before discharge
- Record if another appointment was required and subsequently made
- Signed or initialled by the writer, when completed, and counter-signed by the operator as necessary – computer records can be set to indicate the writer automatically, but this relies on passwords to be accurate

Decontaminate the surgery and instruments

The aspects of infection control and health and safety that are relevant to surgery and equipment decontamination (especially cleaning methods), infection control and sterilisation are fully discussed in Chapters 4 and 12.

In summary, they are as follows:

- All sharps are carefully disposed of in the sharps box – this includes local anaesthetic needles
- All autoclavable items are placed in a washer-disinfector unit or an ultrasonic bath and are decontaminated thoroughly before being placed in the autoclave for sterilisation
- All contaminated waste is placed in hazardous waste sacks or sharps bins
- All surfaces are disinfected using the correct solution

235

10

Unit 310: Provide Chairside Support during Non-surgical Endodontic Treatment

Learning outcomes

1. Be able to prepare the clinical environment for non-surgical endodontic procedures
2. Be able to assist the operator during non-surgical endodontic procedures

Outcome 1 assessment criteria

The learner can:

- Provide the necessary patient's charts, records and images
- Correctly identify the planned treatment
- Select the correct equipment, instruments, materials and medicaments for the different stages of endodontic treatment
- List the different equipment, instruments, materials and medicaments that may be required at each stage of non-surgical endodontic treatment
- List the different materials used in sealing, filling and restoration of the root canal
- List the equipment and instruments that may be required for the isolation of a tooth for non-surgical endodontic treatment

Diploma in Dental Nursing, Level 3, Third Edition. Carole Hollins.
© 2014 John Wiley & Sons, Ltd. Published 2014 by John Wiley & Sons, Ltd.
Companion website: www.wiley.com/go/hollins/dentalnursinglevel3

Outcome 2 assessment criteria
The learner can:
- Assist the operator and support the patient during isolation of the tooth
- Aspirate the treatment area, maintaining a clear field of operation
- Provide equipment and medicaments required for irrigating root canals
- Assist the operator in the measurement and recording of the root canal length
- Correctly prepare materials and medicaments for either temporary or permanent placement in the canals
- List the equipment, instruments, materials and medicaments that may be required during each type of non-surgical endodontic treatment, and their uses

This unit is assessed by:
- observation in the workplace, with examples included in the learner's portfolio
- an appropriate alternative method

Details of various elements of theory and underpinning knowledge are included in Chapter 15, and these are assessed within the written paper.

237

The theory and underpinning knowledge required to understand the scientific principles involved in the management of oral diseases and dental procedures, including non-surgical endodontic techniques, are fully discussed in Chapter 15. This chapter explains the dental nurse's role and responsibilities in relation to these procedures before, during and after they are carried out. Those responsibilities are to the operator (the person carrying out the procedure – usually the dentist, but in some cases it may be the therapist) and also to the patient who is undergoing the procedure, and the patient's guardian where relevant.

Many patients expect that endodontic treatment is a painful procedure, but there is no reason why it should be any more painful than other dental procedures. Nevertheless, some patients will be fearful at the prospect of this treatment and a huge part of the dental nurse's role at these times is to be calming, friendly and supportive, and to anticipate the concerns and needs of the patient throughout the procedure.

Before the procedure

The vast majority of dental workplaces operate on one appointments system or another, so that the working day can be correctly planned and all of the necessary instruments, materials and equipment are known to be available as required. There would be little point in a patient attending for an endodontic procedure, for example, if the workplace had run out of files or paper points. Forward planning is therefore a key element in the successful completion of a busy working day and, along with the skills in the following list, is among the abilities required by a competent dental nurse to provide successful chairside support for non-surgical endodontic procedures:

- Correct identification of the patient
- Correct identification of the procedure
- Knowledge of the records and images required by the operator for the procedure
- Knowledge of the correct setting up of the area for the procedure
- Knowledge of the instruments, materials and equipment that may be required for the procedure
- Knowledge of the actions to take if the dental nurse is unable to fully prepare for the procedure

Correct identification of the patient

The day list will refer to each patient attending that day by name and/or date of birth and/or address, and/ or some kind of patient identification marker – such as a unique computer number or the patient's NHS number.

Whatever the system in place, the dental nurse should be familiar with it and be able to access the patient's records so that a cross-reference check can be made between the notes and the expected procedure to be carried out. So if the notes refer to a tooth to be extracted but the day list indicates that the patient is attending for a first-stage endodontic procedure , one of the following scenarios has occurred which must be checked with the operator and the patient before the procedure begins:

- The records and the day list entry are for two different patients
- The records are incomplete and a change in treatment has been decided without being recorded
- The records are correct and the day list entry is incorrect
- The records are incorrect and the day list entry is correct

Any of these scenarios could quite easily have occurred and the matter should be referred to a more senior colleague (ideally the operator concerned) so that the dental nurse can assist in determining the way forward – to identify the correct patient and the correct procedure to be carried out that day.

The records required may be hard copies in full (i.e. a "pack" of handwritten patient notes, with paper copies of their medical history, previous treatment plans and consent forms, and so on) or they may be fully computerised and only accessible "on screen", or a combination of the two. Whatever their presentation, they should be collected by the dental nurse and presented in the treatment area so that the operator can access them and check their content too.

In large dental workplaces, such as dental schools and hospitals, the dental nurse can check the correct patient identity by asking patients to confirm their name, date of birth and address and that they know why they are attending on the day. The final decision to confirm the patient's identity is the duty of the operator.

In smaller workplaces, many of the patients are recognisable to the staff by sight – some may even be known by their first names – but identity and procedure checks should still always be carried out to avoid any mishaps. Once the patient has been correctly identified, the records and treatment area can be prepared.

The records to be set out will include the following:

- Notes written at the previous appointment or when the decision was made to carry out the particular procedure – these will remind the operator of the reasons for the treatment decisions taken
- Medical history form, to be checked to highlight any potential concerns – for example, is a certain local anaesthetic required, or does the patient have an allergy to latex?
- Consent form, indicating that the patient has given valid consent to the procedure (see Chapter 13)
- Radiographs of the relevant tooth – these will allow the operator to plan the procedure and the technique used and to show any potential difficulties such as curved roots or lateral canals on the tooth involved

The dental nurse can also access the records for the following purposes:

- The notes may refer to the patient's level of anxiety, so the dental nurse is aware of the heightened need to be supportive and helpful to the patient throughout the procedure – the issue should also be pointed out to the operator
- The medical history can be checked and any recognised potential issues pointed out to the operator

- Patients can also be asked to confirm if there have been any changes to their medical history since they were last seen, and these are then recorded appropriately and pointed out to the operator
- The consent form can be checked to ensure it covers the planned procedure and that it has been signed and dated by the patient, or that it requires to be signed and dated by the patient today – any discrepancies can be pointed out to the operator
- The radiographs must be correctly displayed to show the tooth under treatment, either as digital images on the computer or as hard copies on film
- Hard copies must be correctly mounted on the viewing screen:
  ○ Intra-oral views with the pimple facing out (to indicate left from right), and upper teeth with their roots above the crown and lower teeth with their roots below the crown (see Figure 7.13)
  ○ Extra-oral views with the "L" marker in the bottom right-hand corner of the radiograph as it is positioned on the viewing screen, to indicate the patient's left side (see Figure 8.1)

239

Correct identification of the procedure

The patient is attending for one of the procedures in the list that follows – the actual one should be referred to in the notes and on the day list (although some computer software systems are not programmed to allow individual procedures to be booked – they just record a time slot as a "root filling" procedure).

Endodontics is the term used for all forms of root canal therapy and many dental personnel often refer to it as "RCT" or even as "root filling". Non-surgical endodontic treatment includes the following three procedures:

- Pulpectomy – conventional root canal therapy, involving the removal of all the pulp from the tooth and its replacement with a root-filling material
- Pulpotomy – removal of the coronal pulp only, leaving the radicular pulp intact
- Pulp capping – sealing of a small coronal pulp exposure, with no removal of pulp contents

The reasons for carrying out each procedure are discussed in detail in Chapter 15.

The records and images required by the operator in order to carry out the procedure are detailed in the preceding section.

Knowledge of the correct setting up of the area

As with all dental procedures, the treatment area (surgery) must be clean before being set up for a non-surgical endodontic session, and left in a similar condition afterwards, to avoid any possibility of cross-infection occurring. The principles of infection control are discussed in detail in Chapter 12.

Before the surgery is prepared for use, dental nurses must ensure that they do not inadvertently introduce any contamination into the area, and so must undertake the correct hand washing technique before applying the correct personal protective equipment (PPE). As a clinical procedure is to be carried out, the appropriate hand washing technique is as follows:

- Turn on the tap using the foot or elbow control, to prevent contamination of the tap (see Figure 4.4)
- Wet both hands under running water of a suitable temperature
- Apply a suitable antibacterial liquid soap from the dispenser (Figure 8.2) and wash all areas of both hands and wrists thoroughly – this should take at least 30 seconds to carry out thoroughly, and the correct routine is illustrated on the poster that is present at each hand washing station (see Figure 1.3)
- Nail brushes are not advised unless they are autoclavable, as they can become contaminated with repeated use

- Rinse both hands under running water, holding them so that the water does not flow back over the fingers
- Dry the hands thoroughly, using disposable paper towels for single use

The equipment and instruments can now be handled safely, unless the dental nurse has any cuts or abrasions on the hands, in which case the lesion should be covered with a waterproof dressing and a pair of clinical gloves must be worn before any items are handled.

The surgery itself is then made ready as follows:

- The electric and water supplies should be switched on to all static equipment (dental chair, suction unit, etc.) if this has not already been done
- Any portable items not likely to be required for the procedure should be placed in cupboards or drawers, or removed from the surgery, so that the work surfaces are clear of any clutter
- The controls of any large equipment items which are likely to be contaminated during the procedure must be protected by a barrier technique, including:
  - Dental chair controls, if not foot-operated
  - Dental light controls and handles (see Figure 8.3)
  - Computer keyboard, if various screens are in use
  - Bracket table handles and controls
- In some surgery settings, the aspirator pipes and handpiece tubing may also require barrier protection if they are of a design that makes them difficult to wipe down thoroughly (such as corrugated piping)
- The patient records are accessed on the computer, or the paper copies are laid out on an area of the work surface away from the surgical field (to minimise their contamination)
- Relevant radiographs are correctly mounted on the viewing screen, in easy reach of the operator
- PPE is laid out ready for the patient, the operator and the dental nurse:
  - Protective glasses, disposable bib, tissues – for the patient
  - Protective glasses or visor, face mask, gloves – for the operator and dental nurse
- Mouth rinse and cup are made ready for the patient
- Suitable aspirator tips are connected to the suction unit; both a wide-bore and a finer surgical tip should be available
- The correct local anaesthetic equipment and materials are laid out for use, in easy reach of the operator and dental nurse, and covered with a disposable bib until the patient is seated:
  - Topical anaesthetic and cotton wool rolls (where relevant)
  - Syringe (aspirating type if a nerve block is likely)
  - Short or long needle (depending on which tooth is involved)
  - Local anaesthetic cartridges
  - Re-sheathing device
- The local anaesthetic solution should be checked by the operator for suitability before use
- The correct instruments are laid out for the procedure (see later), in easy reach of the operator and the dental nurse, and covered with a disposable bib until the patient is seated:
  - If they are stored within an enclosed tray system, the lid should be replaced once the tray has been checked for all items present
  - If they are within sterile pouches, these should remain sealed until just before their use
- Single-use items, materials and medicaments should be gathered together and made ready for use, and covered with a disposable bib until the patient is seated:
  - Paper points
  - Gutta-percha points
  - Canal medicaments
  - Mixing pad/block and spatula
  - Restorative materials, where relevant

Knowledge of the instruments, materials and equipment required

Pulpectomy

This is the non-surgical endodontic procedure carried out to try and save a fully formed permanent tooth from extraction, once it has suffered from irreversible pulpitis. The procedure is carried out in one or more stages, depending on the level of any infection present associated with the tooth, and on the operator's preference – some operators prefer to complete the full procedure in one appointment; others prefer to remove the pulp contents and dress the tooth at the first appointment, and then complete the root-filling procedure at a second appointment. Familiarity with each operator's preference will allow the dental nurse to set up the surgery accordingly.

The specific root canal therapy instruments required are usually kept together in a lidded tray, with the various instruments likely to come into contact with the pulp (such as broaches and files) being replaced after each use, as single-use items. The various instruments and their particular functions are described in the following table.

Item	Function
Broach	Plain broach to help locate the entrance to each root canal Barbed broach (Figure 10.1a) to remove (extirpate) the pulpal contents from the canal
Gates Glidden drill (Figure 10.2)	Alternative to a plain broach to locate and access the root canal entrance. Some operators also use them to enlarge the root canal
Reamer (Figure 10.1b)	Hand or rotary – to enlarge the root canals in a circular shape laterally, down to the root apex
File (Figure 10.1c)	Hand or rotary – to enlarge the canal in its actual shape laterally, smooth the root canal walls, and remove any residual debris from them
Irrigation syringe (Figure 10.3)	Blunt-ended with a side bevel, to irrigate and wash out debris from the root canal without injecting the syringe contents through the root apex. Solutions used include chlorhexidine, sodium hypochlorite and local anaesthetic solution
Metal ruler	Used with a file in place, to work out the full length of each root canal by comparing to a periapical radiograph view of the tooth to the established working length
Apex locater (Figure 10.4)	To determine the working length electronically
Spiral paste filler (Figure 10.1d)	Used with the slow dental handpiece to spin sealant material into the root canal
Lateral condenser, or finger spreader (Figure 10.5)	Used to condense the root-filling points laterally into each root canal, so there is no space remaining for microorganisms to return. Not required if root-filling material used is inserted while hot and flowable

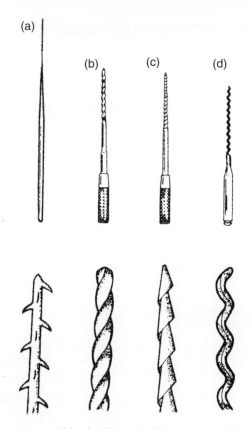

Figure 10.1   Endodontic instruments: (a) barbed broach; (b) reamer; (c) file; (d) spiral paste filler. Source: *Levison's Textbook for Dental Nurses*, 11th edition (Hollins), 2013. Reproduced with permission of Wiley-Blackwell.

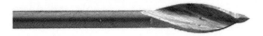

Figure 10.2   A Gates Glidden drill. Source: *Levison's Textbook for Dental Nurses*, 11th edition (Hollins), 2013. Reproduced with permission of Wiley-Blackwell.

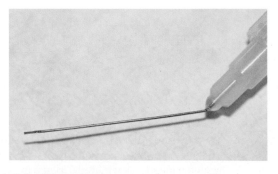

Figure 10.3   An endodontic irrigation syringe.

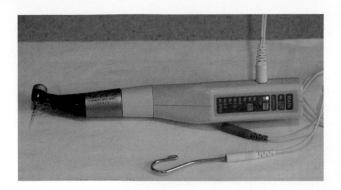

Figure 10.4   An apex locator.

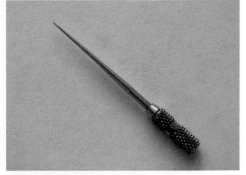

Figure 10.5   A finger spreader.

243

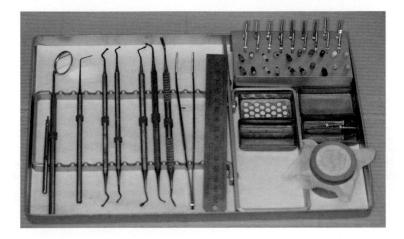

Figure 10.6   An endodontic instrument tray.

In addition, a routine conservation tray will also be required, although these instruments are often also present within the lidded endodontic kit (Figure 10.6).

Many operators also carry out root canal therapy under rubber dam, to provide isolation of the tooth and prevent further contamination of the pulp chamber with microorganisms. The rubber dam kit (see Figure 9.9) contains the items shown in the following table, which also outlines their function.

Item	Function
Rubber dam sheet	A sheet of latex (green) or non-latex (purple or blue) rubber-like material that is used to separate the tooth from the rest of the oral cavity. It is impervious to water and other irrigant solutions, and to blood, and is available on a roll as well as in separate square sheets
Rubber dam punch	The instrument used to punch a hole through the rubber dam so that the tooth undergoing the procedure is visible to the operator. It has a dial device which allows the size of the hole to be varied – e.g. that required for a molar tooth will be much larger than that for an incisor

Item	Function
Clamps	Various shaped metal gripping devices which are placed around the tooth to hold the dam tightly in place, so that the tooth is kept isolated from the rest of the mouth. There are molar and premolar designs, as well as a "butterfly" clamp for use on anterior teeth. The "wings" of this clamp hold the dam material well away from the narrow anterior teeth and give better visibility to the operator
Clamp forceps	This instrument is used to hold the clamp securely while it is placed over the tooth with the dam material beneath it. The blades are inserted into holes on the arms of the clamp, and as the forceps handles are squeezed, the clamp is opened. Once in position on the tooth, the forceps are disengaged and the clamp springs shut around the tooth
Rubber dam frame	A plastic or metal U-shaped frame which holds the dam material taut across the oral cavity, so that the tooth remains isolated and any irrigation fluids can be collected more easily

The materials and medicaments used throughout root canal therapy treatments are as follows:

- **Irrigation solution** – used during root canal preparation to lubricate the instruments and wash out any debris; the solution used is an individual choice among sodium hypochlorite (bleach), chlorhexidine (although some patients may be allergic to this prodcut) and a local anaesthetic solution
- **Antiseptic paste** – non-setting and containing antiseptic anti-inflammatories, this paste is used to dress infected root canals for a time before root filling – an example is Ledermix paste (Figure 10.7)
- **Paper points** – tapered paper points of various diameters that are used to absorb unwanted moisture from within the root canal and to apply medicaments into the canal (Figure 10.8)
- **Cresophene** – medical grade creosote used to dress infected root canals for a time, soaked onto paper points before insertion (Figure 10.9)
- **Lubricating gel** – for use with engine files and reamers (those used with a handpiece) to ensure the instruments do not snag on the canal walls and snap during use – an example is Glyde (Figure 10.10)

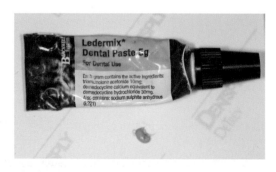

Figure 10.7   Ledermix paste.

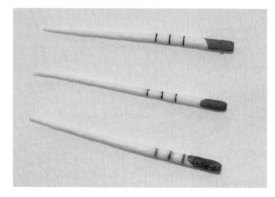

Figure 10.8   Paper points.

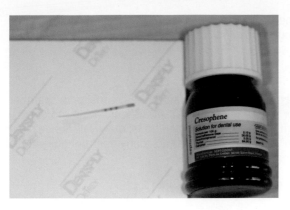

Figure 10.9   Cresophene antiseptic solution.

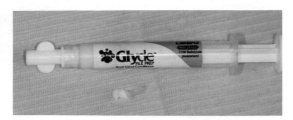

Figure 10.10   Glyde lubricant.

245

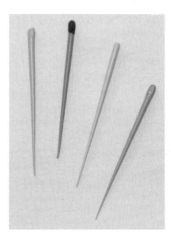

Figure 10.11   Gutta-percha points.

- **Gutta-percha points (GP points)** – tapered rubber points of various diameters that are used to fill (obturate) the root canal system and that follow the same colour-coded width system as files and reamers (Figure 10.11) – so if a "red" (size 25) file or reamer is used as the final canal preparation instrument, then a red GP point must be used to obturate the root canal
- **Sealing cement** – setting cement used to aid the insertion of the GP points and to seal off any residual spaces in the root canal, some contain antiseptics and anti-inflammatories
- **Restorative materials** – used to restore the tooth to full function and appearance after root filling

Pulpotomy

This is a non-surgical endodontic procedure carried out on vital permanent teeth that still have an open apex, because they are recently erupted. The very rich blood supply through an open apex allows healing to occur when the coronal pulp chamber has been breached by caries. So the radicular pulp (within the root) survives once the caries has been treated, and root growth continues to its natural completion. Therefore, pulpotomy involves the removal of the coronal pulp only and this can be carried out using sterile routine conservation instruments (such as an excavator) rather than specialised endodontic instruments.

The only additional material required for the technique is a calcium hydroxide lining material, which is placed over the top of the radicular pulp and allowed to set before being covered with a base material and then a permanent restorative material.

Pulp capping

This technique is performed when an unexpected pinprick exposure of the coronal pulp chamber occurs, either following injury to the tooth or during conservation treatment. Again, no special endodontic instruments are required to carry it out, and the only additional materials are calcium hydroxide liner and a device to act as the "cap" over the exposure site. Many operators use items such as a section of a glass ionomer class V matrix for this purpose.

Knowledge of the actions to take if preparation cannot be completed

If any instruments, materials or items of equipment are not readily available for use immediately before the procedure is scheduled to start, the dental nurse must report the matter to an appropriate person immediately. This may be the operator, a senior dental nurse (or line manager) or the practice manager.

In smaller dental workplaces, if just one set of endodontic or rubber dam equipment and instruments is available for use by several operators, it is the responsibility of reception or administration staff to ensure that similar procedures are not booked at the same time. However, in the unlikely event that a double booking has occurred, the operator and the administration staff must be informed immediately, before the patient undergoes any initial part of the procedure, as the appointment may have to be postponed and rebooked.

The final preparation that the dental nurse must carry out is to check with the patient that any prescribed pre-treatment instructions have been followed correctly. In particular, the following points should be clarified:

- Have all routine medications been taken as requested, including any prescribed antibiotics?
- If the procedure is being carried out under any form of conscious sedation technique, has the patient complied with all of the relevant additional points as requested?
- If the patient is a child or a vulnerable adult, are they in attendance with a suitable adult escort, to look after and see them safely home after the procedure?
- If the patient is frail or excessively nervous, are they in attendance with a suitable adult escort for the same purpose?
- Has the patient (or guardian) read and understood any pre-treatment information provided – are there any further questions?
- Has the patient (or guardian) been given enough information to provide valid consent for the procedure, and has that consent been given?

When it becomes apparent that one or more of these points have not been followed, the dental nurse must report the matter to the operator immediately, and allow them to discuss the situation further with the patient. It is not the role of dental nurses to act beyond their level of competence by making unilateral decisions about any of these issues – the responsibility lies with the operator.

During the procedure

Usually, the dental nurse will collect patients (and their guardians where relevant) from the reception area and escort them to the surgery, rather than the operator. The dental nurse should be welcoming and friendly towards patients (and guardians) and use the time to put them at their ease.

With experience, dental nurses will develop their communication skills and their own style of patter that they can use successfully, and patients will respond positively to a good dental nurse with obvious empathy to their situation. Communication skills are discussed in detail in Chapter 5, and the skills of reflection and developing one's own self in practice are discussed in Chapter 2.

The abilities required by a competent dental nurse to provide support during the procedure include the following:

- Preparation of the patient
- Assistance during the administration of local anaesthesia, where necessary
- Assistance during the placement of rubber dam, where necessary
- Identification and correct handling of the instruments, materials and equipment throughout the procedure
- Adequate provision of moisture control and tissue retraction throughout the procedure, where necessary
- Monitoring and support of the patient

Although forward planning of the procedure should avoid the possibility, it may be necessary for the dental nurse to retrieve unprepared instruments and items during the procedure, especially if an unexpected pulp exposure occurs. If so, then gloves must be removed and replaced with a new pair each time the surgical area is left and re-accessed.

Preparation of the patient

A final check is made by the operator of the patient's identification and consent to undergo the procedure. The dental nurse will then assist patients into the dental chair, and ready them for the treatment start as follows:

- Help them to remove their coat if necessary and hang it up
- Assist them into the dental chair – they may need physical support, for example, or the chair raising or lowering
- Apply their required PPE:
  - Safety glasses – these need to be tinted if the curing light is to be used to set materials
  - Protective bib
  - Some patients like to have a tissue in hand too
- Monitor the patient for signs of anxiety, and notify the operator as necessary
- Reassure the patient in a calm and friendly manner – many appreciate the opportunity of a hand to hold at this point, although this action can be passed to an escort/guardian if appropriate

Assistance during the administration of local anaesthesia

Local anaesthetic will usually be required for non-surgical endodontic procedures, unless the tooth is definitely non-vital. Even then, some patients may prefer to have local anaesthetic administered anyway as an assurance that they will feel no pain, so that they can relax fully during the procedure. The operator and the dental nurse apply their own PPE (safety glasses/visor, face mask, gloves).

The disposable cover used to hide the items while patients enter and settle in the dental chair is removed from the equipment, and the operator must check that the correct items and local anaesthetic are prepared. The topical anaesthetic is applied to a cotton wool roll and handed to

247

the operator for application in the patient's mouth. While this takes effect, the syringe is loaded ready for use, quietly and out of sight of the patient:

- Noisy clattering of metallic items can be particularly unnerving for patients, so items must be handled proficiently at all times
- The local anaesthetic cartridge is loaded into the syringe correctly, with the cap end at the bottom where the needle will be applied
- If an aspirating technique is to be used, any screw-in plunger is locked into the cartridge bung before the needle is added
- The needle is screwed on to the threaded end of the syringe, with the guard in place
- On removal of the topical anaesthetic, the needle guard is loosened but left over the needle and the loaded syringe is offered to the operator (see Figure 8.16)
- As the operator receives the syringe, the dental nurse keeps hold of the loosened needle guard so that it becomes unsheathed as it is transferred over
- The guard is then placed in the re-sheathing device, ready for the operator when the anaesthetic procedure is completed (see Figure 1.29)
- Successive cartridges are handed to the operator as required during the administration procedure
- When the administration is complete, the equipment is re-sheathed by the operator without being handled by the dental nurse (this avoids increasing the likelihood of an inoculation injury)

Assistance during the placement of rubber dam

The rubber dam kit is usually kept in a lidded tray, and the items should be separated out so that they can be picked up more easily. Many operators apply rubber dam without any assistance from the dental nurse, while others will require the hole to be punched and perhaps the clamp forceps to be loaded. Once the dam is successfully in place on the tooth, the dental nurse may assist in applying it to the dam frame and passing additional items such as floss to ensure the tooth is fully exposed (see Figure 9.25).

Some operators prefer to have a saliva ejector placed in the floor of the patient's mouth once the rubber dam is in place.

Identification and correct handling of the instrument

The pulpectomy, pulpotomy and pulp capping procedures are described in detail in Chapter 15.

Conservation trays and endodontic kits are usually kept as pre-set loaded trays, which simply require the lids removing before use and placing within easy reach of the operator and the dental nurse. Items that are stored separately in pouches can be opened and placed on the tray with the other items before treatment begins.

The specialist endodontic instruments tend to be used in the order listed earlier, and a conventional one-stage pulpectomy would proceed as follows:

- The tooth is **isolated** from the rest of the mouth, usually by the application of rubber dam, but good aspiration and the use of cotton wool rolls will also suffice in some cases
- **Access** is gained to the pulp chamber, either through the occlusal surface of a posterior tooth or the palatal/lingual surface of an anterior tooth, using the air turbine handpiece and appropriate diamond burs
- The root canal entrance is opened, using the slow handpiece and stainless steel burs or a Gates Glidden drill, and the pulp tissue is located using a plain broach or the drill
- Pulp tissue is **extirpated** using a barbed broach
- The root canal is debrided and widened using files and/or reamers, and **prepared** to receive the root filling

- Copious **irrigation and lubrication** are used to avoid the possibility of fine instruments becoming jammed and then snapping within the canal
- The canal is dried thoroughly using paper points
- An apex locator or a diagnostic radiograph is used to determine the correct **measurement** of the root canal length to be filled
- Once this is known and the canal has been suitably widened, it is fully **obturated** using GP points and a suitable sealant material
- The sealant material can be spun into the canal using a spiral paste filler, or the points can be coated first and then inserted into the canal
- Occasionally, silver points are used instead of GP, but these can only be used successfully in straight canals as they will not follow root curvature
- The access cavity is sealed with a conventional filling material so that the tooth is **restored** to its normal function

Some operators use engine-driven files and reamers in special endodontic handpieces or dual-purpose apex locators, and the dental nurse may be tasked with loading these with the appropriate file or reamer. Some operators also prefer to have the dental nurse passing items such as paper points and GP points directly to them, rather than picking them up individually themselves. If so, they should be passed safely using a second pair of tweezers and held onto until the operator has a firm hold on the item.

During the procedure, the canal will require regular irrigation and while some operators use local anaesthetic solution for this, others will require a solution such as chlorhexidine or sodium hypochlorite to be drawn up into the irrigation syringe. These solutions should be ready for use, in a suitable pot for drawing up by the dental nurse, as required.

When the operator has finished with an instrument, its either placed back on the tray or should be safely passed back to the dental nurse, who receives it and places it on the tray. During the procedure, the dental nurse is likely also to be aspirating and retracting soft tissues, so the receiving and passing of instruments too will require the use of both hands. Experience will improve this ability with time, but all members of the dental team must develop a routine of never passing items across the patient's face while performing instrument transfer – it only takes one dropped item to permanently scar or blind a patient.

When liquid medicaments such as cresophene are in use, a few drops may be placed on a waxed paper pad or into a plastic well so that the bottles do not require repeat opening and closing by the dental nurse. Pastes and cements should not be set out ready for mixing until their use is imminent, so that they are not exposed to any potential aerosol contamination.

Paste-type sealant materials are used ready mixed from their tube, as necessary, while those medicaments presented as a powder and liquid require conventional spatulation and mixing before their use, using either a glass slab or a waxed paper pad and a spatula.

When any items are handled that are not disposable or able to be sterilised after the procedure, such as bottles and lids, the dental nurse must remove and replace any contaminated gloves to do so. Similarly, when a diagnostic radiograph is required during the procedure, gloves must be changed before and after it is exposed and processed, as necessary.

Once the working length of the root canal has been determined, the dental nurse may be required to pre-set the rubber stops on the canal hand instruments to the correct length, measuring them accurately with the ruler present in the endodontic kit. If a single-stage pulpectomy technique is carried out, the dental nurse will also assist during the restoration of the tooth once the root filling has been placed, in the normal way.

The pulpotomy and pulp capping procedures are less complicated, with the dental nurse assisting in the following ways:

- Good moisture control to avoid contamination of the exposure site with saliva, especially if the operator is working without rubber dam
- Provision and passing of sterile cotton wool balls (pledgets) which are applied to the root canal stump or the exposure site to control bleeding

- Some operators use these soaked in local anaesthetic solution to take advantage of the vaso-constrictor in achieving haemostasis
- Mixing of calcium hydroxide paste to seal the pulp stump, and use of the curing light to set the material where necessary
- Assistance with placing the "cap" device over the exposure site, during pulp capping
- Mixing of base material and assistance in its application
- Assistance during the restoration of the tooth

Adequate provision of moisture control and tissue retraction

When rubber dam is in place for non-surgical endodontic procedures, adequate moisture control and tissue retraction are far easier to achieve for the dental nurse, as the tooth is isolated from the rest of the mouth by the dam. Any handpiece water or canal irrigation fluid can easily be aspirated away by the use of the wide-bore suction tip as it is held against the exposed tooth.

During the procedure the dental nurse will be expected to use the relevant instruments and equipment correctly, to assist the operator in the following techniques:

- **Moisture control** – removal of moisture (saliva, blood, irrigation solution) from the operative area so that adequate vision is possible by the operator and so that the patient is not choking on a mouthful of fluid, using:
  - Wide-bore aspirator for fast fluid removal, as well as some soft tissue retraction
  - Saliva ejector beneath the rubber dam, which may need repositioning from time to time
  - Use of cotton wool rolls and pledgets for precise moisture control around and within the tooth
- **Irrigation** – from the air turbine handpiece during the pulp access procedure, to avoid heat damage to the tooth, as well as irrigation of the root canal during instrumentation
- **Tissue retraction** – to avoid damage to the soft tissues from burs and drills, and to provide good vision for the operator, using:
  - Flanged wide-bore aspirator tips to retract the cheek, lips or tongue
  - Special cheek retractors, although these tend to be reserved for extraction and minor oral surgery procedures
  - Mouth mirror to retract the tongue or lips, and to reflect light and thus illuminate the operative field
  - If rubber dam is in place, the need for tissue retraction is greatly reduced

Retraction of any soft tissues for any prolonged length of time can be quite tiring for the dental nurse, and if they need to stop for a rest or to reposition the retractor, the operator must be fore-warned so that they do not continue drilling or cutting as the soft tissues collapse across the operative field.

Monitoring and support of the patient

Throughout the whole procedure, the patient must be monitored and supported by the dental team, and this duty falls to the dental nurse in particular. The dental nurse must remain calm, friendly and helpful throughout, by taking the following general actions:

- Providing support during mouth rinsing, including helping patients to avoid spillages once the local anaesthetic has been administered, and wiping their mouth as necessary
- Holding a patient's hand if requested to do so, and if it is possible (with particularly fearful patients, especially children, a second person may need to carry out this duty)

- Alerting the operator immediately if they suspect a patient can actually feel pain (see later)
- Constantly reassuring patients in a calm and even tone, and repeatedly encouraging them by saying phrases such as "You're doing really well"
- Avoiding the use of fearful phrases
- Once the procedure is over, congratulating the patient and reassuring them again
- Wiping any blood and debris from a patient's face before discharge
- Removing their PPE when it is safe to do so
- Assisting them from the surgery area when the operator indicates that they can leave

In particular, the dental nurse must constantly assess and monitor patients for pain during the procedure. Signs of pain could be grimacing, wincing or crying and should be pointed out to the operator if they have not noticed – this may be achieved by attracting the operator's attention out of sight of the patient and quietly indicating the fact by facial expressions such as raising the eyebrows and dropping the eyes to the patient several times.

After the procedure

Once the procedure has been completed, patients will require various checks to be made before they are allowed to leave, as follows:

- Check that they have been sufficiently cleaned of blood and debris
- Check that they feel well enough to go home
- Give the relevant postoperative instructions if requested to do so, in relation to allowing the local anaesthetic to wear off and avoiding the use of the tooth as necessary
- Check whether the operator requires a further appointment to be made, and organise the making of the appointment – this may involve notifying reception to make the appointment or actually making it while the patient is still present

Immediately after the procedure has been completed, all dirty PPE should be removed and placed in the hazardous waste sack. The dental nurse can then apply clean gloves to assist patients while they rinse out their mouths or spit out the contents, and then while their facial area is cleaned of all debris.

All the used instruments should be left in situ, either out of the patient's view or covered with disposable bibs until the patient has left the surgery. The dental nurse should escort patients to the reception area if the surgery is not used for making appointments.

The abilities required by a competent dental nurse to provide support after the procedure include the following:

- Hand over the patient to reception for discharge
- Complete the patient records
- Decontaminate the surgery and instruments

Complete the patient records

Some operators prefer to write the patient records themselves, while others will dictate exactly what to write to the dental nurse. As with all records, they must be accurate, legible, avoid the use of any derogatory or slang terms, and refer only to accepted shorthand phrases that can be easily translated if necessary.

If the dental nurse is required to complete the records alone, they should be made available for the operator to check and then sign to say that this has been done – their accuracy is ultimately the responsibility of the operator. The issues of record-keeping and confidentiality are discussed in detail in Chapter 13.

The points that must be included in the records are:

- Written for the correct patient in their records, either on paper or on computer
- Date of procedure and date of writing (if different) – these will be recorded automatically on computer records
- Ideally completed on the day of the procedure, and as soon after its completion as possible
- Identify the operator and the dental nurse – this may be obvious in a small surgery setting, but less so in hospital departments and clinics
- Identify the procedure undertaken
- The charting must be updated to indicate the completion of a root filling and restoration (using the relevant charting notations as necessary – see Chapter 13)
- Note the local anaesthetic used and the number of cartridges (batch numbers tend to be recorded centrally rather than in every set of patient notes)
- Give a brief description of the procedure
- Record the number of canals involved, their individual working lengths, the size of point used to obturate each and the sealant material used
- Record any treatment complications accurately, where relevant – additional local anaesthetic used, difficulty accessing a canal, presence of a pulp stone, and so on
- Record when the patient was notified of a problem, where relevant, such as any reason why the procedure was not completed, and indicate that the patient was informed of this event
- Record any major complications and their outcome, where relevant
- Record if another appointment was required and subsequently made
- Signed or initialled by the writer, when completed, and counter-signed by the operator as necessary – computer records can be set to indicate the writer automatically, but this relies on passwords to be accurate

Decontaminate the surgery and instruments

The aspects of infection control and health and safety that are relevant to surgery and equipment decontamination (especially cleaning methods), infection control and sterilisation are fully discussed in Chapters 4 and 12.

In summary, they are as follows:

- All sharps are carefully disposed of in the sharps box – this includes local anaesthetic needles and all endodontic hand instruments that may have come into contact with pulp tissue
- All autoclavable items are placed in a washer-disinfector unit or an ultrasonic bath and are decontaminated thoroughly before being placed in the autoclave for sterilisation
- All contaminated waste is placed in hazardous waste sacks or sharps bins
- All surfaces are disinfected using the correct solution

252

11

Unit 311: Provide Chairside Support during the Extraction of Teeth and Minor Oral Surgery

Learning outcomes

1. Be able to prepare the patient and the dental environment for extractions and minor oral surgery
2. Be able to support the operator and the patient during extractions and minor oral surgery
3. Be able to support the operator and the patient following extractions and minor oral surgery

Outcome 1 assessment criteria

The learner can:

- Make available the correct patient's charts, records and images
- Prepare and list the equipment, instruments, materials and medicaments that may be required for:
  - Extracting erupted teeth
  - During minor oral surgery
- Check with the patient that they have followed the prescribed pre-treatment instructions, and report any non-compliance promptly to the appropriate member of the team

Diploma in Dental Nursing, Level 3, Third Edition. Carole Hollins.
© 2014 John Wiley & Sons, Ltd. Published 2014 by John Wiley & Sons, Ltd.
Companion website: www.wiley.com/go/hollins/dentalnursinglevel3

Outcome 2 assessment criteria
The learner can:
- Provide the patient with appropriate support during the administration of local or regional anaesthesia
- Aspirate, irrigate and protect the patient's soft tissues
- Monitor the patient, identify any complications and take the necessary actions without delay
- Assist the operator during the:
  - Extraction of erupted teeth
  - Minor oral surgery procedures
- Assist the operator in the placing of sutures (if used), and record the sutures correctly

Outcome 3 assessment criteria
The learner can:
- Provide the patient with appropriate postoperative instructions following the extraction of erupted teeth and minor oral surgery, including access to emergency care and advice
- Complete the necessary charts and records accurately and legibly following the procedure
- Provide information on why it is important to confirm with the operator that the patient is fit to leave the surgery prior to them doing so

This unit is assessed by:
- observation in the workplace, with examples included in the learner's portfolio
- an appropriate alternative method

Details of various elements of the theory and underpinning knowledge are included in Chapter 15, and these are assessed within the written paper.

The theory and underpinning knowledge required to understand the scientific principles involved in the management of oral diseases and dental procedures, including extractions and minor oral surgery techniques, are fully discussed in Chapter 15. This chapter explains the dental nurse's role and responsibilities in relation to these procedures before, during and after they are carried out. Those responsibilities are to the operator (the person carrying out the procedure – usually the dentist, but in some cases it may be the therapist) and also to the patient who is undergoing the procedure, and their guardian where relevant.

Extractions and minor oral surgery tend to be the procedures that patients are most fearful of, probably because of their perceived expectations of feeling pain, seeing blood, having a body part removed, and so on. A huge part of the dental nurse's role at these times is to be calming, friendly and supportive, and to anticipate the concerns and needs of the patient throughout the procedure.

Before the procedure

The vast majority of dental workplaces operate on one appointments system or another, so that the working day can be correctly planned and all of the necessary instruments, materials and equipment are known to be available as required. There would be little point in a patient attending for a minor oral surgery procedure, for example, if the workplace had run out of scalpel blades or sutures. Forward planning is therefore a key element in the successful completion of a busy working day and, along with the skills in the following list, is among the abilities required by a competent dental nurse to provide successful chairside support for extractions and minor oral surgery procedures:

- Correct identification of the patient
- Correct identification of the procedure

- Knowledge of the records and images required by the operator for the procedure
- Knowledge of the correct setting up of the area for the procedure
- Knowledge of the instruments, materials and equipment that may be required for the procedure
- Knowledge of the actions to take if the dental nurse is unable to fully prepare for the procedure

Correct identification of the patient

The day list will refer to each patient attending that day by name and/or date of birth and/or address and/or some kind of patient identification marker – such as a unique computer number or the patient's NHS number.

Whatever the system in place, the dental nurse should be familiar with it and be able to access the patient's records so that a cross-reference check can be made between the notes and the expected procedure to be carried out. So if the notes refer to a tooth to be restored with a filling, but the day list indicates that the patient is attending for an extraction, one of the following scenarios has occurred which must be checked with the operator and the patient before the procedure begins:

255

- The records and the day list entry are for two different patients
- The records are incomplete and a change in treatment has been decided without being recorded
- The records are correct and the day list entry is incorrect
- The records are incorrect and the day list entry is correct

Any of these scenarios could quite easily have occurred and the matter should be referred to a more senior colleague (ideally the operator concerned) so that the dental nurse can assist in determining the way forward – to identify the correct patient and the correct procedure to be carried out that day.

The records required may be hard copies in full (i.e. a "pack" of handwritten patient notes, with paper copies of their medical history, previous treatment plans and consent forms, and so on) or they may be fully computerised and only accessible "on screen", or a combination of the two. Whatever their presentation, they should be collected by the dental nurse and presented in the treatment area so that the operator can access them and check their content too.

In large dental workplaces, such as dental schools and hospitals, the dental nurse can check the correct patient identity by asking patients to confirm their name, date of birth and address and that they know why they are attending on the day. The final decision to confirm the patient's identity is the duty of the operator.

In smaller workplaces, many of the patients are recognisable to the staff by sight – some may even be known by their first names – but identity and procedure checks should still always be carried out to avoid any mishaps. Once the patient has been correctly identified, the records and treatment area can be prepared.

The records to be set out will include the following:

- Notes written at the previous appointment or when the decision was made to carry out the particular procedure – these will remind the operator of the reasons for the treatment decisions taken
- Medical history form, to be checked to highlight any potential concerns – for example, is a certain local anaesthetic required, or does the patient take an anticoagulant drug?
- Consent form, indicating that the patient has given valid consent to the procedure (see Chapter 13)
- Radiographs of the relevant tooth – these will allow the operator to plan the procedure and the technique used and to show any potential difficulties such as curved roots on the tooth involved

The dental nurse can also access the records for the following purposes:

- The notes may refer to the patient's level of anxiety, so the dental nurse is aware of the heightened need to be supportive and helpful to the patient throughout the procedure – the issue should also be pointed out to the operator

- The medical history can be checked and any recognised potential issues pointed out to the operator
- Patients can also be asked to confirm if there have been any changes to their medical history since they were last seen, and these are then recorded appropriately and pointed out to the operator
- The consent form can be checked to ensure it covers the planned procedure and that it has been signed and dated by the patient, or that it requires to be signed and dated by the patient today – any discrepancies can be pointed out to the operator
- The radiographs must be correctly displayed to show the tooth under treatment, either as digital images on the computer or as hard copies on film
- Hard copies must be correctly mounted on the viewing screen:
  - Intra-oral views with the pimple facing out (to indicate left from right), and upper teeth with their roots above the crown and lower teeth with their roots below the crown (see Figure 7.13)
  - Extra-oral views with the "L" marker in the bottom right-hand corner of the radiograph as it is positioned on the viewing screen, to indicate the patient's left side (see Figure 8.1)

Correct identification of the procedure

The patient is attending for one of the procedures in the list that follows – the actual one should be referred to in the notes and on the day list (although some computer software systems are not programmed to allow individual procedures to be booked – they just record a time slot as a "minor oral surgery" procedure).

The procedure list is as follows:

- **Simple extractions** – of roots or whole teeth, where no soft tissue or bone removal is required
- **Surgical extractions** – of roots or whole teeth, where soft tissue alone or with bone has to be removed to gain access to the root or tooth
- **Implant placement** – the replacement of a missing tooth (or teeth) by the surgical placement of a titanium implant into the alveolar bone
- **Apicectomy** – the amputation of a root apex and any associated pathology as a surgical end-odontic procedure
- **Frenectomy** – the surgical removal of the frenal soft tissue attachment between the lip and the alveolar ridge
- **Alveolectomy** – the surgical adjustment and removal of bone spicules from the alveolar ridge after tooth extraction, to produce a smooth base for denture seating (see previously)
- **Soft tissue biopsies** – the partial or complete removal of soft tissue oral lesions for pathological investigation and diagnosis

These procedure are discussed further in Chapter 15, along with other surgical techniques. The last five procedures, along with surgical extractions involving bone removal, are referred to as minor oral surgery (MOS) procedures.

The records and images required by the operator in order to carry out the procedure are detailed in the preceding section.

Extractions

When an extraction is to be performed, the complexity of the procedure will depend mainly on which tooth is involved, how much tooth or root is present, and its position in the jaw bone. The options available for the extraction procedure will then fall into one of the following categories:

- Simple extraction
- Surgical extraction involving dissection of the tooth in its socket and removal in sections
- Surgical extraction involving soft tissue removal to expose an unerupted tooth or buried root
- Surgical extraction involving the raising of a mucoperiosteal flap and bone removal to gain full access to a tooth or root

The equipment and instruments required for each type of extraction will vary slightly, and those surgical techniques involving all but tooth sectioning will be very similar to other MOS techniques.

Knowledge of the correct setting up of the area

As with all dental procedures, the treatment area (surgery) must be clean before being set up for an extraction or MOS session, and left in a similar condition afterwards, to avoid any possibility of cross-infection occurring. The principles of infection control are discussed in detail in Chapter 12.

257

Before the surgery is prepared for use, dental nurses must ensure that they do not inadvertently introduce any contamination into the area, and so must undertake the correct hand washing technique before applying the correct personal protective equipment (PPE). As a clinical procedure is to be carried out, the appropriate hand washing technique is as follows:

- Turn on the tap using the foot or elbow control, to prevent contaminating the tap (see Figure 4.4)
- Wet both hands under running water of a suitable temperature
- Apply a suitable antibacterial liquid soap from the dispenser (Figure 8.2) and wash all areas of both hands and wrists thoroughly – this should take at least 30 seconds to carry out thoroughly, and the correct routine is illustrated on the poster that is present at each hand washing station (see Figure 1.3)
- Nail brushes are not advised unless they are autoclavable, as they can become contaminated with repeated use
- Rinse both hands under running water, holding them so that the water does not flow back over the fingers
- Dry the hands thoroughly, using disposable paper towels for single use

The equipment and instruments can now be handled safely, unless the dental nurse has any cuts or abrasions on the hands, in which case the lesion should be covered with a waterproof dressing and a pair of clinical gloves must be worn before any items are handled.

The surgery itself is then made ready as follows:

- The electric and water supplies should be switched on to all static equipment (dental chair, suction unit, etc.) if this has not already been done
- Any portable items not likely to be required for the procedure should be placed in cupboards or drawers, or removed from the surgery, so that the work surfaces are clear of any clutter
- The controls of any large equipment items which are likely to be contaminated during the procedure must be protected by a barrier technique, including:
  - Dental chair controls, if not foot-operated
  - Dental light controls and handles (see Figure 8.3)
  - Computer keyboard, if various screens are in use
  - Bracket table handles and controls
- In some surgery settings, the aspirator pipes and handpiece tubing may also require barrier protection if they are of a design that makes them difficult to wipe down thoroughly (such as corrugated piping)

- The patient records are accessed on the computer, or the paper copies are laid out on an area of the work surface away from the surgical field (to minimise their contamination)
- Relevant radiographs are correctly mounted on the viewing screen, in easy reach of the operator
- PPE is laid out ready for the patient, the operator and the dental nurse:
  - Protective glasses, disposable bib, tissues – for the patient
  - Protective glasses or visor, face mask, gloves, disposable apron – for the operator and dental nurse
- Mouth rinse and cup are made ready for the patient – a disinfectant solution (such as chlorhexidine) may be required for some surgical procedures
- Suitable aspirator tips are connected to the suction unit; both a wide-bore and a finer surgical tip should be available
- The correct local anaesthetic equipment and materials are laid out for use, in easy reach of the operator and dental nurse, and covered with a disposable bib until the patient is seated:
  - Topical anaesthetic and cotton wool rolls (where relevant)
  - Syringe (aspirating type if a nerve block is likely)
  - Short or long needle (depending on which tooth is involved)
  - Local anaesthetic cartridges
  - Re-sheathing device
- The local anaesthetic solution should be checked by the operator for suitability before use
- The correct instruments are laid out for the procedure (see later), in easy reach of the operator and the dental nurse, and covered with a disposable bib until the patient is seated:
  - If they are stored within an enclosed tray system, the lid should be replaced once the tray has been checked for all items present
  - If they are within sterile pouches, these should remain sealed until just before their use
- Single-use items, materials and medicaments should be gathered together and made ready for use, and covered with a disposable bib until the patient is seated:
  - Bite packs (Figure 11.1)
  - Sterile saline sachets and disposable irrigation syringe, with bowl (where relevant)
  - Haemostatic sponges (Figure 11.2)
  - Suture packs (where relevant)
- A written postoperative instruction sheet or leaflet is available, to be handed to the patient or guardian after the procedure has been completed

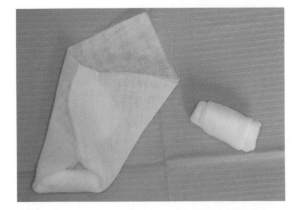

Figure 11.1   Bite pack.

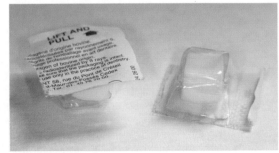

Figure 11.2   Haemostatic sponges.

Knowledge of the instruments, materials and equipment required

The instruments required for a simple extraction may involve forceps, elevators and luxators, and the specific forceps required will be determined by which tooth (or root) is being extracted, as discussed later in this section. The functions of the various instruments are listed in the following table.

Item	Function
Forceps	Range of sterile hand instruments used to grip a tooth or root at its neck before applying appropriate wrist actions to loosen the tooth/root in its socket during the extraction procedure. Various designs are available for use on upper or lower teeth, and for each individual tooth/root, as shown in Figure 11.3
Luxators	Sterile hand instruments used to widen the socket and sever the periodontal ligament attachment as they are pushed towards the apex, lifting the tooth out of the socket (Figure 11.4)
Elevators	Sterile hand instruments used to prise the tooth/root out of the socket. Various patterns are available – Cryer's, Warwick James', Winter's (Figure 11.5)
Fine-bore aspirator	Disposable suction tip used to suck away all blood and maintain good moisture control during the procedure – also useful for sucking and holding tooth debris so that it can be removed from the mouth safely (Figure 11.6)
Haemostats	Gelatine sponges or oxidised cellulose packs, which are inserted into the socket after extraction to aid blood clotting and achieve haemostasis – can be used with or without a suture

259

The commonest patterns of forceps used are shown in Figure 11.3. They can be identified individually by the following descriptions:

- **Upper incisor and canine forceps** are straight with single rounded blades and have both wide and narrow patterns
- **Upper root forceps** are similar in appearance, with narrow, straight blades
- **Upper premolar forceps** have slightly curved handles and single rounded blades
- **Upper left molar forceps** have curved handles, a beaked blade to the right of the instrument, and a rounded blade to the left to grip the buccal roots and the palatal root, respectively (many dental nurses identify upper molar forceps by the mantra "beak to cheek")
- **Upper right molar forceps** have curved handles and the beaked blade is to the left of the instrument
- **Upper bayonet forceps** have extended handles and angled blades to gain access to third molars or have angled pointed blades to gain access to fractured roots
- **Lower anterior forceps** have single, rounded blades at right angles to the handle that are particularly useful for extracting lower premolars
- **Lower root forceps** are similar, with narrow and straight blades that are also particularly useful for extracting small or crowded incisors

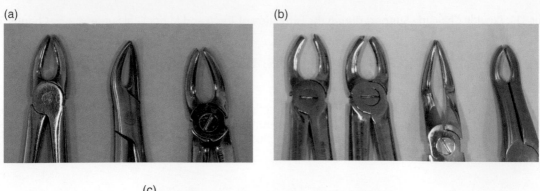

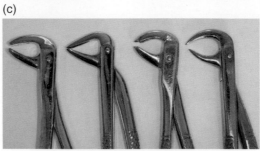

Figure 11.3 Extraction forceps: (a) upper straight, root, premolar; (b) upper left and right molar, bayonets; (c) lower anterior, root, molar, cowhorns.

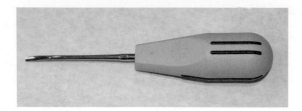

Figure 11.4 A luxator.

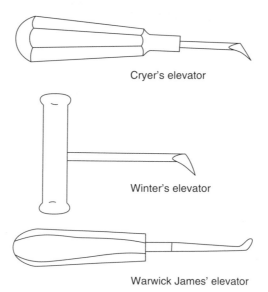

Cryer's elevator

Winter's elevator

Warwick James' elevator

Figure 11.5 Elevators.

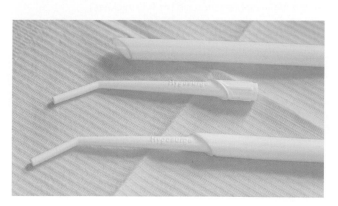

Figure 11.6   A disposable fine-bore aspirator.

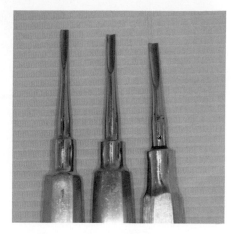

Figure 11.7   Coupland chisels – sizes 1, 2, and 3.

261

- **Lower molar forceps** have beaked blades at right angles to the handles, to grip the furcation of the two roots
- **Lower "cowhorn" forceps** have curved and pointed blades at right angles to the handles, to grip the furcation of lower molar teeth
- **Smaller versions** of most patterns exist, for deciduous tooth extractions

Similarly, elevators are available in a variety of patterns and are used to gradually sever the periodontal membrane and loosen the tooth in the socket (Figure 11.5). They are specifically used to elevate retained roots and impacted teeth, where adequate access to the root or tooth is not possible with conventional forceps, or where the angle of elevation required to loosen the root or tooth is not possible with forceps.

The more common types are as follows:

- **Cryer's elevators** are available as left and right patterns, but can be used on either side of the mouth, depending whether they are engaged mesially or distally – the tips are triangular-shaped and pointed
- **Winter's elevators** have a similar blade design as Cryer's, but have a corkscrew style handle to give more leverage
- **Warwick James' elevators** are available as left, right and straight patterns – the tips are a similar shape to the round blade of forceps

If an extraction procedure is to be carried out that will involve the dissection of a multi-rooted tooth, a set of Coupland chisels should also be available (Figure 11.7). These will be inserted into a drilled notch between the roots and twisted, so that the roots snap apart at the furcation and can be extracted separately.

If a surgical extraction is to be carried out, the relevant forceps and a minor oral surgery kit of instruments should be made available. This kit is the same as that required for other minor oral surgery procedures and should contain the items listed in the following table.

Item	Function
Scalpel blade and handle (Figure 11.8)	To make the initial incision through the full-thickness mucoperiosteum and around the necks of the teeth to create the flap
Osteotrimmer (Figure 11.9)	To raise the corners of the flap off the underlying alveolar bone To scoop out any pathological debris from the bony cavity at the periapical area during an apicectomy procedure
Periosteal elevator (Figure 11.10)	To complete the elevation of the flap off the bone, by pushing the instrument over the bone surface beneath the flap and effectively peeling it off the bone To be held lingually during a lower third molar surgical extraction, to retract the lingual tissue and protect the lingual nerve
Handpiece and surgical burs	To remove any alveolar bone necessary to gain access to the tooth or root (this function may also be carried out using a surgical mallet and bone chisel) To drill a notch between the roots of multi-rooted teeth, so that they can be separated before extraction The handpiece and burs used during implant procedures are specialised for this purpose alone
Irrigation syringe	To irrigate the surgical field with sterile saline or sterile water, although the handpiece often has its own irrigation supply from the bracket table bottle The irrigation system used during implant procedures is supplied as a drip-type bottle of sterile saline, which connects directly to the handpiece
Austin and Kilner retractors	To protect and retract cheeks, lips and tongue from the surgical field, providing clear access for the operator
Rake retractor	To hold and retract the mucoperiosteal flap itself, so that the immediate surgical field is clear
Bone rongeurs	To nibble away bony spicules and produce a smooth bone surface for healing (this function may also be carried out using the handpiece and surgical burs)
Dissecting forceps (Figure 11.11)	To hold the loose flap edges taut during suturing To hold and remove solid debris from the surgical area
Needle holders (Figure 11.12)	To hold the pre-threaded needle firmly while suturing. Some designs also have a dual function as suture scissors
Suture pack (Figure 11.13)	Half-moon shaped needle, pre-threaded with either black braided silk or a resorbable suture material such as vicryl, to suture the flap back into position over the alveolar bone
Suture scissors (Figure 11.14)	To cut the suture ends after each stitch, using the notched blades

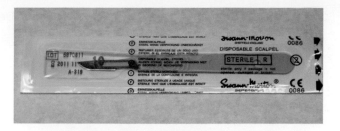

Figure 11.8   Scalpel blade and handle.

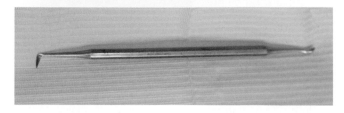

Figure 11.9   An osteotrimmer.

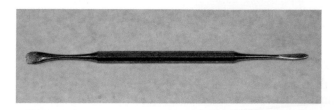

Figure 11.10   A periosteal elevator.

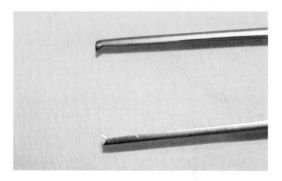

Figure 11.11   Tissue dissecting forceps.

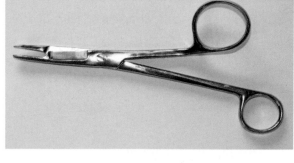

Figure 11.12   A pair of needle holders.

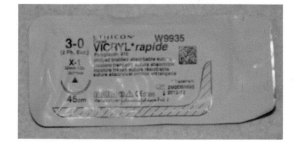

Figure 11.13   A suture pack.

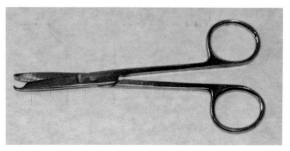

Figure 11.14   Suture scissors.

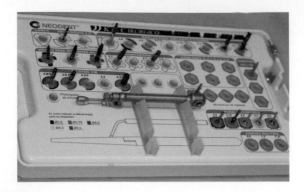

Figure 11.15   An implant kit.

If an implant procedure is to be carried out, the following specialist items will also be required:

● Sterile saline irrigation device connected to the implant handpiece
● Implant drill bits, corresponding titanium implant inserts and torsion adjusting device in a pre-packed kit (Figure 11.15)
● Biosynthetic bone material, with sterile bowl to allow hydration and mixing of the material before use

If an apicectomy procedure is to be carried out, a standard conservation tray of filling instruments will also be required to place the retrograde filling in the root stump.

Knowledge of the actions to take if preparation cannot be completed

If any instruments, materials or items of equipment are not readily available for use immediately before the procedure is scheduled to start, the dental nurse must report the matter to an appropriate person immediately. This may be the operator, a senior dental nurse (or line manager) or the practice manager.

In smaller dental workplaces, if just one set of specialist extraction or MOS equipment and instruments is available for use by several operators, it is the responsibility of reception or administration staff to ensure that similar procedures are not booked at the same time. However, in the unlikely event that a double booking has occurred, the operator and the administration staff must be informed immediately, before the patient undergoes any initial part of the procedure, as the appointment may have to be postponed and rebooked.

The final preparation that the dental nurse must carry out is to check with the patient that any prescribed pre-treatment instructions have been followed correctly. In particular, the following points should be clarified:

● Have all routine medications been taken as requested?
● Have any prescribed antibiotics been taken as requested?
● Has the anticoagulant aspirin been stopped as requested?
● Has the patient had a recent blood test to check their international normalised ratio (INR) if they take warfarin?
● If so, what was the score? (This should be checked by looking at their INR card, and the score must be below 4.0 if the procedure is to be safely carried out away from a hospital setting)
● Has the patient had a light snack within the last 2 hours, to avoid the possibility of a fainting episode?

- If the procedure is being carried out under any form of conscious sedation technique, has the patient complied with all of the relevant additional points as requested?
- If the patient is a child or a vulnerable adult, are they in attendance with a suitable adult escort, to look after and see them safely home after the procedure?
- If the patient is frail or excessively nervous, are they in attendance with a suitable adult escort for the same purpose?
- Has the patient (or guardian) read and understood any pre-treatment information provided – are there any further questions?
- Has the patient (or guardian) been given enough information to provide valid consent for the procedure, and has that consent been given? (This may be given in written form in some instances)

When it becomes apparent that one or more of these points have not been followed, the dental nurse must report the matter to the operator immediately, and allow them to discuss the situation further with the patient. It is not the role of dental nurses to act beyond their level of competence by making unilateral decisions about any of these issues – the responsibility lies with the operator.

265

During the procedure

Usually, the dental nurse will collect patients (and their guardian where relevant) from the reception area and escort them to the surgery, rather than the operator. Patients often use this time to express their level of anxiety (or even fear) at the imminent procedure, and the dental nurse should help to calm them in a friendly manner, without being patronising and dismissive. A thoughtless comment such as, "Oh, don't be silly" or "You need to man up" can destroy their trust and compliance completely, and patients would be fully justified in feeling offended and ridiculed.

With experience, dental nurses will develop their communication skills and their own style of patter that they can use in these situations, often more successfully than some operators, and patients will respond positively to a good dental nurse with obvious empathy to their situation. Communication skills are discussed in detail in Chapter 5, and the skills of reflection and developing one's own self in practice are discussed in Chapter 2.

The abilities required by a competent dental nurse to provide support during the procedure include the following:

- Preparation of the patient
- Assistance during the administration of local anaesthesia
- Identification and correct handling of the instruments, materials and equipment throughout the procedure
- Adequate provision of moisture control, irrigation and tissue retraction throughout the procedure
- Correct handling of body tissues
- Assistance during the placement of haemostats and/or sutures
- Monitoring and support of the patient
- Recognition of complications
- Actions to take in the event of a complication

Although forward planning of the procedure should avoid the possibility, it may be necessary for the dental nurse to retrieve unprepared instruments and items during the procedure. If so, gloves must be removed and replaced with a new pair each time the surgical area is left and re-accessed.

Preparation of the patient

A final check is made by the operator of the patient's identification and consent to undergo the procedure.

The dental nurse will then assist patients into the dental chair, and ready them for the treatment start as follows:

- Help them to remove their coat if necessary, and hang it up
- Assist them into the dental chair – they may need physical support, for example, or the chair raising or lowering
- Apply their required PPE:
  - Safety glasses
  - Protective bib
  - Some patients like to have a tissue in hand too
- Monitor the patient for signs of anxiety, and notify the operator as necessary
- Reassure the patient in a calm and friendly manner – many appreciate the opportunity of a hand to hold at this point, although this action can be passed to an escort/guardian if appropriate

Assistance during the administration of local anaesthesia

The operator and the dental nurse apply their own PPE (safety glasses/visor, face mask, gloves, plastic apron). The disposable cover is removed from the equipment and the operator must check that the correct items and local anaesthetic are prepared. The topical anaesthetic is applied to a cotton wool roll and handed to the operator for application in the patient's mouth. While this takes effect, the syringe is loaded ready for use, quietly and out of sight of the patient:

- Noisy clattering of metallic items can be particularly unnerving for patients, so items must be handled proficiently at all times
- The local anaesthetic cartridge is loaded into the syringe correctly, with the cap end at the bottom where the needle will be applied
- If an aspirating technique is to be used, any screw-in plunger is locked into the cartridge bung before the needle is added
- The needle is screwed on to the threaded end of the syringe, with the guard in place
- On removal of the topical anaesthetic, the needle guard is loosened but left over the needle, and the loaded syringe is offered to the operator (Figure 8.16)
- As the operator receives the syringe, the dental nurse keeps hold of the loosened needle guard so that it becomes unsheathed as it is transferred over
- The guard is then placed in the re-sheathing device, ready for the operator when the anaesthetic procedure is completed (see Figure 1.29)
- Successive cartridges are handed to the operator as required during the administration procedure
- When the administration is complete, the equipment is re-sheathed by the operator without being handled by the dental nurse (this avoids increasing the likelihood of an inoculation injury)

Identification and correct handling of the instruments

The disposable cover is removed from the instruments and equipment, out of sight of the patient. Tray lids are removed, but bagged items are left whole until their use is imminent. The instruments are best laid out in their likely order of use, especially the minor oral surgery kit – this is as listed earlier. Otherwise, unnecessary time is wasted while the dental nurse has to locate each required item.

The operator may choose to pick up the instruments from the surgical kit personally, but those that are bagged will require handling and opening by the dental nurse first. As required, each instrument should be carefully opened without touching it and then handed to the dentist handles first, while holding the tips still within the sterile pouch – this is the "no-touch" technique (Figure 11.16). In this way, infection control is maintained.

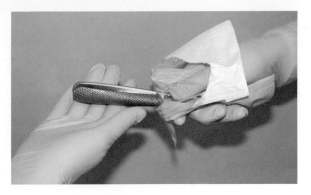

Figure 11.16   No-touch technique of passing bagged items.

When the operator has finished with an instrument, it should be safely passed back to the dental nurse, who receives it and places it on a separate area of the work surface from the unused items in a typical "zoned" layout. The clean items are kept spatially separate from the used and dirty items, to avoid cross-infection.

During the procedure, the dental nurse is likely also to be aspirating and retracting soft tissues, so the receiving and passing of instruments will require the use of both hands. Experience will improve this ability with time, but all members of the dental team must develop a routine of never passing items across the patient's face while performing instrument transfer – it only takes one dropped item to permanently scar or blind a patient.

Adequate provision of moisture control, irrigation and tissue retraction

During the procedure the dental nurse will be expected to use the relevant instruments and equipment correctly, to assist the operator in the following techniques:

- **Moisture control** – removal of moisture (saliva, blood, irrigation solution) from the operative area so that adequate vision is possible by the operator, and so that the patient is not choking on a mouthful of fluid, using:
  - ○ Wide-bore aspirator for fast fluid removal, as well as some soft tissue retraction
  - ○ Fine-bore aspirator for precise blood removal directly at the operative site, as well as collection of small debris particles (pieces of bone, tooth or root)
- **Irrigation** – to avoid heat damage to the bone, as well as to clear the operative field of blood and debris. Modern handpieces tend to have their irrigation supply incorporated into the design, but occasionally the dental nurse provides irrigation by washing the area with sterile saline or water from a disposable syringe:
  - ○ The usual sharp needle can be replaced by a blunt, side bevel needle (such as those used in endodontic treatment) to avoid inoculation accidents
  - ○ Larger syringes (above 10 mL) provide longer irrigation periods
  - ○ The wash solution must be irrigated slowly and consistently, rather than as a fast "squirt"
  - ○ The dental nurse must inform the operator to stop when the syringe needs refilling, so that treatment does not continue without irrigation
  - ○ The dental nurse must also be aspirating at the same time as irrigating, so that the patient does not choke

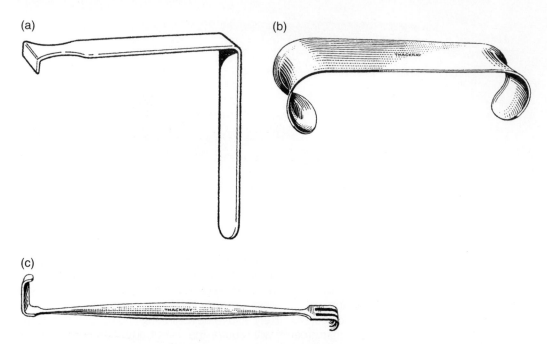

(a)   (b)   (c)

Figure 11.17   Retractors: (a) Austin; (b) Kilner; (c) tissue rake. Source: *Levison's Textbook for Dental Nurses*, 10th edition (Hollins), 2008. Reproduced with permission of Wiley-Blackwell.

- **Tissue retraction** – to avoid damage to the soft tissues from burs and drills, and to provide good vision for the operator, using:
  - Flanged wide-bore aspirator tips to retract the cheek, lips or tongue
  - Special cheek retractors such as the Austin or Kilner designs (Figure 11.17)
  - Tissue rake to hold the mucoperiosteal flap itself (Figure 11.17)
  - Mouth mirror to retract the tongue or lips, and to reflect light and thus illuminate the operative field

Retraction of any soft tissues for any prolonged length of time can be quite tiring for the dental nurse, and if they need to stop for a rest or reposition the retractor, the operator must be forewarned so that they do not continue drilling or cutting as the soft tissues collapse across the operative field.

To achieve adequate moisture control, irrigation, and retraction at the same time may require a second dental nurse to assist the operator.

Correct handling of body tissues

As a tooth or root is extracted by forceps, it is usually passed directly to the dental nurse upon removal from the mouth. Some operators hand over the forceps while still gripping the tooth in the blades, and the dental nurse needs to receive the instrument, too, using gauze or a tissue and without dropping anything. Most operators will check the extracted tissue to ensure that all pieces are accounted for, so the extracted pieces are laid in the dirty zone for inspection rather than being disposed of immediately.

Soft tissue debris, such as clumps of granulation tissue, is also received into gauze or a tissue and placed in the dirty zone. However, when a soft tissue biopsy procedure is being undertaken, the removed tissue must be deposited directly into a pathology pot (usually containing formalin) ready for sending to the pathology department for investigation. This tissue is best not handled by the dental nurse so as not to damage its structure – so the open pathology pot is held carefully to receive the tissue directly from the operator, making sure it is within the operator's reach (so that the specimen can be dropped into the pot) and out of view of the patient. Once the tissue is in the pot, the lid can be replaced.

When a particularly nasty and infected tooth is extracted, some operators prefer that it is immersed directly in a disinfectant bath so that malodours do not permeate the surgery. The bath will have been set up beforehand by the dental nurse and placed in the dirty zone before the procedure began. Again, the tissue can then be inspected by the operator before being disposed of correctly.

Assistance during the placement of haemostats/sutures

As soon as the tooth or root has been extracted, or the surgical procedure completed, patients will be asked to bite onto a pack for a few minutes. This begins the process of haemostasis (stopping the bleeding), allows patients to rest their jaw for a while, and also allows the operator and the dental nurse to rest their arms, hands and fingers.

At this point, the operator and the dental nurse may change their gloves for a new pair each, especially if the procedure has been particularly bloody and sutures still need to be placed. The dirty pairs must be deposited either into the dirty zone or directly into the hazardous waste bin. Similarly, a new disposable aspirator tip can be connected, ready for the suture procedure – this avoids having to continue to use a bloody item, as well as ensuring that the new tip is clear of blockages from blood clots or tissue debris.

If an apicectomy procedure has been carried out, the retrograde filling will be placed at this point in the same way as a conventional filling. The dental nurse must ensure that filling material bottles, syringes and mixing equipment is not contaminated during the procedure, by replacing dirty gloves whenever necessary throughout.

With clean gloves on, the dental nurse can now ready the haemostat sponge and suture for the operator to insert into the extraction or surgical site, as follows:

- The sterile suture equipment is opened and passed as for the other instruments, in the following order:
  - Needle holders
  - Suture pack
  - Dissecting forceps
  - Suture scissors – which the dental nurse will use
- The dental nurse must retract the soft tissues and aspirate again, as necessary
- The haemostat sponge (if used) is passed over within its plastic cell to be picked up with the dissecting forceps or the needle holders and gently pushed into the site by the operator
- The operator will suture the mucoperiosteal flap back into place or the soft tissue edges of the extraction socket together so that healing can occur
- Most operators use an "interrupted suture" technique, where each stitch is placed and tied off separate from the next one
- The dental nurse will cut the ends of the tied suture at the point indicated by the operator when instructed to do so
- The half-moon notch of the scissors is used to cut the suture, and the dental nurse must ensure that no other tissue is between the scissor blades before the cut is made (Figure 11.18)
- A note must be made in the patient's notes of the number of sutures used, for reference when the patient attends again

Monitoring and support of the patient

Throughout the whole procedure, the patient must be monitored and supported by the dental team, and this duty falls to the dental nurse in particular. Extractions and surgical procedures are usually perceived to be fearful events by patients, and the assistance and support they require throughout is often greater than for any other type of dental treatment.

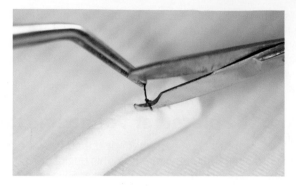

Figure 11.18 Cutting the suture.

The procedure cannot progress if the patient is anxious and uncooperative, and it would be dangerous to proceed in these circumstances. The dental nurse must remain calm, friendly and helpful throughout, by taking the following general actions:

- Providing support during mouth rinsing, including helping patients to avoid spillages once the local anaesthetic has been administered, and wiping their mouth as necessary
- Holding a patient's hand if requested to do so, and if it is possible (with particularly fearful patients, especially children, a second person may need to carry out this duty)
- Alerting the operator immediately if they suspect a patient can actually feel pain (see later)
- Constantly reassuring patients in a calm and even tone, and repeatedly encouraging them by saying phrases such as "You're doing really well"
- Avoiding the use of fearful phrases such as "The pain won't last much longer now", or "Just a bit more bone drilling to go"
- During some extractions, the patient and operator will benefit from the dental nurse supporting the head or jaw during extraction movements – but the patient must be told you are going to do this beforehand, otherwise they may believe they are being held down; this is especially important to avoid with children
- Once the procedure is over, congratulating the patient and reassuring them again
- Wiping any blood and debris from a patient's face before discharge
- Removing their PPE when it is safe to do so
- Assisting them from the surgery area when the operator indicates that they can leave

In particular, the dental nurse must constantly assess and monitor the patient for the following, to avoid serious complications arising, as the operator is often focused entirely on the oral cavity and the procedure in hand and may not notice subtle changes immediately:

- **Pain** – signs of pain in the patient could be grimacing, wincing or crying and should be pointed out to the operator if they have not noticed – this may be achieved by attracting the operator out of sight of the patient and quietly indicating the fact by facial expressions such as raising the eyebrows and dropping the eyes to the patient several times
- **Colour** – this can indicate various problems are about to occur:
  - The patient may feel faint and become pale and clammy, so the procedure must be stopped while action is taken to restore the cranial blood flow (usually by dropping the dental chair so the patient's head is below their feet)
  - The patient's lips may become blue-purple (cyanotic) if the airway is compromised by loose debris and their breathing becomes restricted
  - The patient's skin colour may become pale then grey if there is cardiac arrest

Recognition of complications

Forward planning and risk assessment should highlight the potential for some complications to occur, before the procedure begins. Their avoidance should then be possible by taking the appropriate action beforehand. So patients with known and complicated medical issues should be referred to hospital for their treatment, for example, and radiographic review will indicate the possibility of nerve damage in some cases, so these patients can be referred to a specialist oral surgeon for treatment, and so on.

Complications that may occur unexpectedly during the procedure are:

- Nerve damage – by trauma during instrumentation
- Unexpected tooth fracture – especially if the tooth is heavily filled or root-filled, and this may result in a simple extraction becoming a more complicated one
- Accidental tooth loss – either into the respiratory or digestive tracts or out of the mouth, and as a result of it slipping out of the operator's grip while pushing the tooth out of the socket or lifting it out of the mouth
- Haemorrhage – primary haemorrhage is normal during extraction and surgical procedures, but damage to a local blood vessel may cause unexpected and profuse bleeding
- Oro-antral fistula – due to a perforation of the maxillary sinus, this can occur while extracting the upper premolar or molar teeth, as the maxillary sinus lies over their roots and is often only separated by a membrane which can be easily perforated
- Patient collapse – due to a medical emergency
- Equipment failure – either actual failure or loss of the electricity supply

271

Actions to take in the event of a complication

The senior person during the procedure is the operator, so the final responsibility for the actions taken following a complication lies with them. However, dental nurses have a vital role to play in assisting the operator to successfully manage the complication at the time, and would be expected to do so. If a complication does occur, the one action the dental nurse must try to avoid is to express alarm or shock in front of the patient, as this will be upsetting and may cause them to react unexpectedly and cause further problems still.

The specific actions that the dental nurse can take are as follows:

- Nerve damage – this may be identified as witnessing the actual cutting of the nerve during the procedure by the operator, but it can also occur by careless soft tissue retraction by the dental nurse, causing trauma to the nerve; the actions are:
  ○ Use the correct retraction technique at all times
  ○ Do not remove or adjust the retractor without informing the operator first
  ○ Be prepared to retrieve any additional instruments and equipment that the operator may require
- Unexpected tooth fracture – this will be identified by the snapping of the tooth (often audibly) and its disintegration into pieces; the actions are:
  ○ Collect all loose pieces with the aspirator and remove them from the mouth
  ○ Reassure the patient
  ○ Be prepared to retrieve any additional instruments and equipment that the operator may require
  ○ Be prepared to proceed to a surgical procedure
- Accidental tooth loss – this may be identified as witnessing the actual loss from the operative field at the time; the actions are:
  ○ If it is visible in the mouth, aspirate and remove it from the mouth
  ○ Help to locate it if it was seen to come out of the mouth
  ○ Assist the patient if they begin choking, as the tooth is inhaled
  ○ Monitor the patient to see if they swallow it, and confirm this with them
  ○ Reassure the patient

- Haemorrhage – this will be sudden and either red and spurting if an artery is involved or purple and welling if a vein is involved; the actions are:
  - Apply immediate pressure to the area, using gauze
  - Aspirate to clear the field if possible, while still applying pressure
  - Reassure the patient
  - Be prepared to retrieve any additional instruments and equipment that the operator may require
  - Be prepared to fetch help
- Oro-antral fistula – this will be identified by the sudden visual loss of the tooth from the socket; the actions are:
  - Assist the operator if requested to do so
  - Be prepared to retrieve any additional instruments and equipment that the operator may require
  - Reassure the patient
- Patient collapse – this will be identified by monitoring the patient to notice any skin colour change, any alteration in their breathing, that they have slumped in the chair, that they have become unresponsive; the actions are:
  - Determine the cause of the collapse from the signs and symptoms
  - Carry out the necessary basic life support techniques (see Chapter 13)
  - Be prepared to fetch help
- Equipment failure – this will be identified by the item's malfunction and may be accompanied by electric flashes or burning smells, or be as simple as a blocked aspirator tube; the actions are:
  - Stop using the equipment immediately
  - Switch off the appliance and disconnect it from the mains
  - Reassure the patient and ensure their safety
  - Unblock the aspirator if possible
  - Check to determine if a duplicate portable item can be seconded from elsewhere, or if a spare surgery is available
  - Abandon the procedure if it cannot be safely completed without the item

After the procedure

Once the procedure has been completed, patients will quite often express huge relief and then wish to leave as soon as possible. They must not leave until the following checks have been made and instructions given:

- Check that they have been sufficiently cleaned of blood and debris
- Check that they feel well enough to go home – sometimes a patient may experience nausea or faintness after the procedure, as a result of the release of tension and emotions
- Check that their escort is available to take them home, where relevant – this may involve organising a taxi, as patients must not be expected to walk home and ideally they should not use public transport either
- Check that haemostasis has been achieved and that they have been issued with a spare bite pack (see later)
- Give postoperative instructions, including access to emergency care and advice (see later)
- Check whether the operator requires a further appointment to be made and organise the making of the appointment – this may involve notifying reception to make the appointment, or making it while the patient is still present
- Check with the operator that the patient is fit to leave the surgery (see later)

Immediately after the procedure has been completed, all dirty PPE should be removed and placed in the hazardous waste sack. The dental nurse can then apply clean gloves to assist patients while they rinse out their mouths (if the operator agrees) or spit out the contents, and then while their facial area is cleaned of all blood and debris.

All the used instruments should be left in situ, either out of the patient's view or covered with disposable bibs until the patient has left the surgery. Patients may need to remain in the dental chair until they are discharged, or they may be required to move to a recovery area (this is more likely in the hospital setting) and then discharged from there. The dental nurse should remain with patients until discharge, or hand over to another competent member of staff in the recovery area, as necessary.

The abilities required by a competent dental nurse to provide support after the procedure include the following:

- Provide postoperative instructions
- Complete the patient records
- Discharge the patient
- Decontaminate the surgery and instruments

Provide postoperative instructions

273

Once a tooth has been extracted or a surgical procedure completed, the patient is effectively left with a wound in the mouth that requires care and attention while healing, and it is necessary to avoid any postoperative complications. Complications that may occur after extraction are bleeding and infection of the bony socket. The reasons for the occurrence of these complications are as follows:

- Bleeding – either within hours of the extraction (**reactionary haemorrhage**) due to the blood clot being disturbed and reopening torn blood vessels, or after 24 hours (**secondary haemorrhage**) due to an infection developing at the surgical site
- Infection – between 2 and 4 days after the procedure and following disintegration of the blood clot in the socket, the exposed bony socket walls can become infected – the condition is called **localised osteitis** (dry socket)

It is important that the patient (or their guardian) understands that these postoperative complications can occur because of a disturbance to the blood clot that forms in the area, and that they should therefore avoid this happening wherever possible.

Postoperative instructions are given to advise the patient on how to avoid disturbing the blood clot, and how best to look after the wound to encourage healing, and should include the following points:

- Pain, swelling or bruising may occur after the procedure – this is especially likely after a surgical procedure and is quite normal
- Analgesics (**except aspirin**) may be taken as required – these may be started as soon as the patient arrives home, if required
- Alcohol, hot drinks and exercise should be avoided for 24 hours after the procedure – all of these activities make loss of the blood clot more likely
- Food can be taken once the local anaesthetic has completely worn off, but should be kept away from the wound and should consist of bland foods only on the day of the procedure
- Patients who smoke should be advised to refrain from doing so for at least 24 hours after the procedure – smoking makes the disintegration of the blood clot more likely and then a postoperative infection will occur
- No mouth rinsing should be carried out on the day of the procedure – this will wash out the blood clot and result in reactionary haemorrhage
- Hot salt water mouthwashes should be carried out after each meal, from the day after the procedure for up to 1 week later – these will wash away any food debris from the wound and encourage the soft tissues to heal
- If bleeding does occur, bite onto the moistened spare bite pack or a cotton pack for up to 30 minutes, without removing the pack – in most instances this will succeed in stopping the bleeding

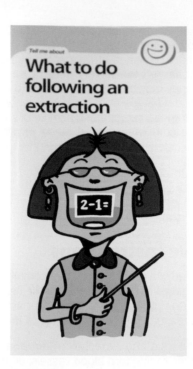

Figure 11.19 Postoperative instruction leaflet.

- Give an emergency telephone number for care and advice if problems occur out of hours, and ensure they have the surgery number in case problems occur during opening hours
- Give details of further appointments if necessary, including suture removal

The postoperative instructions should be given both verbally – so the patient has the opportunity to clarify any points at the time – and in written format so they can be referred back to later in the day (Figure 11.19).

Complete the patient records

Some operators prefer to write the patient records themselves, while others will dictate exactly what to write to the dental nurse. As with all records, they must be accurate, legible, avoid the use of any derogatory or slang terms, and refer only to accepted shorthand phrases that can be easily translated if necessary. So, for example, the accepted use of "LA" for local anaesthesia, "xla" for extraction under local anaesthesia, "xo" for simple extraction, "tooth #" for tooth fracture, and so on.

If the dental nurse is required to complete the records alone, they should be made available for the operator to check and then sign to say that this has been done – their accuracy is ultimately the responsibility of the operator. The issues of record-keeping and confidentiality are discussed in detail in Chapter 13.

The points that must be included in the records are:

- Written for the correct patient in the records, either on paper or on computer
- Date of procedure, and date of writing (if different) – these will be recorded automatically on computer records
- Ideally completed on the day of the procedure, and as soon after its completion as possible

- Identify the operator and the dental nurse – this may be obvious in a small surgery setting, but less so in hospital departments and clinics
- Identify the tooth extracted or the minor oral surgery procedure undertaken
- The charting must be updated to indicate an extraction (using "X" on the outside chart – see Chapter 13)
- There is no manual method of charting MOS procedures (except surgical extractions), but some computer programs may have a code incorporated into their software
- Note the local anaesthetic used and the number of cartridges (batch numbers tend to be recorded centrally rather than in every set of patient notes)
- Give a brief description of the procedure – if an implant was placed, state the details
- Record any treatment complications accurately, where relevant – additional local anaesthetic used, tooth fracture, root apex retained, and so on
- Record when the patient was notified of a problem, where relevant – so if a root apex fractured and was left in situ, indicate that the patient was informed of this event
- Record any major complications and their outcome, where relevant
- Record the type and number of sutures placed, where relevant
- Record that haemostasis was achieved before discharge – "HA achieved"
- Record that postoperative instructions were given before discharge – "POIG to pt"
- Record if another appointment was required, and subsequently made
- Signed or initialled by the writer, when completed, and counter-signed by the operator as necessary – computer records can be set to indicate the writer automatically, but this relies on passwords to be accurate

275

An example of a completed procedure entry is shown in Figure 11.20.

Discharge the patient

This is the ultimate responsibility of the operator, but the dental nurse can assist in the following ways:

- Check the patient feels well enough to leave
- Check the escort is available and transport has been arranged
- Give full verbal and written postoperative instructions
- Check an additional appointment has been made, where relevant
- Check haemostasis has been achieved – carefully remove the bite pack and check that a clot is present, then provide a fresh bite pack for the journey home
- Check any patient questions have been answered or passed on to the operator, where relevant

Once the operator has confirmed that the patient can be discharged, assist them from the surgery.

Decontaminate the surgery and instruments

Whichever technique is used to extract a tooth or root, and whichever minor oral surgery technique has been carried out, the procedure is considered a surgical one, as bleeding will definitely occur and the tissues of the patient's oral cavity will be breached by the instruments used. There is a potential risk of cross-infection during any dental procedure, but more so with these oral surgery events than with any other.

The aspects of infection control and health and safety that are relevant to surgery and equipment decontamination, especially cleaning methods, infection control and sterilisation are fully discussed in Chapters 4 and 12.

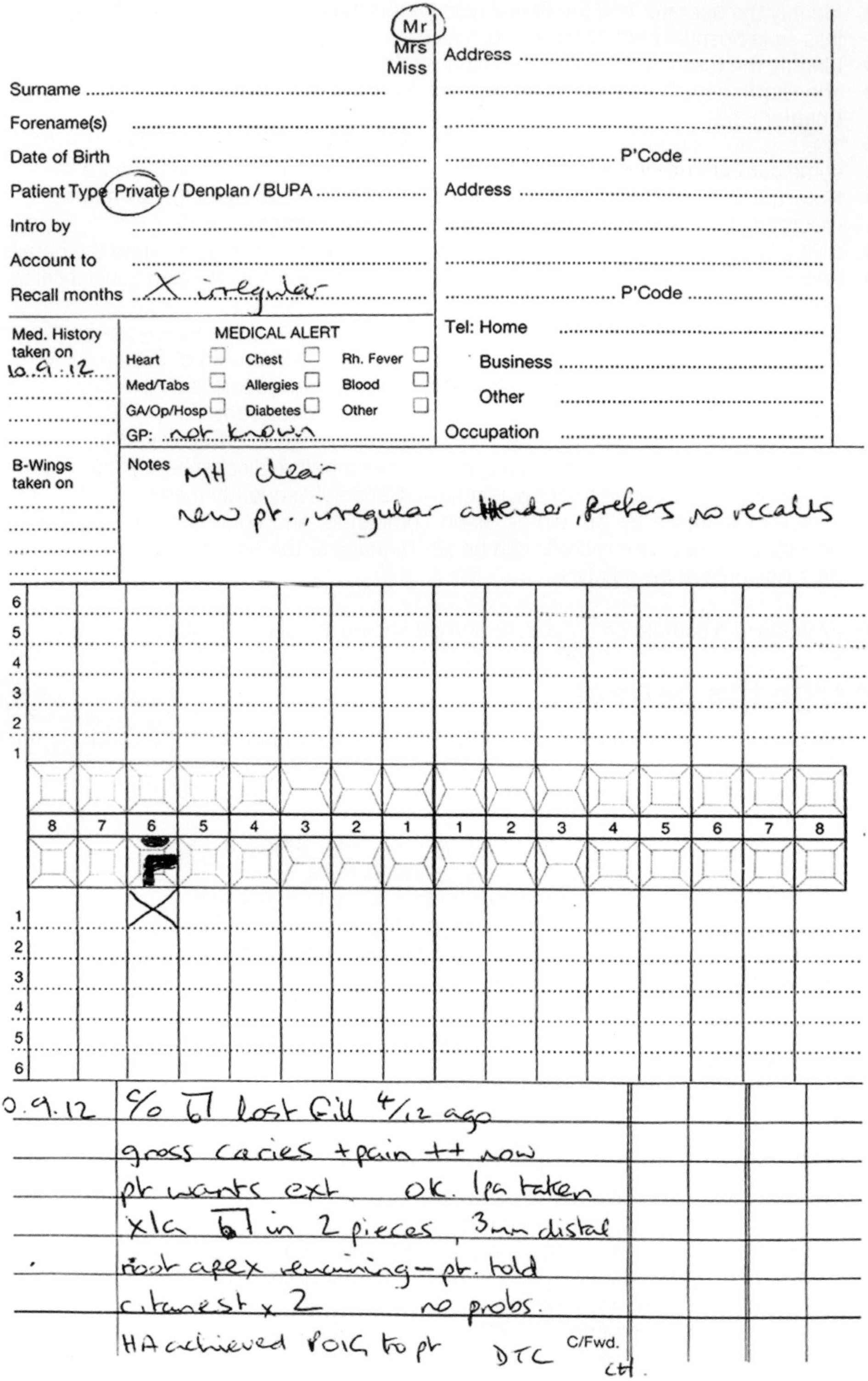

(Mr)
Mrs   Address ....
Miss   ....

Surname ....

Forename(s) ....

Date of Birth .... P'Code ....

Patient Type (Private) / Denplan / BUPA ....   Address ....

Intro by ....

Account to ....

Recall months ... X irregular .... P'Code ....

Med. History taken on 10.9.12	MEDICAL ALERT	Tel: Home ....

Heart ☐ Chest ☐ Rh. Fever ☐   Business ....
Med/Tabs ☐ Allergies ☐ Blood ☐   Other ....
GA/Op/Hosp ☐ Diabetes ☐ Other ☐
GP: not known ....   Occupation ....

B-Wings taken on

Notes   MH clear
new pt., irregular attender, prefers no recalls

10.9.12	⁸⁄₀ 6⎤ lost fill ⁴⁄₁₂ ago
	gross caries + pain ++ now
	pt wants ext ok. lfa taken
	x/a 6⎤ in 2 pieces, 3mm distal
	root apex remaining — pt. told
	citanest x 2 no probs.
	HA achieved POIG to pt DTC C/Fwd. ctl.

Figure 11.20   Handwritten procedure entry.

In summary, they are as follows:

- All sharps are carefully disposed of in the sharps box – this includes local anaesthetic needles
- All autoclavable items are placed in a washer-disinfector unit or an ultrasonic bath and are decontaminated thoroughly before being placed in the autoclave for sterilisation
- All contaminated waste is placed in hazardous waste sacks or sharps bins
- All surfaces are disinfected using the correct solution

Because of the liklihood of blood splatter occurring during surgical procedures, the following additional actions must be taken:

- **PPE for the dental team** – over and above the usual PPE requirements for dental procedures, surgical gowns or single-use plastic aprons will have been used to prevent blood contamination of the uniform; these must be disposed of as hazardous waste
- **Disposable items** – wherever possible, disposable items will have been used to prevent cross-infection, including aspirators, scalpel blades, needles, suture needles, etc.; these must be disposed of as hazardous waste, some of them as sharps
- **Contamination policy** – any single-use items and materials that have been opened but not used during the procedure should be disposed of anyway, to avoid their possible contamination and then spread of infection by resealing and using at a later date
- **Suction equipment** – this must be run through immediately after the procedure with the required disinfectant solution to remove all traces of blood from its inner workings, rather than at the end of the session as usual
- **Operative field** – should be assumed to be blood-contaminated and wiped down thoroughly with sodium hypochlorite (bleach) or another accepted decontaminant, as soon as the patient has left the surgery
- **Equipment coverage** – items such as the dental chair will obviously be reused and are not sterilisable, so they will have been covered before the procedure with a single-use impervious membrane to prevent blood contamination – these barrier covers must be disposed of as hazardous waste

12

Unit 312: Principles of Infection Control in the Dental Environment

Learning outcomes

1. Understand the process of infection control
2. Understand the significance of microorganisms
3. Understand the management of infectious conditions affecting dental patients
4. Know the various methods of decontamination
5. Understand relevant health and safety legislation, policies and guidelines

Outcome 1 assessment criteria
The learner can:
- Describe the causes of cross-infection
- Describe the methods for preventing cross-infection
- Explain the principles of standard (universal) infection control precautions

Outcome 2 assessment criteria
The learner can:
- Describe the main microorganisms in potentially infectious conditions
- Explain the routes of transmission of microorganisms
- Explain the significance of the terms "pathogens" and "non-pathogens"

Outcome 3 assessment criteria
The learner can:
- Describe infectious conditions which affect individuals within the dental environment
- Describe what actions to take to prevent the spread of infectious diseases in the dental environment

Diploma in Dental Nursing, Level 3, Third Edition. Carole Hollins.
© 2014 John Wiley & Sons, Ltd. Published 2014 by John Wiley & Sons, Ltd.
Companion website: www.wiley.com/go/hollins/dentalnursinglevel3

- Explain the importance of immunisation of dental personnel
- Describe how the potentially infectious conditions affect the body systems

Outcome 4 assessment criteria

The learner can:
- Describe the principles and methods of clinical and industrial sterilisation
- Describe the principles and methods of disinfection
- Explain the preparation of a clinical area to control cross-infection
- Explain the procedures used to decontaminate a clinical environment after use
- State the chemical names for decontaminants and where they are used

Outcome 5 assessment criteria

The learner can:
- Identify health and safety policies and guidelines in relation to infection control
- Describe how to deal with a sharps injury
- Explain the use of personal protective equipment (PPE) in the dental environment
- Describe ways of dealing with clinical and non-clinical waste

This unit will be assessed by:
- an assessment paper containing multiple choice and short answers questions

The content is the theory and underpinning knowledge required and links to the information contained in Chapters 1 and 4.

The maintenance of a high standard of cleanliness and the control of infection are topics of huge importance in the dental workplace, as they are in any clinical environment. All members of the dental team have a duty of care to protect their patients and themselves from coming to harm while on the premises, and one potential area of vulnerability is to become contaminated by, or to acquire an infection from, another patient or a member of staff or from a dirty instrument. This contamination is called **cross-infection**.

The methods used to avoid cross-infection are the foundations of good infection control and of the principles of maintaining an adequate standard of cleanliness. The environment, instruments and equipment must all be properly prepared and maintained before, during and after each dental procedure. These preparation and maintenance tasks are two of the main duties of a dental nurse working at the chairside.

The aim of the preparation procedure is to ensure that all of the instruments and equipment to be used are clean and free of contamination by microorganisms from a previous patient or from dental staff. They can then be safely used in the prepared environment (the dental surgery) without the risk of passing on, or cross-infecting, the next patient or staff.

Similarly, the aim of the maintenance procedure is to ensure that all the instruments and equipment used are then disposed of safely, or cleaned to a high enough standard that they can be reused without the risk of cross-infecting the next patient, and so on. Likewise, the environment must also be cleaned thoroughly so that it is safe to be reused.

The risk that the microorganisms pose is that they can spread disease and infection from one person to another, either directly from person to person, or indirectly via contaminated instruments or equipment.

Those microorganisms that are capable of causing disease are referred to as **pathogenic microorganisms**, while those unable to cause disease are called **non-pathogenic microorganisms**.

A full understanding of the principles of infection control involves an understanding of the basics in relation to microbiology and pathology, so that the actions of the microorganisms, the way in which they cause disease and the body's defence mechanisms against them can be appreciated.

Background knowledge of microorganisms

There are four main types of microscopic organisms involved in transmitting disease:

- Bacteria
- Viruses
- Fungi
- Protozoa

Protozoa have little clinical significance in dentistry.

Bacteria:

- They are visible under a light microscope
- They are single-celled organisms
- Their rigid wall determines their shape, and therefore their name; so circular bacteria are called "cocci", rod-shaped bacteria are called "bacilli", and spiral-shaped bacteria are "spiro-chaetes" (Figure 12.1)
- They survive as spores in unfavourable environments (extremes of temperature or very dry conditions, for example)
- Active bacteria are prevented from reproducing and multiplying by **bacteriostatic antibiotics**
- They can also be killed by **bactericidal antibiotics**
- Spores can only be killed by the process of **sterilisation**

Viruses:

- They are so small that they are only visible using an electron microscope (so their correct definition would be an ultra-microorganism)
- They must live within the cells of other organisms (host cells)

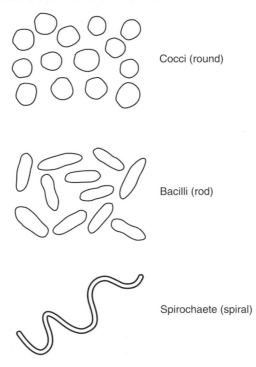

Cocci (round)

Bacilli (rod)

Spirochaete (spiral)

Figure 12.1 Shapes of bacteria.

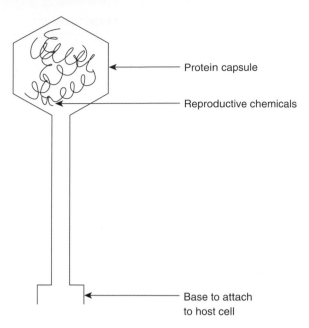

Protein capsule

Reproductive chemicals

Base to attach
to host cell

Figure 12.2   Structure of a virus. Source: *Levison's Textbook for Dental Nurses*, 11th edition (Hollins), 2013. Reproduced with permission of Wiley-Blackwell.

- They exist as a protein capsule containing the necessary chemicals to reproduce within the host cell (Figure 12.2)
- It is this protein capsule that causes our body to react against them and it is unique for each virus
- They are unaffected by antibiotics, but some can be treated using **antiviral drugs**
- **Vaccines** have been developed to provide immunity against some of the more serious viral infections (such as hepatitis, measles, mumps)

Fungi:

- They are larger than bacteria but still only visible with a light microscope
- They are actually a type of microscopic plant similar to mushrooms and toadstools, and reproduce by budding or by spore production
- They grow by producing an extensive branching network across tissues (called hyphae)
- Only one fungus is clinically significant in dentistry, and that is the organism causing oral thrush – *Candida albicans*
- It is unaffected by antibiotics but can be treated with **antifungal agents**

Infections with various microorganisms that are of importance in dentistry include the following:

- **Dental caries** – bacterial infection of the hard tissues of the tooth, especially with *Streptococcus mutans*
- **Periodontitis** – bacterial infection of the periodontium, especially with *Porphyromonas gingivalis*
- **Cold sore** – viral infection of the lip with h**erpes simplex type I**
- **Oral thrush** – fungal infection of the oral soft tissues with *Candida albicans*
- **Hepatitis** – viral infection of the liver with various organisms, including **hepatitis A, B, C, E or non-A-non-B**
- **Chickenpox** – viral infection of certain nerves with **herpes varicella**
- **AIDS (acquired immune deficiency syndrome)** – viral infection of the immune system with **human immunodeficiency virus (HIV)**

281

- **Shingles** – viral infection of certain nerves with **herpes zoster**
- **Meningitis** – bacterial infection of the brain coverings with **meningococci**
- **Glandular fever** – viral infection of the lymph glands with **Epstein–Barr virus**
- **Mumps** – viral infection of the parotid salivary glands with **paramyxovirus**

More recently, the existence of **prions** has been discovered. These are not living microorganisms, but are a type of special protein that is also capable of causing disease. Their associated diseases include "mad cow disease" and the human variation of it, called **Creutzfeldt–Jakob Disease (CJD)**. CJD affects the brain and spinal cord and has no known treatment or cure – it is a fatal illness.

The significance of prions to clinical dentistry is that they cause cross-infection through contaminated nerve tissue, theoretically including that found within the root canals of teeth and referred to as "the pulp".

Prions cannot be killed by the disinfection or sterilisation methods currently used in the dental surgery. For this reason, recent regulatory changes dictate that the dental instruments used to carry out root canal treatments (endodontics) must be regarded as single-use and safely disposed of between patients.

Infection

Infection occurs when pathogenic microorganisms gain entry to the body tissues. In the dental surgery environment, this can happen in a variety of ways:

- **Direct contact** with body fluids – blood, saliva or vomit
- **Airborne droplets** of blood or saliva – from sneezing or coughing
- **Aerosol spray** containing blood or saliva – created during the use of dental handpieces and water sprays
- **Direct entry** through damaged skin or membranes – cuts, grazes, piercing of the eye membrane
- **Inoculation injury** with a contaminated sharp instrument – such as a "needlestick" injury

The methods used in the dental surgery environment to reduce the risk of infection by a pathogenic microorganism will be discussed in detail later in this chapter.

Exposure to these microorganisms does not always result in an infection progressing to become a disease. The body has natural defence mechanisms in place to prevent the microorganisms gaining entry in the first place and to fight the invaders if they do manage to penetrate the body tissues.

Response of the body to infection

The body has three lines of natural defence against infection:

1. An **intact skin and mucous membrane** to prevent the entry of the microorganisms initially, with surface secretions to immobilise them – such as sweat, saliva, and gastric juice produced in the stomach
2. The **inflammatory response** initiated by the body cells if the skin or mucous membranes are breached
3. The **immune response** if infection takes hold, whereby the body's immune system is activated to fight the infection

Inflammatory response

If the microorganisms do gain entry to the body, the tissues involved will become irritated by their presence, and the five classic signs of inflammation will be seen:

- **Heat, redness, and swelling** – due to the increased blood flow to the area
- **Pain** – caused by the pressure of the increased blood flow on the surrounding nerve endings in the tissues affected
- **Loss of function of the affected tissue** – due to the pain and swelling present

When the inflammation and swelling occur quickly and over a short period of time, the condition is very painful and is referred to as **acute inflammation**. A dental example is an acute alveolar abscess. When the swelling is less pronounced and occurs over a longer period, it tends to be far less painful or even painless and is referred to as **chronic inflammation**. A dental example is chronic periodontitis.

In fit and healthy patients, the microorganisms are usually overcome by the body's own inflammatory response. The increased blood flow carries huge numbers of **leucocytes** (white blood cells) to the area and these pass out of the capillaries and into the tissues at the site of the infection. They battle with the invading microorganisms, and **pus** is formed as the various cells die. In addition, **antitoxins** and **antibodies** may be carried to the area in the blood plasma and assist in the attack against the microorganisms.

In the very young, the elderly or those who are ill and debilitated, help is often required to stop the invasion of the body tissues by the microorganisms. This is the role of antibiotics, antivirals and antifungals. These drugs may also have to be prescribed when the microorganisms involved are particularly nasty and strong, or **virulent**.

Immune response

283

Once the body has been exposed to an invasion by a microorganism, our immune system develops **antibodies** to it and **antitoxins** to the poisons they produce. This ensures that if the same microorganism and its toxins attack the body cells in future, they are recognised and the body is able to automatically fight off the infection. This is referred to as **acquired immunity.**

Immunity can also be naturally received from one's mother, or acquired by **vaccination** against an illness without actually suffering from that illness. This method tends to be used to give acquired immunity against more serious illnesses, such as hepatitis B. Unfortunately vaccines have not yet been developed against other serious blood borne diseases that pose a risk to dental staff, such as AIDS.

While working at the chairside, dental staff members are particularly vulnerable to becoming infected by microorganisms from patients – directly from their blood or saliva, by inhalation of contaminated aerosols or airborne droplets, or by contact with infectious lesions in their oral cavity. This is why all dental personnel must be vaccinated against a range of diseases before starting to work at the chairside, why they must always wear PPE when in clinical contact with patients or equipment and instruments, and why they must always follow the infection control policy of the dental workplace at all times.

Occupational hazards – cross-infection and inoculation injury

Cross-infection, especially by inoculation injury, is one of the three major occupational hazards in dentistry; the other two are exposure to ionizing radiation and mercury poisoning. All three concern dental nurses and they must be trained to be aware of the dangers and know how to avoid them. Cross-infection is covered here as its prevention is the purpose of good infection control.

The close nature of dental treatment exposes all surgery staff to a variety of microorganisms on a daily basis, as dental treatment often involves the shedding of blood. Even the smallest blood-stained droplets may contain viruses, and such blood-borne viruses can be sprayed over a wide area of the surgery when using high-speed handpieces and ultrasonic scalers, as an aerosol, and by three-in-one syringes as spatter. In this way, instruments, work surfaces, surgery equipment and surgery staff are all exposed to potential contamination.

The pathogenic microorganisms of particular concern to the dental team are:

- **HIV** – a viral infection that destroys the body's leucocytes, weakening the patient's immune system and leaving them unable to fight off diseases naturally. They eventually go on to develop AIDS, a fatal condition and for which there is no vaccine currently available

- **Hepatitis B** – a viral infection causing liver inflammation, which is often fatal. All dental staff must be immunised against the virus before working in the clinical environment
- **Hepatitis C** – a similar virus to that causing hepatitis B, but much more likely to prove fatal. There is no current vaccination against the virus
- **Herpes simplex type I** – a viral infection affecting the lips and oral cavity in particular. It is not fatal, but is highly contagious when "cold sore" lesions are present on the lips of the sufferer

By always following "standard precautions" (see later) to control infection within the clinical environment, the risk to staff and other patients of being cross-infected from sufferers of these diseases should be minimal. However, it is good practice to take additional precautions when treating patients known to be suffering from any of the first three (the more serious) of these infections (discussed later).

Any patient attending with an active cold sore should not be dentally treated except in an emergency. The lesion will diminish within 10 days, so their appointment can be rebooked as necessary.

In addition, dental staff may come into contact with other diseases during a normal working day, or even be the source of an infection to colleagues or patients if not appropriately vaccinated themselves. It is therefore of great importance that all dental staff receive the following immunisation programme before working at the chairside:

- **Diphtheria** – normally received routinely during childhood
- **Pertussis** – whooping cough, normally received routinely during infancy
- **Poliomyelitis** – normally received routinely during childhood
- **MMR** [measles, mumps and rubella (German measles)] – normally received during infancy
- **Tetanus** – normally received routinely during childhood and can be boosted as required
- **Tuberculosis** – received routinely after giving a negative Heaf test, but may need boosting after 15 years
- **Hepatitis B** – received as an occupationally required vaccine before working in any clinical area, a blood test is required to prove seroconversion and ensure immunity, but boosters are currently not considered necessary
- **Chickenpox** – if not naturally immune due to childhood exposure
- **Meningitis** – normally received routinely as a teenager
- **Influenza and swine influenza** – received as an adult when winter outbreaks are expected

Special care should be taken if child patients have been in contact with viral infections such as **measles**, **mumps** or **rubella** (German measles). The virus is present in saliva before any signs of illness are apparent, and surgery staff may become infected in this way from an apparently fit child. If there is any evidence of contact, appropriate questioning of parents will allow the dentist to assess the risk of infection and decide whether to postpone treatment. Although such infections are usually trivial in children, they can cause serious complications in susceptible adults.

If rubella occurs in the first 3 months of pregnancy, it can affect the unborn child – and this may happen before pregnancy is confirmed. Such a child is likely to have serious physical defects, and in such cases there are strong medical grounds for advising termination of the pregnancy.

Adult males are most at risk from mumps as it may cause sterility. All surgical staff should therefore check their own medical history and vaccination records. They should be immune to common childhood infections previously contracted and are only at risk from any which are not included in these records.

Even such a trivial viral infection as the common cold is infectious. If surgery staff or their patients have a cold, transmission to others can be prevented by wearing protective clothing. Although the effects of a cold are not serious, they often necessitate time off work with the resultant inconvenience caused by staff shortage.

Hepatitis B

Hepatitis B is an inflammation of the liver caused by a virus. Its effect varies from a mild attack of jaundice to a severe or fatal illness. Over 50% of cases are undiagnosed as their symptoms are too mild to indicate the disease. On the other hand, 80% of primary liver cancers are as a result of hepatitis B.

The hepatitis B virus (HBV) is always present in the blood of people suffering from the disease. It may also be present in people who have no symptoms of the disease. Such people are called **carriers**; they may or may not have had any symptoms before and most of them are unaware that they are carriers. About one person in every 1000 of the population is an HBV carrier, so all dentists are likely to treat patients who are carriers at some point in their career.

Hepatitis B is highly infective and is very resistant to destruction. It can survive boiling for up to half an hour, immersion in chlorhexidine disinfectant, and can live outside the body for some weeks. Disinfectants capable of killing HBV include those based on hypochlorite.

Hepatitis B virus has been found in all body fluids, including blood, saliva and breast milk. It is transmitted by people suffering from the disease and by carriers who have no symptoms at all and are unaware of their condition. Diagnosis is by blood test.

In dental practice, the main source of infection is by direct contact with blood containing HBV. This is most likely to occur from an inoculation injury, i.e. accidentally pricking oneself with a syringe needle used on an HBV carrier – a third of such accidents results in HBV infection.

Staff members are also at risk from the use of high speed equipment, such as an air turbine handpiece with water spray, an ultrasonic scaler or a three-in-one syringe. These release a cloud of water and saliva particles into the air which, if contaminated with a carrier's blood, may infect the dentist or dental nurse via the nose, eyes or skin abrasions. Furthermore, adjacent working surfaces become infected too; while inadequate sterilisation procedures may cause infection of other patients. Infection of staff from non-sharp causes may be prevented by protective clothing, as described previously.

Although the risks may seem alarming, all dental nurses and other chairside staff are required to be vaccinated against HBV and should therefore be safe from danger.

285

High-risk groups

Among the general population, the main modes of transmission of HBV are childbirth, the sharing of needles by drug addicts, and sexual contact. Thus certain groups of people are much more likely to be carriers, including:

- Drug addicts
- The sexually promiscuous
- Those who have received long-term regular blood transfusions, such as haemophiliacs, dialysis and transplant patients
- Special needs patients living in institutions, and staff in close contact with them
- Those working or living in institutions, such as prisons or rehabilitation centres for drug addicts and alcoholics
- Partners and close relatives of carriers, not necessarily with sexual contact

Prevention of cross-infection

As the majority of HBV carriers are unaware of their condition, it has been estimated that 400 are treated daily in dental practice. But provided the sterilisation and surgery hygiene procedures in this chapter are adopted, there need be no cause for alarm. However, the existence of high-risk groups emphasises the importance of obtaining an adequate medical history before treatment.

Fortunately all dental staff can obtain protection against hepatitis B by vaccination. This will also protect their patients against HBV infection from dental staff. Vaccination is available under the NHS. It involves a series of three injections, followed by a blood test to check its success. A booster injection may be required at a later date. As vaccination is a requirement for chairside employment, documentary evidence of successful immunisation must be kept. Although vaccination is completely safe, special arrangements are necessary for staff who are pregnant, or who become pregnant, during the course of injections.

Treatment of known carriers

The basic principle of preventing infection with HBV is to avoid contact with the patient's blood. In addition to the sterilisation and surgery hygiene procedures already detailed, the following extra precautions have been recommended for general practice:

- For operations involving extensive loss of blood, such as multiple extractions and minor oral surgery, or if the disease is in an active state, refer the patient to hospital – where full sterile surgical facilities are available
- Reserve the last appointment of the day for treatment of known carriers. This allows more time for infection control procedures before any more patients are seen, but does not excuse non-compliance with the full infection control procedures at other times
- Move all unnecessary equipment and materials away from the chairside. Protect essential working surfaces and equipment controls, such as switches, operating light handle and three-in-one syringe, with plastic bags or cling film
- Take great care to avoid inoculation injuries
- Regard steel burs and matrix bands as disposable. After treatment, flush the aspirator tubing through with hypochlorite, and leave the solution in a collection jar overnight
- Items that cannot be sterilised by heat or hypochlorite should be immersed in a suitable disinfectant for the manufacturer's recommended time
- Launder linen and towels in a hot wash of 90 °C for 10 minutes
- Pregnant staff or those who have not been vaccinated against HBV should not have any contact with known carriers

Hepatitis C

This disease is similar to hepatitis B in the way that it is contracted, transmitted and diagnosed. However, it is a far more dangerous disease with a much higher mortality rate and there is no vaccine for it. In the past, hepatitis C was sometimes transmitted by blood transfusion, but this has not happened since 1993, when screening of donors began.

Nowadays the main sources of infection are drug addiction, tattooing, body piercing and other modes of infected blood-to-blood contact, but sexual transmission is uncommon. The pathogenic microorganism involved is the hepatitis C virus (HCV).

The greatest risk to dental staff is from an inoculation injury, but provided that the safety precautions to prevent this are followed, there is no danger of HCV infection. However, it should be understood that if such a situation does arise, there is a 1 in 30 chance of transmission of the disease.

AIDS

In people with AIDS, the body's natural defence mechanism against infection is seriously impaired. Consequently, AIDS patients succumb to infections that are not normally serious or not normally experienced. The outcome of AIDS is usually fatal as there is no cure, no vaccination and no resistance to infection. However, progress of the disease can be delayed, and life prolonged, by the use of antiviral and other drugs which boost the immune system. The apparent success of these treatments is, unfortunately, having the perverse effect of increasing the number of people contracting the disease. The reason for this is that many people are now ignoring the safety measures that were followed in the past, when AIDS was rapidly fatal.

AIDS is caused by infection with the human immunodeficiency virus (HIV). There are no particular symptoms of AIDS as they depend solely upon whichever chance infection affects the sufferer. Like hepatitis B, the AIDS virus has been found in most body fluids but is transmitted mainly by contact with blood containing the virus. HIV is present in the blood of all infected persons but it usually takes years before they suffer any effects. Furthermore, as there are no specific symptoms, many of those infected with HIV are unaware that they have AIDS. Diagnosis is by blood test.

Infectivity

Unlike HBV, the AIDS virus is not very infective and is not resistant to heat or disinfectants. Although every infected person is potentially infectious, repeated exposure to HIV in blood or body fluids is usually required for transmission of AIDS. Among the general population the usual modes of transmission are sexual promiscuity, the sharing of needles by drug addicts, childbirth and repeated transfusions with contaminated blood.

In dental practice, the main hazard is an inoculation injury, but the infectivity of HIV is so low that a single such accident would only result in a 1 in 300 chance of contracting AIDS. However, no chances can be taken as AIDS is a fatal disease for which there is no cure and no vaccine.

High-risk groups

From the modes of transmission of HIV just described, those most at risk of being carriers are:

- The sexually promiscuous
- Drug addicts
- Haemophiliacs and other patients who have received long-term regular blood transfusions
- Sexual partners of these groups
- Infants born to infected mothers

Prevention

Although no preventive treatment by drugs or vaccination is possible, AIDS is easily avoided. All that is required as far as the general population is concerned is to avoid any form of sexual promiscuity or the sharing of needles with drug addicts.

In dental practice, prevention is the same as for hepatitis B – by correct sterilisation and surgery hygiene procedures. Dentists may be the first health care workers to see the early signs of AIDS, as some very unusual mouth conditions may occur for no apparent reason. As in the case of oral cancer, early referral to a specialist may be a life-saving measure.

Treatment of known carriers

This is the same as for hepatitis carriers. Fortunately HIV has a very low infectivity and is easily destroyed by routine sterilisation procedures. Nevertheless, no chances can be taken as AIDS is fatal and no vaccination is available.

Known carriers of HIV and hepatitis viruses are those who are aware of their condition and have informed the dentist when their medical history is taken. Patient confidentiality is of paramount importance in such cases. Most carriers are either unaware of their condition or unwilling to disclose it in case the information is revealed to unauthorised people. Some are also afraid of being denied dental treatment if they admit to being carriers. When any medical history is taken, it is ethically and legally essential to ensure that it cannot be overheard anywhere else in the practice, and is taken under conditions that give patients the confidence to provide a complete relevant history without embarrassment.

Only a minority of carriers are known to be such, so most are treated without the dentist being aware of their condition. This emphasises the importance of strict adherence to correct procedures for the prevention of cross-infection by all staff within the dental workplace.

New variant Creutzfeld–Jakob disease (vCJD)

This is one of a group of rare, but fatal, related diseases (similar to "mad cow disease") caused by infection with a unique non-microbial source of disease called a **prion protein**. The infection occurs within nerve tissue, affecting both the brain and all nerve tissues throughout the body, including that found within the pulp of the teeth. Its importance is entirely due to the fact that prions cannot be destroyed by normal methods of sterilisation.

Consequently, current recommendations are to consider all endodontic instruments that come into contact with the tooth pulp as single use items, to prevent the transmission of the disease by indirect cross-infection, although the risk is considered to be only theoretical. Therefore broaches, files, reamers and handpiece-driven endodontic instruments must be safely disposed of as infectious hazardous waste (sharps) after a single use.

Inoculation injury

Nearly all dental procedures involve the use of sharp items; these include local anaesthetic needles, sharp instruments, or scalpel blades. All must be handled with great care by staff to avoid an inoculation injury.

Every dental workplace must have a policy in place to avoid a sharps injury and it should ideally include all of the following points:

- The dentist (or therapist or suitably trained hygienist) using a local anaesthetic needle should be the person responsible for its re-sheathing and safe placement in a sharps bin, so that injury to others does not occur as there is no transference of the sharp item from one person to another
- Needle guards should be used when re-sheathing needles, so that they can be placed within their plastic sheath without being held in the fingers (see Figure 1.29)
- Heavy-duty rubber gloves and full PPE should be worn by any staff responsible for instrument cleaning and debridement before sterilization

Although a sharps injury from a sterile, unused instrument may be momentarily painful, it is of no consequence save to reconsider the level of care taken by the staff member involved. However, if a contaminated inoculation injury occurs, the following actions must be carried out:

- Stop all treatment immediately and attend to the wound
- Squeeze the wound to encourage bleeding, but do not suck it
- Wash the area with soap and running water, then dry and cover the wound with a waterproof dressing
- Note the name, address and contact details of the source patient if a contaminated item is involved, so that their medical history can be checked immediately
- Complete the accident book
- Report the incident to the senior dentist/line manager
- The consultant microbiologist at the local hospital must be contacted immediately if the source patient is a known or suspected HIV or hepatitis C carrier, as emergency antiviral treatment must commence within 1 hour of the injury

The contact details for the consultant microbiologist should be readily available within the infection control policy documentation, and updated whenever necessary.

Infection control

Infection control is one of the most important parts of an effective risk management programme to improve the quality and safety of patient care and the occupational health of staff. Control of cleanliness in the dental workplace is imperative because:

- All patients have hundreds of oral bacteria present, even when they are healthy
- When diseases are present, they may also have fungi or viruses
- All instruments and equipment coming into contact with these microorganisms could potentially become contaminated by them
- If the instruments and equipment are not cleaned thoroughly between patients, other patients and staff can easily become cross-infected
- The use of dental air turbines creates an aerosol which falls onto the surrounding work surfaces in the clinical area and contaminates them
- Obviously, if staff are also not personally clean and are taking part in close dental procedures, they themselves can contaminate the patients and other staff members

Basic principles of infection control

A system of **standard precautions** (previously referred to as "universal precautions") has been adopted in healthcare work, which is designed to protect staff from inoculation and contamination risks and to protect patients from being exposed to the risk of cross-infection.

The basic principle is to assume that any patient may be infected with any microorganism at any time, and therefore that they always pose an infection risk to all dental staff and to other patients. A detailed medical history questionnaire, completed at the patient's initial attendance and updated at every appointment thereafter, will identify the majority of problems.

However, patients may be infected with a microorganism without showing any signs of disease, and may therefore be unaware of the risk they pose to others – these patients are called **carriers**. Patients may also choose not to disclose their full medical history to the dental staff, and would then wrongly be assumed to be "safe" to treat, without taking any additional precautions.

So, if all patients are always considered to be a possible source of infection (no matter what their medical history) and treated as such, the infection control techniques used in the dental environment will be good enough to reduce all cross-infection risks to a minimum.

The other basic principles of infection control to be adopted are summarised below:

- Apply good basic personal hygiene with regular appropriate hand washing
- Cover existing wounds with waterproof dressings
- Do not undertake invasive procedures if suffering from chronic skin lesions on the hands
- Wear appropriate gloves at all times when assisting and discard after single use
- Avoid contamination with body fluids by wearing appropriate protective clothing, safety spectacles and masks – referred to as "personal protective equipment"
- Institute approved procedures for decontamination of instruments and equipment
- Apply good basic environmental cleaning procedures
- Clear up blood and other body fluid spillages promptly
- Follow the correct procedure for safe disposal of contaminated waste and sharps
- Ensure all staff are aware of, understand and follow infection control policies and procedures
- Ensure all staff are fully vaccinated against hepatitis B (this is now a legal requirement for all those who work in the clinical environment) and that all childhood immunisations are up to date

In the dental surgery environment, special methods of infection control are now routinely practised in line with recent legislative and regulatory changes, as well as with Department of Health guidelines, in particular the following:

- Correct cleaning of the hands
- Use of PPE
- Correct cleaning of the clinical environment
- Correct cleaning of dental equipment, handpieces and instruments

The terms "cleaning" and "cleanliness" in a clinical context are quite different from a layperson's concept of them, and definitions of the relevant terms used here are as follows:

- **Social cleanliness** – clean to a socially acceptable standard, but not disinfected or sterilised
- **Disinfection** – the destruction of bacteria and fungi, but not spores or some viruses (the technique usually involves the use of chemicals)
- **Sterilisation** – the process of killing all microorganisms and spores to produce asepsis (the technique usually involves the use of special equipment which operates under high temperatures and pressure)
- **Asepsis** – the absence of all living pathogenic microorganisms
- **Decontamination** – the process used to remove contamination from reusable items, so that they are safe for further use on patients and safe for staff to handle – it may also be referred to as "reprocessing", and involves the following four stages:
  - **Cleaning**
  - **Disinfection**
  - **Inspection**
  - **Sterilisation**

Cleaning of the hands

This is the most important method of preventing cross-infection, and the technique used should be that stipulated by the Health and Safety Council. It is now a requirement for the correct hand washing technique to be displayed as a poster in all relevant areas of the dental workplace (see Figure 1.3).

The three levels of hand hygiene recognised are as follows:

- **Social** – to become physically clean from socially acquired microorganisms, using general-purpose liquid soap
- **Clinical/hygienic** – to destroy microorganisms, maintain cleanliness and avoid direct cross-infection using an approved antibacterial hand cleanser
- **Surgical** – to significantly reduce the numbers of normally resident microorganisms on the hands, before an invasive surgical procedure is carried out, using an approved antibacterial hand cleanser

Nails should be kept short and wounds covered with a waterproof dressing to reduce the number of areas for microorganisms to contaminate. The minimum amount of jewellery should be worn by those working in a clinical environment, for the same reason.

The correct procedure for **clinical/hygienic hand washing** is as follows:

- Turn on the tap using the foot or elbow control, to prevent contaminating the tap (see Figure 4.4)
- Wet both hands under running water of a suitable temperature
- Apply a suitable antibacterial liquid soap from the dispenser (see Figure 8.2) and wash all areas of both hands and wrists thoroughly – this should take at least 30 seconds to carry out thoroughly, and the correct routine is illustrated on the poster that is present at each hand washing station (see Figure 1.3)

- Nail brushes are not advised unless they are autoclavable, as they can become contaminated with repeated use
- Rinse both hands under running water, holding them so that the water does not flow back over the fingers
- Dry the hands thoroughly, using disposable paper towels for single use
- Heavy-duty gloves must be worn whenever the cleaning of dirty instruments is being carried out
- Clinical gloves must be worn whenever patients are being treated, and discarded between patients

Whenever a surgical clinical procedure is to be carried out, this hand washing procedure should be extended to include the forearms too, and should be carried out for a minimum of 2 minutes to be completed effectively. Special surgical grade hand wash should be used, with a sterile, single-use scrubbing brush.

At the end of the cleaning, the hands should be held up during rinsing to allow the water to drain off the elbows, and then the hands and forearms should be dried with sterile paper towels. Sterile gloves should then be placed on both hands. This "scrubbing-up" procedure is known as the **aseptic technique of hand washing**.

Social hand washing is that of a general level of cleanliness and should be carried out before preparing food or eating, and especially after using the toilet facilities. It follows a similar technique to that used for clinical hand cleansing, but should not take as long, as it need not include the wrists or forearms. Many suitable antibacterial hand wash liquids are available for both the washroom area and the surgeries.

Use of PPE

This includes items worn to prevent staff from coming into direct contact with patients, their blood and other bodily fluids, and contaminated instruments, by acting as a physical barrier between the staff member and the contamination source.

It is a legal requirement for dental employers to provide the following protective clothing for their staff (see Figure 4.1):

- Gloves of varying quality, as discussed earlier
- High-temperature-wash uniform, to be worn in the work area only
- Plastic apron to be worn over the uniform when soiling may occur during surgical procedures or while cleaning the surgery
- Safety glasses, goggles or visors to prevent contaminated material from entering the eyes
- Face masks of surgical quality should be worn whenever dental handpieces or ultrasonic equipment are in use, to prevent the inhalation of aerosol contamination and pieces of flying debris

Cleaning of the clinical environment

The whole of the dental practice should be cleaned to a socially acceptable standard on a daily basis, and this is usually carried out by a domestic cleaner. In clinical areas, however, a far higher standard of cleaning is necessary because these are the areas where contamination of the environment by body fluids is greatest and where the highest chance of cross-infection is likely to occur.

The standard to be achieved in the clinical environment is that of **disinfection**. This involves the use of various chemicals to inhibit the growth of, or ideally kill, bacteria and fungi. However, most are not effective against bacterial spores or some viruses. Those in common use in the dental workplace include the following (see Figure 1.21):

- **Bleach-based cleaners** – containing sodium hypochlorite and used to disinfect all non-metallic and non-textile surfaces, and to soak laboratory items
- **Aldehyde-based cleaners** – can be used on metallic surfaces and to soak laboratory items
- **Isopropyl alcohol wipes** – to disinfect items such as exposed X-ray film packets for safe handling during processing

- **Viricidal wipes** – as a recommended alternative to alcohol wipes, as they actually kill viruses
- **Chlorhexidine gluconate** – as an irrigating disinfectant during root canal treatments and as a skin cleanser

The dental workplace as a whole should be kept clean, dry and well ventilated. Some workplaces have air conditioning installed, but care should be taken that the system operates without the risk of recirculating the contaminated surgery air. In addition, outbreaks of *Legionella* have been linked to poorly maintained air conditioning systems, and various testing and maintenance techniques must now be carried out on a regular basis where these air control systems are in operation. *Legionella* is a serious, pneumonia-type infection affecting the respiratory system, which can be fatal.

A written protocol for surgery cleaning must be available in all dental workplaces, which lays out the correct procedure to be followed in a logical manner and details how each item should be dealt with. In general, it must include the following points:

- All work surfaces should have the minimum items of equipment out for each procedure, and when these items are not in use they should be stored in drawers or cupboards to prevent their contamination with aerosols
- All stored instruments should be kept in lidded trays or in sealed pouches while in the cupboards or drawers (Figure 12.3)
- Pouches must be date-stamped, with a one year "use by" date indicated on every pouch
- Areas should be designated as "clean" and "dirty" so that dirty used instruments are not placed where clean items should be – this is called **zoning**
- Work surfaces should be cleaned after each session with a detergent solution or a suitable viricidal disinfectant, using a suitable reusable microfibre cloth or ideally single-use paper towels
- Equipment likely to be contaminated during operation such as chair and light controls and headrests should be covered with impervious plastic sheets (such as cling film) and changed between patients – this is called using **protective barriers**
- Dental aspirators that exhaust outside the surgery area will reduce the risk of aerosol contamination; they should be used routinely and flushed through daily with a recommended non-foaming disinfectant (Figure 12.4)
- Clinical records and computer keyboards should not be handled while gloves are being worn, and keyboards should also be protected by an impervious barrier cover
- All non-metallic equipment should be wiped down with a bleach-based preparation, which is particularly effective against viruses, at the end of each day
- Bleach-based disinfectants cannot be used on metallic items as they will corrode the metal
- All intra-oral radiographs should be wiped with an isopropyl alcohol (or suitable alternative) wipe before being handled with clean gloves and taken for processing

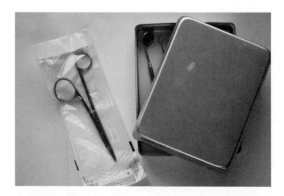

Figure 12.3   Sealed pouch and lidded tray.

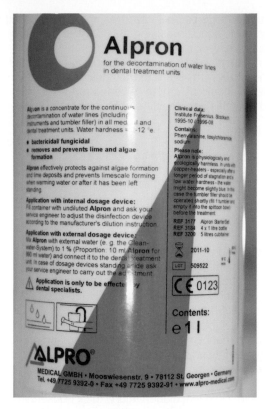

Figure 12.4　A non-foaming aspirator disinfectant.

Cleaning of equipment, handpieces and instruments

These are potentially the most contaminated of all items found in the clinical environment, as they are used in the patient's mouth where microorganisms proliferate. Their potential to cause injury and disease by cross-infection to all dental staff should not be underestimated. All of these items should always be handled carefully and only while wearing the correct articles of PPE, so that staff avoid direct contact while transferring the items for disposal or cleaning.

The risk of cross-infection between patients can be eliminated by the use of **disposable items** that are safely discarded after a single use, rather than being cleaned and reused. For expensive items, such as handpieces and metal hand instruments, this is not feasible and so these items must be **decontaminated** and then **sterilised** to ensure that all microorganisms and bacterial spores have been killed during the cleaning process.

Single-use items are sterilised by the manufacturer using an industrial process, before being made available to the dental workplace. The usual industrial sterilisation method is that of the wrapped and sealed item being exposed to gamma irradiation before despatch.

Any single-use items that are to be disposed of are classed as **hazardous waste** and treated accordingly (see later). Other items are treated as follows:

- All items which are not disposable after a single use should be sterilised in an **autoclave**
- Before placing in an autoclave, all solid debris must be removed from the items, either by manual cleaning, the use of an **ultrasonic bath** (see Figure 4.11), or the use of a **washer-disinfector** (see Figure 4.12)

- Only then should these items be autoclaved, as any residual solid debris left on the items will harbour microorganisms and spores, and shield them from the sterilisation process so that they are capable of causing cross-infection
- Handpieces must not be placed in an ultrasonic bath, and the manufacturer's specific instructions should be consulted with regard to their advice on oiling after sterilisation
- Sterilised instruments should be stored in lidded trays in cupboards or drawers, or in sealed and date-stamped pouches until they are next used, or until they pass the "use by" date and are re-sterilised

Details of cleaning techniques for reusable items

Manual cleaning

This is the simplest method of cleaning reusable items before sterilization, but is the most difficult to validate – i.e. to prove that it has been effective – as it depends entirely on the thoroughness of cleaning by the staff member at the time. By its "hands on" nature, it is also the technique most likely to result in an inoculation injury to the staff member (see later).

Under Department of Health guidelines, manual cleaning is an acceptable method to be used (as long as plans are clearly in place to introduce automated cleaning at some point in the future), but under best-practice guidance it should only ever be used on items where the manufacturer states that automated cleaning is unsuitable.

The basic procedure for safe and effective manual cleaning of items is as follows:

- Wear suitable PPE – to avoid inoculation injury, thick household gloves should be worn whenever any items are cleaned manually, as well as face and eye protection
- Always clean the items as soon as possible after use, to avoid contaminants drying onto their surfaces – this is far more difficult to remove than wet contamination
- Use cold water and a suitable detergent in a dedicated instrument-cleaning sink/bowl – hot water "fixes" contaminants such as blood onto the item surface and makes it far more difficult to remove
- Use nylon bristled, autoclavable scrubbing brushes to remove difficult contaminants, as wire bristles will scratch the metal surfaces and allow corrosion and rusting to occur
- The items should be scrubbed while under the water surface to avoid spraying contaminants into the immediate vicinity
- A separate sink/bowl of distilled or reverse osmosis water should be used to rinse the items after cleaning, in order to remove any detergent and loose contamination
- Tap water must not be used as it will contain unwanted chemicals and its level of "cleanliness" is dependent on the water utility provider rather than on the workplace
- The items should be visibly inspected (ideally using an illuminated magnifier – see Figure 4.10) to ensure that all contamination has been removed – if any is found, the item should be cleaned and rinsed again
- The items should then be autoclaved as soon as possible before they can dry in the air – this can result in corrosion or recontamination otherwise
- Those that are to be bagged before vacuum sterilising should be dried thoroughly first

Ultrasonic bath

These are suitable devices that act to remove debris from items by vibrating at an ultrasonic frequency and transmitting that vibration to the instruments loaded into the bath on the tray (see Figure 4.11). They require the use of special detergents diluted in distilled/reverse osmosis water within the bath to be effective, and the solution should be replaced at the end of each clinical session or when it is obviously heavily contaminated with particles of debris.

Ultrasonic baths should not be used to debride handpieces, as the bearings will become damaged. Manufacturers' instructions should be consulted for any particular operating advice relevant to each machine used in the dental workplace.

The basic procedure to decontaminate items using the ultrasonic bath is as follows:

- Heavy soiling with blood and other visible contaminants should be reduced by briefly soaking the items in cold detergent solution beforehand and then rinsing
- Hinged items (such as extraction forceps) should be opened and assembled items (such as amalgam carriers) should be disassembled
- All items should be placed on the bath tray and be fully immersed beneath the solution, to allow debridement to occur effectively
- The bath should not be overloaded with items, as debridement will not be effective
- The timer should be set according to the manufacturer's instructions, the lid closed on the machine and the programme started – the lid must be closed to prevent aerosol contamination of the vicinity
- When the timer ends, the basket and its contents should be lifted and allowed to drain; the items should then be rinsed in a dedicated sink/bowl of distilled or reverse osmosis water
- The items should be visibly inspected to ensure debridement has occurred and, if debris remains, put through the process again
- Items should be sterilised as soon as possible after being decontaminated, as for manually cleaned items

Maintenance and testing of ultrasonic bath

As with all electrical items that are used to perform certain tasks in the dental workplace, the ultrasonic bath should be maintained on a regular basis by a service engineer or a delegated competent person in decontamination – for many units this is an annual recommendation by manufacturers, as a minimum.

The working efficiency of the bath will also be maintained if regular in-house testing is also carried out, and these daily and weekly duties are often delegated to the dental nurse.

Daily duties are as follows:

- **Strainer/filter cleaning** – remove these items from the bath and clean using a suitable detergent solution and brush, to remove the debris contamination produced during normal operation
- **Tank draining** – the bath solution should be fully drained at the end of the day, or at the end of a busy clinical session, so that contaminants are disposed of rather than transferred to future instruments
- **Cleaning check** – all instruments placed in the bath should be visibly checked at the end of the cycle to ensure that all visible debris has been removed – an illuminated magnifier should be available for use during this procedure (see Figure 4.10)

Additional weekly duties are as follows:

- **Safety check** – ensure that the lid of the bath fits adequately and continues to prevent aerosol contamination of the surroundings during use. Check for signs of any solution splatter around the unit
- **Protein residue test** – use of a special test device to ensure that protein residues are being removed effectively during the ultrasonic cycle, so that items are indeed decontaminated before sterilisation (proteins are present in blood, pulp, tooth and soft tissues and microorganisms)

One final test that can be carried out in-house on a quarterly basis to test the efficiency of the debridement action of the ultrasonic bath is an **activity test using aluminium foil**. Details of this test can be found in the Department of Health's HTM 01-05 document (see later), but basically it involves immersing several strips of aluminium foil in the bath solution and running a normal cycle. On inspection, the aluminium should be eroded off the strips at similar points along their length, indicating that the debridement action occurs similarly throughout the whole tank.

Any variation in the position and extent of the aluminium erosion indicates that the tank is not vibrating uniformly, and instrument debridement will therefore occur in an unsatisfactory "hit and miss" manner.

Washer-disinfector

These devices (see Figure 4.12) are the preferred method of item decontamination under the best-practice guidelines of HTM 01-05, although they are under further review with regard to the possibility of "protein fixing" during the cycle. The washer-disinfector operates in a similar fashion to a specialist dishwasher machine, and some makes are suitable for the safe disinfection of dental handpieces, as well as other dental items and instruments.

Each typical machine cycle goes through five stages during the cleaning and disinfection process, as follows:

- **Flush** – an initial pressure rinse to remove gross solid and liquid debris from items; previously this was using water at high temperatures, but now a temperature below 45 °C is recommended to prevent the possibility of protein fixing and the consequent failure of the disinfection cycle
- **Wash** – use of a recommended detergent and/or disinfectant with water to complete the removal of liquid and solid debris, by both chemical and mechanical actions during the wash process (so the detergent/disinfectant breaks down the debris chemically, and the mechanical action of the solution swishing around in the machine mechanically dislodges the debris from the items)
- **Rinse** – using suitable quality mains water (this will vary across the UK and needs to be clarified with the water provider in the area) or reverse osmosis water to remove all traces of the detergent/disinfectant solution; any evidence of marking, smearing or spotting on the cleaned items indicates that the water quality is inadequate for use in the machine
- **Thermal disinfection** – the temperature used is pre-set at the start of the cycle and can be varied depending on the contents of the load to be disinfected; the chosen temperature is then achieved and held for the required time within the machine
- **Drying** – heated air is pumped into the disinfection chamber so that any residual moisture is removed from all items before the end of the cycle, as wet items will allow microorganisms to recolonise their surfaces more readily

Full training of staff in the correct use of the washer-disinfector is vital to ensure that every cycle produces clean and disinfected items ready for sterilisation. Written records of any training received should be kept by the dental workplace, and the full procedure for the machine use should be included in the infection control policy documentation.

Maintenance and testing of washer-disinfector

As with the ultrasonic bath and other electrical devices, maintenance and testing of the washer-disinfector must be carried out on a regular basis by a service engineer. Intermediate in-house tests are also advised.

Some washer-disinfectors have automatic data-logging devices incorporated into their design that produce printouts of their operational parameters for each cycle (in a similar way to those produced by some autoclaves). This ensures that a validated record is available to prove that each cycle ran efficiently and had produced clean and disinfected items at its end point.

However, daily and weekly in-house efficiency tests should still be carried out, as for the ultra-sonic bath. In addition, on a quarterly basis, the following in-house tests should also be carried out on the washer-disinfector:

- **Automatic control test** – to ensure that the cycle parameters set are actually achieved, with regard to temperature, time, drying, etc.
- **Chemical dosing** – test to ensure that the detergent and/or disinfectant is released into the machine correctly during the cycle and that low levels of either are indicated as necessary
- **Thermometric disinfection test** – using a heavily soiled load, the temperatures achieved during the cycle are tested to ensure that those reached are suitable to ensure disinfection has occurred

Autoclave

Once reusable items have been decontaminated by either manual or automated means, they are ready to be rendered safe for reuse on another patient by undergoing sterilisation. The machines used in the dental workplace to achieve sterilisation are called autoclaves, and there are two basic types – "N" type and "B" type. A third specialised type ("S" type) is available for use, but this is more frequently seen in the hospital environment. The details of the more usual types are given here.

297

"N" type (downward displacement – see Figure 4.13) autoclave:

- Heats to 134 °C and holds for 3 minutes at 2.25 bar pressure (32 pounds per square inch, psi)
- Steam displaces air downwards in the chamber so that it contacts all items
- The cycle lasts for 15–20 minutes, depending on the make of the autoclave and how often it has been in use previously, as it warms up and retains the heat after each use
- It is suitable for unwrapped solid items laid in a single layer on perforated trays
- The machine can hold several trays at a time, cutting the number of cycles required
- The cycle can be set to dry instruments before they are removed from the autoclave
- The door cannot be opened during operation until the cycle is completed

"B" type (vacuum – see Figure 4.14) autoclave:

- Heats to 134 °C and holds for 3 minutes at 2.25 bar pressure
- Air is sucked out of the chamber to create a vacuum so that steam contacts all the items present as it is also sucked through, including the insides of hollow items
- There are various cycles to choose from, depending on the requirements of the loaded items for each cycle
- The cycle can last for up to 45 minutes if a vacuum programme is required
- The vacuum cycle is suitable for wrapped items and those with a hollow lumen, such as handpieces and triple syringe tips
- The machine often has a data-logging device incorporated so that the operating parameters for each cycle are recorded and can be checked (see Figure 4.8)
- The machine can hold several trays at a time, cutting the number of cycles required
- The cycle can be set to dry instruments before they are removed from the autoclave
- The door cannot be opened during operation until the cycle has been completed
- It is more expensive than the "N" type autoclave

However, neither type of autoclave will sterilise items thoroughly unless they have been suitably processed beforehand, and this is one of the most important duties for the dental nurse to complete on a daily basis, as detailed previously.

Handling and storage of sterilised items

The correct handling and storage of items once they leave the autoclave is imperative in ensuring that their sterility is maintained until they are required for use again. The obvious ways of achieving this are as follows:

- Removing from the autoclave and handling while wearing clean PPE
- Drying with a single-use cloth or towel
- Placing within a device to act as a barrier between the items and the general atmosphere to avoid aerosol and microorganism recontamination, such as:
  - Sealed view pouch
  - Lidded tray
  - Sterilisation bag (for use with vacuum autoclave only)

With all autoclaves, the sterilised items must be dry before any further packaging occurs, before storage. Residual moisture allows recontamination of the items with microorganisms, so it must be removed by using the "drying cycle" of the autoclave or by manually drying the items as soon as they are taken out of the autoclave.

Similarly, a damp cloth or towel that is repeatedly used to dry the items is also more likely to become contaminated over time, so single-use towels must be available.

For "N" type autoclaves, all items must be sterilised unwrapped and then dried and wrapped after removal from the machine. As they must therefore be handled to do so, it is currently recommended that the storage packages are date-stamped so that the items are used or re-sterilised within 1 year of this date (see Figure 4.15).

If the items are to be used again during that treatment session, they can be covered rather than fully wrapped.

With vacuum autoclaves, items can complete the sterilisation cycle while enclosed in pouches and lidded trays, and then be dried and further packaged at the end of the cycle. These items should then be date-stamped so that they can be safely reused within the 1-year period.

Once all items have been dried and packaged, they should be stored in their designated place in the dental workplace. While it is acceptable to store packaged items in the clinical area for ease of access, they must be kept within drawers or cupboards until immediately before use, and as far away from the chairside as possible. However, in the clinical area the potential for recontamination is greater than for other areas of the workplace, due to the aerosol scatter created during dental treatment and to the throughput of the patients.

The least contaminated area of the workplace should be the "clean zone" of the actual decontamination area itself, where the sterilised items are produced (see later) and where there is no access to the public. For this reason, best-practice guidelines recommend that all sterilised items are stored within the clean zone of the decontamination room, collected from there by staff when their use is imminent, and taken to the clinical area as required for use.

Maintenance and testing of autoclave

Autoclaves use pressure to ensure sterilisation of the contained items, and this means that they have to comply with various health and safety laws because of the potential danger they pose to staff and patients if they malfunction. The health and safety policy in all dental surgeries must contain written requirements for the correct use of autoclaves, as they are considered to be pressure vessels. The requirements are as follows:

- Daily test carried out on each autoclave, recording the temperature, pressure and time interval for a full cycle – these details must be kept as a written record in a dated log book
- An automatic control test should be carried out daily for all types of autoclave, and the test strip retained within the workplace records – the usual technique is to use a "TST" strip (see

Figure 4.7) or something similar
- A steam penetration test should also be carried out for vacuum autoclaves to ensure that steam does indeed penetrate the inside of any packaging used during the sterilisation cycle – these are usually performed using a Helix or Bowie-Dick test (see Figure 4.9)
- Only purified or reverse osmosis water should be used within the autoclave, never tap water
- Water should be drained from the reservoir and replaced daily
- Door seal and safety devices used to prevent door opening during the cycle must be visually checked on a weekly basis by designated staff
- An authorised engineer must carry out an annual inspection to ensure that each autoclave operates correctly and issue a certificate to that effect
- Each autoclave must also be checked for its conformation with the Pressure Systems Safety Regulations on a regular basis
- The practice's insurance policy must include third party liability cover for the use of autoclaves, in case of explosion and resulting injury to staff or patients
- Any serious accident involving an autoclave, including its explosion, must be reported to the Health and Safety Executive (HSE) under the Reporting of Injuries, Diseases and Dangerous Occurrences Regulations (RIDDOR – see later)

The first six points are very often delegated to a dental nurse, following suitable recorded training.

Other methods of sterilisation

As mentioned previously, some single-use products are provided by manufacturers as pre-packaged sterile items, such as syringes and needles, local anaesthetic cartridges, scalpel blades, swabs and other cotton products, gutta-percha and paper points used in endodontic treatments, and more recently the endodontic hand instruments themselves. These are industrially sterilised within sealed packages after production, by exposure to gamma rays, a type of radiation similar to X-rays. As gamma radiation is highly dangerous, it must be used under strict regulation and in specialised control zones, so it is not suitable for use in dental practice.

The effectiveness of the technique is checked for each batch of items, by carrying out microbiological tests on them before despatch. All industrially sterilised items are considered as single-use and disposable, but any with faulty packaging should also be safely discarded without being used.

In a dental environment in the hospital setting, it is likely that all items to be sterilised are collected and sent for decontamination and sterilisation **centrally**, along with any items from other departments and clinics. This is more efficient when large numbers of items are involved than for each department to operate its own autoclave. The autoclaves used centrally are the specialised "S" type, which tend to operate under high vacuum and are much larger, so that greater loads can be sterilised during each cycle.

Decontamination room

Although the provision of a decontamination room is a requirement only under best-practice HTM 01-05 guidelines, the need for a separate area to process reusable items away from the clinical area is an obvious one, and many dental workplaces have operated with separate facilities for some time.

However, some older dental workplaces may still operate a system of cleaning reusable items within the clinical area and, if so, the following points should be incorporated into the procedure as soon as possible:

- Reprocessing should be carried out between patients, not while patients are present
- The reprocessing area should be as far away from the chairside as physically possible

- Ultrasonic baths and autoclaves must not be in use within the surgery area while the patient is present
- Manual washing of items should not be carried out within the surgery area while the patient is present
- Strict zoning of clean and dirty areas must be followed at all times, to avoid cross-contamination
- Thorough surface decontamination should be carried out between patients, and after each reprocessing activity

Ideally, all reprocessing activities should be carried out in a designated decontamination room, physically separated from the clinical area. The ideal layout is illustrated in Figure 12.5 and its correct operation is as follows:

- The decontamination room must be separated physically from all clinical areas (a separate room is required)
- Ideally, the dirty zone, where items are received for reprocessing, and the clean zone, where the sterilised items are produced, should also be separate rooms – this allows for the maximum possible separation of dirty and clean items, and therefore the minimum possibility of recontamination
- There should be a flow of air from clean to dirty in the decontamination room(s) – this should be an active air flow system provided by an extractor fan sucking air out of the dirty zone to the exterior of the premises, thereby causing clean air to be passively pulled in to the clean zone and across to the dirty zone in a one-way flow system
- A single worktop area should run the length of the room, and be long enough to allow the autoclave to be well away from the cleaning/decontamination area
- The worktop should be sealed along its length and its surface should be easily cleanable (i.e. smooth rather than indented)

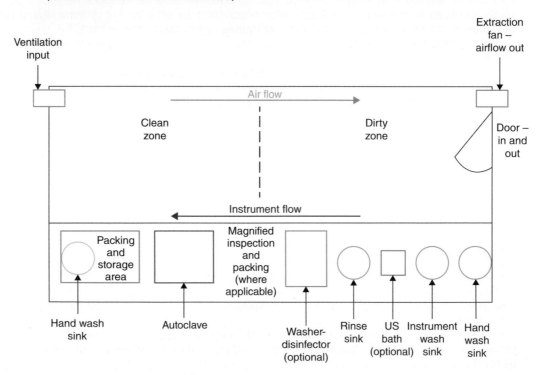

Figure 12.5 Layout and operation of the decontamination room. Source: *Levison's Textbook for Dental Nurses*, 11th edition (Hollins), 2013. Reproduced with permission of Wiley-Blackwell.

300

- The areas should then be set out in the following order:
  - Set-down area for dirty items
  - Hand washing sink
  - Instrument washing sink
  - Ultrasonic bath (if required)
  - Rinsing sink
  - Washer-disinfector
  - Illuminated magnifier for inspection
  - Autoclave
  - Packaging and storage
- The dirty and clean zones should be clearly labelled as such, to avoid cross-contamination between them

Hazardous waste disposal

Recent changes in the legislation and regulation of waste disposal in the UK has led to possible variations in the guidance available for this topic. The information given in this section is correct at the time of writing, but students are advised to check for further information on the relevant legislation affecting waste management in their area on the www.environment-agency.gov.uk website for England and Wales, or their equivalent agencies in Scotland, Northern Ireland, or Southern Ireland. Further information may also be available at www.opsi.gov.uk.

The current legislation and regulations apply to all healthcare waste producers, which includes all dental workplaces. Healthcare waste is of particular concern for environmental and personal safety because, by its nature, it is likely to be contaminated with body fluids or body parts and therefore poses a risk of cross-infecting anyone who handles it. This may be dental personnel or waste management contractors as well as the public, if it is not disposed of safely.

Some types of waste produced in the dental workplace will pose a greater risk of cross-infection than others, while other waste products are hazardous by their chemical nature and possible toxicity. All must be correctly segregated, safely stored and then handed over to a licensed waste contractor to be disposed of in a suitable manner.

Waste classification

Dental workplaces produce a wide range of both hazardous and non-hazardous waste, and in order to segregate the waste correctly, it must first be identified and then classified in line with the current regulatory guidance. The legislation that sets out which wastes must be classed as hazardous is contained in the Special Waste and Hazardous Waste Regulations (2005).

The guidance in current use in England is based on the information contained in Appendix 1 (Waste Disposal) of the Government's "Health Technical Memorandum 01-05" (HTM 01-05). Modified versions of this document are in use in Northern Ireland and Wales, while Scotland has its own system of compliance guidance. In addition, those providing dental treatment in a hospital or a community setting may also be subject to local arrangements for the management of health-care waste, which may have regional variations too.

The current classification of waste produced in the dental workplace is divided into four main areas – non-hazardous waste, offensive waste, trade waste and hazardous waste. The final category is then split further into infectious (clinical) and non-infectious (chemical) waste, with sub-categories for each, as illustrated in the flowchart in Figure 12.6.

All waste from the clinical area of the dental environment is classed as **hazardous waste**, as it is likely to be contaminated by a patient's body fluids – this is usually in the form of saliva or blood, but may include vomit. In addition, any sharp items (including used instruments) can cause an inoculation injury if great care is not taken while handling them.

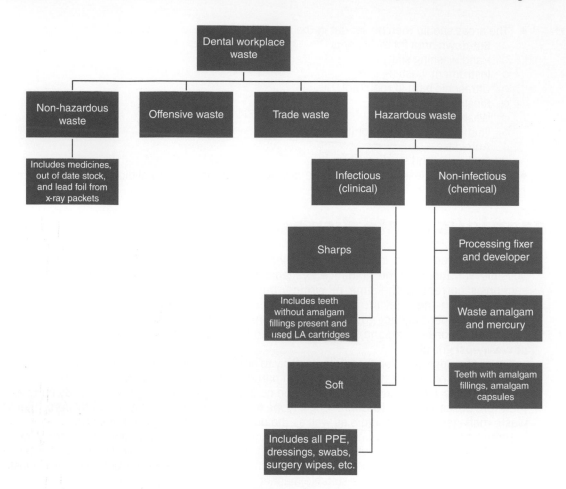

Figure 12.6 Hazardous waste designations. LA, local anaesthetic; PPE, personal protective equipment. Source: *Levison's Textbook for Dental Nurses*, 11th edition (Hollins), 2013. Reproduced with permission of Wiley-Blackwell.

Offensive waste products are defined as "wastes which are non-infectious, do not require specialist treatment or disposal but may cause offence to those coming into contact with it". In the dental workplace this will include any PPE, cleaning towels, X-ray films and other similar items that have not been contaminated with body fluids, medicines, chemicals or amalgam, as well toilet hygiene waste.

Trade waste includes items such as dental equipment (e.g. dental chairs, curing lights, portable suction units), as well as commercial electronic waste such as computer screens, televisions, fluorescent lighting tubes and batteries.

The main change between the old waste classification and the current one is that items that used to be referred to as "special waste" are now categorized as "non-infectious hazardous waste". The exception is the lead foil from X-ray film packets, which is now classed as non-hazardous because the lead is only toxic when present in solution (dissolved in water). The addition of the offensive waste category has occurred in all workplaces.

All dental staff must wear the appropriate PPE while handling any hazardous waste, to avoid direct contact with any contamination.

Relevant health and safety legislation, policies and guidelines

Infection control is a very important topic that is relevant to every member of the dental team, in particular to dental nurses, as its correct management is often delegated to them. Failure to follow the correct procedures relevant to any area of infection control may result in disease, injury or even death of any person on the premises and its importance cannot be over-emphasised. Accordingly, there are several legal Acts, sets of regulations, and Department of Health policies and guidelines to be complied with to ensure the health and safety of all dental personnel, and all other persons who visit the dental workplace at any time:

- Health and Safety at Work Act
- Care Quality Commission (CQC)
- Department of Health guidelines on decontamination in primary care dental practices – HTM 01-05
- Control of Substances Hazardous to Health (COSHH)
- Reporting of Injuries, Diseases, and Dangerous Occurrences Regulations (RIDDOR)
- Special Waste and Hazardous Waste regulations
- Environmental Protection Act (waste disposal)

303

Health and Safety at Work Act

The requirements of this Act and its full relevance to the dental workplace are covered in detail in Chapter 1. The health and safety legislation seeks to protect staff and patients while on the premises by making staff aware of any potential hazards at work and encouraging them to find the best ways of making their particular premises safer for all concerned. In legal terms, the employer has a statutory duty to ensure that, as far as is reasonably practicable, the health, safety and welfare at work of all employees and all visitors (including patients) is protected at all times. In this chapter, the potential hazards to people's safety are the following:

- Cross-infection
- Inoculation injury
- Use of hazardous chemicals to control the spread of infection
- Use of dental equipment that may cause injury during malfunction

As with all health and safety issues in the workplace, a full risk assessment of the potential hazards must be carried out to identify what is the risk, who is at risk, how they are at risk, how to reduce or eliminate that risk, and to record the risk assessment findings.

The methods determined as being necessary to control the risk by reducing or eliminating it will form the basis of the infection control policy of the dental workplace, and a written record of this will mean the information is always available for staff members to follow. Compliance with the policy by all staff members should then ensure the health and safety of everyone on the premises. Failure to follow the workplace policy in any way is likely to increase the potential for someone to suffer harm, or become injured during the routine activities of the workplace. The matter will be investigated by the HSE and the guilty party may face prosecution – the more serious the matter, the more likely it is that this will happen.

All dental personnel must therefore comply with the health and safety policies of the workplace at all times.

Care Quality Commission

The CQC is the independent regulator of health and adult social care services in England, and since the empowerment of the Health and Social Care Act of 2008 it has been the organisation responsible for ensuring adequate standards in premises such as hospitals, nursing homes for the elderly, and care homes for those with a wide range of special needs.

From 1 April 2011, their powers of regulation were extended to include all providers of primary dental care services in England that carry on "regulated activities" (in this case dentistry and oral health care), and all providers, whether NHS or private, have had to become registered with them from this point on.

Registration with CQC has involved every primary dental care provider, as an individual or as an organisation, showing evidence of their compliance with new essential standards of quality and safety in all of its regulated activities. However, it should be noted that CQC registration is relevant in England only, and not in Scotland, Wales or Northern Ireland. Other laws and regulators are likely to perform a similar role in future throughout the UK.

The stated aim of CQC is to "make sure that people get better care". They achieve this by:

- Driving improvement across health and adult social care
- Putting people first and championing their rights
- Acting swiftly to remedy bad practice
- Gathering and using knowledge and expertise, and working with others

In the dental workplace, the relevance of CQC registration is that all primary care providers are expected to comply fully with the essential standards of quality and safety – the vast majority found that they already did so, but that they had little or no evidence in place to prove it, while others found that they did not fully comply. In other words, a standard had been set that every dental workplace must achieve as a minimum to ensure registration. Although initially the registration process was partially a "tick box" exercise for the workplaces, the CQC are currently inspecting those providers who are registered to ensure that there is indeed evidence of their full compliance in all of the essential standards.

The regulations are set out in the Health and Social Care Act 2008 (Regulated Activities) Regulations 2010, and although the full content of the standards and outcomes is beyond the remit of the trainee dental nurse, further information is available for those who are interested at www.cqc.org.uk.

Areas of the essential standards of particular relevance to trainee dental nurses, which they will come across regularly, are as follows:

- The new procedures involved in infection control, such as the bagging and date stamping of all sterilised reusable items
- The necessity of re-sterilising unused bagged items within set time periods to ensure their sterility at the time of use
- The setup and correct use of the decontamination area

In relation to infection control, then, the essential standards expected to be in place by CQC are those set out in the Department of Health's HTM 01-05 document in relation to guidelines on decontamination in primary dental care practices.

Decontamination in primary dental care practices – HTM 01-05

In England, the guidelines applicable with regard to decontamination in general dental practice (primary care dental practices) are covered by the Department of Health document HTM 01-05. Northern Ireland and Wales have their own modified versions of this document, while Scotland has not adopted it but instead has a number of organisations that provide guidance on compliance with decontamination standards.

Further information for students in Wales and Scotland is available at www.dh.gov.uk. Those students working in Northern Ireland are advised to access further specific information at www.dhsspsni.gov.uk.

HTM 01-05 is produced as a guide to decontamination techniques for use in the dental work-place itself and is a "working document" in that it may be updated as evidence of better techniques and systems become available. It is intended to help dental workplaces establish a programme of continuous improvement in their decontamination techniques. Those currently included are listed in two categories:

- **Essential quality requirements** – the basic level of decontamination standards that all work-places will achieve within the first year of implementation of the guidance
- **Best practice** – the "gold standard" to be aimed at in the future (no timescale has currently been set); the additional improvements required to achieve best practice cover the following main points:
  ○ Use of a washer-disinfector to clean instruments
  ○ Separate facility for decontamination tasks, away from the clinical treatment area
  ○ Separate storage area for sterilised items, away from the clinical treatment area (a "clean zone" within the decontamination room would be adequate)

Although it is accepted that many dental workplaces will be unable to achieve full "best practice" status due to the limitations of their building layout, all will need to assess the improvements they can make and have a plan in place to implement what is achievable.

Control of Substances Hazardous to Health (COSHH)

Many of the chemicals and other hazardous substances used in the dental workplace on a day-to-day basis can be harmful to a person's health if they are misused, or if adequate precau-tions are not taken to prevent access by unauthorised persons. However, without these substances, the business of dentistry could not be carried out, so the continued use of the chemicals under safe conditions is the desired outcome.

The determination of the level of risk from any of the chemicals or substances involved, those who may be harmed and the necessary precautions to take are all determined by carrying out a risk assessment. The process to be followed in this case is determined by the COSHH regula-tions, which require all dental workplaces to carry out a risk assessment of all the chemicals and potentially hazardous substances used in the premises, to identify those that could harm or injure staff members.

Harm may be caused if an accident exposes personnel to an unusually large amount of a chemical, if a chemical accidentally enters the body (e.g. by being inhaled), or merely as a result of the dangerous nature of even small amounts of a chemical (e.g. mercury).

The risk assessment process follows the usual steps, but the written report produced must include every potential chemical hazard found and the following specific information:

- The hazardous ingredient(s) it contains
- The nature of the risk, ideally by indicating the risk category using recognised symbols (see Figure 1.10)
- The possible health effects of the hazardous ingredient(s)
- The precautions required for the safe handling of the product
- Any additional hazard control methods required for its safe use
- All necessary first aid measures required in the event of an accident involving the product

The reports are then kept in a COSHH file for quick reference, as necessary, and are updated reg-ularly. They should be available to the whole dental team for reference, and all staff members should sign to say they have read and understood the information. An example of a COSHH assessment sheet is shown in Figure 1.11.

The risk assessment follows the usual steps, with pertinent points to be determined as detailed in the following list for each substance used in dental practices – ranging from specific dental materials to general cleaning agents:

- **Identify those substances that are hazardous** – by reading the manufacturers' leaflets and instruction sheets enclosed with the product, or shown on the label
- **Identify who may be harmed** – this is likely to be anyone who uses the substance, although public access must also be taken into consideration
- **Identify how they may be harmed** – e.g. is the product hazardous on skin contact, or by inhaling fumes, or an eye irritant?
- **Evaluate the risk** – is the substance only harmful if misused, or is it harmful with every use?
- **Determine whether health monitoring is required** – e.g. during exposure to mercury, or nitrous oxide gas used in inhalation sedation as a conscious sedation technique
- **Control the risk** – by ensuring the substance is not misused, by providing suitable PPE, or reduce the risk as far as possible if it is harmful with every use; this may involve changing the product if the potential risk is considered too great
- **Inform all staff of the risks** – through staff meetings and introduction of the COSHH sheets to be read and signed by all team members
- **Record the risk assessment** – keep documented evidence that the assessment has been carried out, with review and update dates recorded as necessary

While the dental nurse is an integral part of the risk assessment procedure as a member of staff, more senior dental nurses may take over the role of maintaining the COSHH files and updating them as necessary, once suitable and documented training has been given. However, all student dental nurses must receive health and safety information covering these issues as part of their induction training with their employer.

In this chapter, COSHH is relevant to the wide range of chemicals used as disinfectants and decontaminants in the dental workplace, including bleach (sodium hypochlorite).

Exposure to many types of disinfectant is the norm throughout the working day for all dental staff. Some disinfectants can irritate the skin, airway and eyes when used carelessly, while others can cause irritation or initiate hypersensitivity or even allergic reactions in staff no matter how low their exposure to the disinfectant. PPE consisting of gloves, mask and glasses should be worn when handling them and working areas must be well ventilated to avoid irritation of the airway. Manufacturers' instructions must always be followed, in particular the first aid advice recorded in the COSHH file in the event of an accident.

Bleach is a powerful disinfectant and is used in many situations in the workplace:

- Fresh solution of 10 000ppm (approximately 1%) to disinfect all non-metallic, non-fabric surfaces within the surgery
- Fresh solution (as above) to disinfect impressions and removable prostheses before transferring between the patient and the laboratory
- Fresh solution (as above) to clean away blood spillages within the surgery

Other disinfectants used for surface and laboratory item decontamination include a variety of antimicrobial and isopropyl alcohol solutions, often also sold as spray solutions or pre-soaked wipes.

Bleach has an unpleasant taste and smell and is a chemical irritant to soft tissues. It can cause tissue damage to the mouth and digestive tract, the eyes and the lungs if strong vapours are inhaled. Appropriate PPE must be worn whenever it is handled, and fresh solutions made daily for the uses indicated in the list should be held in lidded containers, so that the noxious chlorine vapours do not become overpowering.

Disinfectant bottles of any solutions used will show the necessary hazardous substance symbol and give the necessary first aid actions in the event of an accident, in line with COSHH regulations (see Figure 1.22).

Reporting of Injuries, Diseases, and Dangerous Occurrences Regulations (RIDDOR)

Accidents that occur in the workplace fall into one of two categories:

- **Minor accidents** – these result in no serious injury to persons or the premises and are dealt with "in house" and recorded in the **accident book**
- A written record of the minor accident must be made and kept by the workplace in the accident book, under the Notification of Accidents and Dangerous Occurrences Regulations
- Examples of minor accidents include a trip or fall resulting in no serious injury, a clean (non-infectious) needlestick injury, or a minor mercury spillage that can be safely dealt with using the spillage kit
- **Major accidents** – these result in a serious injury to a person or severe damage to the premises
- They are classed as "significant events" and are therefore **notifiable incidents** that must be reported to the HSE under RIDDOR

Notifiable incidents do not include those occurring to a patient while undergoing dental treatment, but do cover all persons on the premises otherwise.

Once notified, the HSE will carry out an investigation into how the incident occurred, to determine whether it was purely an accident or whether the practice or a staff member was at fault. Advice will then be given on how to avoid similar incidents in future, but in serious cases prosecution may follow.

Dental nurses should remember that once qualified and registered with the General Dental Council, they are personally responsible for their own errors and acts of omission under health and safety law – so they could be prosecuted themselves. While in the dental workplace as a student, the trainee dental nurse is under the supervision of a more senior colleague at any one time, and that senior person will be held accountable for any event under RIDDOR. The only exception to this would be if written records proved that the trainee had received the correct training in health and safety issues, but had knowingly and blatantly disregarded them, resulting in the occurrence of the notifiable incident.

The significant events covered by the regulations fall into one of three categories – injuries, diseases, or dangerous occurrences. Further information is available at www.hse.gov.uk/riddor.

As with any other workplace, the occurrence of accidental injuries while on the premises is a rare event in the dental world – but nevertheless they can, and do, happen. Minor injuries, as discussed earlier, are handled "in house" as they result in no serious harm to any persons. However, major injuries do result in serious harm or even death to the casualty.

The **injuries** that must be reported are as follows:

- Fracture of the skull, spine or pelvis
- Fracture of the long bone of an arm or leg
- Amputation of a hand or foot
- Loss of sight in one eye
- Hypoxia (oxygen deprivation to the brain) severe enough to produce unconsciousness
- Any other injury requiring twenty four hour hospital admission for treatment

In this chapter, relevant injuries may occur under the following circumstances:

- Slipping on a wet floor while cleaning is being carried out in the workplace
- Inhalation of fumes from cleaning chemicals, causing respiratory distress and hypoxia

The dental team may be exposed to common diseases in the workplace on a daily basis from patients (such as those with simple colds or chest infections), or they may be exposed away from the workplace – in this case they are at risk of transmitting the infection to others in the workplace themselves.

Dental personnel are also at risk of exposure to more serious pathogens by direct contact with infected blood and saliva from patients, and particularly by receiving an inoculation injury.

The risk of infection by airborne diseases is increased significantly when the workplace is inadequately ventilated or poorly temperature-controlled, and by cross-infection when the workplace is inadequately cleaned.

The **diseases** that must be reported under RIDDOR are any that cause acute ill health by infection with dangerous pathogens or infectious materials, such as:

- Legionella – causing Legionnaires' disease
- Hepatitis B or hepatitis C infection – both linked to the development of liver cancer
- HIV – causing AIDS

In the hospital environment or in those with poor personal hygiene, dental personnel may also be exposed to, or even transmit, other dangerous pathogens, such as methicillin-resistant *Staphylococcus aureus* (MRSA – referred to as one of the "superbugs" by the lay public) or *Clostridium difficile* (an intestinal microorganism associated with diarrhoea and tetanus).

A dangerous occurrence is a significant event that could result in a serious injury or death to anyone on the premises at the time that it happens. It would result in the attendance of the emergency services (ambulance, fire and/or police) as well as specialists in service provision, depending on the cause (gas, electric, service engineer, environmental health officer, etc.)

The **dangerous occurrences** that must be reported are as follows:

- Explosion, collapse or burst of a pressure vessel (an autoclave or compressor)
- Electrical short circuit or overload that causes more than a 24-hour stoppage of business
- Explosion or fire due to gases or inflammable products that causes more than a 24-hour stoppage of business
- Uncontrolled release or escape of mercury vapour due to a major mercury spillage
- Any accident involving the inhalation, ingestion or absorption of a hazardous substance that results in hypoxia severe enough to require medical treatment

In this chapter, relevant dangerous occurrences include the following:

- The explosion or bursting of an autoclave during its routine use to prevent cross-infection
- An event that allows the release of dangerous fumes from cleaning chemicals, such as a large spillage
- An event that results in someone ingesting or absorbing a cleaning chemical and requiring medical treatment due to hypoxia

Special Waste and Hazardous Waste Regulations

The current classification of waste products is shown in Figure 12.6, and while the term "special waste" is no longer in use, much of the waste produced in the dental workplace is classed as hazardous. To enable its safe storage, handling and disposal by licensed contractors, hazardous waste must be correctly segregated while on the premises.

In this chapter, the relevant category of waste is that referred to as "infectious hazardous waste" and includes any item that may cause cross-infection if not handled safely. It includes all of the following:

- **Soft waste** – all items of used PPE, tissues, paper towels, rinsing cups, used X-ray film packets, used plastic barrier shields, any other non-sharp waste that may be contaminated by body fluids by use on a patient
- **Sharps waste** – needles, blades, matrix bands, burs, teeth without amalgam fillings present, local anaesthetic cartridges, any other sharp items that may cause injury if mishandled

Environmental Protection Act

In accordance with the Environmental Protection Act, the duty of care is with the dental work-place to ensure that healthcare waste is managed and disposed of safely and correctly. To comply fully, all dental workplaces must ensure that they:

- Have a written healthcare waste policy in place which identifies a named person as respon-sible for waste management on the premises (referred to as the "registered manager" in HTM 01-05)
- Provide staff access to the policy and give recorded training in correct waste management methods
- Segregate waste in accordance with Figure 12.6 and store it safely while on the premises, away from public access
- Use the correct storage containers for each waste category – see later
- Only use licensed waste collectors for the removal from the premises and disposal of the waste at an authorized disposal site
- Accurately describe the container contents of all non-hazardous waste on transfer notes, which must be kept for a minimum of 2 years from the date of collection
- Accurately describe the container contents of all hazardous waste on consignment notes, which must be kept for a minimum of 3 years from the date of collection
- Receive and keep the quarterly "consignee returns" documentation which records the final destination of the hazardous waste consignment and its disposal details
- Register with the Environment Agency as a hazardous waste producer if more than 500 kg of hazardous waste is produced annually

For quick and easy identification of each category of waste produced in the dental workplace, various colour-coded containers are used to help segregate the various items. In addition, on all documentation, the European Waste Catalogue (EWC) codes should be used – however, details of these codes are not relevant to the student dental nurse.

In this chapter, the relevant storage containers to be used are:

- **Soft infectious (clinical) hazardous waste** – orange sack, no more than three-quarters full and tied at the neck (see Figure 1.25)
- **Sharps infectious (clinical) hazardous waste** – all yellow rigid container, no more than two-thirds full (see Figure 1.26)

13

Unit 313: Assessment of Oral Health and Treatment Planning

Learning outcomes

1. Understand the various methods of dental assessment
2. Know the clinical assessments associated with orthodontics
3. Understand the changes that may occur in the oral tissues
4. Know the medical emergencies that may occur in the dental environment
5. Know the basic structure and function of oral and dental anatomy

Outcome 1 assessment criteria

The learner can:

- Describe methods of recording soft tissue conditions
- Explain methods of recording periodontal conditions using periodontal charts
- Describe the reasons for taking radiographs and photographs during assessment and treatment planning (include reasons for the monitoring of dental practices)
- Describe the uses of the different materials used within dental assessment (include impression materials for study models)
- Describe the methods of measuring pulp vitality and their advantages and disadvantages
- Explain the legislation and guidelines relating to patients' records and confidentiality
- Explain the importance of informed consent and its relevance prior to any treatment undertaken
- Explain the workplace policies relating to complaints and their role throughout

Diploma in Dental Nursing, Level 3, Third Edition. Carole Hollins.
© 2014 John Wiley & Sons, Ltd. Published 2014 by John Wiley & Sons, Ltd.
Companion website: www.wiley.com/go/hollins/dentalnursinglevel3

Outcome 2 assessment criteria
The learner can:
- Describe the classifications of malocclusion
- Describe the types of orthodontic appliances in relation to treatment required
- Explain pre- and postoperative instructions for orthodontic procedures
- Explain the role of the dental nurse in providing support during orthodontic assessment and treatment

Outcome 3 assessment criteria
The learner can:
- Explain diseases of the oral mucosa
- Describe the effects of ageing on the soft tissue
- Identify the medical conditions that may affect the oral tissues

Outcome 4 assessment criteria
The learner can:
- Identify medical emergencies that may occur in the dental environment and how to deal with them

Outcome 5 assessment criteria
The learner can:
- Describe the structure, morphology and eruption dates of the primary and secondary dentition
- Describe the structure and function of gingivae and supporting tissue
- Describe the position and function of salivary glands and muscles of mastication
- Describe the structure of the maxilla and mandible, and movements of the temporo-mandibular joint
- Describe nerve and blood supply to the teeth and supporting structures
- Describe the structure and function of teeth and gingivae, including the number of roots
- Explain common oral diseases including both malignant and potentially malignant lesions, and methods for their diagnosis, prevention and management
- Describe the diagnosis and management of diseases of the oral mucosa, other soft tissues, and the facial bones and joints

This unit is assessed by:
- An assessment paper containing multiple choice and short answer questions

The content is the theory and underpinning knowledge required and links to the information contained in Chapters 3, 6 and 7.

Oral health assessments

Oral health assessments are carried out each time that a patient attends the dental workplace, usually at the time of undergoing a dental examination. Some patients attend more or less frequently than others by their own personal choice, and some require more frequent attendance than others, in the dentist's professional opinion. The dentist's opinion is based on the known risk factors of various oral diseases and the patient's frequency of exposure to these risk factors.

The two main purposes of carrying out the oral health assessment are:

- Prevention of disease by regular opportunities to reinforce oral health education messages
- Early detection and diagnosis when disease is already present

If disease is already present, regular oral assessment will detect it at an earlier stage and allow the necessary treatment to be carried out so that a full recovery is more likely. If a serious and potentially life-threatening disease is present, such as oral cancer, regular inspection will identify it earlier and allow the patient to be referred for urgent specialist care, with a better chance of successful treatment and recovery.

Although the oral health assessment should detect an abnormality in any of the areas assessed, the obvious oral diseases that are particularly looked for are dental caries, chronic gingivitis and chronic periodontal disease.

The whole dental team has an important role to play in this assessment and prevention process, as follows:

- **Dentist** – makes the initial diagnosis, formulates a treatment plan and carries out all treatments restricted to the dentist only
- **Hygienist** – works under the prescription of the dentist to carry out scaling and oral hygiene instruction
- **Therapist** – works under the prescription of the dentist to carry out suitable treatments as necessary
- **Dental nurse** – assists the dentist during the assessment by accurately recording all the information as necessary; assists the other dental team members while treating the patient; and reinforces all the oral hygiene messages given to the patient

Assessment of oral health is carried out in the following areas:

- Extra-oral soft tissues
- Intra-oral soft tissues
- Periodontal tissues
- Occlusion
- Deciduous and mixed dentition of children
- Permanent dentition

Methods used to carry out assessment

The main methods available to carry out oral health assessments are the following:

- **Visual inspection** to detect visible abnormalities, such as size and colour changes
- **Manual inspection** to feel abnormalities, such as a lump where none should be present
- Use of **mouth mirrors** for intra-oral soft tissue and tooth charting assessments
- Use of various **dental probes** for tooth inspections and charting
- Use of **periodontal probe** for periodontal assessment
- Use of various **radiograph** views to determine both the presence and absence of various structures or pathology
- Use of **photographs** to record the visible appearance of a structure at that time and for comparison with earlier or later views
- Use of **study models** to record the occlusion of the teeth and the individual appearance and position of each tooth
- Use of **vitality tests** to determine if an individual tooth is alive, dying or dead (non-vital)

Extra-oral soft tissue assessment

Dentists will often be visibly assessing the extra-oral soft tissues (those outside the mouth) of patients while meeting and greeting them into the surgery area, and chatting to them before

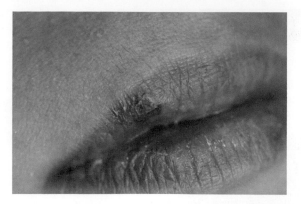

Figure 13.1   A "cold sore" lesion on upper lip.

beginning the intra-oral assessments. In particular, they will be looking and palpating the following structures for any signs of abnormality:

- **External facial signs** – checking for skin colour, facial symmetry and the presence of any blemishes, especially moles and "cold sores"
- **The lips** – checking for any change in colour or size, the presence of any blemishes, and palpated for any abnormalities
- **The lymph nodes** – lying under the mandible and in the neck, these are palpated to detect any swellings or abnormalities, the presence of which may indicate an infection or a more sinister lesion

Variations in skin colour between patients do occur, especially in different ethnic groups. Some patients are naturally pale and others are naturally ruddy. However, an unusual facial appearance can sometimes indicate problems, such as nervous patients becoming pale and clammy as they are about to faint, or the unnatural ruddiness of a patient with hypertension.

Facial asymmetry (where one side of the face is shaped differently from the other) could indicate the presence of a swelling or problems with the nerve supply or muscular control of that area, all of which require further investigation.

The sudden appearance of unusual skin blemishes, especially moles, may indicate the presence of an early skin cancer (**melanoma**), which will need urgent referral for treatment.

Similarly, the lips are examined and details recorded of blemishes, such as the presence of a "**cold sore**" (Figure 13.1) indicating infection with the herpes simplex type 1 virus, or the presence of minor salivary gland cysts (mucoceles). Lips that are generally tinged bluish-purple indicate some degree of chronic heart failure, which needs noting before local anaesthesia and traumatic dental procedures are carried out.

Lymph nodes are part of the body's immune system and are present in certain areas of the body. Any enlargement of those accessible to the dentist in the head and neck region indicates that the body is fighting infection or some other disease process and requires further investigation.

Intra-oral soft tissue assessment

This is carried out at each dental examination and in a systematic manner, so that no areas are missed out and all lesions are investigated:

- **Labial, buccal and sulcus mucosa** – checked for their colour and texture, the presence of any white patches (especially affecting the buccal mucosa, as shown in Figure 13.2), and the moisture level is noted

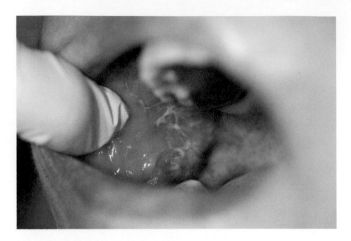

Figure 13.2 A white patch on buccal mucosa.

- **Palatal mucosa** – both the hard and soft palates, the oropharynx and the tonsils (if present)
- **Tongue** – checked for colour and texture, symmetry of shape and movement, the level of mobility; all surfaces are checked, especially beneath the tongue, as this is one of the commonest sites for oral carcinoma to develop
- **Floor of mouth** – checked for colour and texture, the presence of any white or red patches, and the presence of any swellings under the tongue

Low moisture levels in the mouth can indicate problems with the functioning of the salivary glands, such as **Sjögren's syndrome**, or **xerostomia** (dry mouth) due to age-related changes to the glands or as a side-effect in those taking certain medications. Saliva has important functions with regard to defence, cleansing and dental disease initiation, and any indication of reduced flow levels is of great importance to the dental team, with regard to maintaining a healthy oral environment for the patient.

The more likely areas for oral cancers to develop are on the borders of, or beneath, the tongue and in the floor of the mouth, and these areas will be particularly well examined in patients with known risk factors, such as smoking and excessive alcohol consumption. All findings can then be recorded on a suitable assessment sheet (see Figure 6.5). In addition, photographs can be taken at the time and retained for comparison at a later date, while any benign lesions are kept under observation.

Periodontal assessment

The periodontal tissues are those acting as **supporting tissues** around the tooth – the gingivae, the periodontal ligament and the underlying alveolar bone forming the tooth socket. These tissues can undergo disease processes to varying degrees, and in the worst-case scenario healthy teeth can be lost due to periodontal disease. Periodontal disease is the commonest dental disease found in adult patients and its presence can easily be missed or remain undetected for many years due to its slow onset and painless nature.

As with tooth charting, a system has been developed whereby the presence of periodontal disease can be quickly recorded during routine oral assessment, by dividing the mouth into sextants and recording the presence and depth of any unnatural spaces down the side of the teeth – these are called **periodontal pockets**.

This recording technique is called a **basic periodontal examination (BPE) assessment** and is noted as shown in Figure 13.3.

Healthy periodontal tissues appear pink, firmly attached to the necks of the teeth with a gingival crevice no deeper than 3 mm, and they do not bleed when touched. Teeth are firmly held in

Upper teeth

18–14	13–23	24–28
48–44	43–33	34–38

Lower teeth

Figure 13.3   Division of mouth into sextants for recording of the basic periodontal examination (BPE).

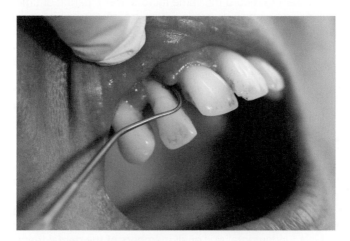

Figure 13.4   Periodontal pocket probing procedure. Source: *Levison's Textbook for Dental Nurses*, 11th edition (Hollins), 2013. Reproduced with permission of Wiley-Blackwell.

their sockets by the periodontal supporting tissues and no plaque is present on the tooth surfaces.

Specially designed periodontal probes (such as a BPE probe – see Figure 6.21) are used to record the presence and depth of any periodontal pockets discovered in each sextant of the dental arches. The probe has a ball end, so that it does not pierce the soft tissues when inserted into the pocket, and graduated marks along its shank at 3.5, 5.5 and 7 mm. These graduations are easily visible to the dentist during the periodontal pocket probing procedure (Figure 13.4) so that a universal coding system can be used as follows:

- **Code 0** – healthy gingival tissues with no bleeding on probing
- **Code 1** – pocket no more than 3.5 mm, bleeding on probing, no calculus or other plaque retention factor present
- **Code 2** – pocket no more than 3.5 mm but plaque retention factor detected (such as subgingival calculus or a filling overhang)
- **Code 3** – pocket present up to 5.5 mm deep
- **Code 4** – pocket present deeper than 5.5 mm but less than 7 mm
- **Code *** – gingival recession or furcation involvement present, pocket present deeper than 7 mm

A typical completed BPE chart is shown in Figure 6.3.

Higher codes therefore indicate a more serious periodontal problem, such as that shown in Figure 13.4 where the 7 mm graduation mark is no longer visible during pocket probing. Where codes greater than 3 are recorded, a full pocket depth record will be made of each tooth in that sextant so that specific problem areas can be identified and intensive periodontal treatment can be initiated. A full detailed periodontal recording is made in these cases using a chart such as that shown in Figure 6.4, which can be used to record individual pocket depths at various points around each tooth, as well as areas of recession and tooth mobility. In addition, the presence and extent of any plaque found can be recorded on these detailed charts.

Tooth mobility is graded as follows:

- **Grade I** – side-to-side tooth movement less than 2 mm
- **Grade II** – side-to-side tooth movement more than 2 mm
- **Grade III** – vertical movement present

By using this type of chart to record the same factors over a period of time, a record is built up of active periodontal lesions as well as areas where treatment has been successful and pockets have not increased in depth.

All of these assessments can be recorded manually, either in long hand directly onto the patient's record card, or on a pre-printed full periodontal chart that is kept as an insert in the patient's records, or directly into the relevant files of a computerised record system.

The standard of oral hygiene can be graded as excellent, good, fair, or poor, and should be recorded at each oral health assessment so that patient motivation and compliance can be monitored.

Tooth charting

Accurate tooth charting is one of the most important skills acquired by dental nurses in their role as an assistant to the dentist, both during oral health assessments and during the provision of dental treatment.

Inaccuracies in the charting can result in catastrophic consequences for the patient, such as the wrong classification or type of restoration that is being provided, or even the wrong tooth being extracted. It is a fundamental skill of all members of the dental team to record and follow a tooth chart correctly.

Charting is used as a style of "dental shorthand" to quickly and accurately record a patient's dentition as it appears at the time of the oral health assessment. Dental nurses are referred to the definitive "Charting Booklet" produced by the National Examining Board for Dental Nurses (NEBDN) at www.nebdn.org. This describes the approved current charting notations used both for teeth and for periodontal conditions, following the three styles currently in use:

- **Palmer notation** – for tooth charting
- **International Dental Federation (FDI) notation** – for tooth charting
- **Basic Periodontal Examination (BPE)** – for periodontal charting

Although many dental workplaces are now computerised, the software systems in use for tooth charting vary enormously and very often cannot actually distinguish the finer points of the written notation, which may lead to errors. Therefore, it is necessary for trainee dental nurses to be taught tooth charting using written records, so that they are standardised upon qualification.

With tooth charting, a two-grid system is used (forensic notation) which separates the current dental status from any treatment required. Each anterior tooth charted diagrammatically is shown with four surfaces and an incisal edge or canine cusp, and each posterior tooth with five surfaces, as shown in Figure 6.18.

The teeth are recorded from the centreline backwards for both the deciduous and the permanent dentition, and the charting grid is arranged as follows:

- Inner grid – shows current dental status and dental treatment already present in the mouth
- Outer grid – records all dental treatment that needs to be carried out

For the purpose of tooth charting, current dental status refers to the following notations only:

- The presence or absence of a tooth
- The presence of a root
- The notation of any tooth that is stated as unerupted – charted as "UE"
- The notation of any tooth that is stated as partially erupted – charted as "PE"
- The position of a tooth in relation to the normal dental arch – may be stated as "instanding" or "buccal to the arch", for example

The condition of the teeth and the presence of any restorations can then be charted in a code form on the inner grid, and work to be carried out is recorded in the outer grid. Examples of some of the recognised charting notations are shown in Figure 6.2, but readers are again advised to consult the Charting Booklet produced by NEBDN for the full range of current definitive notations.

The notable exception to the usual rules of inner grid versus outer grid is the charting of a fracture to a tooth. A fracture can range from a minimal incisal edge chip to a tooth, which requires no treatment (and is therefore charted on the inner grid, as it represents "current dental status"), or it can be a full fracture of the crown of the tooth from its root at gingival level (and is therefore charted on the outer grid, as it represents "dental treatment that needs to be carried out").

The charting symbol in both these instances of a fracture is "#", so the dental nurse must be careful to determine if an indication is made as to whether the tooth is to be restored or not, as this will determine which grid should be used for the notation.

Palmer notation

This is based on the division of the dentition into four quadrants when looking at the patient from the front: upper right and left, and lower left and right. Using either the letters representing the deciduous dentition or the numbers representing the permanent dentition (see later), each tooth can then be written and identified individually. With the increased use of computers to record the patient's dental records, including tooth chartings, the use of the quadrant symbol has been superseded by the following:

- UR for upper right
- UL for upper left
- LL for lower left
- LR for lower right

So, individual teeth are charted as, for example, UR6 (upper right first permanent molar) and LLE (lower left second deciduous molar), and so on.

The Palmer system relies on the use of the English language for its correct interpretation, and a more international system of tooth charting is also available that is not language-dependent, but is based on numbers only. This is the FDI system.

Two-digit FDI notation

This system replaces the quadrant symbol or use of UR, UL, etc. with a quadrant number as well as a tooth number, as follows:

- Upper right – permanent quadrant 1, deciduous quadrant 5
- Upper left – permanent quadrant 2, deciduous quadrant 6
- Lower left – permanent quadrant 3, deciduous quadrant 7
- Lower right – permanent quadrant 4, deciduous quadrant 8

The quadrant number forms the first digit while the second identifies an individual tooth as 1 to 8 in the same way as the Palmer system. Reading clockwise from the upper right third molar, all

32 permanent teeth and 20 deciduous teeth have their own two-digit number indicating their quadrant (first digit) and identity (second digit) as shown:

18 17 16 15 14 13 12 11   21 22 23 24 25 26 27 28
48 47 46 45 44 43 42 41   31 32 33 34 35 36 37 38

For deciduous teeth:

55 54 53 52 51   61 62 63 64 65
85 84 83 82 81   71 72 73 74 75

The lower left second premolar, for example, is written as 35 and pronounced "three-five", not thirty-five, and the upper right deciduous first molar would be written as 54 and pronounced "five-four", and so on.

While examining the teeth, the dentist will also record any evidence of non-carious tooth surface loss that is evident – **erosion, abrasion or attrition.** This information will be linked in with other information (such as diet, tooth brushing habits) provided during medical, social and dental history-taking (see Chapter 15).

The dental instruments normally used to carry out the tooth charting assessment are:

- **Mouth mirror** – used to reflect light on to the tooth surface, to retract the soft tissues to provide clear vision, and to protect the soft tissues during the assessment
- **Angled probe** – used to detect soft tooth surfaces and margins on existing restorations
- **Tweezers** – used to hold cotton wool pledgets to wipe tooth surfaces dry or to place cotton wool rolls
- **Briault probe** – two-ended probe specially designed to detect interproximal caries, either mesially or distally (see Figure 6.14)

Use of radiographs

Dental radiography is an important diagnostic tool used in dentistry and medicine to help the clinician to see within the body tissues and help diagnose the cause of dental and medical problems. The theory and underpinning knowledge of the principles of dental radiography are discussed in Chapter 14.

In oral health assessment and treatment planning, dental radiographs are used to detect and diagnose the following lesions and structures:

- **Dental caries** – this shows up as a dark area of destruction extending inwards from the enamel surface (Figure 13.5)
- Presence and extent of **periodontal disease** – this shows up as a loss of the lamina dura forming the crest of the alveolar bone, loss of height of the alveolar bone, and a widening of the periodontal ligament space (Figure 13.6)
- Periodontal and periapical **abscesses** – chronic alveolar abscesses show up as a dark circular area at the apex of an affected tooth, caused by destruction of the apical lamina dura and spongy bone (see Figure 7.14)
- **Cysts** affecting the dental tissues – these can show up as enlarged darker areas surrounding other structures, and can sometimes be seen to be pushing tooth roots out of their normal positions
- **Iatrogenic problems** – i.e. those caused by the dentist; such as overhanging restorations (Figure 13.7), or tooth perforations by posts
- To detect **supernumerary** teeth and **unerupted** teeth (Figure 13.8) or to determine the **congenital absence** of unerupted teeth
- To diagnose **hard tissue lesions**, such as bone cysts and tumours, salivary calculi and jaw fractures

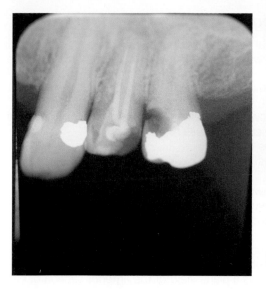

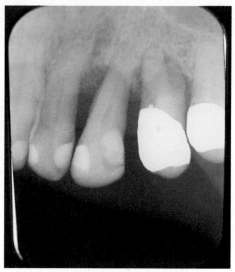

Figure 13.5   Radiograph showing dental caries.

Figure 13.6   Radiograph showing periodontal disease.

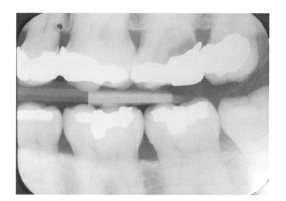

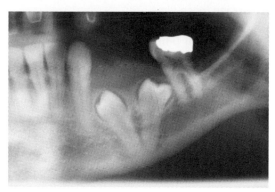

Figure 13.7   Radiograph showing filling overhangs UL6 and UL7.

Figure 13.8   Radiograph showing unerupted teeth.

In addition, radiographs are used during the provision of dental treatment to avoid problems occurring, to ensure that the treatment is successful and to monitor the health of the tooth – examples are:

- To aid in the provision of **endodontic** treatment
- To monitor the health of the tooth after endodontic treatment
- To determine the number and position of tooth roots before **extraction**
- To ensure the health of a tooth before it undergoes **crown or bridge** preparation
- To monitor the health of the tooth after crown or bridge treatment
- To ensure the health of a tooth before it is used as an abutment during **denture construction**

Types of views used in dental radiography

There are various types of film used in dental radiography, depending on the reason for taking the dental image, but all are either those taken within the oral cavity (**intra-oral films**) or those taken outside the oral cavity (**extra-oral films**).

The intra-oral views that can be produced using these films are:

- **Horizontal bitewing** (see Figure 6.6) – shows the posterior teeth in occlusion, and is taken to view:
  ○ Interproximal areas and to diagnose caries in these regions
  ○ Restoration overhangs in these areas
  ○ Recurrent caries beneath existing restorations
  ○ Occlusal caries
- **Vertical bitewing** (see Figure 7.2) – shows an extended view of the posterior teeth, from mid-root of the uppers to mid-root of the lowers as a minimum, and are taken to view:
  ○ Periodontal bone levels of the posterior teeth
  ○ True periodontal pockets
- **Periapical** (see Figure 6.7) – shows one or two teeth in full length with their surrounding bone, and is taken to view the area and the teeth in close detail
- **Anterior occlusal** (see Figure 7.3) – shows a plane view of the anterior section of either the mandible or the maxilla, and is used especially to view the area for unerupted teeth, super-numerary teeth and cysts

Extra-oral films are used to produce much larger images showing many structures and are supplied in cassettes that are used outside the oral cavity. The extra-oral views that can be produced using these films are:

- **Dental panoramic tomograph (DPT)** (see Figure 6.8) – shows both jaws in full and their surrounding bony anatomy, and is taken for orthodontic and wisdom tooth assessments, as well as to help diagnose pathology and jaw fractures
- **Lateral oblique** – shows the posterior portion of one side of the mandible, including the ramus and angle and the lower molar teeth, and is an alternative to a DPT to view the position of unerupted third molar teeth (these are used infrequently now, as the image produced on a well-aligned DPT is far superior)
- **Lateral skull radiograph** (see Figure 6.9) – this is a view of the side of the head, taken in a specialised machine called a **cephalostat** (which may be present as an attachment to a DPT machine, or as a "stand alone" device), and is used to monitor jaw growth and determine orthognathic surgery techniques in complicated cases of malocclusion

When DPTs initially became widely available to the dental profession, they were called "orthopan-tomographs" and referred to as OPGs or OPTs – these abbreviations are still in current use in some areas.

Use of photographs

These can be taken to record various aspects of the dentition or soft tissues, for future reference. They can be produced using conventional cameras (especially "Instamatic" types), digital cameras with "macro" lenses for close-up shots, or by using specialist intra-oral digital cameras. Specialised computers and equipment are required for this last technique.

Photographs are useful for the following:

- To record soft tissue lesions to aid diagnosis
- To record the extent of injury following trauma

- To record before and after views of dental treatment
- To record potentially sinister lesions that can be emailed to specialists immediately, to aid a speedy diagnosis

Use of study models

In some situations, it is necessary for the dentist to consider the patient's occlusion before being able to decide on any treatment necessary, for example when providing partial dentures or orthodontic treatment. Impressions are taken of both dental arches using alginate impression material (see Chapter 15) and then cast up to produce a set of study models (see Figure 6.10).

Study models are useful in the following cases:

- Occlusal analysis in complicated crown or bridge cases
- Orthodontic cases, to determine if extractions are required and which type of appliance is necessary
- Occlusal analysis where full mouth treatment may be necessary, to determine the functioning of the dentition
- Where tooth surface loss is evident, either by erosion from acidic foods and drinks, or by attrition due to tooth grinding, so that the progression of the tooth wear can be monitored and treatment determined

321

Vitality tests

These are sometimes necessary to help in determining whether a tooth is vital (alive) or non-vital (dead), and the tests available are:

- Cold stimulus with **ethyl chloride** (Figure 13.9)
- Hot stimulus with warmed **gutta-percha** (Figure 13.10)
- Electrical test with **electric pulp tester**

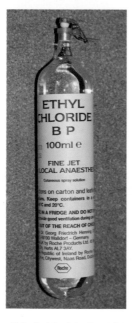

Figure 13.9   Ethyl chloride liquid in container.

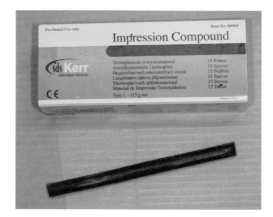

Figure 13.10   Greenstick compound for vitality testing. Source: *Levison's Textbook for Dental Nurses*, 11th edition (Hollins), 2013. Reproduced with permission of Wiley-Blackwell.

The first two techniques are used to diagnose toothache where the symptoms include pain with cold or heat, whereas electric pulp testers are more accurate in determining the "degree" of vitality of a tooth, as follows:

- Normal response – healthy pulp
- Increased response – early pulpitis present
- Reduced response – pulp is dying, or tooth has heavily lined deep restoration present so the voltage cannot be adequately transmitted to the pulp
- No response – pulp tissue is dead

Patients will vary in their response to electric pulp testers, so it is always advisable to test several apparently healthy teeth to establish what their "normal" response is, before testing the suspect tooth.

Electric pulp testers are either battery-operated or mains-operated and they work by sending an increasing voltage into the tooth until the patient is aware of a tingling sensation in that tooth. The point at which the patient indicates a sensation is recorded numerically on a scale, so that the "degree" of vitality can be determined in relation to "test" teeth.

Ethyl chloride is a liquid that vaporises quickly at room temperature, leaving ice crystals which provide a cold stimulus when touched by the skin or onto a tooth. This cold sensation is detected particularly well by a hypersensitive tooth, and can help to indicate which one requires dental treatment.

Gutta-percha is a natural rubber-like product with several uses in dentistry. As a compound of greenstick (Figure 13.10), it can be warmed in a flame and placed on a pulpitic tooth to determine a hypersensitivity reaction to heat, indicating which one requires dental treatment. The teeth to be tested should be dried in both cases first, and a thin smear of petroleum jelly placed before applying the warm greenstick compound to avoid the substance sticking to the tooth and causing pain to the patient.

The advantage of all these testing techniques is that a positive response enables the dentist to correctly determine which tooth requires treatment at that time, rather than having to treat several adjacent teeth in a quadrant before the correct one is identified by the cessation of symptoms. The disadvantage of all is that the patient often has to experience a painful stimulus before the correct tooth is identified.

Materials used in oral assessments

Materials that may be used to carry out oral assessments are:

- **Alginate impression material** – consisting of calcium and alginate salts which are mixed with water at room temperature and loaded into trays for insertion into the mouth so that accurate impressions can be taken
- **Dental stone** – a yellow-coloured, hardened calcium sulphate plaster mixed with water and used to produce a study model cast
- **Dental plaster** – a white-coloured calcium sulphate plaster mixed with water and used to make a base for the dental stone cast
- **Ethyl chloride** – a liquid which vaporises easily and produces a cold sensation on doing so, and can be applied to teeth as an aid to detecting dental problems
- **Gutta-percha as greenstick** – a compound which can be heated and applied to a tooth to aid in the detection of dental problems

Legislation and guidelines in relation to patient records and confidentiality

While an oral health assessment is being carried out and a treatment plan is being formulated for the patient, the dental nurse will be recording the various findings and points made in the patient's records. The purpose of dental records is to provide an up-to-date case history of each patient's condition, and includes the examination findings and treatment given on each attendance at the surgery. By referring back to previous visits, the dentist can assess the results of earlier courses of treatment and thereby decide the best line of treatment on future occasions. Adequate records also facilitate the transfer of patients between dentists in the practice when absence or staff changes occur. When recorded correctly, another dentist should be able to determine all previous treatments for a patient and continue that care safely, without any risk of errors or omissions due to incomplete information.

In effect, the records are a communication tool that allows anyone reading them to determine what treatment was carried out, when and by whom, and how it was achieved. So the completeness and accuracy of the records is required for:

- Patient safety
- Evaluation of treatment
- Basis for patient accounts
- Monitoring of the provision of care
- Probity enquiries

Recording methods will be either manual or on computer, and the amount of detail recorded may vary considerably from practice to practice, but patients' records essentially consist of personal and clinical information. They should include all of the following:

- Patient name, address, date of birth and telephone numbers
- Doctor's details and contact information
- Full medical history
- Dental history
- Contemporaneous clinical notes of each attendance (i.e. written at the time or as soon as possible afterwards, so that they are in date order)
- Tooth and periodontal chartings
- Soft tissue assessments
- Details of all appointments with other staff, such as the hygienist, therapist and oral health educator
- All legally required NHS or private paperwork
- Consent forms
- Copies of all referral letters and response correspondence
- Correctly identified and mounted radiographs
- Photographs
- Laboratory slips
- Records of all payment transactions
- Copies of all patient correspondence
- Information on failed or cancelled appointments

Where there are two or more patients with the same name or date of birth, the record should be clearly marked to alert all readers that this is the case – otherwise, there is a risk that one patient will receive the treatment that is required by another.

For new patients, the personal details, reason for attendance and medical and dental history are all conveniently recorded by giving or sending a medical history form, such as the British Dental Association (BDA) Confidential Medical History Form, for completion at home before their first visit. At that visit it would be assessed by the dentist, signed and dated, and placed in the patient's file. Clinical details of the visit, and subsequent ones, are entered on a dental chart and kept in the file.

Importance of records

Accurate dental records are essential to ensure that patients receive necessary, appropriate and safe treatment. Poor record-keeping often forms the basis of patient complaints that cannot be defended, and dentists are ultimately responsible for their errors and omissions unless the notes were written to record treatment provided by a dental care professional. Errors or omissions in recording information may result in incorrect treatment being carried out, or failure to provide necessary treatment to maintain oral health. The dental nurse must accurately record information given by the patient or dictated by the dentist, ensuring that records are filed properly, made available at each appointment, and signed as necessary by the patient and the dentist.

Dental records are also extremely valuable as a means of establishing identity. In fatal accidents where facial features are destroyed, the teeth are often unaffected and can be compared with dentists' records to identify a victim.

Proper records allow correct treatment planning and provide a check on details of past treatment. They form the basis on which fees are calculated and accounts rendered to patients. Failed appointments and refusals of treatment are noted and the patient's attitude to oral health, as well as any risks factors to good oral health, can be assessed. Appropriate recall arrangements can then be made for each patient, in line with guidelines of the National Institute for Health and Clinical Excellence (NICE).

Adequate records allow the practice to run with the greatest efficiency for all concerned and should be retained for at least 11 years after completion of treatment, or to the age of 25 years in the case of children's records. Many difficulties concerning individual patients can be prevented altogether if complete records are available of all attendances at the practice, while no time is wasted in putting such information at the dentist's disposal. Recording and filing systems may vary considerably in different practices, but whichever method is used, records must always be accurate, legible, comprehensive and easily accessible.

Clinical records

Clinical records consist of the past and present appointment and day books, as well as records of each patient attending the practice, and contain the information specific to the delivery of oral health care to that patient. They include the medical history (see later), dental history, present oral health status (including chartings), treatment received on each date, and then the required estimate, consent and account paperwork. The relevance of the information to be recorded is discussed in the following sections.

Dental history

Diagnosis of the present condition and determination of the treatment plan may depend on details of earlier dental disorders and their treatment. Knowledge of previous difficulties, such as excessive bleeding, poor response to anaesthetics, difficult extractions, allergy to dental materials, latex gloves or rubber dam, or any other complications will help the dentist to avoid their reoccurrence.

Present oral health status

The present condition of the teeth is recorded on the dental chart, and any other conditions, such as the state of existing restorations and dentures, level of oral hygiene, periodontal disease, malocclusion and tooth discoloration, that may affect treatment are also noted. The dentist can then assess the patient's general attitude towards their oral health and accordingly advise the most appropriate treatment. Much of this information is conveniently set out in the Oral Health Assessment documents that are currently being piloted before NHS contracts change again in the near future and can be used as prompts to gather the required information.

Pertinent questions are asked and responses recorded about all issues that may affect the patient's oral health, especially diet, alcohol consumption and tobacco usage.

Treatment

Full details of dental treatment received and the date on which it was provided are recorded on the dental chart and in the notes. These will include the results of any special procedures carried out or events that happened, such as:

- Radiographs, vitality tests, periodontal status, oral cancer check and orthodontic study models
- Local anaesthesia, type of filling and lining, shades used for fillings, artificial teeth and crowns
- Drugs and dosage, and any prescriptions issued
- Complications that occurred, e.g. excessive bleeding or retained roots after extractions
- Treatment plans and options, cost estimates and the patient's choice of treatment
- Missed appointments and refusals of treatment
- Any accidents or complications, such as retained roots following extractions or breakage of an instrument (e.g. a root canal file), must be explained to the patient and its occurrence recorded, together with the measures and options offered, and emergency treatment arrangements

National Health Service records

The NHS provides a large number of forms for detailing treatment plans, costs, emergency visits, orthodontic and periodontal treatment, exemption from payments and many other aspects of NHS procedure. Currently, the most commonly used forms include:

- A standard chart (Form FP 25) for recording patient visits, and treatment required and provided, together with a folder (Form FP 25 a) to hold subsequent treatment forms and details
- Form FP17 DC/GP17DC is given to the patient. It outlines treatment required and the NHS charges, as well as the details and costs of any agreed private treatment
- The Dental Estimates Form FP17 is used by practitioners to record details of treatment required, and subsequently given, and provides a form of account for payment claimed
- Form FP10D, for prescriptions

With the expected introduction of the new NHS contract over the next few years, the details of this paperwork may well change.

Many practices are now partially or fully computerised with regard to patient records, but all the information held must be accessible to the dental team, the authorities and the patient, as necessary. Several software systems are available for use and the NHS records detailed in the list are compatible with many of them. Whichever system is used, and whether manual or computerised, the records must be written, handled and stored in full accordance with all the relevant legislation. A good knowledge of the use of computers and information technology is required by, and expected of, the modern dental nurse.

Confidentiality of patient records

All members of the dental team have both an ethical and legal duty to keep patient information gained in the course of their professional relationship confidential, and not to release it to others without the patient's permission, or in accordance with strict protocols if they do so without their permission.

As with the setting of minimum standards in clinical issues within the NHS under clinical governance requirements, a similar quality assurance process has been introduced recently in relation to record-keeping and maintenance of record confidentiality. This is referred to as information governance and is discussed later.

The specific legislation that applies to issues of patient health information and confidentiality consists of:

- Data Protection Act 1998
- Access to Health Records Act 1990
- Freedom of Information Act

The Data Protection Act aims to protect the confidentiality of sensitive personal data (including the personal health information held by the dental workplace) by placing obligations on the data controller (the dentist or organisation responsible for the data) only to make third party disclosures under the conditions of the Act, and to keep the data secure otherwise.

Data may be legally shared with certain organisations such as the Business Services Authority, the dental department of the local hospital or the salaried community dental services, but only on a "need to know" basis. It must also only be shared in order to provide the patient with appropriate care and treatment, and for the provision of general health services.

The data must be kept for no longer than is necessary, and although NHS regulations require dental records to be retained for only 2 years (6 years in Northern Ireland), medico-legally they should be held for 11 years or to the age of 25 with child patients – whichever is the longer.

When in the dental workplace, all dental staff must adhere to the workplace confidentiality policy, but inadvertent breaches involving patients' health information can occur all too easily if common sense is lacking. Examples of ways to avoid these non-deliberate breaches include the following:

- Patients must not be discussed in front of other patients – even when names are not used, some unusual or unique circumstance may make it possible to deduce a patient's identity, so conversations must never take place in hearing of others
- Privacy must be maintained when discussing any personal matters with patients – this may involve taking them away from the reception area if other patients are around, and using another room for private discussions
- Attendance at the practice is private and cannot be revealed to other patients, to employers or to schools – so phone calls asking for confirmation of a patient's attendance by an employer or a school must not be responded to by the staff; an appointment card may be issued to the patient to confirm the details instead
- All written communications with patients should be sent in sealed envelopes – this includes examination reminders that traditionally were sent on postcards, as they reveal the confidential fact that the patient attends a certain practice
- Dental records must be kept for the correct length of time by the practice and not be destroyed beforehand, either partially or wholly

Disclosure without patient consent

Under normal circumstances, information about a patient can only be disclosed to a third party with the patient's written consent. However, there are some circumstances under which the dentist has a statutory obligation to disclose the necessary information, or a legal right to do so, as follows:

- To assist in the identification of a person involved in a road traffic accident where facial trauma prevents identification otherwise – disclosure is allowed under the Road Traffic Act 1988
- When requested to do so by the Dental Practice Division of the Business Services Authority (formerly known as the Dental Practice Board) – this is when an audit of patient records is to be carried out, rather than when a course of treatment is underway
- To provide information about a child to a parent or legal guardian – although issues of age of consent to disclosure must also be considered (see later)
- When it is in the public's interest, such as with suspected or known criminals

- When disclosure is requested by court order, under the Prevention of Terrorism Act 1989 or under the Police and Criminal Evidence Act 1984
- When disclosure is necessary to a solicitor or debt-collecting agency, to enable them to pursue a legal claim against the patient on behalf of the dentist

Access to health records

Patients also have the right of access to their own manual or computerised health records, under the Access to Health Records Act 1990 and the Data Protection Act 1998. This covers all their medical and dental records written since November 1991, with the following provisos:

- Only the dentist, as the record holder, can approve access
- The patient request must be made in writing and there may be a fee to cover administration costs (usually around £10)
- The dentist must respond within 40 days of the fee payment
- The patient identity must be checked before releasing their records, and must be released to the patient only, or their legal representative
- Once viewed, the patient can request that any inaccuracies in their records are amended
- Any dental terminology, abbreviations or jargon must be explained on request

Dental nurses must therefore not release any records or parts of records themselves, or alter them in any way before they are to be released. They must be true, accurate, contemporaneous (as written at the time) and contain no derogatory comments. If the dental nurse is responsible for writing the notes, these should be written exactly as dictated by the dentist and not altered in any way. However, it is the responsibility of the dentist to check that they have been recorded accurately.

There are certain instances when the dentist can refuse to disclose the patient records to the patient (or a legal representative of the patient's next of kin), as follows:

- When disclosure would cause serious harm to the patient
- When a second person is mentioned by name and has not given consent for disclosure (does not include the dental team)
- When access to their records after their death has specifically been refused by the patient beforehand

The Freedom of Information Act excludes health records as a source of information that can be made available to a person on request, in contrast with other government-held information. The Access to Health Records Act allows patients or their legal representative to gain access to these records, while preventing third parties from doing so.

General Dental Council (GDC) Standards Guidance and confidentiality

The professional codes of practice and the ethical standards that the dental nurse must follow are contained in the General Dental Council's 'Standards for the Dental Team' documentation, which has recently been updated and extended from six key principles with accompanying guidance booklets into 9 core ethical principles of practice, with guidance provided within just the one document (see Figure 2:5).

The GDC Standards documentation can be downloaded directly from the GDC website at; www.gdc-uk.org.

327

The nine core ethical principles of practice are;

1. Put patients' interests first
2. Communicate effectively with patients
3. Obtain valid consent
4. Maintain and protect patients' information
5. Have a clear and effective complaints procedure
6. Work with colleagues in a way that is in patients' best interests
7. Maintain, develop and work within your professional knowledge and skills
8. Raise concerns if patients are at risk
9. Make sure your personal behaviour maintains patients' confidence in you and the dental profession

Each principle has a set of standards attached which must be followed and met by every GDC registrant. Failure to meet the standards is likely to result in their professional registration with the GDC to be at risk of suspension or even erasure. The standards to be followed by the dental team are based on the reasonable patient expectations of the dental professionals that they come into contact with during their treatment.

The booklet now contains considerable guidance to enable registrants to meet the standards, or to be able to use their own judgement and insight when necessary to justify any variation from the guidance. However, it clearly states that when the word **'must'** is used, the duty is compulsory and is therefore not open to interpretation or variation. Only where the word **'should'** is used will it be accepted that the duty may not apply in all situations, and that alternative action may be appropriate.

The fourth key principle states that members of the dental team must "maintain and protect patients' information", and it covers patients' expectations with regard to the personal and clinical information that the workplace holds for them. They do not expect any third party to be able to gain access to their personal information without their knowledge or agreement (although legal precedents do exist), but they do expect to be able to access their own information if necessary – clinical records should not be kept secret from the patient themselves. With this in mind, it is therefore obvious why the accuracy of the records is of paramount importance to the dental team, and that no defamatory or derogatory comments are ever included – this is grossly unprofessional.

Information governance

This is a quality assurance system that has been implemented to ensure the safety and appropriate use of personal and patient information. It brings together all the legal rules, guidance and information on best practice that apply to the handling of information. Compliance with information governance (IG) requirements by organisations should then show that they can be trusted to maintain the confidentiality and security of personal information.

For healthcare organisations, including dental workplaces providing NHS care for their patients, the Department of Health has developed a set of IG requirements in the form of a toolkit, which enables NHS organisations to measure the level of their own compliance.

These requirements cover the following areas:

- Data protection and confidentiality
- Information security
- Information quality
- Health records management
- Corporate information (where relevant)

The main points are that every NHS workplace must have a named IG lead person on the premises, who takes responsibility for:

- Registering the workplace on the IG toolkit website
- Accessing the toolkit requirements and completing them on behalf of the workplace's current systems of data security and maintenance

- Using the underpinning procedures and processes of the toolkit to develop the IG policy for the workplace
- Ensuring all other staff are aware of the organisation's approach to IG and where further information can be found, including the IG policy itself – this should be as a hard copy file kept securely on the premises, but accessible to all staff
- The lead must aim for best practice by reviewing the policy and compliance with the requirements of the toolkit annually and updating it as necessary
- Where amendments have been made during this review process, they must be signed off by a senior person in the organisation
- Confirm the named person at the Primary Care Trust who acts as the Caldicott Guardian for the workplace – this is a person with specialist knowledge in the area of confidentiality and information governance issues, who can give help, support and advice to the workplace in matters of patient protection and confidentiality

Templates are available from the website to download and use as the basis of the organisation's IG document, or they can develop their own.

The IG policy must contain the following information:

- Why the policy is required – this may be stated as "to ensure patient and data confidentiality, and the safe handling of sensitive information"
- Give an overview of how information should be handled in the workplace, including:
  - Storage of data
  - Consent to view data
  - Maintenance of patient confidentiality
  - Situations where information disclosure may be required
- Give a description of the accountability and responsibility for the policy:
  - Name of the IG lead
  - Job roles of support staff
- State the process of policy monitoring
- State the staff duties and their responsibilities in relation to IG
- Describe how areas of the policy link together
- Actions to take if the policy is breached:
  - Sanctions against staff involved
  - Remedial work for those responsible for IG procedures, to avoid future breaches

Further information is available at www.igte-learning.connectingforhealth.nhs.uk.

Consent to treatment

No matter what information an oral health assessment reveals and therefore what dental treatment a patient requires, the dental team must gain consent from the patient before that treatment can be provided.

The law concerning issues of consent to treatment is complicated and subject to change, so this chapter merely provides a simplified overview of the topic and the issues it raises in relation to dental professionals and their working lives. The main points to be clarified here are:

- What is consent?
- The key definitions of consent
- Who can give consent?
- GDC *Standards Guidance* on patient consent

Consent is effectively the patient, or their legal guardian, giving permission to the dental professional for treatment or physical investigation to be carried out. It is a legal and ethical principle that consent must be first given, and reflects the right of patients to decide what happens to their own bodies. It cannot be assumed that their attendance at the workplace is a signal for any type of "hands on" treatment to be carried out – indeed, without gaining consent to do so before touching the patient is considered assault. The GDC would consider this occurrence as serious professional misconduct and may suspend or remove the dental professional from the register.

To gain consent to proceed with a dental procedure, three key principles must be addressed:

- **Informed** – the patient must be given enough information to be able to make a decision, and in issues of treatment options this must include a host of information, as discussed later
- **Voluntary decision** – the patient alone must make the decision to proceed, without coercion or threat
- **Ability** – the patient must actually have the ability to make an informed decision

These principles form the basis of the guidance issued by the GDC, and they are discussed in more detail later.

Key definitions

Legally, there are various definitions used depending on the type of consent required, and the three that are of relevance in this text are:

- **Informed consent** – patients must be given full information about the treatment offered to be able to make an informed decision as to whether they wish to proceed or not:
  - The nature of the treatment (e.g. filling, crown, extraction)
  - The purpose of the treatment (e.g. restore function, alleviate pain, remove infection source)
  - The risks of the treatment (e.g. what can go wrong, what further treatment may be required)
  - The consequences of not having the treatment (e.g. effect on oral health, effect on general health)
  - The risks and benefits of any alternative treatment available
  - The longevity of success – will further treatment be required in weeks or months, or not for years, if at all?
  - The cost of the treatment, whether NHS or private
- The information must be given in a way that the patient understands, and this could involve the use of visual aids, an interpreter, or sign language
- Patients must have all of their questions answered in a way that is understandable, without the use of dental terminology if it is not appropriate (communication skills are discussed in detail in Chapter 5)
- **Specific consent** – this is the consent gained expressly for each stage of the treatment, and not just consent assumed to be for a full course of treatment without the patient being aware of what is involved at each stage. Thus, in the case of a symptomatic fractured tooth that is to be restored initially with a filling, but which may require endodontic treatment, and then restoration with a crown within 6 months, the patient must give specific consent for each stage before it is carried out
- **Valid consent** – for consent to be considered valid, it must be:
  - Informed
  - Specific
  - Given by the patient or their parent or guardian (if too young to give informed consent)

Consent does not have to be given in writing, especially for minimal and non-invasive procedures, but for more complicated treatment plans and for treatment provided under conscious sedation, a signed consent form is appropriate. Oral consent is adequate otherwise.

Although dental staff can be very helpful in assisting discussions to help the patient make a decision about whether to proceed with treatment or not, it is the responsibility of the dentist alone to obtain that consent from the patient. It is not the duty of the dental nurse, or any other dental care professional (DCP) to do so. Where a patient is receiving prescribed treatment from a dentist by a hygienist or a therapist, the dentist must first obtain the consent and then the DCP must check with the patient before starting the treatment that they are still happy to proceed.

Who can give consent?

For consent to be valid, it must be both informed and specific. However, for consent to be informed, the patient must:

- Be able to understand what is wrong
- Be able to understand that it requires treatment to make it right
- Be able to understand the consequences of both undergoing or declining the treatment
- Be able to communicate their decision (not necessarily verbally)

Under these circumstances, then, it is perfectly feasible for some children under the age of 16 to be able to give informed consent for their own treatment. This is called "**Gillick competence**" and is accepted by law as the right of the child to make the decision to proceed with treatment, and cannot be overruled by the parent or guardian. A child under 16 may also be perfectly capable of refusing to undergo treatment in contradiction to the wishes of their parent or guardian, but this can be overruled by the parent.

Similarly, children under the age of 16 who are judged by the dentist to be mature and intelligent enough to understand the situation, and competent to make their own decisions, can also refuse the disclosure of their health records to their parent or guardian.

Children over the age of 16 and of sound mind can legally consent to undergo any treatment and cannot be overruled by their parent or guardian, but theoretically they can be overruled if they refuse treatment. However, in view of the complexity of the legal issues involved, the dentist would be advised to make an application to a court for a decision in these cases. Alternatively, where a parent or guardian refuses treatment that is in the child's best interests, a court can be asked to make an order for the treatment to be carried out anyway, and lawfully.

In Scotland, the Age of Legal Capacity (Scotland) Act 1991 is quite specific and provides that a person under 16 who, in the dentist's opinion, is capable of understanding the nature and possible consequences of the procedure or treatment shall have legal capacity to consent on his or her own behalf to any dental procedure or treatment. In Northern Ireland the age of consent for medical and dental treatment is 16 years anyway.

Once a person reaches the age of 18 years and also has the capacity to reach decisions on their own behalf, that person is judged to be a **competent adult** and can give or withhold consent. "Capacity" in this context means the patient has the ability to:

- Be able to understand, believe and retain the information provided about treatment
- Consider the information appropriately in order to choose whether or not to proceed

No one else is able to consent to treatment on behalf of a competent adult, and all adults must be assumed to be competent and able to make their own decisions unless they demonstrate otherwise. Indeed, this does happen and there are some adult patients who may not have the capacity to give informed consent – these patients are referred to as "**incompetent adults**".

Incompetent adults are those who, for reasons of mental incapacity or illness, cannot give informed consent to treatment because they do not have the capacity to reach an informed decision on their own behalf. However, not all mentally ill or incapacitated patients are incompetent, and the dentist has to assess the patient at that time and determine the validity of any consent that the patient has given. Sometimes the opinion of a second professional is required to determine the validity.

Whatever the decision, the dentist carrying out the treatment must always act in the best interests of the patient, and they must be able to justify their actions if necessary. Further information should be sought by viewing the provisions available under the Mental Capacity Act 2005.

In summary then, those who can give consent are:

- Parent or guardian of a child to the age of 16
- "Gillick competent" child to the age of 16 in England and Wales
- Scottish equivalent
- 16- to 18-year-old of sound mind, in England and Wales
- 16-year-old in Scotland and Northern Ireland
- Competent adult
- Dentist on behalf of an incompetent adult, when in the patient's best interest and with an agreeing second opinion from another professional

GDC Standards Guidance *and patient consent*

One of the nine key principles of the GDC *Standards Guidance* document states that dental professionals must "obtain valid consent" and accept the patient's right to be asked if they wish to proceed with the treatment they require.

The guidance says that all dental professionals must treat patients politely and with respect, in recognition of their dignity and rights as individuals. So, dental professionals must not ignore patients' wishes when offering or undertaking to provide dental treatment – they must not be overbearing or bombastic in their manner, with a "doctor knows best" attitude towards the patient when they do not wish to take the advice on offer. It is particularly frustrating for dental professionals when patients do not wish to follow their advice, especially when the known result otherwise will be damaging to their oral health, but it is the patient's right to choose to refuse treatment and the team must accept that. They must also continue to support the patient to maintain their oral and general health in the meantime, and to the best of their abilities.

The guidance also says that the team must recognise and promote patients' responsibilities for making decisions about their bodies, their priorities and their care, and do nothing without their consent.

The guidance does not attempt to give any legal advice and the dental professional must seek this advice from other sources, such as a dental defence organisation. Finally, the guidance reminds all dental professionals that it is their own personal responsibility to stay up-to-date with all the laws and regulations that affect their work, in this case with regard to the issue of consent.

Patient complaints

All dental workplaces undertaking NHS dental treatment for their patients must handle complaints about NHS care according to a formal procedure that complies with the regulations. Also, dental professionals offering both NHS and/or private treatment must comply with the GDC's guidance on complaints handling. Which is discussed at the end of this section.

A complaint is any expression of dissatisfaction by a patient about a service or treatment, whether it is justified or not – so a complaint often results from the patient feeling that their expectations have not been met. Complaints can be about any part of the service the workplace provides, and many may well not be about the technical skill of the dentist or the quality of care that has been received. When patients feel that their expectations of a good level of service have not been met, more often than not it is merely due to a lack of communication. Good communication skills are discussed in detail in Chapter 5.

A general overview of what is required from an "in house" complaints procedure is given here, as it is relevant to the level of knowledge required for dental nurses. Further information in greater detail can also be requested from the following sources, if required:

- **England** – information from "The Local Authority Social Services and National Health Service Complaints (England) Regulations 2009"
- **Wales** – information from "Complaints in the NHS – A Guide to handling complaints in Wales 2003"
- **Scotland** – information from "Directions to Health Boards, Special Health Boards and the Agency on Complaints Procedures 2005"
- **Northern Ireland** – information from "The Health and Social Care Complaints Procedure Directions 2009"

"In house" complaints procedure

333

The GDC requires all dental practices (NHS and private) to have an "in house" patient complaint handling procedure, which should aim to fully resolve any complaint received to everyone's satisfaction, and as quickly as possible. Ideally, the matter should be resolved without the need for other authorities, such as the Primary Care Trust (or their replacement body after April 2013) or the GDC, becoming involved.

The procedure should include the points listed in the following table.

Procedure point	Action and necessity
Responsibility	A "responsible person" must be delegated within the workplace who ensures that the complaints procedure is followed correctly – this should be a senior dentist
	A complaints manager should also be delegated to receive any complaints on a day-to-day basis – this can be a dental care professional who liaises with the responsible person, or both roles can be carried out by the same person
Acknowledgement	Receipt of a complaint should be acknowledged within a few working days, and the complainant must then be kept informed of how the complaint will be dealt with, who will be involved and the expected timescale
Investigation	Obviously a thorough investigation must be carried out, and the essential point to consider is "What is the complaint about?"
	Gathering this information may involve a meeting with the complainant to discuss the details, a meeting with those staff involved, and reading all relevant patient records
	A resolution meeting with the complainant and the relevant member of staff present together may be very useful, and with someone else present to take notes Notes from the meeting should then be confirmed with all concerned afterwards
Timescale	The whole procedure should be completed promptly, and if delays occur due to the involvement of a defence organisation, the complainant should be kept informed of any likely extensions to the timescale

Procedure point	Action and necessity
Report	A written report should be sent by recorded delivery to the complainant when the investigation is complete
	It should contain the following information:
	• How the complaint was considered
	• Conclusions reached:
	○ No basis for the complaint
	○ No blame attributable, but explain what happened and why (e.g. regulations prevented a different course of action)
	○ Blame attributable, explain what happened and apologise, indicate measures taken to prevent a recurrence, offer reasonable redress (e.g. re-do treatment for free)
	○ Make it clear that the offer of redress is not an admission of liability, but is a goodwill gesture only
Appeal	If the complainant is not satisfied, information should be given of the bodies to which a formal complaint can be made:
	• Primary Care Trust (or future NHS commissioning body after April 2013)
	• Health Service Ombudsman for NHS patients
	• Dental Complaints Service for private patients
Records	Full written details of the procedure followed must be kept, from the point at which the complaint was made onwards
	These records should be kept in a secure central complaints file, not in the patient's records
	Make a note in the patient's records that a complaint was received on a certain date As always, the records must be contemporaneous, legible, accurate and remain unaltered in any way
	Complaint reports must be submitted to the commissioning body on an annual basis in England, Wales and Scotland, and quarterly in Northern Ireland

Any patient complaint, if not spurious in nature, can be used by the dental team as an opportunity to review and change workplace procedures if necessary, with the aim of improving the standard of service being offered to the patients.

Even if the workplace does not receive any complaints or negative comments, it is a very good idea to encourage patients to comment on the care and service they have received, using a patient survey or feedback process. The professional relationship desired, with patients as customers, requires that complaints are answered satisfactorily so that the matter can be put right, and the information provided is used to improve the service and therefore the patient's future dental experience.

Good communication skills and an open, honest approach are important when dealing with a complaint, and a sympathetic and understanding manner will often diffuse what could be a tense situation. All complaints should be resolved at the earliest opportunity, and often all that is required by the patient is an apology. This can be given without fear of admitting liability or negligence.

GDC Standards Guidance *and complaints handling*

One of the nine key principles of the GDC *Standards Guidance* document states that dental professionals must "have a clear and effective complaints procedure".

The guidance says that all dental professionals must give a timely and helpful response to a patient when they make a complaint, and that the right of the patient to complain must be respected. The team member must follow the complaints procedure of the workplace and co-operate fully with any formal inquiry into the treatment of the patient.

The guidance is set out to provide a checklist to follow when a complaint has been received and reiterates all of the guidance and information given earlier in this section:

- Respect the patient's right to complain
- Checklist to cover the following points:
  - That a complaints procedure is in place and is suitable for purpose
  - That it follows certain regulatory requirements
- The framework in place identifies who to contact when making a complaint, and that all team members are familiar with the complaints procedure
- The process to be followed when handling a complaint
- How to deal with the complaint correctly and constructively
- Try to learn from the complaint

Summary of oral assessment

335

For each patient that attends the dental workplace, an oral health assessment will guide the dentist towards diagnosing the presence of an oral disease and help to formulate a treatment plan where necessary, or to refer on for specialist tests and treatment in some cases. Not every patient will have to undergo every assessment method described, and the dentist will use professional knowledge and discretion in each case to assist in the assessment, diagnosis and treatment planning that is required.

The role of the dental nurse is to understand the need for the various assessments and to be able to assist the dentist and patient while they are carried out, as well as to accurately record all of the findings in each case. In particular the dental nurse must be able to:

- Support and reassure the patient throughout the assessment
- Have all the necessary instruments, materials and equipment ready for use
- Make accurate clinical records as required
- Be proficient in the use of:
  - Soft tissue record sheets
  - Tooth charts
  - Periodontal charts
- Complete a full medical history form with the patient
- Assist the dentist as necessary throughout the assessment

In addition, the dental nurse must understand the relevance of any necessary legislation, guidelines and workplace policies in relation to the carrying out of oral assessments and the formulation of treatment plans, and must abide by them at all times.

Orthodontic clinical assessment

One of the factors that the dentist considers during an oral assessment of a new adult patient or a child is the way that their teeth bite together – their **occlusion**. When normal occlusion is not present, the patient is described as having a type of **malocclusion**, and the treatment of malocclusions forms the basis of orthodontics.

Occlusion is the term used to describe the situation when the mouth is closed and the teeth of both jaws interlock together so that their occlusal surfaces are in contact. When each jaw is of a

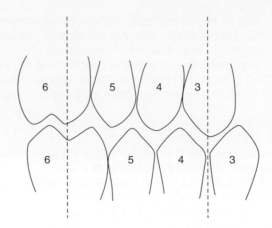

Figure 13.11 Class I molar and canine relationship. Source: *Levison's Textbook for Dental Nurses*, 11th edition (Hollins), 2013. Reproduced with permission of Wiley-Blackwell.

normal size in relation to the other, and they have developed during childhood in the correct relationship to each other, the cusps of the teeth in one arch should interdigitate with the fissures and interproximal areas of the other.

In normal occlusion, all the teeth are well aligned and there is no crowding, no protruding teeth and no undue prominence of the chin. Upper incisors slightly overlap the lowers vertically and horizontally and special names are given to this overlap: vertical overlap is called **overbite** and horizontal overlap is called **overjet** (see Figure 6.26). With the mouth closed and the teeth touching in occlusion, the position of the first molars and the canines in each jaw determines ideal occlusion and malocclusion. This is called Angle's classification.

Ideal **class I occlusion** occurs where the mesiobuccal cusp of the upper first molar lies in the buccal groove of the lower first molar (Figure 13.11). The ideal overjet is 2–4 mm and the ideal overbite is 50%.

For teeth to erupt into normal occlusion, the jaws must be in correct horizontal and vertical relationship to each other and of sufficient size to accommodate their full complement of teeth. The teeth can then erupt into a normal position of balance between the pressures exerted by the lips and cheeks on their outer side, and the tongue on the inner side of the dental arches.

Types of malocclusion

The basic types of malocclusion are caused by a combination of any of the following:

- Crowding
- Protruding upper incisors
- Prominent lower jaw.

Crowding

Crowding is caused by insufficient room for all of the teeth to erupt in line and occurs in jaws which are too small to accommodate 32 permanent teeth. The teeth become crooked and overlapping as the permanent dentition erupts, and those which are normally last to erupt cannot take up their proper position in the dental arch as there is insufficient room left. Thus the upper canines are usually displaced buccally, the lower second premolars lingually and the lower third molars are impacted within the bone of the mandible at the ramus.

Early extraction of carious deciduous molars also contributes to the crowding in these cases. The gap left by an extraction soon closes, as the remaining posterior tooth drifts forward and takes up some of the space required for the permanent successor.

Protruding upper incisors

Many children attend for orthodontic treatment because their upper front teeth protrude (procline) between their lips. This condition usually arises from a jaw relationship in which the upper teeth are too far forward relative to the lowers. It is commonly associated with an open lip posture and is called a **class 2 division 1 malocclusion** (Figure 13.12).

This tends to occur because the mandible is too far behind its normal position, and not because the maxilla is too far forwards, as may be thought. The maxilla is a fixed bone of the facial skeleton and cannot alter its position during growth, whereas the mandible is the only moveable bone of the skull and its position can alter markedly as it grows and develops.

When the mandible is not so far posterior to its normal position, so that the jaw relationship is not quite so severe, the upper incisors become trapped behind the tightened lower lip and erupt upright, or even pulled back (retroclined). This is called a **class II division 2 malocclusion** (Figure 13.13).

337

Prominent lower jaw

This condition, in which the chin is unduly prominent, is caused by a jaw relationship in which the mandible and the lower teeth are too far forward relative to the maxilla and the upper teeth. It usually results in the incisors biting edge to edge; or with the lowers in front of the uppers, instead of behind them. This is called a **class 3 malocclusion** (Figure 13.14).

Orthodontic appliances

Orthodontic appliances are used to align (straighten) crooked teeth, so that the patient is able to carry out effective oral hygiene techniques and prevent caries or periodontal disease from developing. Two basic types of appliance are used:

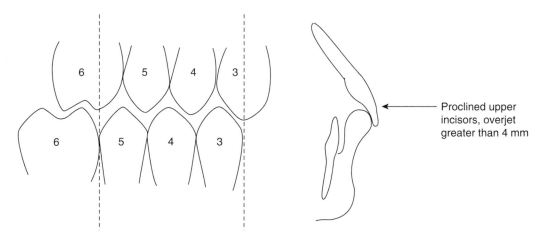

Figure 13.12   Class II division 1 malocclusion. Source: *Levison's Textbook for Dental Nurses*, 11th edition (Hollins), 2013. Reproduced with permission of Wiley-Blackwell.

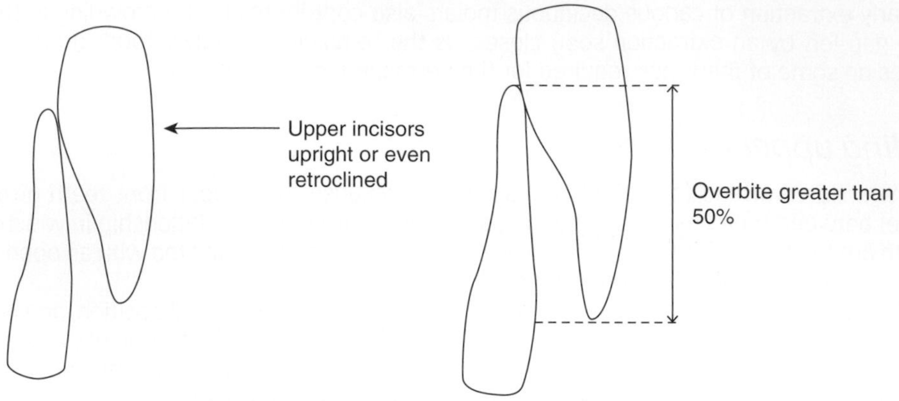

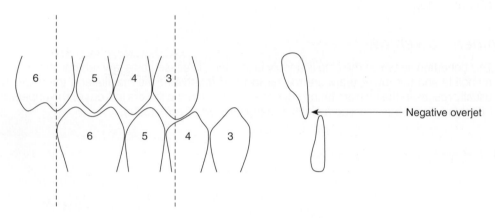

Figure 13.13 Class II division 2 malocclusion. Source: *Levison's Textbook for Dental Nurses*, 11th edition (Hollins), 2013. Reproduced with permission of Wiley-Blackwell.

Figure 13.14 Class III malocclusion. Source: *Levison's Textbook for Dental Nurses*, 11th edition (Hollins), 2013. Reproduced with permission of Wiley-Blackwell.

- **Fixed appliance** – composed of individual metal or ceramic components bonded onto each tooth and connected together by an archwire, they cannot be removed from the mouth by the patient
- **Removable and functional appliances** – composed of an acrylic base with stainless steel clasps and springs (in both the upper and lower jaws for functional appliances), these can be removed from the mouth for cleaning, eating and adjustment

Greater and more complicated forces can be applied to the teeth using fixed appliances, and the range possible for both types of appliance is as follows:

- Movement of teeth forwards or backwards in each arch – removable and fixed
- Movement of jaws in relation to each other – functional and fixed
- Alignment of slightly misplaced teeth in arch – removable and fixed
- Alignment of severely misplaced teeth in arch – fixed
- Derotation of teeth – fixed
- Guided eruption of unerupted teeth – fixed
- Guided reduction of deep overbite – removable and fixed

Fixed orthodontic appliances

These consist of separate stainless steel or ceramic components called brackets that are individually bonded onto each tooth, using an orthodontic light-cured resin material. Molar teeth often have a circular metal device placed instead, called an orthodontic band, and these can be cemented with any type of luting cement.

The fitting procedure, called bonding, is carried out in the surgery with no laboratory input required except to cast up the preoperative and postoperative study models required. Bonding of the components causes no tooth damage and they are "snapped off" at the end of the treatment harmlessly, using special orthodontic instruments.

The equipment and instruments required for the monitoring and adjustment of the fixed appliance once it has been initially bonded are shown in the following table.

Item	Function
Archwire (see Figure 9.23)	Flexible nickel titanium or stainless steel wires, to fasten into the brackets or bands
End cutters	Right-angled cutters to trim the ends of the archwire after replacement
Alastiks	Rubber bands to hold the archwire into the slots of each bracket
Alastik holders	Ratcheted holders (similar to artery forceps) to apply the alastiks to the brackets
Brackets (see Figure 9.23)	Metal or ceramic components to attach to each tooth, if any have been lost since last appointment
Bands (see Figure 9.23)	Metal rings to attach to molars especially, although bands are available for all teeth and were the only attachments available before brackets were developed
Bracket holders	To hold and position each bracket to the centre of the tooth, if any replacements are required
Bracket and band removers	To remove brackets, bands and any residual bond material before replacing, if necessary
Bonding materials	Acid etch and orthodontic resin bond material, to hold brackets onto the tooth
Band cement	Any luting cement material, to hold bands onto the molar teeth

Patient advice for fixed appliances

Every tooth is incorporated into a fixed appliance, so the number of stagnation areas, and the potential for oral damage to occur, is far greater than for individual fixed prostheses. Routine twice-daily tooth brushing alone is insufficient to maintain adequate standards of good oral hygiene, and special instructions and techniques are recommended for patients undergoing fixed orthodontic therapy:

- Careful manual tooth brushing should be carried out after each meal
- Good quality electric toothbrushes, such as Sonicare and Oral B, may be safely used instead

- Use of fluoridated toothpaste
- Daily use of **interdental brushes** to clean around each bracket individually
- Avoidance of cariogenic and acidic food and drinks for the full period of treatment
- Avoidance of sticky foods for the full period of treatment
- Use of **fluoride mouthwash** daily to minimise the risk of decalcification
- Regular use of **disclosing tablets** to highlight problematic areas where plaque is being retained, in order to minimise the risk of decalcification

Removable orthodontic appliances

These are similar to dentures in construction, in that alginate impressions of both arches and a wax bite registration are taken and sent to the laboratory, along with a work ticket detailing the exact design of appliance required. Usually, the technician involved in the appliance construction is one who specialises in orthodontic devices, as various of the components used are specific to this dental discipline and are not used with other prostheses.

A set of both study models and working models are cast from the impressions, and the latter set are used to construct the acrylic bases for each appliance, or for just one appliance if treatment is being carried out in one arch only. The additional components that can then be added to the acrylic base are:

- **Adams cribs** to retain the appliance in the mouth, usually to fit onto molar or premolar teeth and made of stainless steel (Figure 13.15)
- **Springs** in a variety of designs to move the teeth along the arch as required (Figure 13.16)

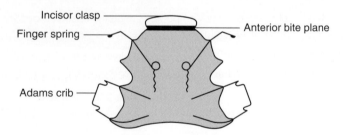

Figure 13.15 Removable upper orthodontic appliance. Source: *Levison's Textbook for Dental Nurses*, 11th edition (Hollins), 2013. Reproduced with permission of Wiley-Blackwell.

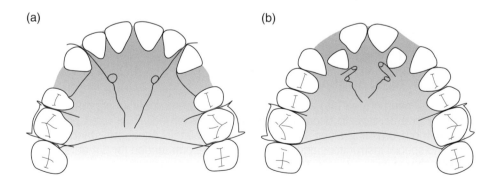

Figure 13.16 Types of spring: (a) palatal finger spring; (b) "Z" spring.

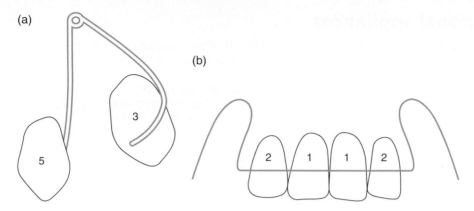

Figure 13.17   Types of retractor: (a) buccal canine retractor; (b) Roberts retractor.

- **Retractors** to push one or several teeth backwards (Figure 13.17)
- **Expansion screws** to move several teeth or each half of the upper arch outwards

The equipment and instruments required for the monitoring and adjusting of the appliance are shown in the following table.

Item	Function
Adams crib pliers (see Figure 9.21)	To adjust all metal springs and retractors, as necessary
Straight handpiece and acrylic trimming bur (see Figure 9.22)	To adjust all acrylic areas of the appliance, as necessary
Measuring ruler	To record any measurable tooth movement, such as the overjet
Expansion screw key	To count the number of turns applied to the screw between visits, to ensure compliance by the patient

Patient advice for removable appliances

As with removable prostheses, orthodontic appliances are capable of acting as stagnation areas and holding food debris and plaque against the teeth and gingivae, unless a good standard of oral hygiene is maintained.

Although some dentists prefer patients to wear appliances during meals, it is possible that more acrylic breakages will occur if this is the case. The instructions necessary for patients wearing removable appliances are as follows:

- Wear as directed by the dentist
- Clean the appliance and teeth after each meal, using a toothbrush and toothpaste
- Avoid cariogenic and acidic foods and drinks, as advised
- Attend all dental appointments for the necessary adjustments
- Contact the surgery immediately if any breakages or loss of the appliance occur
- Expect the appliance to feel tight initially after each adjustment
- Contact the surgery if any prolonged or excessive symptoms occur
- If the appliance is to be removed for meals, ensure it is placed safely in a rigid container to avoid breakages during mealtimes

Functional appliances

These are a specialised type of removable orthodontic appliance made of acrylic and stainless steel components and worn in both arches at the same time, the commonest one currently being a "**Twinblock**" (Figure 13.18)

They are used to correct skeletal class II discrepancies, where the mandible is further back from the ideal position, and work by holding the mandible forwards in the ideal class I position and allowing mandibular growth to occur and correct the malocclusion naturally. As their success depends on the growth of the mandible, they can only be used while the patient is still growing but after the premolars have erupted (these teeth are required for retention of the appliance), so the ideal age is up to 14 years old.

The materials, instruments and patient advice are as for removable orthodontic appliances.

The wearing of any type of orthodontic appliance demands a high degree of motivation and cooperation from patients. Their diet has to be restricted to minimise the risk of caries developing –in the teenage years this is often unacceptable to patients and their motivation will wane. This is more likely to happen with prolonged courses of treatment.

Cooperation and motivation need to be assessed at each adjustment appointment, and reinforced as necessary by both the dental nurse and the dentist. Warning signs of reducing cooperation include:

- Failed appointments for appliance adjustment
- Recurrent breakages of the appliance, either brackets dislodging or springs and acrylic being fractured
- Continual reporting of problems wearing appliances which cannot be detected by the dentist, which have resulted in non-wear
- Falling standards of oral hygiene or evidence of carious damage
- Obvious disinterest during adjustment appointments
- Requests for early removal of fixed appliances, before treatment has been completed
- Failure to wear removable or functional appliances during the daytime, so that, because they are only worn at night, little improvement is achieved

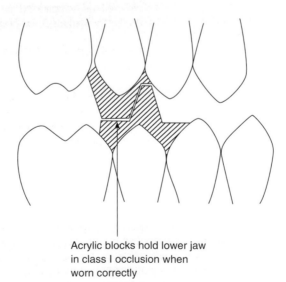

Acrylic blocks hold lower jaw
in class I occlusion when
worn correctly

Figure 13.18   Functional appliance. Source: *Levison's Textbook for Dental Nurses*, 11th edition (Hollins), 2013. Reproduced with permission of Wiley-Blackwell.

Any combination of these signs should alert the oral health team that the treatment may fail, so cooperation must be reinforced and improvement seen to happen, otherwise the decision must be taken to abandon the treatment.

A system of discontinuation of treatment must be in place so that patients are aware that failure to comply will result in the early removal of the appliance and incomplete treatment. This may mean that malocclusions remain as they were for life, with all of the consequences that that will infer to the patient. If a patient persistently fails to wear the appliance or to attend appointments for adjustment and review, treatment is best discontinued at an early stage before too much surgery time has been wasted.

Patients who have discontinued treatment once and who then re-present for continuation should be treated with great caution, as the likelihood of a second failed course is greater still.

Role of the dental nurse during orthodontic assessment and treatment

As with any other dental procedure, the dental nurse must support both the clinician and the patient during the provision of orthodontic assessment and treatment sessions. The clinician may be the dentist or the orthodontic therapist, and the patient may be a child or an adult.

In summary, the role includes all of the following:

- Have a good understanding of the procedure to be carried out
- Be aware of the position in the dental team for the procedure – this may be as the chairside nurse assisting directly with the procedure, or as a second nurse available to comfort the patient, mix materials, load impression trays and pass instruments as necessary
- Have all the patient records available, including any blank assessment sheets for the assessment appointment
- Have all the patient records, charts, radiographs, study models, orthodontic appliance and consent forms available for the treatment appointment
- Be aware of the correct equipment, instruments and materials to be used, and mix any material accordingly when directed
- Communicate effectively with the patient throughout the procedure, inspiring confidence and trust – this is especially important when impressions are being taken, as many patients find the procedure unpleasant
- Monitor the patient throughout the procedure, ensuring their comfort and well-being, giving assurance as necessary, and assisting them if they are unfortunate enough to vomit during impression taking
- Anticipate and pass instruments etc. to the dentist in the correct order during the procedure
- Record the accurate assessment details into the patient's records as necessary
- Follow the infection control policy in relation to the safe handling of any impressions taken
- Follow the infection control policy to fully decontaminate the surgery after use, especially in relation to clearing away vomit
- Follow the health and safety policy with regard to hazardous waste disposal
- Ensure that all records, charts and so on are correctly and securely stored for future use after being completed by the clinician, maintaining patient confidentiality at all times

Disease-related changes of the oral tissues

During an oral assessment, some patients may present with a lesion affecting their oral mucosa that indicates they are suffering from a disease or that they have a medical condition that affects the oral tissues in some way. The natural process of ageing also has an effect on the normal appearance of the oral soft tissues. The changes to the oral tissues that may be seen are discussed here.

Diseases of the oral soft tissues

Oral ulceration is probably one of the commonest soft tissue lesions that are seen in the dental workplace, and they have many causes and vary considerably in appearance:

- **Recurrent ulceration** – these affect around 20% of the population and are so called because they occur again and again in the same patient, usually with no diagnosed cause, although they are linked to nutritional deficiencies in some patients:
  - ○ **Minor aphthous ulcers** – small, shallow, painful ulcers that heal within 14 days and cause no scarring
  - ○ **Major aphthous ulcers** – larger, painful ulcers that take weeks or months to heal and cause scarring
  - ○ **Herpetiform aphthous ulcers** – very small multiple ulcers that occur sometimes up to 100 at a time
- **Ulceration due to systemic disease** – various diseases affecting the digestive system often exhibit oral ulceration, although the patient is likely already to have been diagnosed with the overlying disease before being seen by the dental team, and this should be noted in the medical history:
  - ○ **Crohn's disease**
  - ○ **Ulcerative colitis**
  - ○ **Coeliac disease**
  - ○ **Inflammatory bowel disease**
- **Ulceration due to viral infection** – two viral diseases in particular are associated with, and often diagnosed by, the presence of specific oral ulceration:
  - ○ **Herpes simplex** – as the primary infection of the patient with this virus, causing ulceration of most of the oral soft tissues and recurring throughout later life as herpes labialis ("cold sores")
  - ○ **Coxsackie virus** – hand, foot and mouth disease in childhood, with small ulcers present in all these areas at the same time, and specifically on the soft palate and back of the mouth in the oral cavity
- **Ulceration due to skin disorders** – the relevant condition in this category is that of **lichen planus**:
  - ○ An inflammatory skin condition that often causes oral ulceration in sufferers
  - ○ Oral lesions are recognised as being **premalignant** – i.e. they can undergo cell mutation and develop into malignant (cancerous) lesions
  - ○ Ulcers appear orally with white striae (stripes) around them
- **Malignant ulceration – squamous cell carcinoma** is the predominant manifestation of oral cancer and usually develops as an ulceration in the floor of the mouth or on the sides of the tongue:
  - ○ Painless ulcer with no obvious cause, such as trauma from a sharp tooth, and which does not heal within 2–3 weeks of its first appearance
  - ○ Aphthous-like ulcer with a "punched out" floor and rolled edges – this is the classic appearance of an advanced malignancy
  - ○ Very usually (but not always) diagnosed in smokers, users of other tobacco products and heavy drinkers (of alcohol)
  - ○ More detailed information is given at the end of this section

Oral white and red patches

Oral white patches can occur as transient or persistent lesions and have several causes.

- **Oral candidiasis** – commonly occurring infection with the fungus *Candida albicans*, producing a transient white patch which can be wiped off the oral mucosa to leave a raw-looking area beneath:

- Often occurs following the use of broad-spectrum antibiotics, which disturbs the normal microorganism balance in the body and allows the overgrowth of the fungus
- Also occurs in immune-compromised patients and those who are seriously ill with systemic disorders
- Can occur in patients using long-term steroid inhalers, such as asthmatics
- **Leukoplakia** – a white patch that has no obvious local cause, such as chronic trauma from a sharp tooth, and cannot be removed from the mucosa by wiping:
  - Often appears as white striae on the buccal mucosa or tongue, similar to lichen planus
  - Regarded as a potentially **premalignant** condition, although it sometimes has no sinister consequences
  - Particularly associated with smoking, and also with heavy alcohol intake
- **Erythroplakia** – a red patch on the oral mucosa, in isolation or sometimes adjacent to an area of leukoplakia, and regarded as a sinister sign of **premalignancy** of the soft tissues involved

Inflammatory disorders

Inflammation may affect any of the oral mucosal tissues – it is often not a result of infection with microorganisms but is related to underlying disorders instead:

345

- **Stomatitis** – a general inflammatory condition affecting the oral cavity:
  - Often occurs in the elderly and in denture wearers
  - Mucosa appears red and inflamed and often has an overlying *Candida* infection present
  - Responds well to improved oral and denture hygiene in most cases
  - Can be due to general debilitation and malnutrition, especially in the elderly
- **Angular cheilitis** – inflammation at the corners (angles) of the mouth:
  - Often occurs in the elderly and in denture wearers, as an extension of stomatitis
  - Appears as red and inflamed angles, often with cracking of the surface on mouth opening
  - Often due to a loss of facial height, which allows saliva pooling in the area
  - Wet conditions produced allow infection with common skin microorganisms, such as *Staphylococcus aureus*
- **Glossitis** – inflammation of the tongue which appears as red and smooth, and is sore:
  - Often seen in iron deficiency anaemia
  - Also occurs when extensive *Candida* infection is present in debilitated patients
  - May also indicate vitamin B deficiencies
- **Burning mouth syndrome** – usually occurs in elderly women and is described as the oral cavity feeling "as though on fire":
  - Usually no physical abnormality is found on examination
  - Considered psychogenic in many cases, due to depression, fear of cancer or of other serious disorders

Diseases affecting the teeth and supporting structures are discussed later.

Effects of ageing on the soft tissues

The number of people living longer is steadily increasing in the UK as medical treatment improves and healthier lifestyles predominate. A greater proportion of the population is being made up of those over the age of 70 years – the elderly. Dentally, as oral health has become understood and methods of maintaining good oral health have been developed, these patients are also keeping their natural teeth for longer, but because of age-related changes to the oral tissues, their dental treatment is different in some aspects from those who are younger and is classed separately as "gerodontology".

The changes to the oral tissues with age, and their relevance to dentistry, are summarised here.

Skin:

- Has less underlying fat and elasticity
- This gives increased tissue fragility and the likelihood of soft tissue trauma and bruising postoperatively

Bone:

- Tends to be more brittle, especially in postmenopausal women, who may have some degree of osteoporosis present
- The jaw bones are therefore at increased risk of fracture during extraction
- In particular, those elderly female patients who take bisphosphonates to counteract the debilitating effects of osteoporosis are likely to require referral for tooth extraction, as the risk of postoperative bone necrosis is high
- The natural resorption of the jaw bones following tooth extraction makes denture retention more difficult to achieve

Oral mucosa:

- Is thinner and less elastic
- It is therefore easier to traumatise during routine treatment
- The alveolar ridge areas are less tolerant of bearing dentures, with discomfort and ulceration more likely
- Gingival recession will be more pronounced, which increases the risk of root caries developing

Salivary glands:

- Undergo an alteration of the salivary components and volume, especially with certain drugs
- More likely to suffer from a dry mouth (xerostomia)
- This leads to an increased caries rate, as the self-cleansing action of saliva is reduced
- It may also cause problems with swallowing, speech and denture retention, as well as an increased incidence of localised periodontal conditions

Teeth:

- Undergo a gradual darkening in colour, making shade matching of anterior restoratives more difficult to achieve
- Narrowing and sclerosis of the pulp chamber lead to difficulties in gaining access to the root canals during endodontic treatment
- Have a reduced sensitivity

Medical conditions that affect the oral tissues

Various medical conditions can have a detrimental effect on the oral tissues, either directly as an effect of the disease itself or as a side-effect of drugs used to treat it.

Oral cancer

Oral cancer can affect various areas of the mouth, the soft tissues, the salivary glands or the jaw bones. Ninety per cent of oral cancers affect the soft tissues initially, as a lesion called **squamous cell carcinoma** (SCC). The suggested causative factors are as follows:

- **Tobacco habits** – all tobacco products contain chemicals capable of causing cancer (**carcinogens**)
- **High alcohol consumption** – alcohol acts as a solvent for the carcinogens and allows them easier entry into the soft tissues
- **Tobacco and alcohol** – smokers who also drink to excess are at most risk of SCC
- **Sunlight** – in fair-skinned people, sunlight is associated with SCC affecting the lower lip
- **Diet** – research is ongoing into links between SCC and diets high in fats and red meat, or low in vitamin A and iron intake
- **Genetics** – some people are genetically predisposed to developing SCC, as with other types of cancer

The signs and symptoms of SCC may be any of the following and will be specifically looked for during routine oral examination and assessment by the dentist:

- Painless ulcer that has no obvious cause and fails to heal fully within 2–3 weeks – obvious "normal" causes of these types of lesion are trauma from denture flanges, chipped restorations or vigorous tooth brushing, or even burns from hot foods and drinks
- In particular, an ulcer occurring beneath or on the side of the tongue, or on the floor of the mouth, as these are the oral areas where more sinister lesions develop
- Obvious oral ulcer with raised and rolled edges, which has no obvious cause
- Presence of a white or red patch of oral mucous membrane that is associated with the ulcer (these are called leukoplakia and erythroplakia, respectively)

The risk factors shown previously make the occurrence of the signs and symptoms far more serious in certain individuals, and any suspicious lesions must be referred to an oral surgery hospital department for investigation immediately. Even then, the 5-year survival rate from SCC is only around 55% and is very dependent on early detection and aggressive treatment.

The aggressive surgical treatment will be carried out by maxillofacial surgeons, and often involves the removal of large sections of the jaw and facial bones and their surrounding soft tissues, depending on the position of the cancer and the depth and area of its spread.

Years ago, the typical oral cancer sufferer was a 60+ male, usually from a lower socioeconomic background, who was a lifelong smoker and drinker. In recent years, this has changed and those being diagnosed with oral cancer are more likely to be much younger patients (even in their 20s), both male and female, usually smokers and especially binge drinkers, and also those who use sunbeds or sunbathe with little ultraviolet protection for their lips. Obviously this last group will also be at much greater risk of developing skin cancer (melanoma).

The dental team has a vital role to play not only in early detection of SCC, but also in patient education of the risk factors, especially in these high-risk patients. This is especially important with smoking and tobacco usage, whether with cigarettes, cigars or pipes, and including the habitual chewing of betel nuts and tobacco paan in some Asian societies.

Herpes

This group of viruses can affect the oral tissues in three specific disease conditions:

- **Herpes simplex type I** – as a primary infection in childhood which takes the form of an acute inflammation of the oral soft tissues, called gingivostomatitis, and appearing as multiple painful ulcers within the oral cavity
- **Herpes labialis** – the recurrent condition that occurs after the initial primary herpes simplex infection, commonly called a "cold sore" and occurring on the lip
- **Herpes zoster** – shingles, which occurs as a re-activation of the virus in patients previously infected with chickenpox (herpes varicella), and can affect the area supplied by the trigeminal nerve (the oral cavity), as well as the skin of the torso

Human immunodeficiency virus (HIV)

This virus is the causative agent of the fatal condition known as acquired immune deficiency syndrome (AIDS), and the progressive immune-deficiency conditions that it causes may well present as an oral lesion:

- **Oral candidiasis** – usually as an extensive fungal infection of the oral cavity, with heavy coatings of the white "thrush" lesions over the tongue and palate
- **Herpes zoster** – shingles, but typically affecting more than one body area, so the trigeminal nerve region may be affected at the same time as areas of the torso
- **Kaposi's sarcoma** – this is a characteristic tumour of AIDS sufferers that may occur as a purplish brown lesion on the palate, as well as in the skin
- **Oral hairy leukoplakia** – this is an oral white patch that has a distinct microscopic appearance at biopsy, is always associated with HIV infection and is premalignant

Hepatitis

Cross-infection following a needlestick injury is a very real occupational hazard for the dental team, but carriers or patients suffering from hepatitis are not likely to be easily identified unless they give a truthful medical history. There are no specific oral lesions associated with the medical condition of hepatitis.

Diabetes

This refers to a group of disorders affecting the pancreas that are characterised by a raised concentration of glucose in the blood – it results in an inability of the body cells to metabolise glucose correctly. The two types of diabetes are referred to as type 1 (insulin-dependent) and type 2 (non-insulin-dependent). The effects of the disease on the oral cavity are the same for both types of diabetes:

- **Xerostomia** – some degree of dry mouth is experienced by most patients, so the cleansing and lubricating effects of saliva will be reduced and they are more at risk from developing dental caries
- **Poor wound healing** – the peripheral blood supply is reduced in all areas of the body, including the oral cavity, and patients tend to heal poorly and be more prone to conditions such as chronic periodontal disease
- **Infection** – peripheral vascular disease and peripheral neuropathy result in reduced blood flow and nerve sensation in the oral cavity, so infections are more likely and can often develop more readily into abscesses and more serious conditions in these patients

Epilepsy

This is a condition where the electrical activity in the brain becomes suddenly and temporarily disrupted, resulting in a seizure. The usual drug used to control the occurrence of the seizures has the side-effect of causing gingival tissue overgrowth – **gingival hyperplasia**. This can make adequate plaque removal difficult for the patient as the overgrown gingival tissue covers it and prevents its routine removal by tooth brushing. The patient may have to undergo regular gingivectomy procedures to remove the worst gingival overgrowths.

Eating disorders

Bulimia is an emotional disorder in which the sufferer, usually a young adult female, follows bouts of compulsive overeating with periods of self-induced vomiting or fasting. The regular vomiting has the following oral effects:

- **Enamel erosion** – often severe pitting and enamel loss are present on many teeth, due to the acidic nature of the stomach contents present in the vomit; the palatal surfaces of the upper anterior teeth are particularly affected
- **Soft tissue burns** – the acidic vomit will also cause a burnt, reddened appearance to the oro-pharynx region at the back of the mouth

Anorexia is a psychological disorder characterised by "voluntary starvation" of the sufferer, induced by an obsessive wish to lose weight to the point of becoming life-threateningly emaciated. When forced to eat food, the sufferer will also self-induce vomiting to avoid putting weight on and will consequently experience the same oral effects as a bulimic.

Digestive disorders

The oral cavity forms the first part of the digestive system, so it is not surprising that several digestive system disorders manifest with oral lesions:

- **Crohn's disease** – a chronic inflammatory disease that can affect any part of the gastrointestinal tract, and shows up orally as ulceration throughout the oral cavity
- **Ulcerative colitis** – a chronic inflammatory disease that affects the colon and rectal areas only of the gastrointestinal tract, and shows orally as aphthous ulcers
- **Coeliac disease** – an absorption disorder of the small intestines, which have an intolerance to the cereal protein gluten; it shows up orally as ulceration, glossitis and stomatitis

Medical emergencies

Medical emergencies can occur anywhere, at any time, but some may be more likely to occur in the dental workplace setting due to the nature of dental treatment and the anxiety it evokes in some patients. The anxiety that some patients experience may have the following effects:

- Lowers the pain threshold so that "discomfort" is experienced as "pain", producing an agitated or even uncooperative patient
- Perception of being about to feel pain, so that stress levels and the anxiety state are raised – this can then put a huge strain on the patient's body, especially the heart and circulatory system
- Fear and anxiety at the prospect of dental treatment may worry patients enough to prevent them from eating beforehand, for fear of vomiting – they will then have a low blood sugar and be more prone to fainting; in diabetic patients, this low blood sugar is likely to precipitate a hypoglycaemic attack

In addition, the following points also have to be considered by the dental team:

- Many dental treatments involve the injection of a local anaesthetic, and these drugs may interact with some common patient medications
- Any of the dental materials, antibiotics or local anaesthetics used in dentistry have the potential to cause an allergic reaction in the patient, the worst-case scenario being a full anaphylactic reaction
- Many dental treatments are carried out with the patient lying **supine** (flat) in the dental chair, and this leaves their airway potentially vulnerable to foreign object inhalation, choking and a full respiratory obstruction emergency

The dental team can do much to reduce the anxiety levels of their patients merely by creating a friendly, welcoming and pleasant atmosphere within the workplace. Showing sympathy to an anxious patient helps to reduce stress levels and alleviates their concerns over appearing "foolish" to the staff and to other patients. For those patients whose anxiety is so great that it borders on **phobia** (an exaggerated and illogical fear), all methods of pain and anxiety control techniques should be considered by the dental team, and offered where appropriate. This ensures that these patients will still attend and undergo dental treatment routinely.

However, the patients who pose the greatest concern with regard to medical emergencies are those with diagnosed risk factors, such as:

- Heart conditions – any abnormality or disorder of the heart may potentially allow unexpected problems to arise during stressful episodes, such as when undergoing dental treatment
- Hypertension (high blood pressure) – anxiety often raises the systolic blood pressure, which can then put a considerable strain on an already malfunctioning heart
- Liver or kidney disorders – both these organs are responsible for eliminating waste products and toxins from the body, and any amount of malfunction due to disease could result in drugs not being detoxified and removed adequately
- Diabetes – uncontrolled diabetes or failure to take medications accurately may result in a hypoglycaemic attack. In addition, diabetics tend to heal poorly and be more prone to infections, including those involving the oral cavity

- Allergies – these patients are often sensitive, or even allergic, to more than one allergen, so great care must be taken to avoid the use of known potential allergens in the dental workplace, such as latex and penicillin-based antibiotics
- Certain medications known to react with some local anaesthetics – these are drugs that can be potentiated by adrenaline-containing local anaesthetics, and include medications such as some types of anti-depressants, thyroxine, and any medication that may cause hypertension, such as some contraceptives and hormone replacement therapy
- Previous history of complications during dental treatment – depending on the complication and its cause, it is possible for some to be a regular occurrence with the same patient
- Long-term steroid treatment – this treatment tends to override the body's own production of the hormones required to react to and survive stressful events, resulting in shock and a potentially fatal crash in the patient's blood pressure when stressful events do occur

These patients will be identified by the accurate completion and recording of a medical history at the time of their oral health assessment, before dental treatment begins. This medical history can then be stored with the patient records (either computerised or paper, or both) and updated at the beginning of every course of treatment.

The correct recognition of the cause of any emergency is vital if the casualty is to be correctly treated and their life supported until the emergency services can attend. This is done by being able to recognise the "**signs**" and "**symptoms**" of an emergency.

The signs are what the rescuer can see with regard to the casualty, such as:

- Skin colour – is it pink, grey, red, pale?
- Breathlessness – are they gasping, breathing quickly, struggling to inhale or exhale?
- Suddenness of any collapse – did the casualty fall straight to the ground, or did they slowly slump down?
- Actions before collapse, such as clutching the chest
- Condition of the pulse – is it fast, slow, weak, absent?

At the same time, the casualty will feel symptoms, which may be asked about if they are not unconscious, such as:

- Any pain – is it sharp, dull, throbbing, made worse by anything?
- Location of pain – where is it felt exactly?

- Nausea – does the person feel sick, or have they vomited?
- Drowsiness – do they feel sleepy (are they struggling to respond to verbal commands)?
- Difficulty breathing – are they struggling to breathe in or out, or both?
- Dizziness – do they feel like they will fall over; is the room spinning?

By assessing the casualty and noting the signs and symptoms exhibited, the rescuer can determine the next course of action. Often this will be to reassure the conscious casualty and to summon more experienced help. If the patient has become unconscious, they are said to have collapsed.

Causes of collapse

The various causes of the collapse of a casualty must be known and understood by dental nurses, so that they can usefully assist in the emergency treatment of these individuals should the need arise. While knowing and understanding the functions of the emergency equipment that all dental surgeries must hold, dental nurses would not be expected to administer any of the drugs available, except as a last resort where they are the only rescuer and the casualty is likely to die otherwise, before specialist help arrives.

It is therefore imperative for students to learn the various signs and symptoms of the medical emergencies and their correct treatment thoroughly, so that on qualification they could deal with a medical emergency effectively.

The following medical emergencies are all potentially life-threatening events and are discussed in the following sections:

- Asthma attack
- Anaphylaxis
- Epileptic seizure
- Diabetic hypoglycaemia or coma
- Angina attack that may lead to myocardial infarction
- Choking that may lead to respiratory arrest

In addition, the simple faint (vasovagal syncope) is such a common occurrence in the dental workplace that it is important that the dental nurse can recognise and treat this event successfully too, and it is therefore included in the following text.

All the medical emergencies in the preceding list (except choking) may require the administration of specific emergency drugs to enable the casualty to survive the episode, and the dental nurse must be able to recognise and draw up these drugs ready for the dentist to administer. The details of the emergency drugs that should be present in all dental workplaces, their doses and routes of administration, are shown in the following table.

Emergency	Drug and dose	Route given
Asthma attack	Salbutamol metered dose 0.1 mg Oxygen	Inhaler Face mask
Anaphylaxis	Adrenaline 1:1000 Oxygen Hydrocortisone 100 mg Chlorphenamine 10 mg/mL	IM injection Face mask IM injection IM injection
Epileptic fit	Oxygen if possible Midazolam buccal gel if fit is prolonged	Face mask Oral

351

Emergency	Drug and dose	Route given
Hypoglycaemia	Conscious – Glucogel Unconscious – glucagon 1 mg	Oral IM injection
Angina	GTN metered dose 0.4 mg Oxygen	Sublingual Face mask
Myocardial infarction	Aspirin 300 mg Oxygen	Oral Facemask

GTN, glyceryl trinitrate; IM, intramuscular.

Source: *Levison's Textbook for Dental Nurses*, 11th edition (Hollins), 2013. Reproduced with permission of Wiley-Blackwell.

Faint

This is a brief loss of consciousness due to a temporary reduction in oxygenated blood to the brain (**hypoxia**), and is the likeliest medical emergency to be encountered in the dental surgery.

Signs – pale and clammy skin, weak and thready pulse, loss of consciousness

Symptoms – dizziness, tunnel vision, nausea

Treatment:

- If **unconscious** – lie casualty flat with the legs raised above the head to restore blood flow to the brain (see Figure 3.17)
- Maintain airway and loosen tight clothing
- Provide fresh air flow or oxygen
- If **conscious** – sit casualty with the head down, loosen tight clothing, provide fresh air
- Give glucogel or dextrose tablet when consciousness returns to restore the blood sugar levels

Asthma attack

Asthma is a pre-diagnosed hypersensitivity condition affecting the respiratory airways. They narrow in response to exposure to inhaled particles, so that exhaled air has to be forced out of the respiratory system and the casualty has difficulty breathing. The same response can occur in stressful or fearful situations, or with exercise, especially if the casualty has a respiratory tract infection.

Signs – breathless with wheezing on expiration, cyanosis (blueness of lips), restlessness

Symptoms – difficulty in breathing, sensation of suffocating or drowning

Treatment:

- Administer **salbutamol inhaler** from emergency drug box (Figure 13.19)
- Give **oxygen**
- Calm and reassure the casualty
- Call 999 if the casualty does not make a rapid recovery

Anaphylaxis

This is a severe allergic reaction by the casualty's immune system to an allergen, such as with an allergy to penicillin, latex or food products such as nuts. The immune system overreacts to the allergen, causing severe swelling of the head and neck in particular, and a sudden fall in blood pressure (**hypotension**), causing collapse.

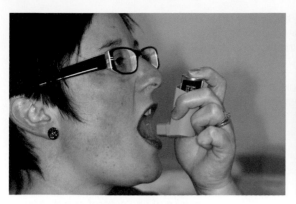

Figure 13.19   Inhaler administration.

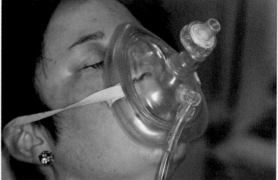

Figure 13.20   Giving oxygen using mask.

353

Signs – rapid facial swelling, formation of a rash, gasping, collapse
Symptoms – sudden onset of breathing difficulties, becoming severe, tingling of extremities
Treatment:

- Call 999 urgently
- Trained rescuer to administer **adrenaline** from emergency drug box
- Also **steroid** and **antihistamine** if necessary
- Maintain airway and give **oxygen** (Figure 13.20)
- Perform **basic life support** (BLS) if necessary until specialist help arrives

Epileptic fit

This is a pre-diagnosed condition, where there is a brief disruption of the normal electrical activity within the brain, causing a fit. The fits can occur mildly (**petit mal**) and the casualty may appear to be daydreaming, or they may occur in a major form (**grand mal**).

Signs – sudden loss of consciousness, followed by "**tonic-clonic**" seizure, possible incontinence. Tonic phase – casualty becomes rigid; clonic phase – casualty convulses

Symptoms – casualty may experience an altered mood (**aura**) just before the fit begins, dazed on recovery, with no memory of the fit

Treatment:

- Protect the casualty from injury, but make no attempt to move them
- Remove onlookers from the area and maintain the casualty's dignity
- Allow their recovery, then ensure they are escorted home
- If no recovery within 7 minutes, call 999
- Trained rescuer to administer **midazolam** buccal gel from emergency drug box

Hypoglycaemia and diabetic coma

These two conditions may occur in pre-diagnosed diabetics who either have not followed their insulin regime correctly or have not eaten at the correct times. The resulting drop in blood glucose levels can be catastrophic and cause collapse. The timing of dental appointments involving local anaesthesia is crucial for these patients, as they will be unable to eat without traumatizing their oral soft tissues until the anaesthetic has worn off. The dental team must therefore ensure that appointment times fit around the diabetic patient's normal insulin and meal regimes.

Signs – trembling, cold and clammy skin, becoming irritable to the point of being aggressive, drowsy, slurred speech, may mistakenly appear to be drunk

Symptoms – confusion, disorientated, blurred or double vision

Treatment:

- If conscious, give **glucogel tube** orally from emergency drug box (Figure 13.21)
- If unconscious, trained rescuer to administer **glucagon** from emergency drug box
- Maintain airway and give **oxygen**
- Call 999 if no recovery

Angina

This usually occurs in pre-diagnosed patients suffering from coronary artery disease, where these blood vessels supplying the heart are narrowed due to the presence of cholesterol or a thrombus (blood clot). During times of stress or anxiety, or while exercising, the reduced oxygenated blood supply to the heart is insufficient to allow full functioning and the casualty will experience chest pains ranging in severity from indigestion to a heart attack.

Signs – congested facial appearance, casualty clutching chest or left arm, irregular pulse, shallow breathing

Symptoms – crushing chest pain that may travel into left arm or jaw, nausea, breathlessness

Treatment:

- Administer **GTN spray** (glyceryl trinitrate) under tongue, from emergency drug box (Figure 13.22)
- Give **oxygen**

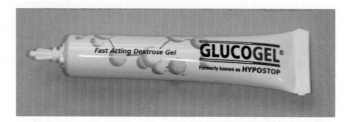

Figure 13.21   Glucogel tube from an emergency kit.

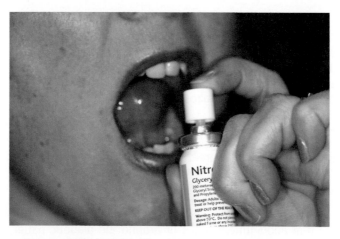

Figure 13.22   Sublingual glyceryl trinitrate (GTN) spray administration.

- Keep sitting upright, but maintain airway
- Calm and reassure the casualty
- Call 999 urgently if no recovery or consciousness is lost – suspect cardiac arrest

Myocardial infarction

This usually occurs in patients with a history of heart disease, especially angina, where either their drug regime has not been followed correctly or they have been exposed to anxiety or stress.

During an angina attack, the turbulence caused by the increased coronary artery blood flow may be sufficient to dislodge any blood clots present, and these may lodge and completely obstruct the blood vessel. This will prevent oxygenated blood from supplying that section of the heart muscle, which will then die.

Signs – sudden clutching of chest, grey appearance, possible collapse
Symptoms – sudden crushing chest pain that is not relieved by GTN spray
Treatment:

- Call 999 urgently
- Administer **aspirin** from emergency drug box
- Give **oxygen** and keep casualty sitting upright
- Maintain airway
- Calm and reassure casualty
- Perform **BLS** if necessary until specialist help arrives

Choking in adults

Like the simple faint, choking is an emergency that may well occur in the dental surgery from time to time, due to the nature of dental treatment. However, unlike the simple faint, choking is a very serious situation that could result in the death of the casualty if not dealt with promptly. It can occur in both the conscious and unconscious casualty, by the partial or full blockage of the respiratory tract causing lack of blood oxygenation. The body tissues will become **hypoxic**, which can be catastrophic when the brain or heart is affected.

Signs – sudden coughing or wheezing, laboured breathing, inability to speak, blue lips
Symptoms – aware of respiratory obstruction, breathing difficulties, dizziness
Treatment:

- Calm and reassure the casualty
- Support them in leaning forward and encourage coughing
- Give five **back slaps** between the shoulder blades to dislodge the obstruction (see Figure 3.14)
- Begin **abdominal thrusts** (**Heimlich manoeuvre**) to cause artificial coughing if the obstruction is still present (see Figure 3.15)
- If the casualty becomes unconscious, clear and open the airway as for **BLS**
- Call 999 if this is unsuccessful

The technique of giving abdominal thrusts is as follows:

- Stand behind the casualty
- Rescuer wraps their arms around the casualty, just below their ribcage
- A fist is formed with one hand and this is grasped by the other, positioning both in the upper abdomen
- Both hands are pulled in sharply, to cause an artificial cough
- Air will whoosh out at each thrust, hopefully dislodging the obstruction as it does so

Choking in young children

The signs and symptoms of choking in a young child will be as for an adult casualty, and they are more likely to experience this emergency due both to their lack of awareness of danger and their tendency to put objects into their mouths without realising the consequences.

The procedure to follow is very similar to that for an adult but with less force, and depends on whether the young child is conscious or not. The important point is that rescue breathing should only be carried out on an unconscious child, as their airway often becomes clear as their muscles relax during their loss of consciousness, and rescue breaths may not be necessary.

The procedure in a choking conscious child is as follows:

- Keep calm and keep the casualty (and any attending parent) calm
- Get the child to cough to try to expel the obstruction
- If unsuccessful, give five back slaps and recheck the mouth
- If unsuccessful, give five chest thrusts from behind against the breastbone, then recheck the mouth
- If unsuccessful, send for help then repeat the back slaps and recheck the mouth
- If unsuccessful, give up to five abdominal thrusts but with less force than that used for an adult, then recheck the mouth
- Continue alternating all three techniques until the obstruction is cleared, the child loses consciousness or specialist help arrives
- If successful, have the child medically checked for any signs of respiratory system damage

If the choking episode is severe and prolonged, or the obstruction is complete, the child will collapse and become unconscious. The rescue procedure is as follows:

- Check the mouth for any obstruction and remove, then open the airway
- Try five times to give two rescue breaths; if the chest rises successfully then carry out chest compressions to circulate the oxygen around the body
- If the chest fails to rise, give five back slaps followed by five chest compressions if the child is still choking
- Re-check the mouth and open the airway, then give another five rescue breaths
- If unsuccessful give another five back slaps followed by five abdominal thrusts
- Continue the cycle until specialist help arrives or the obstruction is removed

Choking in babies

Babies are easier for the rescuer to handle during a choking episode, as they can be held face down for back slaps and carried towards help while still being aided, rather than having to be left. Obviously, the force used to attempt to dislodge an obstruction must be significantly less than that used for a young child. Also, under no circumstances should abdominal thrusts be attempted on a baby, as the internal organs would be easily damaged by this technique.

Again, as with a young child, rescue breathing should not be attempted unless the baby is unconscious. If the baby is conscious and choking, the procedure is as follows:

- Check the mouth for any obvious obstruction and remove it
- With the baby held face down along the rescuer's arm, give five back slaps using fingers only (see Figure 3.16)
- Turn the baby face up and remove any obstruction
- If unsuccessful, give five sharp chest compressions (as for BLS)
- If unsuccessful, call for specialist help and continue the cycle until the obstruction is removed or the baby becomes unconscious

If the baby becomes unconscious:

- Recheck the mouth and open the airway
- Try five times to give two rescue breaths
- If the chest rises, continue chest compressions to circulate the oxygen
- If not, give five back slaps followed by five chest compressions
- Recheck the mouth for any obstruction and open the airway, then repeat the cycle until specialist help arrives

Cardiac arrest and respiratory arrest

When the heart has stopped beating completely, the patient is said to have "arrested" or be in cardiac arrest, and similarly when a patient makes no effort to breathe spontaneously they are said to be in respiratory arrest.

Respiratory arrest can occur while the patient's heart is still beating, so the patient will require assistance by rescue breathing only. However, when the heart stops beating in cardiac arrest, respiration also stops and the patient will require assistance by cardiopulmonary resuscitation (CPR) – they will require both heart compressions and rescue breathing to try to save them. This technique is referred to as basic life support, or BLS.

All members of the dental team are expected to hold a BLS certificate if working with patients, and to undergo the necessary core continuing professional development requirements to update their medical emergencies knowledge as laid down in the GDC's *Standards Guidance* documentation.

The two signs that should prompt any rescuer to begin BLS immediately are:

- **Unconsciousness**
- **Abnormal or absent breathing**

These two signs indicate that the casualty's life is at risk; as sudden unconsciousness may indicate that the heart has stopped beating (**asystole**) or is beating ineffectively (**fibrillating**), and abnormal breathing indicates a compromised airway and possible lack of oxygen to the brain (**hypoxia**). The presence of any of these signs may result in the death of the casualty if not dealt with quickly by the rescuer.

The aim of BLS is to maintain a flow of oxygenated blood to the casualty until one of the following happens:

- They recover and begin to circulate oxygenated blood by breathing unassisted
- Life support is handed over to specialists, usually paramedics
- The rescuer is too physically exhausted to continue
- The casualty's death is confirmed by an authorised practitioner, such as a doctor at the scene

Oxygen is the atmospheric gas that is vital for life. It is breathed into the respiratory system through the nose and mouth, and then passes down the trachea to the two bronchi which enter the right or left lung.

In the lungs, the oxygen passes out into the circulatory system during external respiration and is transported around the body in the arterial blood stream by the continual pumping action of the heart. Where required, the oxygen passes out of the blood vessel and into the body tissues during internal respiration, where it is used to provide energy for the cells to work.

The actions of the respiratory system in taking up oxygen from the atmosphere and absorbing it into the blood, and of the circulatory system in transporting that oxygen around the body to the

357

cells are carefully controlled by the brain. If any one of these three vital organs fails, the other two will also fail shortly afterwards.

Without oxygen, the cells (and therefore the body) cannot function and death will occur. After only 3–4 minutes without oxygen, the brain cells can suffer irreversible damage which, if not fatal, will lead to some degree of permanent brain damage. The quicker the need for BLS is established and it is begun, the better the chances of survival for the casualty – and ideally this should be within seconds of their life support system failing.

So, the fundamental aims of BLS are to maintain the life of the casualty by achieving the following:

- Provide oxygen to the lungs – by some form of **rescue breathing**
- Circulate the oxygen to the body tissues – by **external chest compressions** to mimic the pumping action of the heart

Immediate assessment of the casualty

Unconsciousness indicates that the casualty is unresponsive to all stimuli and that the heart may have stopped beating – they have gone into cardiac arrest. There is no instance where the heart can have stopped beating and a person remain conscious, as the body cells (especially the brain) will become starved of oxygen very quickly and will be unable to function.

Abnormal breathing, such as infrequent noisy gasps, indicates that there is a possible obstruction in the casualty's respiratory system which is making normal breathing difficult. This will gradually reduce the oxygen supply to the body cells, and once breathing ceases completely, the oxygen supply is cut off immediately. The casualty's skin colour will change from pink to pale to blue or grey as the body tissues become starved of oxygen.

This is more difficult to determine in those with darker skin tones, so the lips, nail beds and mucous membranes of the mouth may also be checked for signs indicating lack of oxygenation (hypoxia).

The actions that may be required to help the casualty cannot be determined until the rescuer has fully assessed the situation, and although swift action is necessary to avoid brain damage or death, the following questions must be quickly considered by the rescuer in an effort to realise the correct medical emergency:

- **Why has the individual become unconscious?** Are there any external causes such as trauma, electrocution, poisonous fumes, drowning?
- **How is unconsciousness established?** Is the person alert or moving, responsive to noise or voices, responsive to pain, completely unresponsive?
- **Is breathing abnormal?** Are they gasping, coughing, or even clutching at their throat?
- **Are there any breath sounds?** How is this established?
- **What does the rescuer do next**? At what point should help be summoned and what actions are required immediately?

The accepted order to follow when assessing an emergency situation and determining whether BLS is required can be summarised and easily remembered by the following code:

- **D** for **Danger**
- **R** for **Response**
- **S** for **Shout for help**
- **A** for **Airway**
- **B** for **Breathing**
- **C** for **Circulation**

This is best remembered as **DRSABC** (referred to as "doctors – a – b – c").

DRSABC in detail

Danger

Check the immediate area for possible dangers, such as electric wires running through pooled water, punctured gas canisters, spilt chemicals giving off strong fumes. If hazardous chemicals are suspected of being involved in the emergency situation, the workplace Control of Substances Hazardous to Health (COSHH) file must be consulted at some point for information on first aid actions that may be necessary. This action is best delegated to a spare rescuer, while BLS is being carried out by others.

If possible, any dangers should be made safe by the rescuer before approaching the casualty, but not at the risk of endangering themselves in the process. Ideally, this should not involve moving the individual except in extreme circumstances, such as rising water levels that may cause drowning. This is to prevent any further injury being caused.

Response

The level of responsiveness will determine whether or not the casualty is unconscious. Call loudly to them, asking if they can hear you or if they are all right, while gently shaking them. Their responsiveness can quickly be assessed and determined by a system referred to as the AVPU code:

- **Alert** – the casualty is fully conscious and able to communicate fully and spontaneously
- **Verbal** – the casualty is not fully conscious, but is able to respond to verbal commands and prompts
- **Painful** – the casualty is semi-conscious at best, but able to respond to painful stimuli such as a gentle pinch
- **Unresponsive** – the casualty shows no response to verbal prompts or painful stimuli; they are unconscious and unable to be roused

If casualties show no response whatsoever, they are in need of urgent help. Wherever possible, the level of responsiveness should be determined without moving individuals from the position in which they were found, to avoid any further injury.

Shout

If the casualty is unresponsive and therefore unconscious, the rescuer will need help with any attempt at BLS if it is required, as well as to summon specialist help if necessary. If only one rescuer remains to aid the individual while help is being sought, that person may need to continue BLS for a prolonged period of time, and ultimately this may result in their physical exhaustion. If attempts at BLS have to then be abandoned before specialist help arrives, the casualty is likely to die.

Shout very loudly to alert anyone else in the vicinity that an emergency situation has arisen. In the workplace, there may be internal communication systems in place for just such an event, such as intercoms, alarm bells or coded calls, and these must be known about and used appropriately by the rescuer.

Airway

The airway needs to be checked for any obstruction, such as vomit or debris or the tongue itself, which may have fallen back and blocked it. Any loose obstruction should be removed by rolling the casualty's head to the side to encourage it to drop out of the mouth. In the dental surgery there will also be electrically operated suction equipment available at the chairside, or a manually operated suction device within the emergency kit that all dental workplaces have to have on the premises (see Figure 3.4).

However, these must only be used by those rescuers who have been trained to do so, as they can push debris further down the airway or cause soft tissue injury if not used correctly.

The casualty's airway can then be opened to allow breathing to occur. This can be achieved by tilting the head back by placing the palm of one hand on the casualty's forehead and lifting the chin with the fingers of the other hand at the same time (see Figure 3.5).

However, this technique must never be used when an individual has a suspected neck or spinal injury, as to do so would almost certainly cause further damage to the spinal cord. This could result in permanent paralysis of the individual.

In these cases, the airway can be opened by thrusting the lower jaw forward with both hands, without any head tilting occurring (see Figure 3.6). This should avoid any further neck or spinal injury.

Breathing

With the airway open, breathing is assessed quickly over a 10-second period. The rescuer needs to determine if any spontaneous breathing attempts are being made, and their quality, by checking for the following:

- **Look** to see if the chest is rising and falling
- **Listen** to any breathing sounds
  - Are they regular or infrequent?
  - Are they quiet or noisy?
  - Are they normal or gasping in nature?
- **Feel** for air flow by placing the cheek close to the casualty's mouth (see Figure 3.7)

If breathing is absent or abnormal, the emergency services must be called, as specialist help is required. Ideally a second person can be sent to do this, but if necessary the lone rescuer must leave the casualty and go to call for emergency help.

If it is now decided that BLS is required to maintain the casualty's life until specialist help arrives, the person may require moving to a position where this can be carried out effectively. This is usually achieved by very carefully rolling the individual onto their back with a firm surface beneath them, in a safe area and with enough room to manoeuvre as necessary, as BLS may need to be carried out correctly for a prolonged period until specialist help arrives.

Circulation

Any residual oxygenated blood within the casualty now needs to be quickly pumped around the person's body to the brain, and this is achieved by the rescuer carrying out chest compressions on the individual. These will only be effective if the heart is adequately compressed between the breastbone (sternum) and the spine, on a firm surface, and at a sufficient rate to actually cause the blood to flow through the circulatory system as required, rather than just swishing backwards and forwards (see Figure 3.9).

If any spinal or neck injuries are suspected, ideally casualties should not be moved from the position in which they were found, to avoid further injury. However, this may not always be possible, especially if their position prevents successful BLS from being carried out. Ideally, several helpers should be used to very carefully roll the casualty onto their back on a hard surface, keeping their head in line with their spine at all times – this is often referred to as a "log roll" technique.

In the dental surgery, dental chairs are designed to be firm enough to carry out chest compressions without having to move the casualty onto the floor.

The correct point to apply the compressions is quickly located as follows:

- Kneel at the side of the casualty, or stand if the person is still on the dental chair
- Run a finger along the lower border of the individual's ribcage, towards the midline
- Once in the midline, the breastbone will be felt with the finger
- Place the heel of the other hand adjacent to the finger, towards the head of the individual
- Interlock the fingers of both hands over this compression point (see Figure 3.10)
- Lean over the individual, keeping the arms straight and the elbows locked (see Figure 3.11)

Thirty compressions can now be given at a rate of 100/minute, by compressing the chest by 4–5 cm and then releasing to allow the heart to expand and refill with blood. Once the initial 30 compressions have been administered, two rescue breaths can be given by the lone rescuer, or ideally by a second rescuer.

Rescue breathing

Once the first 30 compressions have been administered, any residual oxygen in the blood will have been used up by the body tissues, and especially the brain. To maintain life, the oxygen now has to be regularly replaced before being distributed around the body again by the chest compressions, and this is achieved by artificial ventilation or rescue breathing.

The atmosphere contains about 21% oxygen, but that which is expired (breathed out) only contains 16%, as our body tissues use up the 5% difference to produce energy for the cells to work. In an emergency situation, rescue breaths are usually given by breathing expired air into the casualty in a mouth-to-mouth technique. If there are facial injuries affecting the mouth, it may be necessary to use a mouth-to-nose technique instead, and with small children or babies the rescuer will breathe into the casualty's mouth and nose together.

The use of emergency oxygen supplies, such as that held by all dental practices, will increase the amount of available oxygen for rescue breathing when given using a pocket mask or a ventilation bag, but the technique can only be successfully used by those who are trained to do so (see Figure 3.12).

The airway will already have been cleared of obstructions during the DRSABC procedure, but will need to be held open now to administer rescue breaths, again using the head tilt/chin lift or jaw thrust technique. Two rescue breaths are then given as follows:

- Maintain the head tilt to keep the airway open
- Pinch the nostrils closed, with the fingers of the hand being used to press onto the forehead
- Support the chin with the other hand while holding the mouth open
- Take a deep breath, then seal the mouth over that of the individual to ensure no air escapes (see Figure 3.13)
- Breathe with normal force into the person's open mouth for about 2 seconds, watching from the corner of the eye to ensure that the chest rises
- With the airway still held open, move away from their mouth and watch the chest fall as the air comes out
- Repeat the rescue breath
- If given successfully, follow with another 30 chest compressions as a BLS cycle

Sometimes problems will be experienced while attempting rescue breathing, the commonest one being that the chest does not rise. In the absence of an obstruction this is usually due to the airway not being fully opened, and the head tilt procedure should be repeated until successful. Otherwise, ensure that the nostrils are fully closed and that a good mouth-to-mouth seal is being achieved.

If the abdomen is seen to rise while the breath is being given, air is being blown into the stomach, rather than the lungs, by being too forceful or too prolonged. The rescue breath should stop once the chest stops rising, usually after just two seconds at a normal breath force.

BLS modifications

The BLS protocols described are to be used for adults and children over the age of 8 years. Babies and young children require less force to be used while carrying out both chest compressions and rescue breathing, to avoid injuring their bodies.

The weight of the foetus in a pregnant woman will also hinder BLS attempts if she is lying on her back, and the usual technique has to be modified for these groups of casualties.

Babies and young children

Anatomically these age groups are different to adults in the following ways:

- They have narrower air passages in the respiratory system
- These air passages are more prone to blockages
- The trachea is more flexible and so it is easily blocked if airway opening attempts are too severe
- They have a relatively larger tongue than an adult, which is more likely to obstruct the airway when the baby or young child is unconscious

Cardiac arrest in these younger casualties is rarely due to heart problems, as in an adult, but is far more likely to be caused by lack of oxygen to the brain due to airway obstruction.

As the DRSABC code is being followed, it will soon become apparent if the young casualty is unresponsive and having breathing difficulties or not breathing at all, and it is imperative that rescue breathing is commenced **BEFORE** starting chest compressions. This is because the likely cause of their collapse will be a shortage of oxygen to their vital organs and any reserves will have been quickly used up by their young bodies and must be replenished as soon as possible.

So the full modified BLS sequence of events in cases involving a baby or a young child is as follows:

- **Danger** – check for dangers as usual
- **Response** – less reliable in younger casualties, so merely determine whether they are unresponsive only
- **Shout** – summon help from anyone in the vicinity, without leaving the casualty
- **Airway** – check the airway for obstruction, especially the tongue, then carefully open the airway, taking care not to overextend the head tilt and so block the trachea
- **Breathing** – look, listen and feel for signs of spontaneous breathing for 10 seconds, and if they are absent **GIVE FIVE RESCUE BREATHS USING THE MOUTH TO MOUTH-AND-NOSE TECHNIQUE**
- **Circulation** – give 30 chest compressions, using two fingers for a baby or one hand for a young child, aiming to compress the chest by one-third of its depth at a rate of 100/minute
- The lone rescuer must continue BLS for a full minute before going for specialist help

Pregnant women

Any premenopausal woman who collapses and requires BLS could potentially be pregnant. In some cases it will be known or obvious that they are pregnant, but otherwise it should always be considered a possibility, especially if BLS attempts are failing for no other obvious reason.

In a heavily pregnant woman lying on her back, the uterus (womb) tends to lie over the major blood vessels that return blood from the lower body to the right side of the heart (the inferior venae cavae). If this casualty collapses and requires BLS, the rescuer has the added difficulty of forcing blood through these squashed blood vessels during chest compressions, and the rescue attempt is likely to fail.

Instead, the pregnant casualty should be laid slightly on the left side with some form of support under the right buttock so that these major blood vessels are not squashed by the uterus. BLS can then be carried out in the normal way, while maintaining this angled position of the woman throughout.

Basic structure and function of oral and dental anatomy

To fully understand the topics of oral health and the diseases that can affect the oral cavity, the dental nurse must also have knowledge of the anatomy and normal functioning of the oral structures. Without this knowledge, comparisons cannot be made between health and ill-health, and advice on prevention and management of oral diseases cannot be disseminated to the patients.

The oral and dental structures to be discussed are as follows:

- Teeth – primary and secondary dentitions
- Supporting structures – gingivae, periodontal ligament, alveolar bone
- Salivary glands – parotid, submandibular, sublingual and minor glands
- Muscles of mastication – temporalis, medial and lateral pterygoids, masseter
- Maxilla, mandible and temporo-mandibular joint
- Nerve and blood supply to the teeth and supporting structures

Teeth

The teeth are the anatomical structures within the oral cavity that are of the greatest relevance to the dental team, as their development, health, disease and restoration are the fundamentals of dentistry. The teeth have the following functions:

- To cut up and masticate food into suitably sized portions before swallowing
- To expose the food surfaces to enzymes and allow digestion to begin
- To support the oral soft tissues of the cheeks and tongue, and therefore enable clear speech

Humans have two sets of teeth – the primary (deciduous) teeth of childhood, and the secondary (permanent) teeth of adulthood. The number and type of teeth in each set differ, although the shape of the common ones is the same.

The detailed anatomical shape of each tooth, and its function, is called **tooth morphology**.

The four types present in the secondary dentition, from the midline of the mouth posteriorly, are:

- **Central and lateral incisors**
- **Canine**
- **First and second premolars**
- **First, second and third molars**

The primary dentition has just two molars and is made up of just three different types of teeth – there are no premolars present. Each tooth of all types, and in both sets, has three sections: the **crown**, the **neck** and the **root(s)**.

The **crown** is the section of the tooth visible in the oral cavity, following its eruption from the underlying alveolar bone. The **neck** is the section where the tooth and the gingival tissues are in contact with each other at the point where the tooth emerges through the gums, and the **root** is the (usually) non-visible section that holds the tooth in its bony socket.

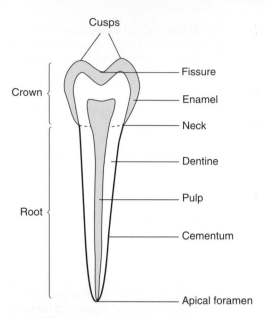

Cusps

Crown

Root

Fissure

Enamel

Neck

Dentine

Pulp

Cementum

Apical foramen

Figure 13.23   The structure of a tooth. Source: *Levison's Textbook for Dental Nurses*, 11th edition (Hollins), 2013. Reproduced with permission of Wiley-Blackwell.

All teeth are composed of the same four tissues:

- **Enamel** – a highly calcified tissue covering the whole crown of the tooth
- **Dentine** – a less calcified tissue than enamel that forms the inner bulk of the crown and root
- **Cementum** – a thin calcified covering of the root dentine only
- **Pulp** – the inner neurovascular tissue of the tooth, within the central pulp chamber

The structure of a typical tooth is shown in Figure 13.23.

Microscopic structure of the teeth

The differences in the microscopic structure of the four layers of the teeth are what determine how they function, how they disease develops within them, how they are treated for that disease and how they are restored or extracted by the dental team.

Enamel

This is the highly calcified, protective outer covering of the crown and is the hardest substance in the body. Its properties and microscopic structure are as follows:

- It is made up of 96% mineral crystals (inorganic) arranged as **prisms** in an organic matrix called the **interprismatic substance**
- The main mineral crystals are **calcium hydroxyapatite**
- The prisms lie at right angles to the junction with the next tooth layer, the **dentine**
- The junction between these two layers is called the **amelodentinal junction** (ADJ)
- Enamel is formed before tooth eruption by the **ameloblast cells**, which lie at the ADJ
- It contains no nerves or blood vessels and therefore cannot experience any sensation

- It is a non-living tissue that cannot grow and repair itself, so progressive damage caused by injury or tooth decay is permanent
- It can, however, remineralise its surface after an acid attack, by taking in minerals from saliva and from oral health products such as toothpaste and mouthwash
- The crystal structure can also be altered without undergoing acid attack, by the exchange of hydroxyl ions in the hydroxyapatite with **fluoride**, to form **fluorapatite crystals** – these make the enamel surface harder and more resistant to acid attack
- The enamel layer is thickest over the biting surface of the tooth (the occlusal surface or the incisal edge) and thinnest at the neck of the tooth – the cervical margin
- It is translucent in appearance, so the shade of a tooth is determined by the colour of the underlying dentine

Dentine

This tissue forms the main bulk of a tooth and occupies the interior of the crown and root. It is also mineralised, but to a lesser extent than enamel, and is covered by enamel in the crown of the tooth and by cementum in the root of the tooth. Its properties and microscopic structure are as follows:

- It consists of up to 80% inorganic tissue, mainly **calcium hydroxyapatite** crystals
- It is composed of **hollow tubes** that originally surrounded the cells within the dentine structure as it was first being formed
- In a fully formed tooth, these **odontoblast** cells lie along the inner edge of the pulp chamber only, but are present throughout life and can lay down more dentine as required
- In this way, it can repair itself by laying down secondary dentine
- This type of dentine is also formed as part of the natural ageing process, and its formation gradually narrows the pulp chamber
- The hollow tubes contain sensory nerve endings called **fibrils**, which run from the nerve tissue within the pulp chamber
- Dentine is therefore a living tissue and can transmit sensations of pain and thermal changes to the brain
- Its hollow structure allows it a degree of elasticity so that it can absorb normal chewing forces without breaking
- However, it also allows tooth decay (**caries**) to spread more rapidly through its hollow structure
- Dentine is a yellowish colour, and gives teeth their individual shade

Cementum

This is the calcified protective outer covering of the root and is similar in structure to bone. Cementum meets enamel at the neck of the tooth, and normally lies beneath the gingivae. Its properties and microscopic structure are as follows:

- Around 65% mineralised, with calcium hydroxyapatite crystals
- The crystals lie within a matrix of fibrous tissue, with the ends of collagen fibres from the periodontal ligament inserted into the outer layer of the cementum
- This allows the attachment of the root to the periodontal ligament, and therefore to the walls of the tooth socket
- The cementum is formed by cells called **cementoblasts** and they can continue laying down more tissue layers when required
- The thickness of cementum may vary at different parts of the root, and changes throughout life, depending on the forces exerted on individual teeth
- The cementum contains no nerves or blood vessels itself, so it receives nutrients from the periodontal ligament

Pulp

Unlike enamel, dentine and cementum, the pulp contains no mineral crystals and is composed purely of soft tissue. It lies within the very centre of every tooth, from the crown as the coronal pulp and into each root as the radicular pulp. The radicular pulp is often referred to as the "root canal" of the tooth. The properties and microscopic structure of the pulp are as follows:

- The pulp contains sensory nerves and blood vessels
- The sensory nerves are end sections of the trigeminal nerve (fifth cranial nerve), either as the inferior dental nerve for the lower teeth or one of the superior dental nerves for the upper teeth
- They allow the tooth to feel hot, cold, touch and pain by the stimulation of its sensory nerve endings which run as fibrils in the hollow dentine tubules
- These pulp tissues enter the tooth through the **apical foramen,** lying at the root apex of every tooth
- The pulp chamber itself is lined by the odontoblast cells which form dentine
- The chamber gradually narrows with age, so that it can become completely obliterated in older patients, making endodontic treatment very difficult
- It can also become blocked by **pulp stones** which are formed by lumps of calcium-containing crystals
- The point where the cementum and the root dentine are in contact with each other is called the **dentinocemental junction**
- Some teeth have additional contact between the pulp and the surrounding periodontal ligament via accessory canals, the presence of which can make successful endodontic treatment of the tooth very difficult to achieve

Tooth morphology

All people have two sets of teeth: the first or **deciduous teeth**, and the second or **permanent teeth**. All have different appearances or **morphology**, which depends on the set and the individual teeth themselves. Their morphology enables each tooth to be individually identified by any trained member of the dental team, this identification being based on the tooth shape and size, the number of cusps present, and the number of roots present. Curvature of the roots will also help to indicate whether a tooth is from the right or the left side of the dental arch.

Primary dentition (deciduous teeth)

The primary teeth are the first set and are also known as milk, temporary or deciduous teeth (Figure 13.24). Their details are as follows:

- Total set of **20 teeth**, 10 in each jaw
- They begin developing in the jaws of the early embryo, around 6 weeks after conception

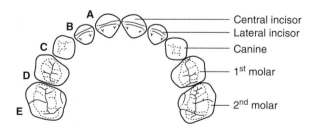

Figure 13.24 Primary dentition. Source: *Levison's Textbook for Dental Nurses*, 11th edition (Hollins), 2013. Reproduced with permission of Wiley-Blackwell.

- They are referred to in dentistry by letter – **A, B, C, D and E** – starting from the midline of the jaw
- They are **smaller** than permanent teeth and **whiter** in colour
- Their roots are **resorbed** by the underlying permanent teeth, as the deciduous teeth gradually loosen and fall out – this is called **exfoliation**
- The roots of the deciduous molars are splayed out to accommodate the presence of the underlying permanent premolar teeth, so the roots are described as **divergent**
- They have a **larger pulp chamber** than the permanent teeth, with **thinner enamel**, which makes them more prone to the development of dental caries
- They begin erupting at around 6 months of age and are usually all present by about 29 months, although individual variation does occur

The five deciduous teeth present in each quadrant of the oral cavity are the **central and lateral incisors**, the **canine**, and the **first and second molars**. There are no premolar teeth in the primary dentition. Their tooth and root morphology is summarised in the following table.

Tooth	Letter	Number of roots	Number of cusps (where applicable)
Uppers			
Central incisor	A	One	N/A
Lateral incisor	B	One	N/A
Canine	C	One	N/A
First molar	D	Three	Four
Second molar	E	Three	Five
Lowers			
Central incisor	A	One	N/A
Lateral incisor	B	One	N/A
Canine	C	One	N/A
First molar	D	Two	Four
Second molar	E	Two	Five

The three roots of the upper molars are arranged as a tripod, with the developing permanent premolar teeth lying within this area, while the two roots of the lower molars lie one in front of the other in the alveolar bone of the mandible. The average eruption dates of the deciduous teeth are shown in the following table.

Tooth	Letter	Uppers (months)	Lowers (months)
Central incisor	A	10	8
Lateral incisor	B	11	13
Canine	C	19	20
First molar	D	16	16
Second molar	E	29	27

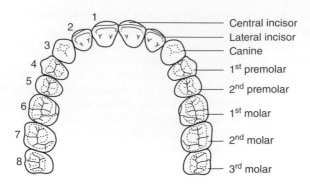

Figure 13.25   Secondary dentition. Source: *Levison's Textbook for Dental Nurses*, 11th edition (Hollins), 2013. Reproduced with permission of Wiley-Blackwell.

The usual eruption pattern of the deciduous dentition is the lower central incisors first, followed by the other incisors, then the first molars followed by the canines, and finally the second molars.

The dentition begins changing again at about 6 years of age, when the permanent teeth begin to erupt by resorbing the roots of their deciduous predecessors and causing their exfoliation.

Secondary dentition (permanent teeth)

Permanent teeth are the second and final set, and are also called the adult teeth (Figure 13.25). Their details are as follows:

- Total set of **32 teeth**, 16 in each jaw
- They begin developing in the jaws just before birth, and continue for many years afterwards
- They are referred to in dentistry by number – **1, 2, 3, 4, 5, 6, 7 and 8** – starting from the midline of the jaw
- They are of very similar morphology to the deciduous teeth, with eight extra teeth called **premolars** present, two in each quadrant
- They are **larger** in size and **darker** in colour than deciduous teeth, with relatively **smaller pulp chambers**
- The three permanent molar teeth in each quadrant develop behind the deciduous teeth, using the space created as the jaws grow during childhood and the teenage years
- So the **deciduous molar teeth** are succeeded by the **permanent premolar teeth**
- It is relatively common for some adult teeth to be **congenitally missing** from the dentition, especially the third molars
- They begin erupting at around 6 years of age, and all except the third molars are usually present by the age of 13 years
- The third molars may be congenitally missing, present but unerupted due to lack of jaw space, or they may erupt from the age of 18 years onwards

The eight permanent teeth present in each quadrant of the oral cavity are the **central and lateral incisors**, the **canine**, the **first and second premolars**, and the **first, second and third molars**. Their tooth and root morphology is summarised in the following table.

Tooth	Number	Number of roots	Number of cusps (where applicable)
Uppers			
Central incisor	1	One	N/A
Lateral incisor	2	One	N/A
Canine	3	One	N/A
First premolar	4	Two	Two
Second premolar	5	One	Two
First molar	6	Three	Five
Second molar	7	Three	Four
Third molar	8	Three	Four
Lowers			
Central incisor	1	One	N/A
Lateral incisor	2	One	N/A
Canine	3	One	N/A
First premolar	4	One	Two
Second premolar	5	One	Two
First molar	6	Two	Five
Second molar	7	Two	Four
Third molar	8	Two	Four

Again, the three roots of the upper molars are arranged as a tripod, and the two roots of the lower molars lie one in front of the other in the alveolar bone of the mandible. The two roots of the upper first premolar teeth lie across the maxillary alveolar bone. The average eruption dates of the permanent teeth are shown in the following table.

Tooth	Number	Uppers (years)	Lowers (years)
Central incisor	1	7–8	6–7
Lateral incisor	2	8–9	7–8
Canine	3	10–12	9–10
First premolar	4	9–11	9–11

Tooth	Number	Uppers (years)	Lowers (years)
Second premolar	5	10–11	9–11
First molar	6	6–7	6–7
Second molar	7	12–13	11–12
Third molar	8	18–25	18–25

Permanent teeth erupt before their roots are fully grown. About two-thirds of their root length has formed when permanent teeth erupt and the apex is still wide open. It takes another 3 years before root growth is complete and the apex closes. The only exceptions are canines and third molars, which do not erupt until root growth is complete.

To enable the dental team to describe and discuss individual teeth and the treatment they may require, each surface of every tooth has its own name in relation to the midline of each jaw, and the anatomical structures that they sit against. It is this **tooth surface nomenclature** that allows the charting of every patient to be recorded accurately – a key task of the dental nurse.

Tooth charting is discussed earlier in this chapter, as it forms an important part of oral health assessment techniques. The general terminology in use for describing the tooth surfaces is summarised here:

- **Labial** – surface adjacent to the lips, applies in both arches and relates to incisor and canine teeth
- **Buccal** – surface adjacent to the buccinator muscle of the cheeks, applies in both arches and relates to premolars and molars
- **Palatal** – surface adjacent to the palate, applies to all maxillary teeth (see Figure 6.19)
- **Lingual** – surface adjacent to the tongue, applies to all mandibular teeth
- **Occlusal** – biting surface of posterior teeth, applies to both arches and relates to premolars and molars
- The sharply raised points of these surfaces are called **cusps**, and the crevices between them are the **fissures**
- **Incisal** – biting edge of anterior teeth, applies to both arches and relates to incisors (canines have a cusp rather than an edge)
- **Mesial** – interdental surface of all teeth closest to the midline of each arch, so the front interdental surface
- **Distal** – interdental surface of all teeth furthest from the midline of each arch
- **Contact point** – the point where the mesial and distal surfaces of adjacent teeth are in contact with each other (see Figure 6.20)
- **Cervical** – the neck region of any tooth, on the buccal, labial, palatal or lingual surface

Using these named surfaces, the anatomy of individual teeth can now be described in detail.

Anatomy of individual teeth

A collection of extracted teeth in good condition is a great help in learning dental anatomy and tooth morphology, but they are more difficult to acquire nowadays due to infection control issues. The secondary dentiton is shown diagrammatically for clarity in Figure 13.26, and various extracted teeth are shown in Figure 13.27.

In the primary dentition there are five teeth in each quadrant of the mouth; central and lateral incisors, a canine, and first and second molars.

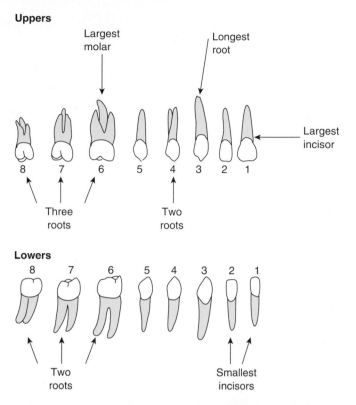

Figure 13.26   Illustrated tooth anatomy. Source: *Levison's Textbook for Dental Nurses*, 11th edition (Hollins), 2013. Reproduced with permission of Wiley-Blackwell.

In the secondary dentition there are eight teeth in each quadrant: central and lateral incisors, a canine, first and second premolars, first, second and third molars. The morphology and function of the similar teeth in each dentition is the same.

Central incisor:

- Chisel-shaped crown with an incisal biting edge
- Single root
- Palatal or lingual surface has a raised area called the **cingulum**
- Upper permanent central incisor is the **largest** of all incisors
- Lower central incisor is the **smallest tooth**
- Functions are to:
  - Cut into food and separate bite-size chunks from the food product
  - Assist the tongue in making certain speech sounds ("th")
  - Assist the lips in making certain speech sounds ("f")

Lateral incisor:

- Narrow, chisel-shaped crown with an incisal biting edge
- Single root
- Lower lateral incisor sometimes has a second (lingual) root canal, especially if the root has split into two

371

372

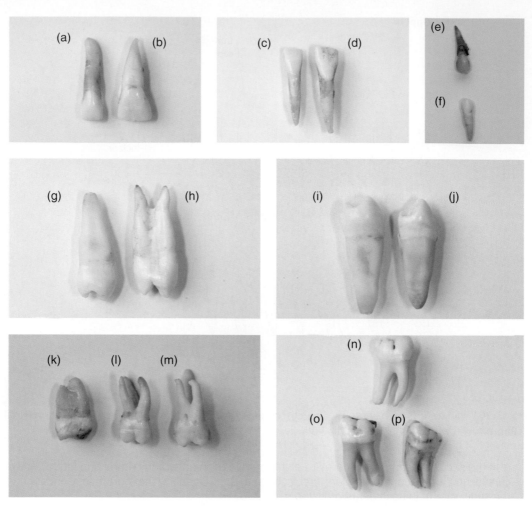

Figure 13.27 Features of individual teeth: (a) upper right lateral incisor; (b) upper right central incisor; (c) lower left central incisor; (d) lower left lateral incisor; (e) upper right canine; (f) lower left canine; (g) upper right second premolar; (h) upper right first premolar; (i) lower left second premolar; (j) lower left first premolar; (k) upper right third molar; (l) upper right second molar; (m) upper right first molar; (n) lower right first molar; (o) lower left second molar; (p) lower left third molar. Source: *Levison's Textbook for Dental Nurses*, 11th edition (Hollins), 2013. Reproduced with permission of Wiley-Blackwell.

- Palatal or lingual surface has a cingulum
- Function is to bite in a scissor action with the upper incisors, and break off separate bite-size portions
- Uppers can be congenitally absent, or develop as abnormally small teeth – often called "**peg laterals**"

Canine:

- Robust tooth forming the "corner" of each dental quadrant
- Incisal edge is sloped to a sharp cusp tip that lies more mesially than distally
- Single root and the **longest** of all teeth

- Root apex sometimes curves distally slightly
- Upper and lower canines have a cingulum, the upper is joined to the cusp tip by a palatal ridge
- Functions are to:
  - Pierce food and tear into it
  - Support the oral soft tissues at the "corners" of the oral cavity
  - Provide "guidance" for normal occlusion, especially when the mandible is moved sideways

First premolar:

- Not present in primary dentition
- The permanent successors to the deciduous first molars
- Has occlusal surface arranged as two cusps lying bucally and palatally, or buccally and lingually (upper or lower)
- Cusps are of equal height in uppers, but lingual is always smaller in lowers
- Mesial and distal edges of all are raised into **marginal ridges**
- Upper has two roots lying in the same orientation as the cusps
- Root apices sometimes curve distally
- Concavity between the roots mesially is called the **canine fossa**, and can be a harbour for microorganisms and calculus in patients with periodontal disease
- Lower first premolar has one root
- Functions are:
  - Cusps assist canine to pierce and tear food
  - Occlusal surface assists molars to grind food
  - To help maintain the shape of the mouth
- Usual tooth to be extracted for orthodontic reasons, as it lies midway along the dental arch and can therefore relieve either anterior or posterior crowding

Second premolar:

- Not present in primary dentition
- The permanent successors to the deciduous second molars
- Has occlusal surface arranged as two cusps, like the first premolars
- Cusps are of equal height in all
- Mesial and distal edges are raised as marginal ridges
- Upper is usually slightly smaller tooth than the first premolar
- Lower is usually slightly larger than the first premolar
- Single root, apex sometimes curves distally
- Root apex of uppers can lie very close to the floor of the maxillary antrum
- Functions are as for first premolars
- Lowers are sometimes congenitally absent
- Can become impacted in either arch, following the early loss of their deciduous predecessor and the eruption of the permanent first molars, so that the arch space for the second premolars is lost

First molar:

- Primary first molars are succeeded by the first premolars and are the smaller of the deciduous molars
- Widely divergent roots present in deciduous molars, with the crown of the developing first premolar lying contained by them
- Permanent first molars are the **largest of all teeth**
- Upper has occlusal surface arranged as four cusps: two buccally and two palatally
- Fifth palatal cusp of uppers may develop as the "**cusp of carabelli**"
- Lower has five cusps: three buccal and two lingual
- Mesial and distal edges are raised as marginal ridges

373

- Uppers have three roots arranged as a tripod: large palatal, shorter mesiobuccal and distobuccal – apices of latter two are sometimes curved distally
- Lowers have two roots arranged as mesial and distal, apices are sometimes curved distally
- Junction of the roots beneath the crown is called the **furcation area** and can be a harbour for microorganisms when periodontal disease is present
- Function is to grind and masticate food chunks so that they can be swallowed
- Root apices of uppers can lie close to, or even penetrate, the floor of the maxillary antrum

Second molar:

- Primary second molars are succeeded by the second premolars and are the larger of the deciduous molars
- Widely divergent roots present in deciduous molars, with the crown of the developing second premolar lying contained by them
- Crown of both upper and lower is smaller than that of the first molar
- Has occlusal surface arranged as four cusps
- Mesial and distal edges are raised as marginal ridges
- Uppers have three roots, arranged as for the first molar and sometimes curved distally
- Lower has two roots, arranged as for the first molar and sometimes curved distally
- Furcation area present in both
- Functions are as for the first molar
- Root apices of the upper can also lie in close proximity to the floor of the maxillary antrum

Third molar:

- Not present in the primary dentition
- Not always present in the secondary dentition
- Referred to as "**wisdom teeth**"
- Morphology varies widely
- Smaller crown size than the second molar usually
- Has occlusal surface arranged as three or four cusps, with marginal ridges present
- Uppers usually have three roots, but not always
- Lowers usually have two roots, but not always
- Furcation area present unless the roots are fused together
- Function as for the first and second molars
- Often extracted if involved with recurrent bouts of disease, or if impacted and associated with pericoronitis

Normal occlusion

When the upper and lower teeth are closed together, they are said to be in **occlusion**. The arch of the upper teeth is larger than the lower, so upper teeth overlap the lowers on the buccal side. Lower buccal cusps accordingly bite into the fissure between upper buccal and palatal cusps (Figure 13.28).

The mesial edges of upper and lower central incisors form one straight vertical line. This is called the midline. As lower central incisors are much narrower than uppers, all the remaining lower teeth occlude with two upper teeth – their corresponding upper tooth and the one in front.

From this explanation of **normal occlusion**, it is clear that:

- The mesial cusp of the upper first molar bites into the fissure between mesial and distal cusps of the lower first molar
- The lower canine bites in front of the upper canine

The mesial edges of the upper and lower central incisors form one straight vertical midline.

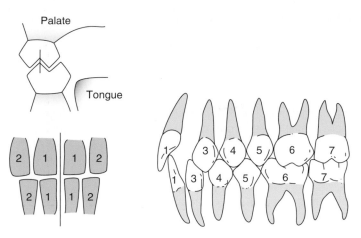

Figure 13.28   Normal occlusion. Source: *Levison's Textbook for Dental Nurses*, 11th edition (Hollins), 2013. Reproduced with permission of Wiley-Blackwell.

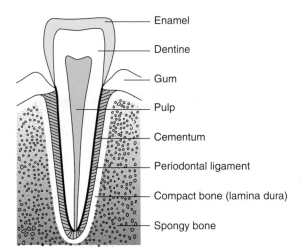

Figure 13.29   Supporting structures of a tooth. Source: *Levison's Textbook for Dental Nurses*, 11th edition (Hollins), 2013. Reproduced with permission of Wiley-Blackwell.

Supporting structures

The supporting structures are collectively referred to as the periodontium, and are those lying around the roots of the teeth which hold them in their sockets (Figure 13.29). Their hold on the teeth is not a rigid one; rather, it allows the teeth to "bounce" in their sockets so that there is some shock absorption effect when the teeth are used for chewing. This prevents fracture of the tooth under normal occlusal forces.

The four supporting structures are as follows:

- **Alveolar bone** – specialised ridge of bone over the bony arch of each jaw, where the teeth sit in their sockets
- **Gingiva** – specialised soft tissue covering of the alveolar processes, which are also in attachment with the teeth at their necks

- **Periodontal ligament** – connective tissue attachment between the tooth and the alveolar bone
- **Cementum** – hard tissue covering of the root that anchors the periodontal ligament to the tooth (discussed previously)

Alveolar bone

The maxilla and the mandible both contain a horseshoe-shaped ridge of bone called the alveolar process. It is here that the teeth form during the growth of the foetus and later the child, and from where they erupt into the mouth at various ages. The properties of the alveolar bone are as follows:

- It is a specialised bone found only in the jaws
- Its outer layer is made of hard, **compact bone**, the outer surface of which is called the **lamina dura**
- The inner layer is called **cancellous bone** and is sponge-like in appearance, to allow the passage of the various nerves and blood vessels that supply the jaws, teeth and surrounding oral soft tissues
- The sole purpose of the alveolar bone is to support the teeth, and it is gradually lost when a tooth is extracted as the bone slowly resorbs away
- The teeth lie within individual **sockets** in the alveolar bone, each one being lined by lamina dura which shows on dental radiographs as a continuous white line – its absence indicates the presence of dental disease
- The outer surface of the alveolar bone is covered in specialised **alveolar mucosa**, which forms the **gingivae** (gums) around the necks of the teeth
- Destruction of the alveolar bone occurs in **periodontal disease**

Gingiva

This is the correct anatomical term for the gums (plural – gingivae). It is a continuous layer of specialised epithelium found only in the oral cavity and which is firmly attached to the underlying alveolar bone as a **mucoperiosteal layer** of tissue. This layer is raised as a flap during oral surgical procedures, to expose the bone below.

There are three distinct areas of gingival coverage, as follows (Figure 13.30):

- **Attached gingiva** – that covering the majority of the alveolar process, which is firmly attached to the underlying bone as the **mucoperiosteum**
- **Marginal gingiva** – that forming the gingival margin of the teeth, which is free from the underlying bone and follows the shape of each tooth in the arch, as well as extending between the teeth in the contact areas; the level at which these two areas meet is called the **free gingival groove**
- **Junctional tissues** – the specialised gingival tissue lying within the gingival crevice and forming the anatomical junction between the teeth and the oral epithelium; this point is called the **junctional attachment**, and the tissues are called the junctional epithelium

The junctional attachment is the point where the integrity of the periodontium has to be maintained in order to avoid the devastation of periodontal disease and the resultant tooth loss that can occur. It provides a mechanical barrier between the oral cavity and the deeper periodontal tissues, preventing microorganisms from gaining entry and causing disease. The main method of maintaining the health and functionality of the whole gingival area is to carry out good levels of oral hygiene on a daily basis.

During a periodontal examination, the gingival crevice should be less than 3 mm deep when probed, with the periodontal probe contacting the junctional attachment at its deepest point.

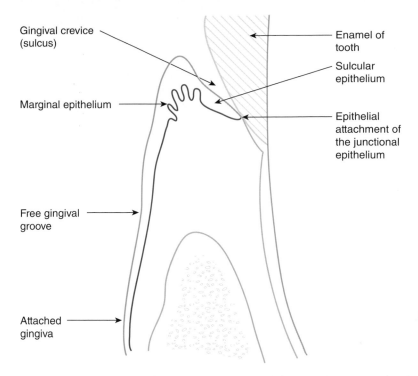

Gingival crevice (sulcus)

Enamel of tooth

Sulcular epithelium

Marginal epithelium

Epithelial attachment of the junctional epithelium

Free gingival groove

Attached gingiva

377

Figure 13.30   The three gingival areas. Source: *Levison's Textbook for Dental Nurses*, 11th edition (Hollins), 2013. Reproduced with permission of Wiley-Blackwell.

The properties of the gingiva are as follows:

- When healthy, the gingivae fit around the neck of every tooth like a tight cuff
- The **gingival crevice** exists as a shallow space of less than 3mm between the tooth surface and the gingival margin, and contains the junctional epithelium
- A natural mound of gingival tissue occurs between each tooth and is called the **interdental papilla**
- In health, the gingivae are pink in colour with a stippled surface, like orange peel
- Inflammation of the gingivae is called **gingivitis**; it affects the marginal gingivae and occurs in the presence of **dental plaque** due to poor oral hygiene control
- Gingivitis appears as red and shiny gingivae that are swollen due to their inflammation and that bleed easily on touching – either during tooth brushing or during dental examination
- The swollen appearance of the inflamed gingivae presents as "**false pockets**" when probed, giving the impression that the gingival crevice is deeper than 3mm – in fact, the junctional attachment is still present and the underlying periodontal tissues are unaffected by the inflamed condition of the gingivae
- The gingiva can also be stimulated to overgrow and become **hyperplastic** as a side-effect of various drugs being taken by the patient, including some antihypertensives (such as nifedipine) and some drugs used to control epilepsy (such as phenytoin)

Oral diseases, including gingivitis and periodontitis, are discussed in detail in Chapter 15.

Periodontal ligament

The periodontal ligament is a specialised fibrous tissue that attaches the teeth to the alveolar bone and the surrounding gingivae. It acts as a shock absorber to the teeth during chewing and its main fibres run between the alveolar bone and the cementum covering the root of the tooth. Other fibres run between the necks of the teeth, and from the cementum into the surrounding gingivae.

The various periodontal ligament fibre groups and their functions are summarised below, and illustrated in Figure 13.31:

- **Alveolar crest fibres** – run from the alveolar bone crest to the cementum at the neck of the tooth; they prevent tooth movements in (intrusion) and out (extrusion) of the socket, as well as resisting tilting and rotation
- **Horizontal fibres** – run horizontally from the alveolar bone to the cementum, just below the crest fibres; they resist tilting and rotation of the tooth
- **Oblique fibres** – run at an angle from the alveolar bone down to the cementum; they prevent intrusion and rotation of the tooth
- **Apical fibres** – occur at the root apex and run between the bone and cementum; they prevent extrusion and rotation of the tooth
- **Transeptal fibres** – run between the cementum of adjacent teeth through the interdental region; they maintain the gingival attachments between the teeth and therefore their positions in the dental arch
- **Free gingival fibres** – run from the cervical cementum into the gingival papillae; they maintain the gingival cuff around each tooth

The properties of the periodontal ligament are as follows:

- Its fibres are made up of a protein called **collagen**
- They run in various directions, the end result being that the teeth are held in their sockets but can "bounce" under normal chewing forces – this prevents tooth fracture and pain during normal occlusal loading and chewing actions
- When excessive occlusal forces are applied, the resultant pain experienced by the patient tends to stop further overuse from occurring

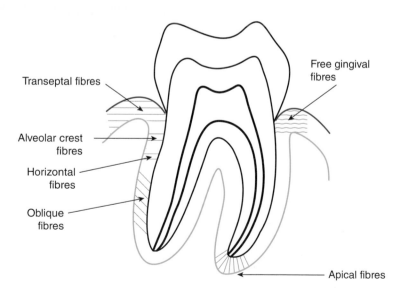

Figure 13.31   Fibre groups of the periodontal ligament. Source: *Levison's Textbook for Dental Nurses*, 11th edition (Hollins), 2013. Reproduced with permission of Wiley-Blackwell.

378

- The ligament has a sensory nerve supply which transmits pressure, pain, touch and temperature changes – the ability of the tooth to detect and transmit these sensations is called **proprioception**
- Inflammation of the ligament is called **periodontitis** and occurs during periodontal disease

Salivary glands

The salivary glands are present in the oral cavity as either numerous minor glands dotted throughout the lining membrane of the oral mucosa, or as one of the three pairs of major salivary glands (Figure 13.32):

- **Parotid salivary glands** – located between the ramus of the mandible and the ear, and deep to the muscles in that area
- **Submandibular salivary glands** – located in the posterior area of the floor of the mouth, beneath the mylohyoid muscle
- **Sublingual salivary glands** – located in the anterior area of the floor of the mouth, above the mylohyoid muscle

The function of all the salivary glands is to produce the secretion **saliva**, which is deposited from the glands into the oral cavity only – this does not occur anywhere else in the body. The saliva is transported to the oral cavity through tube-like structures called ducts, so the salivary glands are classed as **exocrine glands**.

Other structures elsewhere in the body are classed as **endocrine glands** – their secretions pass directly into the adjacent blood vessels (without travelling through ducts) and are transported to their area of action by the circulatory system. Examples are certain glands within the pancreas, the stomach, the liver and the adrenal glands, which lie over the kidneys.

Both types of glands have their secretions controlled by the effects of motor nerve transmission, via the autonomic nervous system.

Parotid gland

The parotid gland lies partly over the outside and partly behind the ramus of the mandible, in front of the ear. It is the largest of the three major salivary glands and the only one to be affected by the viral infection **mumps,** which is caused by a paramyxovirus.

The tube connecting the gland to the oral cavity, the **Stenson duct**, passes forwards across the surface of the masseter muscle and then inwards through the cheek to open into the buccal

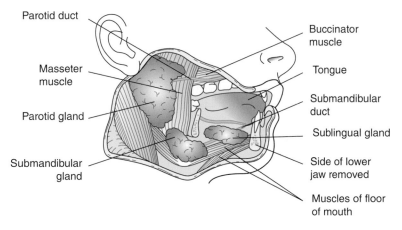

Figure 13.32   Salivary glands. Source: *Levison's Textbook for Dental Nurses*, 11th edition (Hollins), 2013. Reproduced with permission of Wiley-Blackwell.

sulcus opposite the upper second molar. The parotid gland is innervated by the glossopharyngeal nerve (ninth cranial nerve) and is the commonest salivary gland to be associated with both benign and malignant tumours.

Submandibular gland

The submandibular gland lies in the posterior region of the floor of the mouth below the mylohyoid line, against the inner and lower surface of the body of the mandible and near the angle. The submandibular duct (**Warton duct**) passes forward in the floor of the mouth to open at the midline, beside the lingual frenum. It is the longest of the salivary ducts and the most likely to become blocked by salivary stones (calculi). The submandibular gland is innervated by the facial nerve (seventh cranial nerve).

Sublingual gland

The sublingual gland also lies in the floor of the mouth, but above the mylohyoid line and much further forward than the submandibular gland. There are several sublingual ducts, and these open into the floor of the mouth just behind the orifice of the submandibular duct (Figure 13.33). The sublingual gland is also innervated by the facial nerve.

Functions of saliva

Although saliva appears as a watery fluid in the mouth, it contains many different components which differ between each salivary gland. The various components are shown in the following table.

Component	Function or role
Minerals – sodium, calcium, potassium and their electrolytes – such as phosphates	Neutralise dietary acids Buffering to maintain stable pH in the oral cavity Also allow mineralisation of plaque to form supragingival calculus
Salivary amylase	Digestive enzyme that begins starch digestion, before food is swallowed Also called ptyalin
Antibodies	Immunoglobulins (especially immunoglobulin A, IgA) present to fight infections, such as periodontal disease Promotes wound healing IgA is the commonest antibody of the immune system
Leucocytes	White blood cells, as a defence mechanism against oral infection and disease
Mucus	From the mucous secretory cells – to aid lubrication and allow speech and swallowing to occur
Other enzymes	Antibacterial enzymes – to aid in the defence of the oral cavity against disease Promote wound healing
Water	Carrying agent for other components Aids with lubrication for speech and swallowing Dissolves food particles to allow taste sensation Cleansing action by dislodging food particles from around the teeth

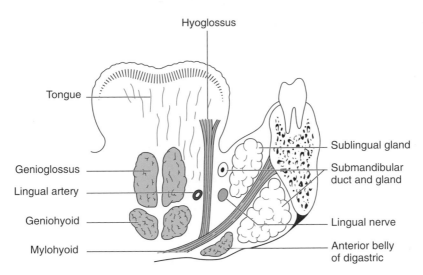

Figure 13.33   Floor of the mouth in cross-section. Source: *Levison's Textbook for Dental Nurses*, 11th edition (Hollins), 2013. Reproduced with permission of Wiley-Blackwell.

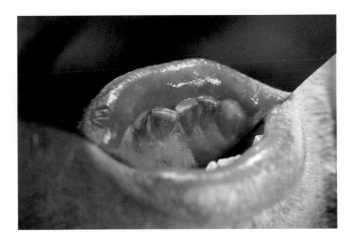

Figure 13.34   Lingual supragingival calculus.

Patients with low mineral content, mainly watery saliva tend to develop little calculus but have a higher caries incidence than patients with high mineral content saliva. Those with a high mineral content tend to have thick, stringy saliva and develop calculus more readily, in the absence of adequate oral hygiene. They also tend to have a lower incidence of caries, often despite adequate dietary sugar control.

The position of the salivary ducts against the upper molars and the lower incisors allows dental calculus to build up easily in these areas, and can be seen as particularly heavy deposits when patients attend for scaling treatment (Figure 13.34).

Saliva is slightly alkaline, due to its electrolyte components, but maintains the oral cavity at a neutral pH of 7 between meals. When the pH falls below 7 following the intake of food, the mineral content of saliva acts to neutralise the acidic environment produced and raises the pH again.

If the pH of the oral cavity falls to the critical level of 5.5, enamel demineralisation will occur.

Disorders of the salivary glands

Xerostomia

This is the uncomfortable condition of having a constantly dry mouth due to the decreased production of saliva. It is relatively common and has several causes:

- **Irradiation** – of the head and neck area, usually as radiotherapy treatment for cancer in this area
- **Medications** – any that affect the nerve supply to the salivary glands to reduce their salivary flow, or that act as a diuretic and stimulate fluid loss, as well as certain drugs such as tricyclic antidepressants which cause dry mouth as a side-effect
- **Sjögren's syndrome** – a syndrome that occurs in conjunction with an autoimmune disorder, such as rheumatoid arthritis, where the body's defence system attacks itself and destroys its own glandular tissues, including the salivary glands and the lacrimal glands in the eye

As all dental professionals know, saliva has many functions in the oral cavity and any reduction in its production will have serious oral consequences, including any of the following:

- Increased incidence of **dental caries**, as the self-cleansing ability is lost
- Increased risk of **oral infections**, as the defence capability is reduced
- Increased risk of **oral soft tissue trauma**, as the protective mechanism is reduced
- **Problems with speech, swallowing and chewing**, as the lubrication effect is reduced
- **Poor taste sensation** and lack of food enjoyment, as the taste buds cannot function correctly in a dry field

Other than to change the patient's drug regime where possible, there is little else that can be done to ease this condition. The use of salivary stimulants and artificial saliva sprays may help in some cases, and research is currently ongoing into salivary gland tissue transplant.

Dental patients suffering from xerostomia should be advised by the dental team as follows:

- Frequent recall attendance to monitor for the onset of caries and other oral problems
- Use of artificial saliva sprays or constant sipping of plain water
- High standard of oral hygiene, and especially the use of topical fluoride products to strengthen teeth against caries
- Dietary advice to avoid cariogenic products
- Avoidance of oral health products containing alcohol, as these tend to worsen the drying effect

Ptyalism

Excessive salivation, or ptyalism, is a symptom associated with an underlying disease rather than a disorder in its own right. It can occur due to any of the following disorders:

- Periodontal disease
- Oral soft tissue injury, or trauma, including that caused by sharp-edged dental appliances
- Oesophagitis and other conditions causing acid reflux
- Disorders affecting the nervous system, including Parkinson's disease and mercury poisoning

Treatment is focussed on the causative disease and the relief of its symptoms, although some drugs may be used to directly reduce the salivary gland secretions as well. In particular, the drug **atropine** may be used during oral and maxillofacial surgery to significantly reduce saliva flow and provide a clear, dry operating field for the surgeons.

Muscles of mastication

These are the four sets of muscles connected between the mandible and the skull (either on the base of the cranium or on the face – Figure 13.35), which act to allow chewing movements and mouth closing to occur:

- **Temporalis**
- **Masseter**
- **Lateral pterygoid** ("p" is silent, so pronounced "terygoid")
- **Medial pterygoid**

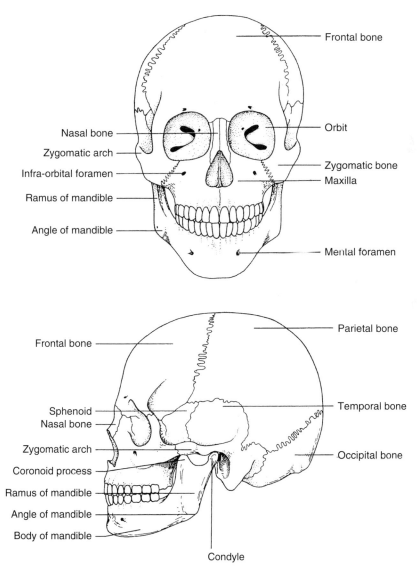

Figure 13.35   The skull in detail. Source: *Clinical Anatomy*, 13th edition (Ellis), 2013. Reproduced with permission of Wiley-Blackwell.

They all receive nerve impulses from the fifth cranial nerve (trigeminal nerve) which cause them to contract so that the length of the muscle shortens. This then causes the various movements of the mandible associated with mouth closing, jaw clenching and chewing, as described previously. The muscles of mastication **do not cause mouth opening** – this is controlled by a different group of muscles called the **suprahyoid muscles**. Each set of the muscles of mastication is connected to the cranium or the face at one end (called their **point of origin**) and at their other end to the mandible (called their **point of insertion**). The contraction of individual sets of muscles, or of just one of the lateral pterygoid muscles alone, shortens their length between these two points. As the mandible is the only movable bone of the temporo-mandibular joint, this muscle shortening causes the movement of the mandible into various positions to allow closing and chewing actions to occur. These actions are summarised as follows.

Temporalis:

- Point of origin – **temporal bone** of the cranium
- Point of insertion – **coronoid process** of the mandible, passing under the zygomatic arch
- Action – **pulls the mandible backwards and closed**

Masseter:

- Point of origin – outer surface of **zygomatic arch**
- Point of insertion – outer surface of **mandibular ramus and angle**
- Action – **closes the mandible**

Lateral pterygoid:

- Point of origin – **lateral pterygoid plate** at the base of the cranium
- Point of insertion – **head of the mandibular condyle** and into the temporo-mandibular joint meniscus
- Action – **both muscles contracting brings the mandible forwards** to bite the anterior teeth tip to tip; **one muscle contracting pulls the mandible to the opposite side**

Medial pterygoid:

- Point of origin – **medial pterygoid plate** at the base of the cranium
- Point of insertion – inner surface of **mandibular ramus and angle**
- Action – **closes the mandible**

When the teeth are clenched together, the temporalis and masseter muscles can be felt by placing a hand on the side of the head and face, respectively. They form the superficial layer of the muscles of mastication, while the medial and lateral pterygoid muscles form the deep layer. The superficial muscles are shown in Figure 13.36, along with some of the suprahyoid muscles, and also the muscles of facial expression.

Other relevant muscle groups

Suprahyoid muscles

As their name suggests, one end of all these muscles is attached to the horseshoe-shaped hyoid bone, which lies suspended in soft tissue beneath the mandible, in the throat. They all lie above this bone, as opposed to a separate group of muscles lying beneath the bone called the infrahyoid muscles.

The suprahyoid muscles are responsible for mouth opening and swallowing actions.

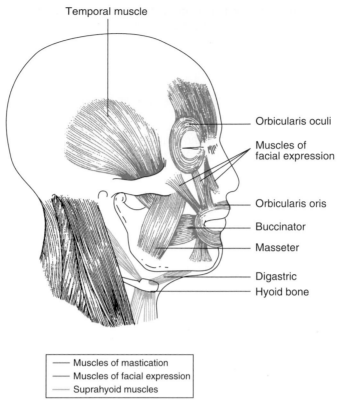

Temporal muscle

Orbicularis oculi

Muscles of
facial expression

Orbicularis oris

Buccinator

Masseter

Digastric

Hyoid bone

- Muscles of mastication
- Muscles of facial expression
- Suprahyoid muscles

Figure 13.36   Oral musculature. Source: *Levison's Textbook for Dental Nurses*, 11th edition (Hollins), 2013. Reproduced with permission of Wiley-Blackwell.

Muscles of facial expression

These are the muscles concerned with performing the numerous facial expressions that humans are capable of showing – smiling, frowning, winking, pursing the lips, and so on.

In contrast to the muscles of mastication and the suprahyoids, those of facial expression are not involved in producing skeletal movement and most are only attached at one end to the skull. Their other ends are inserted into the deep layer of the facial skin only, so that their contraction causes skin movement alone.

All of the muscles of facial expression are innervated by the motor branch of the facial nerve (seventh cranial nerve). For the sake of simplicity, they can be grouped according to the facial region that their actions involve:

- The scalp
- The eyes and surrounding area
- The mouth and surrounding area

Only the last group are of relevance to the dental nurse.

The main muscle of the eye is a ring of tissue called the **orbicularis oculi,** and that of the mouth is the **orbicularis oris**. Thin straps of muscle run between these rings and into the surrounding tissues, to allow movement of the eyelids, lips, mouth and nostrils.

The cheek muscle is called the **buccinator**, and is attached above and below to the outer surface of the alveolar process of each jaw. It connects to the muscular wall of the throat behind, and to the orbicularis oris in front. The buccinator helps with chewing movements by helping to keep ingested food within the confines of the teeth, while the jaw actions cause the teeth to cut and shred the food before swallowing.

Anatomy of the skull

The skull is effectively what a patient would refer to as "the head", and can be divided into three anatomical regions (Figure 13.37):

- **The cranium** – enclosing the brain and forming the largest part of the skull
- **The face** – supporting the eyes and nose and their surrounding structures
- **The jaws** – supporting the teeth and the tongue, and providing openings for the respiratory and digestive tracts

Like most bones in the body, the skull develops in the foetus as **cartilage**, which is gradually converted to bone as the body grows and develops. The outer layer of all bone is called **compact bone**, with anatomical holes (**foramina**) present to allow the passage of blood vessels and nerves from structures outside the bone to within it, and vice versa. The inner layer is called **cancellous bone** and is of a spongy appearance to reduce the overall weight of the bone and to allow the progression of the nerve and blood vessels within.

The **cranium** is made up of six plates of bone:

- Frontal bone – forming the forehead region
- Two parietal bones – joined at the top midline of the skull and forming its upper sides behind the forehead
- Two temporal bones – forming the lower sides of the skull in the region of the ears
- Occipital bone – forming the back of the skull

The six bony plates interlock with each other at the coronal sutures, which are a type of joint between each of them that allows the growth and expansion of the brain during childhood.

The large foramen at the base of the skull through the occipital bone is called the **foramen magnum**, and is where the brain stem becomes the spinal cord within the spinal column.

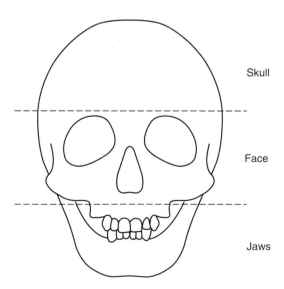

Figure 13.37   The three regions of the skull.

386

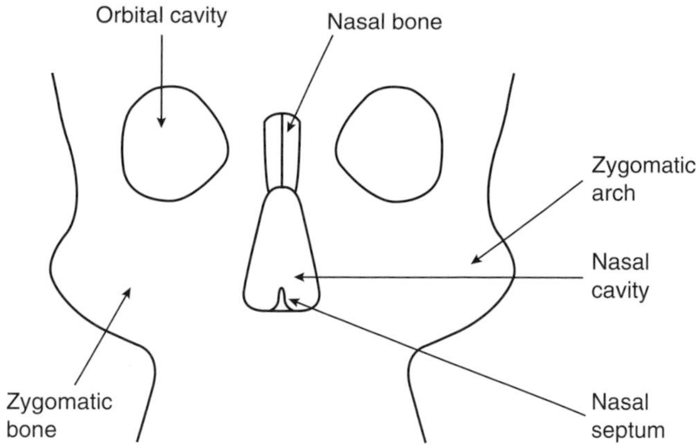

Figure 13.38   The face in detail.

The **face** is composed of many bones, but the six which are relevant to dentistry are as follows:

- Two zygomatic bones – joining the upper jaw to the cranium
- Two zygomatic arches – forming the cheekbones
- Two nasal bones – forming the bony bridge of the nose

These six main bones also form parts of the orbital cavities, enclosing the eyeballs, and the nasal cavity of the nose, containing the nasal septum and the turbinate bones (Figure 13.38).

Jaws – maxilla and mandible

There are two jaws, the upper (**maxilla**) and the lower (**mandible**). Although, strictly speaking, the jaw bones are actually part of the facial skeleton, they are considered separately, as they are of such importance to the dental team. The two jaws are each made up of a pair of bones that are fixed solidly in their midlines:

- **Maxilla** – pair of bones forming the upper jaw, the lower border of the orbital cavities, the base of the nose, and the anterior portion of the hard palate
- **Mandible** – appears as a single horseshoe-shaped bone forming the lower jaw, with its posterior vertical bony struts articulating with the cranium at the temporo-mandibular joint

Maxilla and palatine bones

The maxilla effectively forms the middle third of the face, and as with various other cranial bones, it has several foramina and bony projections that are dentally relevant.

The maxilla is made up of two bones which are separated above by the nasal cavity. They join together below the nose as the front section of the **hard palate**. The back section of the hard palate is formed by the palatine bones, and the whole palate forms the floor of the nose and the roof of the oral cavity, or mouth.

Each side of the maxilla forms part of the eye socket, the nose and the front of the cheekbone. The two maxilla bones themselves are hollow within, because if they were solid bones they would be too heavy to allow the head to be lifted up. Each hollow space is called the **maxillary antrum** or **sinus**, and lies just above the root apices of the upper molar and second premolar teeth (Figure 13.39). This hollow space can be easily perforated during the extraction of these teeth, causing an unwanted connection between the mouth and the antrum called an **oro-antral fistula**. A natural connection between the nasal cavity and the antra exists to allow drainage of the sinuses to occur and to give resonance to the voice.

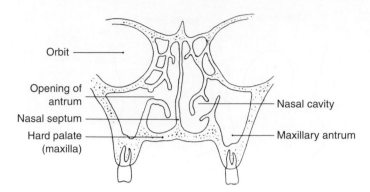

Orbit

Opening of antrum

Nasal septum

Hard palate (maxilla)

Nasal cavity

Maxillary antrum

Figure 13.39   Facial bones and air spaces. Source: *Levison's Textbook for Dental Nurses*, 11th edition (Hollins), 2013. Reproduced with permission of Wiley-Blackwell.

Inflammation of these air spaces (sinusitis) due to a respiratory infection often mimics dental pain in these teeth, or conversely a dental infection can be mistaken for sinusitis.

The two maxilla bones join together in the centreline of the face at the intermaxillary suture, and the lowest portions of these two sections form the alveolar process. This horseshoe-shaped structure is where both sets of upper teeth develop before birth, and later erupt as the upper primary and then secondary dentition.

The back end of each side of the alveolar process is called the **maxillary tuberosity**, and this can be fractured off during difficult upper wisdom tooth extractions.

The maxilla and palatine bones (Figure 13.40) are perforated by several foramina to allow the passage of the nerves and blood vessels supplying the upper teeth and their surrounding soft tissues, the four main ones being:

- **Infra-orbital foramen** – beneath the eye sockets, through which the nerves supplying the upper teeth and their labial soft tissues pass
- **Greater and lesser palatine foramina** – at the back of the hard palate, through which the nerves supplying the palatal soft tissues of the upper posterior teeth pass
- **Incisive foramen** – at the front centre of the hard palate, through which the nerves supplying the palatal soft tissues of the upper anterior teeth pass

Mandible

The mandible is also made up of two bones, joined together in the centreline at the **mental symphysis** to create a single horseshoe-shaped structure, and with its two back ends bent up vertically to the horseshoe. The vertical section is called the **ramus of the mandible**, the horizontal section is called the **body of the mandible,** and the point at which they join is the **angle of the mandible** (Figure 13.41).

The mandible's only connection with the rest of the skull is at the two **temporo-mandibular joints**, where the bone is able to move as a hinge joint and allow the mouth to open and close. The point at which the mandible connects with the temporal bone at the temporo-mandibular joint is the **head of condyle** (Figure 13.42). The muscles of mastication, which allow jaw closing and chewing movements, all connect between the cranium and various points on the mandible.

The mandible also has an **alveolar process** running around it, which supports all the lower teeth. Below this process, on the inner side of the body of the mandible, lies a ridge of bone called the **mylohyoid ridge,** where the mylohyoid muscle attaches to form the floor of the mouth. A bony ridge also lies on the outer surface of the ramus of the mandible, called the **external oblique ridge**, which marks the base of the alveolar process in this area.

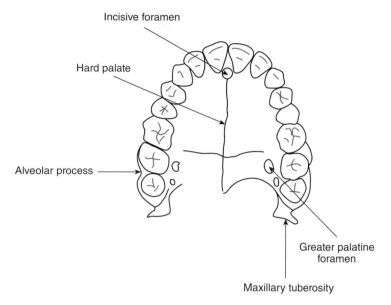

Incisive foramen

Hard palate

Alveolar process

Greater palatine foramen

Maxillary tuberosity

Figure 13.40 Palate and maxillary teeth. Source: *Levison's Textbook for Dental Nurses*, 11th edition (Hollins), 2013. Reproduced with permission of Wiley-Blackwell.

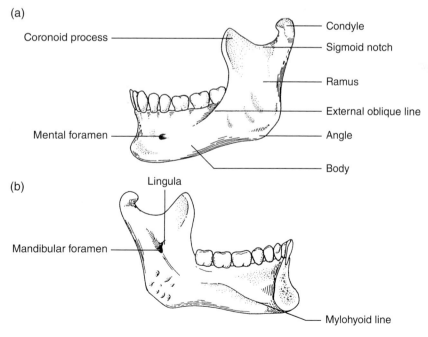

(a)

Coronoid process

Condyle

Sigmoid notch

Ramus

External oblique line

Mental foramen

Angle

Body

(b)

Lingula

Mandibular foramen

Mylohyoid line

Figure 13.41 The mandible: (a) outer side; (b) inner side. Source: *Levison's Textbook for Dental Nurses*, 11th edition (Hollins), 2013. Reproduced with permission of Wiley-Blackwell.

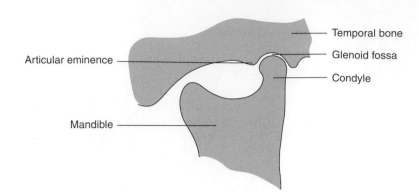

Figure 13.42   Temporo-mandibular joint. Source: *Levison's Textbook for Dental Nurses*, 11th edition (Hollins), 2013. Reproduced with permission of Wiley-Blackwell.

The front edge of the ramus rises up to the **coronoid process**, and the dip between it and the head of condyle at the back of the ramus is called the **sigmoid notch.** When the mouth is closed, the coronoid process slots under the zygomatic arch of the face.

The two foramina in the mandible that are of interest to the dental nurse are:

- **Mandibular foramen** – halfway up the inner surface of the ramus and protected by the bony lingula, and through which the nerve supplying the lower teeth and some of their surrounding soft tissues enters the mandible
- **Mental foramen** – on the outer surface of the body of the mandible, between the positions of the premolar teeth, through which the same nerve exits the mandible

Temporo-mandibular joint and chewing movements

This joint is formed between the condyle of the mandible and the temporal bone at the base of the skull. When the mouth is shut, the condyle rests in a hollow region of the temporal bone called the **glenoid fossa**. The front edge of the glenoid fossa is formed into a ridge called the **articular eminence**.

So the mandibular surface of the joint consists of the condyle, and the temporal surface consists of the glenoid fossa and articular eminence. Between these two surfaces there is a disc of fibrous tissue called the **meniscus**, which prevents the two bones from grating against each other during jaw movements. When the meniscus slips in front or behind its normal position during opening and closing of the mouth, the patient experiences the effect as "jaw clicking". This disarrangement of the joint is called **subluxation**.

During normal jaw movements, the joint allows three basic types of mandibular movement to occur:

- **Gliding movement** – mainly occurs when the disc and the condyle together slide up and down the articular eminence, allowing the mandible to move forwards and backwards
- **Rotational movement** – occurs when the condyle rotates anteriorly and posteriorly over the surface of the disc itself, which remains static, allowing the mandible to move down and up
- **Lateral movement** – this occurs when one joint glides alone, so that the other condyle rotates sideways over its disc, swinging the mandible on the side opposite from the gliding action

As already described, the first stage of opening the mouth is a hinge-like opening of the mandible to separate the incisors. The condyle remains in the glenoid fossa during this stage.

As the mouth opens further, the condyle slides downwards and forwards from the glenoid fossa along the slope of the articular eminence. When the condyle reaches the crest of the articular eminence, the mouth is open to its fullest extent and the incisors can grasp food between their cutting edges. For the closing movement, which produces the shearing action of the incisors, the condyle returns to its rest position in the glenoid fossa, as the mandible moves backwards and closes. This produces a shearing action of the incisors, which thereby cut the food into smaller pieces ready for chewing. It is similar to the cutting action of a pair of scissors. Chewing is brought about by rotational movements of the mandible, which swings from side to side, crushing food between the cusps of opposing molars and premolars.

Sometimes the condyle slips too far forward and gets stuck in front of the articular eminence. When this happens, it cannot move back and the joint is said to be **dislocated**. It is recognised by an inability to close the mouth. It can be resolved by pressing down on the lower molars to force the condyle downwards and backwards into the glenoid fossa – but sedation or a general anaesthetic may be necessary to allow the muscles of mastication to relax fully and allow treatment to be carried out.

The opening movements of the mandible are due to the actions of the **suprahyoid muscles,** which lie in the floor of the mouth and in the throat. The closing and chewing actions of the mandible are due to the actions of the **muscles of mastication,** which run between the mandible and the cranium or facial bones.

Disorders of the temporo-mandibular joint

The temporo-mandibular joint and muscles of mastication may be subjected to excessive strain from seemingly trivial causes, and these can produce a variety of effects, ranging from spasm of the muscles of mastication to degenerative changes in the joint. They result in a wide range of symptoms, but the commonest are pain or tenderness over the joint, clicking noises and restricted movement of the mandible.

As with any joint, the temporo-mandibular joints can also be affected by osteoarthritis and require the use of anti-inflammatories or steroids to relieve the painful symptoms. In extreme cases involving younger patients, the joints can even be replaced by artificial prostheses, such as with hip replacements and knee replacements.

Abnormal, or parafunctional, habits of the patient, especially habitual clenching and grinding of the teeth over long periods, are common findings by the dental team. These habits tend to exhaust the joint musculature and cause pain and discomfort, and the parafunctional action is called **bruxism**. Most patients are unaware that they perform these habitual movements, often doing so in their sleep.

Sufferers will experience any or all of the following symptoms:

- **Trismus** – involuntary painful contracture of the joint musculature, resulting in the inability to open the mouth fully
- **Face and/or neck pain** – often worse in the morning following a night of bruxing, and eased by relaxation and the use of anti-inflammatories
- **Attrition** – enamel wear facets on the teeth, due to the constant grinding of the occlusal and incisal surfaces of each arch against the other
- **Restorative failure** – repetitive fracture and loss of dental restorations, with or without tooth fracture, due to the excessive and prolonged occlusal forces produced
- **Sore mouth** – especially the tongue and cheeks, where cheek ridges and tongue scalloping develop as the tongue is thrust against the teeth and the cheeks are bitten (Figure 13.43)

Similar symptoms are often seen in patients who chew gum excessively.

Following diagnosis and advice on the particular cause of the bruxism, which can often be in relation to stress, treatment involves counselling, use of anti-inflammatories and muscle relaxants, muscle exercises and physiotherapy, and sometimes the provision of night guards or splints to wear as necessary. While not preventing the bruxing action, these devices will hold the jaws open slightly and relieve the tension on the joint musculature. In some cases involving stress as the causative factor, life changes may be necessary.

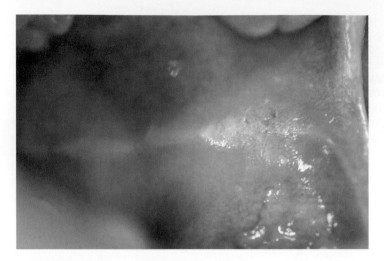

Figure 13.43 Effects of cheek biting.

Trismus may also occur when a patient is suffering from pericoronitis (acute inflammation of the operculum of an erupting lower wisdom tooth), following the surgical extraction of these teeth or during a bout of the viral disease mumps (acute infection of the parotid salivary glands).

Nerve supply to the teeth and supporting structures

The head is supplied by 12 pairs of **cranial nerves**. They all branch off from the brain, one from each pair supplying the left side, while the other supplies the right.

The nerves that make muscles and glands work are called **motor** nerves, and they carry electrical impulses from the brain to effect contraction of the muscles or secretion from the glands. Those nerves that convey pain and other sensation are called **sensory** nerves and they carry electrical stimulation from the body tissues (including teeth) to the brain. Cranial nerves are either motor or sensory, or a combination of the two types, and those relevant to dental nurses are as follows:

- **Trigeminal nerve** – the fifth (V) cranial nerve, supplying the teeth and surrounding soft tissues, and the muscles of mastication
- **Facial nerve** – the seventh (VII) cranial nerve, supplying some taste sensations, some salivary glands and the muscles of facial expression
- **Glossopharyngeal nerve** – the ninth (IX) cranial nerve, supplying some taste sensations, the parotid salivary glands and the muscles of the pharynx
- **Hypoglossal nerve** – the twelfth (XII) cranial nerve, supplying the muscles of the anterior two thirds of the tongue

The nomenclature used to name the various nerves follows that used in other areas of anatomy; so **anterior** and **posterior** refer to front and back, respectively, and **superior** and **inferior** refer to upper and lower, respectively. The areas of supply, in relation to the teeth and their surrounding soft tissues, follow the dental terminology used in naming tooth surfaces.

Trigeminal nerve

The name of this nerve indicates that it splits into three divisions, each of which has several branches. The three divisions are:

- **Ophthalmic division** – sensory supply of the soft tissues around the eye and the upper face
- **Maxillary division** – sensory supply of the upper teeth, the maxilla and the middle area of the face

- **Mandibular division** – sensory supply of the lower teeth, the mandible and the lower area of the face, and motor supply to the muscles of mastication and some of the suprahyoids

The maxillary and mandibular branches of the trigeminal nerve are of most importance to the dental nurse, as together they relay sensory information from the whole of the oral cavity to the brain and provide the motor supply to the muscles of mastication, to effect jaw closing and chewing movements, and to some of the suprahyoid muscles to effect jaw opening.

Maxillary division

The maxillary division of the trigeminal nerve splits further, into five branches, all of which are sensory (Figure 13.44). By definition, then, they transmit sensations (such as heat, cold, pressure and pain) from this area to the brain, including from the upper teeth. It is these branches that have to be anaesthetised before painless dental treatment can be carried out on the upper teeth. The five branches are as follows:

- **Anterior superior dental (alveolar) nerve** – supplies sensation from the upper incisor and canine teeth, and their labial gingivae. In addition, it supplies sensation from the soft tissues of the upper lip and around the nostrils of the nose
- **Middle superior dental (alveolar) nerve** – supplies sensation from the upper premolar and the anterior half of the upper first molar teeth and their buccal gingivae
- **Posterior superior dental (alveolar) nerve** – supplies sensation from the posterior half of the upper first molar and the second and third molar teeth and their buccal gingivae
- **Greater palatine nerve** – supplies sensation from the palatal gingivae of the upper molar, premolar and posterior half of the canine teeth
- **Naso-palatine nerve** – previously called the **long sphenopalatine nerve**, this supplies sensation from the palatal gingivae of the upper incisor and anterior half of the canine teeth

393

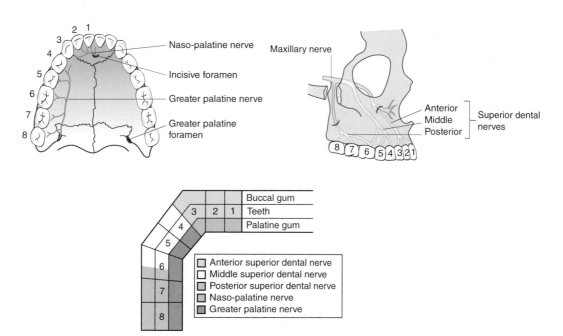

Figure 13.44 Nerve supply of the upper teeth. Source: *Levison's Textbook for Dental Nurses*, 11th edition (Hollins), 2013. Reproduced with permission of Wiley-Blackwell.

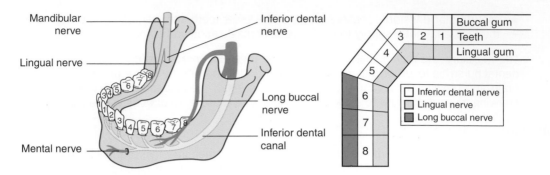

Figure 13.45 Nerve supply of the lower teeth. Source: *Levison's Textbook for Dental Nurses*, 11th edition (Hollins), 2013. Reproduced with permission of Wiley-Blackwell.

Mandibular nerve

The mandibular division of the trigeminal nerve emerges from the skull through the foramen ovale and splits into four branches which carry both sensory and motor components (Figure 13.45). The sensory branches of this nerve require anaesthetising before painless dental treatment can be carried out on the lower teeth. The four branches are as follows:

- **Inferior dental (alveolar) nerve** – supplies sensation from all of the lower teeth, and from the buccal or labial gingivae of all **except** the molar teeth. In addition, it supplies sensation from the soft tissues of the lower lip and the chin
- **Lingual nerve** – supplies sensation from the lingual gingivae of all of the lower teeth, the floor of the mouth, and touch sensation from the anterior two-thirds of the tongue
- **Long buccal nerve** – supplies sensation from the buccal gingivae of the lower molar teeth
- **Motor branch** – supplies stimulation to the muscles of mastication, to effect jaw closing and chewing movements

Trigeminal neuralgia

This is a condition affecting the sensory nerves of either the maxillary or mandibular divisions only of the trigeminal nerve, with no known cause. The sufferer experiences sudden-onset, severe pain in various facial trigger zones, accompanied by muscle spasms in the area.

The neuralgia can be initiated by touch, chewing movements or even speaking, and episodes are usually of short duration. Treatment is difficult without a known cause, and often drastic measures are taken, such as the surgical or chemical destruction of the sensory section of the nerve, to relieve the debilitating symptoms.

Facial nerve

This is a combination nerve, carrying both sensory and motor fibres. Its sensory component carries taste sensation from the anterior two-thirds (front part) of the tongue, while its motor components supply the muscles of facial expression and the saliva secretions of both the submandibular and sublingual salivary glands. Temporary paralysis of this nerve (left or right) gives rise to the condition known as **Bell's palsy.**

Glossopharyngeal nerve

Again, this is a combination nerve. Its sensory component carries taste sensation from the posterior one-third of the tongue, while its motor component supplies the muscles of the pharynx and the saliva secretions of the parotid salivary gland.

Hypoglossal nerve

This nerve has a motor component only, and supplies the muscles of the tongue to effect its complicated movements during speech, mastication, swallowing and so on.

As with all the cranial nerves, the electrical transmissions of these dentally relevant four can be affected by many disorders affecting the brain, including tumours. Dental patients who complain of altered taste sensations or the sudden loss of facial sensations with no obvious cause require rapid neurological investigations to rule out any sinister causes. The dental team has a significant role to play in detecting these aberrations and referring patients for more specialist investigation and diagnosis.

Blood supply to the head and neck

The blood vessels involved tend to run alongside the nerves of the area as **neurovascular bundles**. This arrangement tends to occur throughout the body and, conveniently for the medical professions, ensures that the vessels can be more easily located than if they all ran along their own courses. Similarly, they may also enter and leave the bony cavities of the skull through the same foramina and fissures as do the nerves.

The names of the various blood vessels of the oral cavity are not required knowledge for dental nurses, but, as a general rule, they tend to follow the nerve nomenclature covered previously by being named after their area of supply. Thus the artery supplying the maxillary portion of the face is, unsurprisingly, the **maxillary artery**, while the vein associated with the same area is the **maxillary vein**, and so on.

The major arteries carrying oxygenated blood to the head and neck region are the **common carotid arteries**, which are direct branches from the arch of the aorta as it leaves the left ventricle. These travel up the left and right sides of the neck and are palpable against either side of the larynx as the carotid pulse, often taken by professional resuscitation personnel during medical emergencies.

Around this position of palpation, the common carotids divide into the following major arteries:

- **External carotid artery** – supplying all of the head outside of the cranium, including the face and the oral cavity
- **Internal carotid artery** – supplying all of the inner cranial structures, including the brain, and the eyes

Once the usual gaseous exchange has occurred in the capillary beds of the head and neck region, deoxygenated blood tends to flow from small venules into gradually widening veins until they reach the main venous vessels of the area:

- **External jugular vein** – draining a small area of extra-cranial tissues only
- **Internal jugular vein** – draining the brain and the majority of the head and neck tissues

These veins run on and eventually join the superior vena cava and enter the right side of the heart, where the deoxygenated blood that they carry is pumped to the lungs for reoxygenation.

The flow of deoxygenated blood from the head and neck region is not always in one direction, as occurs in other areas of the body. This is because the veins of this area usually do not contain the one-way valve system present in the majority of these vessels, so blood can flow forwards and backwards depending on changes affecting the local pressure.

Generally, then, it is easier for localised infections to spread in the head and neck regions than elsewhere in the body. The seriousness of this statement is compounded further by the fact that

395

the blood travels through the most important organ of the body, the brain, and that pathogens may enter the area in a variety of ways:

- Inhaled through the nose or mouth
- Ingested through the oral cavity
- Carried by the circulatory or lymph systems
- Traumatically deposited through the soft tissues, such as during dental treatment, local anaesthetic injection or following head and neck injury

The need for the maintenance of high standards of infection control in the field of dentistry is therefore of paramount importance and of great concern to the whole oral healthcare team.

Common oral diseases

The majority of the oral diseases of relevance are covered previously in this chapter and include all of the following:

- **Ulceration** – due to underlying disorders, viral infection and premalignant or malignant conditions
- **Oral candidiasis** – due to infection with the fungus *Candida albicans*
- **Red and white patches** – often as premalignant lesions and usually associated with cancer risk factors, such as smoking and high alcohol intake
- **Inflammatory lesions** – affecting any area of the oral soft tissues and often responding well to improved oral hygiene
- **Viral infection** – specifically with herpes type I virus, and also with HIV
- **Salivary gland disorders** – due to disorders affecting their secretion potential, and also benign and malignant tumours
- **Osteoporosis** – this is a metabolic bone disease that involves an enlargement of the inner bone cavities and results in thinned, brittle bones which are prone to fracture

Osteoporosis has particular significance to the dental team, as not only can it affect the jaws and therefore result in fractures during tooth extraction, but the medication often used to slow down the bone loss resulting from the condition has also been linked to **osteonecrosis** of the jaw.

The group of drugs involved is called **bisphosphonates** and a thorough medical history will highlight the patients at risk – usually elderly and postmenopausal women with hormone-related osteoporosis – although the drugs are also used in the treatment of some cancers. Osteoporosis may also occur in patients who are treated for various medical conditions with long-term steroids, and they are also at risk of developing osteonecrosis (localised bone death) if they are prescribed bisphosphonates.

Patients at risk of osteonecrosis should avoid tooth extraction wherever possible, and undergo the procedure in hospital when this treatment has to be carried out. Those about to receive bisphosphonates for cancer treatment should undergo dental examination and complete any dental treatment required before the medication is started. A high standard of oral hygiene must also be maintained throughout their therapy.

14

Unit 314: Dental Radiography

Learning outcomes

1. Know the regulations and hazards associated with ionising radiation
2. Know the different radiographic films and their uses
3. Understand the imaging process and the different chemicals used
4. Understand the importance for stock control of radiographic films

Outcome 1 assessment criteria

The learner can:
- State the principles of the IRMER regulations
- Explain the safe use of X-ray equipment
- Explain the role of dental personnel when using ionising radiation in the dental environment
- Identify the hazards associated with ionising radiation
- Explain their organisation's practices and policies relating to ionising radiation and the taking of dental images

Outcome 2 assessment criteria

The learner can:
- Explain the uses of different intra-oral radiographs
- Explain the uses of different extra-oral radiographs
- State the reasons for using digital radiography
- Explain the purpose of intensifying screens in dental radiography
- Explain the concerns that patients may have regarding dental imaging

Outcome 3 assessment criteria

The learner can:
- Explain the manual, automatic and digital processing of radiographs
- Describe the faults that may occur during the taking and processing of radiographs
- Explain how processing chemicals should be handled, stored and disposed of safely
- Explain how a spillage of processing chemicals should be dealt with

Diploma in Dental Nursing, Level 3, Third Edition. Carole Hollins.
© 2014 John Wiley & Sons, Ltd. Published 2014 by John Wiley & Sons, Ltd.
Companion website: www.wiley.com/go/hollins/dentalnursinglevel3

- Explain what action to take in the event of equipment failure
- Explain why it is important to protect the processing environment from accidental intrusion, including the use of safe lights

Outcome 4 assessment criteria
The learner can:
- Explain the importance of rotating film stock
- Explain the methods of accurately mounting radiographs, and the consequences of not mounting radiographs correctly
- Describe the storage of radiographs and why X-ray films should be stored away from ionising radiations
- Describe suitable quality control recording systems
- Explain why film stock that has deteriorated should not be used
- Explain the purpose of quality assuring dental radiographs

This unit is assessed by:
- an assessment paper containing multiple choice and short answer questions

The content is the theory and underpinning knowledge required and links to the information contained in Chapters 1, 6 and 7.

Use of ionising radiation in dentistry

Dental radiography is an important diagnostic tool used in dentistry and medicine to help the clinician to see the body's internal tissues and to help diagnose the cause of dental and medical problems. In dentistry, radiographs are used to detect and diagnose the following lesions and structures:

- **Dental caries** – this shows up as a dark area of destruction extending inwards from the enamel surface (see Figure 13.5)
- Presence and extent of **periodontal disease** – this shows up as a loss of the lamina dura forming the crest of the alveolar bone, loss of height of the alveolar bone, and a widening of the periodontal ligament space (see Figure 13.6)
- Periodontal and periapical **abscesses** – chronic alveolar abscesses show up as a dark circular area at the apex of an affected tooth, caused by destruction of the apical lamina dura and spongy bone (see Figure 7.14)
- **Cysts** affecting the dental tissues – these can show up as enlarged darker areas surrounding other structures, and can sometimes be seen to be pushing tooth roots out of their normal positions (Figure 14.1)
- **Iatrogenic problems** – i.e. those caused by the dentist, such as overhanging restorations or tooth perforations by posts (see Figure 13.7)
- To detect **supernumerary** teeth and **unerupted** teeth (see Figure 13.8) or to determine the **congenital absence** of unerupted teeth
- To diagnose **hard tissue lesions**, such as bone cysts and tumours, salivary calculi and jaw fractures

In addition, radiographs are used during the provision of dental treatment to avoid problems occurring and to ensure that the treatment is successful – examples are:

- To aid in **endodontic** treatment
- To determine the number and position of tooth roots before **extraction**
- To ensure the health of a tooth before it undergoes **crown or bridge** preparation
- To ensure the health of a tooth before it is used as an abutment during **denture construction**

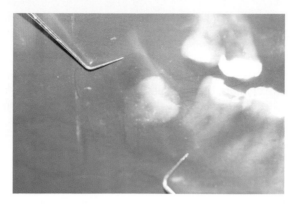

Figure 14.1 Dentigerous cyst surrounding unerupted lower right third molar tooth – margins indicated by probes.

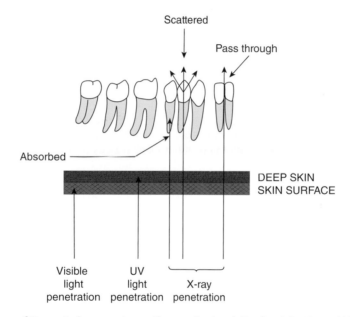

Figure 14.2 Passage of X-rays in human tissue. Source: *Levison's Textbook for Dental Nurses*, 11th edition (Hollins), 2013. Reproduced with permission of Wiley-Blackwell.

For examination purposes, dental nurses are not expected to interpret radiographs, but they should be able to describe both normal and abnormal radiographic appearances of common dental conditions.

Nature of ionising radiation

Ionising radiation is commonly referred to as "X-rays". It is a type of electromagnetic radiation that possesses energy, as are ultraviolet light and visible light. The radiation types differ from each other in the amount of energy they possess; X-rays have more energy and are capable of passing through matter such as human tissue. When they do so, one of three events will occur (Figure 14.2):

- X-rays pass cleanly between the atoms of the matter and are **unaltered**
- X-rays hit the atoms of the matter and are **scattered**, releasing their energy as they do so
- X-rays hit the atoms of the matter and are **absorbed**, releasing their energy as they do so

With larger atoms of matter, such as some metals (including calcium), most of the X-rays are absorbed or scattered; these are **radiopaque** substances. Those that allow the majority of the X-rays to pass through unaffected are called **radiolucent** substances, and include the soft tissues

As bone and enamel have a high calcium content, and dentine and cementum also contain calcium hydroxyapatite crystals, these tissues are variably radiopaque to X-rays. They show up on processed radiographs as varying shades of white/grey images, the more radiopaque structures being the whitest.

Effect of ionising radiation on the body cells – radiation hazards

The energy released when the X-rays interact with human tissue is capable of causing **tissue damage**, and it is this effect that requires that X-rays are used only as necessary and at the lowest dose possible, to reduce the amount of energy released and therefore reduce the amount of tissue damage which occurs.

Tissue damage may occur when the X-rays hit the atoms of the tissue cells and are either scattered or absorbed, because of the energy that is released during these events. The tissue cells contain chromosomes which are made up of our DNA – the building blocks of life that determine exactly the organism we are – and if the energy hits the chromosomes it can damage them and cause them to undergo change (**mutation**) or even die.

This ability of X-ray exposure to cause cell death is used in medicine to treat some types of cancer during radiotherapy treatment. The cancer cells can be accurately targeted by the ionising radiation beam so they are killed outright, or so the cancerous tumour is reduced to a size that can be surgically removed. High doses of X-rays are used for this treatment, and tissue cells that divide and grow rapidly, such as skin cells and the body cells of children, are more easily affected.

When exposed to high levels of ionising radiation, the skin appears reddened and inflamed, similar to sunburn. Higher levels still may cause destruction of the cells of the immune system, resulting in leukaemia and "radiation sickness" before death eventually occurs.

However, these effects of cell death are undesirable during the production of dental images. As there can be no "safe" level of exposure to ionising radiation (i.e. there is always some amount of cell damage caused by X-ray exposure), strict legislation and guidelines have been introduced to ensure the following when X-rays are used in dentistry:

- All use of dental imaging has to be **clinically justified** – so there must be a clinical reason why the patient is being exposed to the X-rays; this will be one of the diagnostic or treatment reasons listed earlier
- The dose of X-rays used must be kept **as low as reasonably achievable (ALARA)** – so the minimum dose of X-rays must be used, for the shortest time, and aimed at the smallest area of tissue possible to produce a functional image
- This technique is now more usually referred to as being **as low as reasonably practicable/possible (ALARP)**
- Only the patient should be exposed to the X-ray beam – all staff and family members must be outside the **controlled zone** during the exposure (the only exception being when a parent assists a small child during exposure)
- Machines must be well maintained and serviced regularly
- No untrained personnel can be involved in radiation exposure procedures
- **Quality assurance (QA) systems** must be operated to ensure that the dental images produced are to a consistently high standard

Ionising radiation regulations

X-rays cannot be seen, heard or felt, and therein lie the dangers as it can easily be forgotten that they are potentially hazardous to health. There is no "safe" level of use – every exposure can cause some amount of tissue damage in the patient, or anyone else in the imaging area who is exposed to the X-ray beam. An overdose can cause serious health effects, ranging from a mild burn to leukaemia and even death.

For this reason, specific legislation is in place to ensure full compliance with the health and safety aspects of ionising radiation by all dental workplaces, under the following regulations:

- **Ionising Radiation Regulations 1999 – IRR99**
- **Ionising Radiation (Medical Exposure) Regulations 2000 – IR(ME)R 2000**

While IRR99 is concerned with the protection of staff and IR(ME)R with the protection of patients, the aim of both sets of regulations is to keep the number of X-ray exposures, and their dose levels, to the absolute minimum required for clinical necessity at all times.

This ALARA/P principle, defined in the preceding section, applies not only to the actual direct X-ray beam that is fired at the patient during the film exposure, but also to the "scattered radiation" that inevitably occurs during this process. Scattered radiation, as its name suggests, is radiation that bounces off tissue cells during exposure in an uncontrolled manner, and can result in the patient being exposed several times over, thereby increasing the actual radiation dose.

In the dental workplace, three simple factors required for the ALARA/P principle to be achieved have helped to reduce the amount of scattered radiation created during a dental exposure by 40%:

- **Use of "fast" films** – F speed intra-oral films are currently available and require the shortest possible exposure time to create the radiographic image, once processed
- **Short exposure time** – achievable with a combination of modern X-ray machines, fast films and fast intensifying screens in extra-oral cassettes
- **Rectangular collimator tubes** – these have replaced the old plastic aiming cones of intra-oral machines, and produce a parallel X-ray beam rather than a disorganised "spray" effect with lots of scattered rays. The rectangular tube end has the same dimensions as a standard intra-oral film (Figure 14.3).

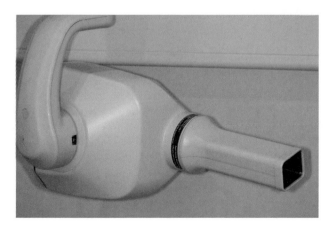

Figure 14.3 X-ray machine rectangular collimator tube.

Compliance with IRR99

This set of regulations is concerned with the safety of staff in the dental workplace where ionising radiation is used, as well as the correct functioning of the radiation equipment, and the initial act of compliance is to inform the Health and Safety Executive of its use on the premises. This must be carried out whenever a dental workplace uses ionising radiation for the first time, and with each change of ownership thereafter.

Three formal appointments must then be made by the workplace owner:

- **Legal person** – a designated person who is to ensure the workplace's full compliance with both sets of regulations (this is usually the employer)
- **Radiation protection adviser (RPA)** – a medical physicist who is appointed in writing by the dental workplace and is available to give advice on staff and public safety in relation to both sets of regulations
- **Radiation protection supervisor (RPS)** – a designated person in the workplace who can assess risks and ensure precautions are taken to minimise them, in accordance with IRR99 (this is usually a senior dentist or a dental care professional with a post-registration qualification in dental radiography)

The role of the RPA is to give advice on the actions the workplace must take to comply with both sets of regulations and will cover the following points:

- The correct installation of all new X-ray machines
- The regular maintenance and certificated checks that are required for each X-ray machine to ensure that the minimum exposure to radiation occurs
- The **contingency plans** that need to be in place in case of an X-ray machine malfunctioning
- The investigation of any malfunction of an X-ray machine
- The designation of a 1.5-metre **controlled area** around each X-ray machine and within the primary beam direction, where no one but the patient may be present during an exposure
- Advise on **risk assessments** with regard to restricting staff and patient exposure to ionising radiation, and review the assessments every five years
- Advise on the necessary **staff training** required so that designated duties are carried out competently and safely
- Assess staff protection with regard to the number of exposures carried out on the premises; if more than 150 intra-oral films or 50 dental pantomographs are taken weekly, staff are **legally required** to wear a personal monitoring badge
- Advise on the appropriate action to take if analysis of the badges indicates excessive exposure to any staff
- Advise on the running of **QA programmes** so that the principle of ALARA/P is maintained at all times

The legal person is responsible for organising a 3-yearly assessment of radiation safety in the workplace. This involves arranging for an inspection by a competent authority such as the Radiation Protection Division of the Health Protection Agency (which has replaced the previous authority, the National Radiological Protection Board) or using the workplace's own X-ray machine and processing test kit to carry out the necessary checks and then sending them to the competent authority for analysis.

In addition, the legal person must draw up a set of **local rules,** which have to be displayed at each X-ray machine, so they can be referred to by all staff. The local rules must give all of the following information:

- The name of the designated RPS and RPA
- The identification of each controlled area to all staff and patients, to limit unauthorised entry during exposure – this is usually an area of 1.5 metres from the machine head and the patient and directly in the primary beam of the radiation during exposure

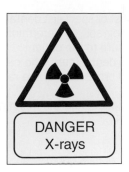

Figure 14.4 A radiation warning sign. Source: *Levison's Textbook for Dental Nurses*, 11th edition (Hollins), 2013. Reproduced with permission of Wiley-Blackwell.

- The designation of a 2-metre safety zone from the machine head will ensure that only the patient remains within the 1.5-metre controlled area during X-ray exposure (see Figure 1.28)
- Show the standard warning sign at each controlled area, indicating the use of ionising radiation – this is a black sign on a yellow background (Figure 14.4)
- A summary of the correct working instructions for each controlled area, including a "no entry" rule for the designated 2-metre safety zone around the X-ray machine head
- A summary of the contingency plan to be followed in the event of a machine malfunction
- Details of the dose investigation level
- The use of a red light and an audible buzzer to indicate the actual exposure time
- The arrangements in place for the safety of pregnant staff

The role of the RPS is to carry out the following:

- Ensure all staff members have suitable training according to the level of their legal responsibility
- Carry out risk assessments with regard to restricting radiation exposure
- Ensure the local rules remain current, updating as necessary
- Maintain the contents of the necessary "radiation protection file" (see later)
- Organise and run QA programmes in relation to the safe use of ionising radiation
- Organise and run quality control tests or delegate the tests to suitably trained members of staff
- Can also be made responsible for ensuring that all staff receive the necessary hours of continuing professional development (CPD) in relation to dental radiography, as it is one of the core subjects for all qualified staff working in the dental surgery environment

Compliance with IR(ME)R 2000

This set of regulations is concerned with the safety of patients in the dental workplace and their protection during exposure to ionising radiation. They are of most concern to those dental personnel who have the qualifications and legal right to expose the patient to ionising radiation – i.e. the dentist and any dental care professional holding a recognised dental radiography qualification. The regulations are therefore of less importance to trainee dental nurses, and consequently only the basics relevant to them are covered here.

Roles and responsibilities

The regulations set out the responsibilities of the various dental personnel who may be involved in taking and processing radiographs within the dental workplace, and restrict those responsibilities by referring to each category with specific appointment titles:

- **Referrer** – the dentist who refers the patient for radiation exposure, either to themselves or to another dentist or specialist dental radiographer who can carry out that exposure

- **IRMER practitioner** – the dentist or specialist dental radiographer who takes responsibility for **justifying** the taking of the radiograph, by determining that the diagnostic benefits gained will outweigh the risks of the exposure to the patient
- **Operator** – any member of the dental team who carries out all or part of the practical duties involved with the exposure and processing of the radiograph, including:
  - Patient identification
  - Positioning of the film, the patient and the machine tube head
  - Setting the exposure controls
  - Pressing the exposure button
  - Processing the film
  - Evaluating the quality of the radiograph
  - Carrying out test exposures for QA purposes
  - Running QA programmes

Except in the hospital setting, then, only a dentist can be a referrer and/or an IRMER practitioner. Therapists and hygienists are likely to have undertaken study and qualification in dental radiography as part of their training course and will therefore be able to carry out all of these duties as operators. With suitable and authenticated training, or a dental radiography qualification, the dental nurse can also carry out a variety of duties under the title of "operator", as shown in the following table.

Duty	Radiography qualified dental nurse	NEBDN qualified dental nurse	NVQ qualified dental nurse	Trainee dental nurse
Patient ID	X	X	X	X
Positioning	X	NO	NO	NO
Setting exposure	X	NO	NO	NO
Pressing exposure button	X	X In the presence of the "set up" operator	X In the presence of the "set up" operator	X In the presence of the "set up" operator
Processing	X	X	X	X
Quality audit	X	X	X	X
QA test exposures	X	X In the presence of the "set up" operator	X In the presence of the "set up" operator	X In the presence of the "set up" operator
QA programmes	X	X	X	X

NEBDN, National Examining Board for Dental Nurses; NVQ, National Vocational Qualification.

Hence a registered dental nurse who also holds the dental radiography post-registration qualification is able to carry out all the duties in relation to positioning, setting, exposing and processing a dental radiograph, on prescription from the dentist. No other category of dental nurse shown is able to position the patient and film or set the exposure control on the X-ray machine. These tasks require specialist knowledge of the principles of dental ionising radiation to be carried out safely.

The exposure button of the machine may be pressed by any dental nurse category shown, following suitable recorded training to do so, and once the patient and machine have been correctly set up by the qualified dental radiography person. This applies whether the exposure is of a patient or a test film for QA purposes.

The ability of suitably trained personnel to "press the button" during radiation exposures is of great help in reducing cross-infection risks, as the "set up" operator would otherwise contaminate the exposure button unless they repeatedly removed and replaced their gloves between setting up and retrieving each film from the patient's mouth.

Patient protection

The IR(ME)R is mainly concerned with the protection of patients while undergoing ionising radiation exposure in the dental workplace, to ensure they are not exposed unnecessarily and that all exposure levels are as low as possible in order to reduce the chance of any tissue damage occurring.

The key points covered are summarised here:

- **Patient identification** – this is of particular importance when the referrer is not also the IRMER practitioner, as occurs when patients are referred to hospital; to avoid the wrong patient being exposed, name, address and date of birth should be used as a minimum, and some workplaces may also operate a patient ID number
- **Referrer and IRMER practitioner** – can only be dentists (unless the patient is referred to a specialist dental radiographer), as only they have the training to determine when an exposure is required for diagnosis and treatment, and when the exposure is justified
- **Justification** – the benefit of exposing the patient should outweigh the risk of causing tissue damage, and so every exposure should be expected to provide new information to help the patient's treatment or prognosis as a minimum requirement, otherwise it should not be undertaken
- **Optimisation** – the dose of radiation should be in line with ALARA/P principles at all times
- **Pregnant patients** – routine dental exposure techniques do not irradiate the pelvic area and involve such low doses that pregnancy is not considered a contraindication to undergoing irradiation; for similar reasons, lead aprons are not required to be used
- **Staff training** – written evidence of all necessary training pertinent to ionising radiation techniques must be kept for all personnel in the radiation protection file (see the next section), as documented proof of their competence in the duties that they undertake
- **Quality assurance** – QA programmes and audits provide a valuable tool for determining whether the systems in place to protect patients (and staff) from any potential harm from ionising radiation are actually working, by looking at the procedures in place and the results achieved, and analysing any problems encountered so that policies and techniques can be suitably adjusted and updated where necessary
- **Accidental exposure** – all X-ray machines must have an isolation switch outside the controlled area, an illuminated control panel or switch to indicate when the mains power is on, and an additional light and an audible buzzer that are activated during the exposure time itself. If a machine malfunctions during use, it will then be obvious by the lights and buzzers, and the mains power can be switched off without the operator having to enter the controlled area

Radiation protection file

Effectively, this acts as a summary document that holds as much information as possible about the procedures in place to ensure radiation protection within the particular workplace. It should be reviewed and kept updated annually to ensure that it remains relevant and effective.

It should contain all of the following information, and have references included for any information that is kept elsewhere (such as qualification and relevant training details that are kept in personnel files):

- Formal appointments of staff on the premises – including referrers, IRMER practitioners and all operators (with details of the range of their duties)
- Reference to the initial risk assessment carried out by the legal person, in consultation with the RPA
- Local rules for each X-ray set on the premises
- Procedures for ensuring patient protection, as required under IR(ME)R
- Information on how ALARA/P is achieved
- Details of protocols followed in relation to justification and authorisation of exposures (usually referenced to the FGDP booklet *Selection Criteria for Dental Radiography*)
- Details of protocols followed in relation to clinical evaluation of radiographs (written notes are kept in the patients' records of each radiograph taken and what the findings were)
- Details of QA programmes to ensure consistently accurate radiographs, including their frequency and the named persons who run them

Principles of dental radiography

As stated previously, there are many sound clinical reasons for dental radiographs to be taken in the dental workplace, and their use is particularly invaluable as a diagnostic tool in dentistry.

However, to avoid their indiscriminate use, guidelines have been drawn up for the safe prescription of dental radiographs in dental practice as follows, and these must be adhered to by all:

- A history and a clinical examination must be performed before any radiograph is taken, otherwise the justification for the exposure is unclear
- Only new patients with clear evidence of some dental disease should have full mouth radiographs taken, rather than carrying them out on every new patient indiscriminately
- Regularly attending child patients in the mixed dentition stage who have orthodontic problems developing can be radiographed as necessary, but each exposure must be justified – such as monitoring the progress of development of an unerupted tooth
- Recall patients with a low caries risk should be radiographed no more frequently than every 18 months, using horizontal bitewings
- Those with a moderate caries risk should be radiographed every 12 months, using horizontal bitewings
- Those with a high caries risk should be radiographed at 6-monthly intervals, using horizontal bitewings, and gradually reducing this rate as the caries is brought under control
- Patients exhibiting evidence of periodontal disease can have selective radiographs taken of problem areas, either vertical bitewings or periapical views, as necessary
- Edentulous patients should only have selective radiographs taken if there are any clinically suspicious areas (such as retained roots or hard tissue lesions) – the view used will depend on the area to be assessed

Views used in dental radiography

There are various types of film used in dental radiography, depending on the reason for taking the dental image, but all are either those taken within the oral cavity (**intra-oral films**) or those taken outside the oral cavity (**extra-oral films**).

Intra-oral films are supplied in child- and adult-size packets that contain the following (Figure 14.5):

- Plastic envelope to protect the contents from saliva contamination
- Wrap-around black paper to prevent exposure of the film to light

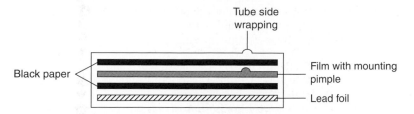

Figure 14.5 Contents of an intra-oral film packet. Source: *Levison's Textbook for Dental Nurses*, 11th edition (Hollins), 2013. Reproduced with permission of Wiley-Blackwell.

- Film – which is exposed to the ionising radiation and produces the dental image once processed or loaded onto the computer (digital imaging)
- Lead foil to prevent scatter of the ionising radiation past the film packet
- Raised pimple marker on the film and packet side towards the X-ray tube, which is used to correctly determine the left and right sides of the image produced (the film is mounted with the pimple towards the observer)

The intra-oral views that can be produced using these films are:

- **Horizontal bitewing** (see Figure 6.6) – shows the posterior teeth in occlusion, and is taken to view:
  - Interproximal areas and diagnose caries in these regions
  - Restoration overhangs in these areas
  - Recurrent caries beneath existing restorations
  - Occlusal caries
- **Vertical bitewing** (see Figure 7.2) – shows an extended view of the posterior teeth, from mid-root of the uppers to mid-root of the lowers as a minimum, and is taken to view:
  - Periodontal bone levels of the posterior teeth
  - True periodontal pockets
- **Periapical** (see Figure 6.7) – shows one or two teeth in full length with their surrounding bone, and is taken to view the area and the teeth in close detail
- **Anterior occlusal** (see Figure 7.3) – show a plane view of the anterior section of either the mandible or the maxilla, and are used especially to view the area for unerupted teeth, supernumerary teeth, and cysts

Extra-oral films are used to produce much larger images showing many structures, and are supplied in cassettes that contain the following:

- Cassette case that is loaded into special imaging machines for use
- Intensifying screens in both sides of the cassette, to reduce the dose of radiation exposure required to produce a dental image
- Film, of a compatible type with the intensifying screens, to produce the dental image once exposed and processed
- Marker to correctly determine the left and right sides of the image produced

Extra-oral film is packed differently from intra-oral films. The latter are individually packed in light-proof wrappers but extra-oral films are not. Packets of extra-oral film only contain unwrapped film and can only be opened in a darkroom or within the light-protected chamber of an automatic processor. On removal from the packet in one of these areas, the film is placed immediately in the special light-proof container or **cassette**, which is then kept closed ready for use.

A typical cassette opens like a book and the film is placed in the middle. On each inside cover of the cassette there is a white plastic sheet called an **intensifying screen**, and the film is sandwiched between the two screens when the cassette is closed ready for use. The screens **fluoresce** on exposure to X-rays, and the brightness of the fluorescence creates the image on the film itself, rather than being produced by the actual X-ray beam. This allows the patient's exposure time to X-rays to be reduced, making the technique safer.

The extra-oral views that can be produced using these films are:

- **Dental panoramic tomograph (DPT)** (see Figure 6.8) – shows both jaws in full and their surrounding bony anatomy, and is taken for orthodontic and wisdom tooth assessments, as well as to help diagnose pathology and jaw fractures
- **Lateral oblique** – shows the posterior portion of one side of the mandible, including the ramus and angle and the lower molar teeth, and is an alternative to a DPT to view the position of unerupted third molar teeth (these views are used infrequently now, as the image produced on a well-aligned DPT is far superior)
- **Lateral skull radiograph** (see Figure 6.9) – this is a view of the side of the head, taken in a specialised machine called a **cephalostat** (which may be present as an attachment to a DPT machine, or as a stand-alone device), and is used to monitor jaw growth and determine orthognathic surgery techniques in complicated cases of malocclusion

When DPTs initially became widely available to the dental profession, they were called "orthopantomographs" and referred to as OPGs or OPTs – these abbreviations are still in current use in some areas.

Radiographic techniques

Any dental image is produced by the correct placing of the film on the far side of the area to be exposed from the X-ray machine. In other words, the radiation beam passes from the machine through the area to be exposed and then hits the film inside either the plastic envelope or the cassette.

Intra-oral films are held in the correct position by the use of film holder devices where possible, as shown in Figures 14.6 and 14.7. These are correctly loaded with the film packet and placed inside the oral cavity for the patient to bite upon so that the radiograph can be produced (Figure 14.8). If a digital imaging technique is used, the film is replaced by a special sensor that is positioned in exactly the same way, but instead of an exposed film being produced which is then chemically processed, the digital image is transmitted directly to a computer screen where it can be viewed immediately.

Intra-oral films can be exposed in one of two angulations, depending upon which is the best technique for the given clinical situation. They are called the "**paralleling technique**" and the "**bisecting angle technique**".

The paralleling technique holds the film exactly parallel to the long axis of the tooth being exposed, so that the image produced is exactly the same size as the actual tooth. This is especially important during endodontic procedures, when the correct diagnostic length of the tooth has to be determined to ensure accurate root filling of the canal (Figure 14.9)

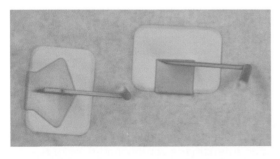

Figure 14.6   Bitewing holders – loaded.

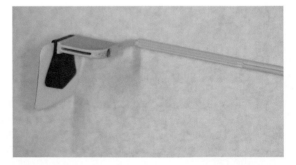

Figure 14.7   A posterior periapical holder – loaded.

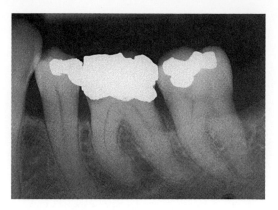

Figure 14.8 A posterior periapical radiograph. Source: *Levison's Textbook for Dental Nurses*, 11th edition (Hollins), 2013. Reproduced with permission of Wiley-Blackwell.

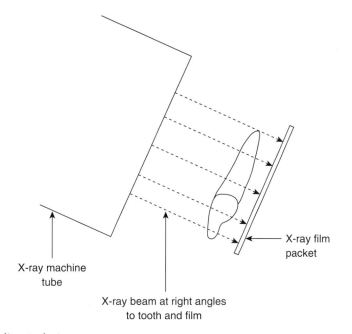

X-ray film
packet

X-ray machine
tube

X-ray beam at right angles
to tooth and film

Figure 14.9 Paralleling technique.

Sometimes the film cannot be placed parallel to the tooth, because of the size restriction of the patient's mouth. In these situations, the bisecting angle technique is used. The film is placed intra-orally and the angulation of the long axis of the tooth against the film is determined by the operator. This angle is then halved (bisected) and the collimator of the tube head is angled to be at right angles to it (Figure 14.10) before the film is exposed.

Anterior occlusal views are produced using the bisecting angle technique, with the patient holding the actual film packet between the teeth anteriorly, as illustrated in Figure 14.11.

Lateral oblique cassettes are held in position by the patient's hand, on the far side of the head from the radiation machine, and angled so that the X-ray beam passes up through the angle of the jaw on that side, so that the third molar teeth on that side only are exposed (Figure 14.12).

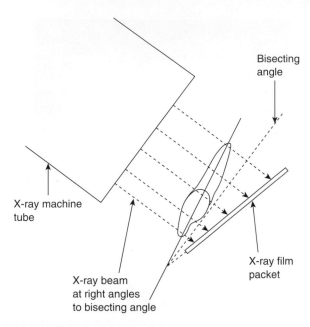

Figure 14.10   Bisecting angle technique.

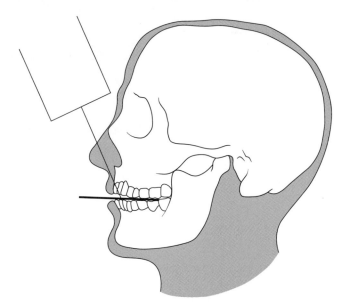

Figure 14.11   Maxillary anterior occlusal positioned. Source: *Levison's Textbook for Dental Nurses*, 11th edition (Hollins), 2013. Reproduced with permission of Wiley-Blackwell.

Extra-oral DPT film cassettes are loaded into their special radiation machines, and then the patient is accurately placed within the machine and the cassette is revolved around the patient's head during the exposure process (see Figure 14.13). Both types of extra-oral film are processed in the same way as the intra-oral films, either manually or by the use of an automatic processing machine, as described later.

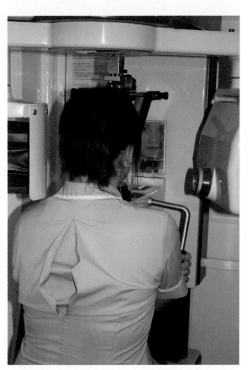

Figure 14.13 Dental panoramic tomograph machine with the patient in position.

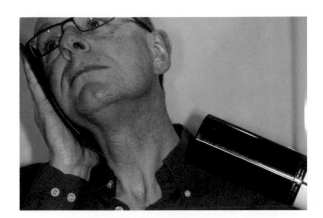

Figure 14.12 Lateral oblique position.

Digital radiography

Conventional X-ray techniques rely on the use of a chemically coated plastic film being exposed to the X-ray beam and then processed in a darkroom or in an automatic processor, using special chemicals to fix the image permanently on to the film.

Digital radiography avoids the use of both the chemically coated plastic film and the need for processing it, as the X-ray beam is fired at a special sensor plate instead (see Figure 7.5), which then relays the image directly to a computer screen on the surgery worktop (Figure 14.14). The reusable intra-oral sensor plate is used instead of film and the radiation dose is far less than with ordinary film. It is a technique similar to the use of digital cameras to produce photographic images which can then be loaded onto the computer from a memory card or a scanner.

The sensor plate is the same size as whichever intra-oral view is being taken – bitewing, periapical or occlusal. It is positioned in exactly the same way in the patient's mouth, using holders so that a paralleling technique is possible. The plate is connected directly to the computer via a cable and the image produced is visible on the screen within seconds.

Extra-oral digital views can also be taken with specialised radiography equipment, but their size and cost are considerable and they are usually only found in hospital radiography departments or specialist orthodontic practices.

The digital image produced on the computer screen can be treated in the same way as digital photographs from a camera, as follows:

- It can be stored on the computer hard drive or transferred to a storage device (disc or flash drive)
- It can be printed on paper and stored as a hard copy in the patient's record card
- It can be sent via e-mail to be viewed by other colleagues

411

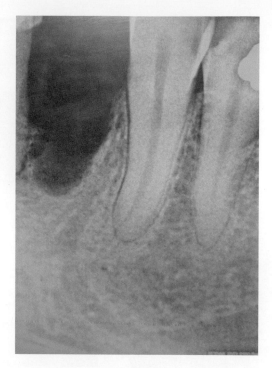

Figure 14.14   Digital image on computer screen.

However, as with digital photographs, the image can be adjusted and edited on the computer screen, and this raises issues in dento-legal situations where an image can be enhanced to make a clinical case look better than it actually is, or the image can be selectively deleted so that poor-quality treatment is not so apparent. Fortunately, computer experts would be able to detect that alterations had been made by examining the hard drive of the computer.

Digital radiographic techniques are now popular, but have not fully superseded conventional techniques in the dental workplace, and many still rely on X-ray films that have been processed either manually or with an automatic processor, such as a Velopex machine. The advantages and disadvantages of digital radiographs are outlined here.

Advantages:

- Financial savings of not having to buy film packets and processing chemicals and equipment
- Avoidance of health and safety issues surrounding Control of Substances Hazardous to Health (COSHH) and the handling of the waste processing chemicals
- Help towards achieving ALARA/ALARP, as the use of the sensor always ensures a lower dose of radiation compared with conventional film
- The image is produced in seconds at the chairside, rather than several minutes in the processing area
- Patients are able to view the magnified image on the computer screen at the chairside and with the dentist, whereas they can only view the actual size conventional radiograph on the light box viewer
- The magnified image can give greater clarity in some instances
- The same sensor can be used over and over again, as long as adequate infection control techniques are in place to avoid cross-infection, by encasing the sensor in a single-use plastic sheath before each exposure

Disadvantages:

- The issue of adequate infection control to avoid cross-infection, although this should be manageable using the sheaths described and wiping the plate with a compatible disinfectant wipe after each use (e.g. isopropyl alcohol wipes)
- Costs of buying the computer with suitable specifications for use with the digital radiography software, the computer software itself (including any updates) and the sensor plates and their attachments
- The ability to alter the image without detection raises dento-legal concerns in complaint and fraud cases, unless an expert is employed to examine the computer hard drive

Formation of the conventional image

An intra-oral X-ray film packet contains a celluloid film coated with light-sensitive silver bromide salts in an emulsion, surrounded by black paper to protect it from unwanted light, and enclosed in a waterproof plastic packet. On one side of the film is a lead foil which prevents the emulsion coat being exposed twice, by absorbing scattered radiation during the actual exposure to X-rays.

The passage of the X-rays through the tissue causes the energy release discussed earlier, and an exact pattern of the tissue is produced within the chemicals on the film itself, as a **latent** (hidden) image, with radiopaque tissues causing the most energy release and therefore a clearer (white) image. Unless a digital imaging technique is used, the latent image can only be seen on the film by the use of special chemicals to make it visible during the processing procedure, in much the same way that conventional photographs from a camera are developed before being able to be viewed as prints.

413

Film processing

As discussed earlier, intra-oral digital images are transmitted directly to the computer and can be viewed within seconds on the computer screen. All other films require chemical processing to convert the latent image to a visible image for viewing, and this can be done using an **automatic processing machine** or by **manually** processing the film, passing it through the chemical tanks by hand and in the correct sequence.

Automatic processing

The machine used consists of a base containing the chemical and water tanks, with conveyor belt-style rollers that carry the film through the machine during processing (see Figure 7.9). These are all beneath a removable, light-tight lid which has hand entry ports so that the film packet or cassette can be put into the light-tight chamber before being opened. If the film is exposed to visible light before being processed, the image will be permanently lost.

The automatic processing procedure is as follows:

- Observe the warning light system to check that the chemical and water levels are adequate, and that the temperature is correct for processing (see Figure 4.6)
- When the temperature is correct, the warning light will go out and the machine is ready for use
- Intra-oral film packets are taken into the machine through the hand ports, while wearing clean gloves
- Extra-oral cassettes are placed into this section by lifting and replacing the lid, and then they can be opened and handled via the hand ports
- The rollers become operational once the processing start button within this first chamber is pressed
- The film packet is carefully opened and the plastic envelope, black paper and lead foil are all dropped to the base of the tank, for removal later
- The film is then held by its sides only, as finger marks on the surface will damage the image

- The film is carefully inserted into the entrance to the rollers, and it will be gently tugged into the machine to be processed
- Once the film has passed through the machine, processed and dried, it will reappear at the delivery port and can be safely handled and viewed

Manual processing

Although the vast majority of dental workplaces use automatic processing machines or digital radiography techniques, it is important for dental nurses to have knowledge of the manual processing technique, so that it can be carried out safely and effectively whenever necessary.

Manual processing follows the same procedure as that occurring in an automatic processor, but is carried out by hand and in a "darkroom" – this is a light-tight, lockable room containing the processing chemicals and water tanks that is heated and maintained in the temperature range 18–22 °C.

Four tanks will be present, as follows (see Figure 7.10):

- **Lidded developing tank** – containing the alkaline developing fluid that produces the initial **latent image**, the lid is only removed during developing as the solution will deteriorate in air
- The image is still unstable in visible light at this point
- **First water tank** – to wash off the developing solution after the correct developing time, using tap water
- **Fixing tank** – containing the acid fixing solution which permanently fixes the image on to the celluloid film, so that it can be viewed in visible light
- **Second water tank** – to wash off the fixing solution after the suitable fixing time, again using tap water

Some vision is required within the room rather than it being completely dark, so an orange or red **safe light** will be present under which the processing can be carried out without exposing the film to actual visible light, and thereby ruining the image. The room must be lockable from within so that the door cannot be opened by anyone else during the processing procedure, as this would result in the accidental exposure of the film to light and the destruction of the image before it has been fully processed.

The manual processing procedure is as follows:

- Check that the chemical and water levels are adequate
- Check the temperature of the solutions and determine the developing and fixing times required from the chemical manufacturer's guidelines provided
- Check that a timing clock and suitable film hangers are available in the room
- Wipe surfaces dry of any previously spilt chemicals or water, if necessary
- Lock the door and switch off all lights except the safe light
- Open the film packet or cassette, locate the film and clip it to one of the hangers available, carefully handling the film by its edges only, to avoid spoiling it with fingerprints
- Remove the developer lid, immerse the hanger in the solution so that the film is completely covered by the solution and start the timer
- When the timer sounds, remove the hanger and film and immerse in the first water tank, agitating the hanger to ensure thorough washing occurs
- Shake off excess water, then fully immerse the hanger and film in the fixer solution, and start the timer
- Replace the developer lid to prevent the solution being weakened by exposure to air, which would allow oxidation to occur otherwise
- When the timer sounds, remove the hanger and film and immerse in the second water tank, agitating the hanger to ensure thorough washing occurs

- Switch on the ordinary light
- Shake off excess water and dry the film – a slow-running hairdryer is suitable for this, as the radiograph must not be dried too quickly

Once dry, the films can be correctly mounted as necessary and returned to the dentist for viewing.

Mounting and viewing films

Once the films have been successfully processed, they will be viewed by the dentist so that diagnoses can be made and treatment plans formulated. Ideally, a light box and magnifier will be available for viewing the films (see Figure 7.11), but it is imperative that they are mounted and positioned correctly, otherwise the left teeth will be viewed as the right, the uppers as lowers, and vice versa.

Extra-oral cassettes are marked with an "L" to indicate the patient's left side, and unless the cassette has been placed upside down in the machine, the film is easily orientated on the viewer so that it is viewed as if looking at the patient from the front (see Figure 8.1).

Various plastic envelope designs are available to mount all types of intra-oral film nowadays, but they must be loaded correctly by the dental nurse first. All intra-oral films have a raised pimple in one corner which must be facing out to view the film correctly, and not back to front. It does not matter which corner of the film the pimple appears in, but it must face out towards the person viewing the radiograph.

Dental nurses should also use their knowledge of oral anatomy to check for themselves – molar teeth are posterior to all other teeth, so correct mounting of bitewing films, for instance, should result in the molar teeth appearing on the outer side of both films, with their pimples palpable in one corner (see Figure 6.6). Upper periapical films should be mounted with the roots above the crowns of the teeth, as they are in the patient's maxilla (see Figure 7.12), lowers with their roots below the crowns, and so on.

Dental workplaces are likely to use one of the various different methods of patient identification and storage of the films, and dental nurses have to be aware of the methods in use in their workplace and use them appropriately. These may include any of the following:

- Digital images will be stored on computer or downloaded onto disks, and they will be individually saved to the patient's own file
- Intra-oral films may be mounted in plastic envelopes, with patient identification details written on in indelible ink
- These may be stored within each patient's record card and filed
- If clinical notes are computerised, there may be a separate filing system used exclusively for films
- Extra-oral films may be too large to store within the record cards, so may also have their own exclusive filing system

Whichever system is used, all films must be marked with the patient's identification details (such as name, date of birth, personal computer number), the date the image was taken, and a note of the view used, before being stored or filed.

Care of processing equipment and film packets

One of a dental nurse's many duties will be to care for all processing equipment, once trained adequately to do so. This is a vital role with regard to patient safety; poorly maintained equipment will lead to poor-quality radiographs that may need to be retaken, causing unnecessary X-ray exposure for the patient. And, as stated previously, there is no "safe level" of X-ray exposure – each one can cause cell damage. The following list summarises the points that should be included in any care and maintenance protocol:

- Ensure adequate training in processing techniques has been given, with a written record kept in the radiation protection file
- Always carry out the pre-processing checks correctly

415

- Always wear suitable personal protective equipment (PPE) when handling all processing chemicals, as they are toxic
- Follow the surgery policy on topping up and changing spent solutions – normally all will require full replacement on a monthly basis
- Dispose of all waste solutions as **non-infectious hazardous waste**, under the health and safety policy (see Chapter 4)
- Follow the training given and the manufacturer's guidelines on cleaning the processing area or the automatic processor, to avoid film contamination
- This is especially important with regard to the roller system in automatic machines, as films can stick to dirty rollers and their images will be destroyed

Be aware of the correct functioning of the equipment, so that failures can be recognised, the equipment switched off safely and the matter reported to the necessary person for repair.

Therefore, if the warning lights on the automatic processor do not go off after the usual remedial action has been taken (such as the low solution level indicator light staying on after the solutions have been topped up), the machine is malfunctioning and should be disconnected from the electricity supply. An "out of use" sign should be displayed on the machine so that other staff members are aware of the malfunction, and the workplace policy must be followed with regard to the person to whom the fault should be reported. This could be the employer, a senior dentist or the practice manager.

In addition, poor-quality or unreadable radiographs will be produced if old film stock is used or if the stock has not been stored correctly. Films can still deteriorate before their expiry date if stored in hot or damp places or if they are kept too near an X-ray set.

Unexposed film packets must be stored as follows:

- Away from all sources of radiation
- Away from all heat sources, and ideally at room temperature
- Away from all liquids that may penetrate the packets and destroy the films before use
- In stock rotation, so that older films are used first

If an expiry date is given on a packet of film, it should not be used beyond that date. Any remaining films should be discarded, as old film will not expose correctly and the image produced will be of poor quality, or possibly unreadable. This will result in the patient having to be re-exposed to produce the same image, which is in direct contravention of the principles of ALARA/P.

Radiograph exposure, handling and processing faults

Exposure faults

Although many dental workplaces have abandoned manual processing in favour of automatic methods, it is still necessary for all dental nurses to understand what happens to a film during exposure and processing. This will help them to run QA systems that will trace any causes of error and help to prevent the need for retakes.

Faults that occur during exposure are the responsibility of the operator taking the view.

Any part of a film exposed to X-rays or daylight is turned black and opaque by the developer solution. The remaining unexposed part is still sensitive to light and appears green and opaque. Fixer dissolves away the unexposed green part, leaving it completely transparent and no longer sensitive to light. Some common faults that occur during **exposure** are outlined in the following table (see also Figure 14.15).

Fault	Reason
Elongation of image (Figure 14.15a)	Collimator angulation is too shallow, producing a long image
Foreshortening of image (Figure 14.15b)	Collimator angulation is too steep, producing a squat image
Coning (Figure 14.15c)	Collimator angulation is not central to the film, so film is only partly exposed
Blurred image	Patient or collimator moved during exposure
Transparent film, or faint image with overlying pattern (Figure 14.15d)	Film placed the wrong way round to the collimator for exposure, with the lead foil pattern superimposed onto the film – this may not always appear as the traditional "herringbone" pattern
Fogged film	Exposed to light before X-ray exposure (this may occur with extra-oral films, as they are being loaded into the cassette)
Blank film	X-ray machine not switched on, although this is unlikely to happen with modern machines, as they have exposure lights and audio signals installed

(a)   (b)

(c)   (d)

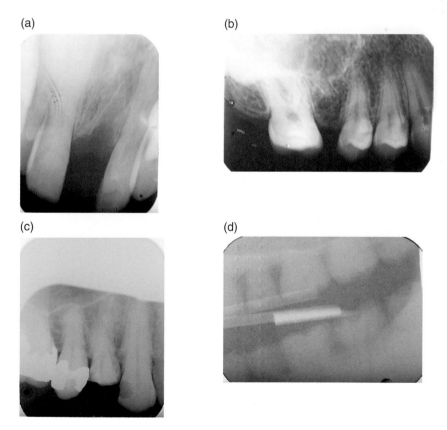

Figure 14.15   Radiograph exposure faults: (a) elongation; (b) foreshortening; (c) coning; (d) reversed film. Source: *Levison's Textbook for Dental Nurses*, 11th edition (Hollins), 2013. Reproduced with permission of Wiley-Blackwell.

Handling faults

Faults can also occur due to a poor handling technique or by poor preparation of the processing equipment – these are both the responsibility of the dental nurse tasked with processing the exposed film. All of these faults are avoidable by adequate training and by following procedures accurately. Some common handling faults are outlined in the following table (see also Figure 14.16).

Faults	Reasons
Scratches or fingerprints (Figure 14.16a)	Catching the film on the tank side during immersion Not holding the film by the edges
Blank spots (Figure 14.16b)	Film splashed with fixer before developing
Black line across film	Film bent or folded during processing
Brown or green stains	Inadequate fixing due to old solution
Crazed pattern on film (Figure 14.16c)	Film dried too quickly over a strong heat source
Presence of crystals on film (Figure 14.16d)	Insufficient washing after fixing

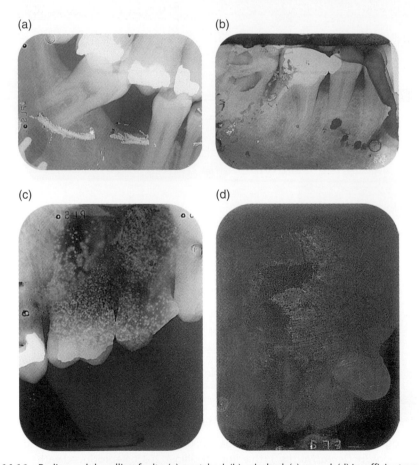

(a) (b) (c) (d)

Figure 14.16 Radiograph handling faults: (a) scratched; (b) splashed; (c) crazed; (d) insufficient washing.

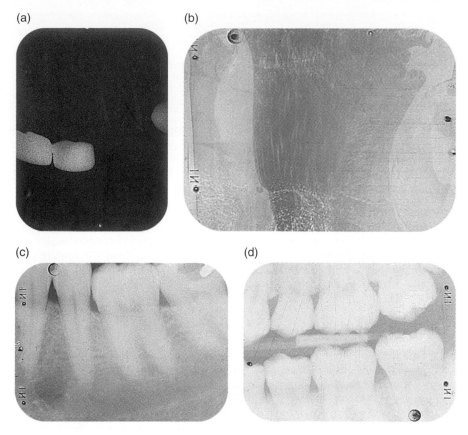

Figure 14.17 Radiograph processing faults: (a) dark film; (b) blank film; (c) fogged film; (d) faint film.

Processing faults

Poor quality radiographs can also be produced due to **equipment preparation faults**, and especially by lack of solution preparation and maintenance of the automatic processor. As the massive majority of film processing will be undertaken by the dental nurse in the workplace, knowledge of the faults, their occurrence and avoidance, and correct processing techniques, should be basic topics of study and understanding for every dental nurse throughout their career.

Some common processing faults are outlined in the following table (see also Figure 14.17).

Faults	Reasons
Dark film (Figure 14.17a)	Developer solution too concentrated Developer solution temperature too high Over developed
Blank film (Figure 14.17b)	Film placed in fixer solution before developer solution, so the image is destroyed
Partly blank film	Film partially immersed in developer solution
Fogged film (Figure 14.17c)	Processing room or machine is not light-tight, so the film is exposed to light before processing

Faults	Reasons
Faint image (Figure 14.17d)	Developer solution too weak Developer solution temperature too low Under-developed
Fading image	Inadequate fixing time so image is not permanently held on the film
Loss of film	Film stuck in roller system due to poor cleaning and maintenance of automatic processor
Visible artefacts	Film contaminated with solution spillages, in cassettes or on work surfaces

Every radiograph must not only be clinically justified but also of diagnostic value, so that an accurate diagnosis can be made and treatment planned accordingly. There should be no need for retakes because of faulty exposure or handling techniques, or poor processing skills. Retakes mean unnecessary additional exposure of patients and staff to X-rays. To ensure perfect results, the films must be in good condition, exposed correctly, processed carefully and mounted properly.

Quality assurance of films

All of the faults that may occur during the taking or processing of a radiograph, which may result in the patient having to undergo a retake, are avoidable. However, it may not be realised by the dental team that there is a recurring problem unless radiographs are regularly checked for quality, and this is especially the case in large, multi-dentist workplaces. A processing fault may affect the radiographs of several dentists, but unless someone is analysing the radiographs from all surgeries, it can easily be overlooked. This is the purpose of a QA system – where all radiographs are analysed and scored according to a universal system of quality so that commonly occurring problems will be identified.

With suitable training, a QA system of radiograph analysis can easily be carried out by the dental nurse, the aim being to reduce all faults to a minimum or to eliminate them completely. Indeed, in line with the relevant ionising radiation legislation and with clinical governance, having a QA system in dental workplaces is now a legal requirement.

To protect both patients and the dental team from unnecessary ionising radiation exposure, it is everyone's duty to ensure that the occurrence of the faults described in the preceding section are either kept to a minimum or eliminated completely. To do this involves assessing the quality of the films processed to determine the following:

- How readable is the film?
- Is a fault present?
- What is the fault?
- How has it occurred?
- How can it be prevented from recurring?
- Is re-exposure of the patient necessary?

When run correctly, the QA system should achieve the following:

- Involve a simple-to-use scoring system that is understood and followed by all staff
- Easily identify any areas of concern
- Develop solutions to the problems identified

- Limit the number of patient exposures to the minimum required for clinical necessity
- Achieve ALARA/ALARP

A simple-to-use scoring system set out in clinical governance guidelines is as follows:

- **Score 1 – excellent** quality radiograph with no errors present
- **Score 2 – diagnostically acceptable** quality, minimal errors present that do not prevent the radiograph from being used for diagnosis
- **Score 3 – unacceptable quality**, where errors present prevent the radiograph from being used for diagnosis, and will therefore involve a retake

Score 1 should be at a minimum of 70% of all exposures, while score 3 should be at a maximum of 10%. The results need to be easily recorded after every exposure so that they can be analysed on a regular basis and any problems identified. A typical recording system is shown in the following table.

Date	Operator	Patient ID	Radiograph	QA score	Details
4.4.12	DTH	4173	L/R BWs	1 and 1	N/A
4.4.12	JM	854	PA UL6,7	2	Coned, unable to use holder
5.4.12	TNL	1559	DPT	1	N/A
5.4.12	DTH	6212	PA UR2	1	N/A
5.4.12	CSH	377	AO-maxilla	2	Elongated but canines visible
6.4.12	JM	5458	L/R BWs	1 and 2	R BW coned
6.4.12	TNL	905	PA UL4	3	Missed apex for endo - retake
6.4.12	TNL	905	PA UL4	1	N/A

Details of the view taken are shown in the fourth column, with the QA score of 1, 2 or 3 in the fifth column. When 2 or 3 is scored, a note on the fault found must be made in the final column to show that analysis has taken place. Obviously, all films that score 1 require no further detail to be added.

All columns require completion for every radiograph analysis, otherwise patterns of faults between operators and views cannot be determined. For example, one operator may not routinely use film holders when taking periapicals, so a pattern of scores 2 and 3 may emerge for these views, and for this operator only. Analysis will conclude that the operator has no faults with other views, so it is safe to assume that the fault lies with attempting to align the periapicals without a holder, and that a holder must therefore be used routinely in future.

A similar QA system can be set up to monitor other areas of dental radiography, such as equipment, working procedures and staff training.

Handling of chemicals

When the dental workplace uses a manual or automatic processing technique for radiographs, rather than a digital system, various chemicals will be required to be used, stored and disposed of in accordance with health and safety and environmental protection legislation, and in compliance with waste disposal regulations. The duties involved are usually assigned to a dental nurse, so it is important that they are aware of the safe handling of these chemicals, and the health and safety issues involved. As with all other chemicals used on the premises, a COSHH assessment will have been carried out for them, and these should be accessed by any staff member involved in their handling and use.

The developer solution is provided in plastic bottles, either ready diluted for use (Figure 14.18) or as a concentrate which requires dilution on the premises. The solution itself is alkaline (pH > 7) and has a pungent odour that may irritate the respiratory system if used in an enclosed space. Similarly, the fixer solution may be ready to use (Figure 14.19) or require dilution, and it is acidic (pH < 7) with a lighter colour and pungent odour.

When diluting solutions, filling or topping up the processor tanks, or draining the tanks when the solutions require replacement, adequate PPE must be worn and the correct equipment used to avoid accidents, including spillages, as follows:

- Gloves should be worn to prevent skin contamination from splashed chemicals, which may be irritant – heavy-duty gloves rather than surgery gloves would be ideal
- Eye protection should also be worn for the same reason
- The chemicals should not be handled in an enclosed space, so an extractor fan should be in use in small areas
- A mask should be worn to reduce the inhalation of the vapours as far as possible – a visor alone is not sufficient in these circumstances
- A disposable plastic apron should be worn to prevent splashes on the uniform
- Full bottles of either chemical might be too heavy to lift for some staff, so a plastic jug might be required to carry smaller volumes safely
- If one jug is provided, it must be thoroughly rinsed and dried between chemicals to avoid contamination of one solution with the other

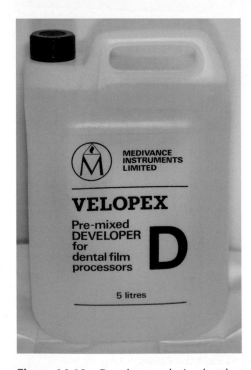

Figure 14.18   Developer solution bottle.

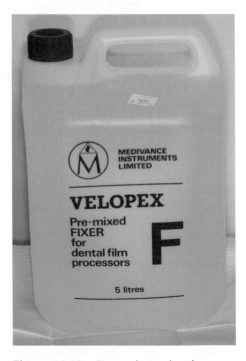

Figure 14.19   Fixer solution bottle.

- When filling or topping up the processor tanks, step ladders may be required to allow the staff member to stand safely above the machine and enable them to see clearly into the various tanks
- A plastic funnel must be used to pour the solutions accurately into the tanks and avoid spillages, and again it must be rinsed and dried between chemicals
- It may require a colleague to assist by holding the funnel firmly while the solutions are being poured, to avoid spillages
- Any spilled chemicals should be wiped away or mopped up immediately and the area washed with a detergent solution to prevent staining of the work surface by the chemicals
- All PPE and used disposable cloths should be disposed of appropriately as non-infectious hazardous waste

When the processing chemical tanks are to be drained so that the solutions can be replaced and the machine cleaned, the waste solutions are usually collected into separate large storage drums (see Figure 1.27).

These are very heavy and should not have to be moved by staff members once they are in use, unless appropriate handling equipment (such as a sack trolley) is available. Ideally, they should be able to remain in place during use and then only handled by the hazardous waste contractor when they require removal and replacement.

423

Storage and waste collection

As with all chemicals stored and used in the dental workplace, processing solutions are subject to the conditions of the Special Waste and Hazardous Waste Regulations (2005), including that they must be held in a secure area where only staff members have access, so that patients, their children, and any visitors to the premises cannot come to any harm. Every member of staff has a duty of care to ensure that this is the case in their workplace. All health and safety policies and procedures must be followed by all staff, especially those that involve the security of chemical storage areas.

Stocks of fresh processing chemicals should be retained in their original containers until ready for use, and these should be kept out of direct sunlight in a locked storage area or cupboard at room temperature.

Again, full PPE should be worn during the drainage and replenishment process of the tanks, as detailed earlier. Most processing machines have removable drain plugs and pipes from each tank to assist the procedure and avoid spillages, and these should run directly into the individual waste storage tanks. As discussed previously, waste solutions should stay in their storage drums in situ, so the processing area should only be accessible by staff members.

The waste solutions must only be collected and removed from the premises by licensed waste contractors, as disposal of the chemicals must follow strict environmental legislation, in accordance with the Environmental Protection Act.

Spillages

If a spillage does occur, the procedure to follow is:

- Wear suitable PPE before handling any of the chemicals
- Although the vapours may be irritant to some staff, especially in an enclosed space, they are not toxic
- The chemicals themselves are harmful, particularly if they are splashed into the eyes or ingested, so eye protection must always be worn and common sense should dictate that no chemical used in the dental workplace is ingested by anyone

- If splashes to the eye or ingestion do occur, the COSHH file must be consulted for the correct emergency first aid treatment to be provided to the casualty
- If a spillage occurs, it should be covered with paper towels to minimise the release of vapours and soak up the majority of the liquid
- Wash down the spillage area with a warm detergent solution and then dry thoroughly with more paper towels or a mop, or allow evaporation to take place
- Any wet floor area should be highlighted to staff and workplace visitors using the necessary signage (see Figure 1.2)
- A risk assessment should be carried out to determine the cause of a large spillage, so that appropriate action can be taken to avoid a similar incident in the future

15

Unit 315: Scientific Principles in the Management of Oral Health Diseases and Dental Procedures

Learning outcomes

1. Know the common oral diseases
2. Understand the methods for the prevention and management of oral diseases
3. Know how to manage and handle materials and instruments during dental procedures
4. Understand the purpose and stages of different dental procedures

Outcome 1 assessment criteria
The learner can:
- Describe the aetiology and progression of caries
- Describe the aetiology and progression of periodontal disease
- Explain the development of plaque and its composition
- Describe the inflammatory process and effects of the disease process

Outcome 2 assessment criteria
The learner can:
- Describe the main types and causes of oral diseases
- Explain the different oral hygiene techniques used to prevent oral diseases

Diploma in Dental Nursing, Level 3, Third Edition. Carole Hollins.
© 2014 John Wiley & Sons, Ltd. Published 2014 by John Wiley & Sons, Ltd.
Companion website: www.wiley.com/go/hollins/dentalnursinglevel3

- Describe how diet and social factors can affect oral health
- Explain the different forms of fluoride and its optimal level
- Explain the methods of communicating information about the prevention of oral diseases

Outcome 3 assessment criteria

The learner can:

- List and state the functions of different equipment, instruments, materials and medicaments used in:
  - Preparation, restoration and finishing of cavities
  - Periodontal therapy and their functions
  - Different stages of endodontic treatment
  - Crowns, bridges and veneers
  - Complete, partial and immediate dentures
  - Different stages of orthodontic treatment
- Describe the advantages/disadvantages and hazards associated with:
  - Restorative materials
  - Lining materials
  - Different types of etchants
  - Different types of bonding agents
  - Curing lights
- Explain the uses, manipulation, disinfection and storage of different impression materials
- Explain the hazards associated with amalgam and how to deal with a mercury spillage
- Explain the importance of matrix systems, and the equipment and instruments that may be used
- Describe the types of equipment used in the administration of local and regional anaesthesia

Outcome 4 assessment criteria

The learner can:

- Explain the different stages in cavity preparation for:
  - Permanent teeth
  - Deciduous teeth
- Explain the purposes of permanent and temporary crowns, bridges and veneer techniques
- Explain the different stages in making complete and partial prostheses, including advice and after care
- List the different types of non-surgical endodontic treatment
- Explain which type of appliance may be used for the different orthodontic treatments
- List the benefits of the treatments available for replacing missing teeth

This unit is assessed by:
- an assessment paper containing multiple choice and short answer questions

The content is the theory and underpinning knowledge required and links to the information contained in Chapters 1, 5, 8, 9, 10 and 11.

Common oral diseases

The three main oral diseases of concern to the dental team are as follows:

- **Dental caries** – the bacterial infection of the mineralised tissues of the tooth
- **Gingivitis** – the inflammation of the gingival tissues at the neck of the tooth
- **Periodontitis** – the inflammation of the supporting structures of the tooth

Their prevalence throughout the world, especially that of caries in developed countries, provides the vast majority of the day-to-day work of dental team members during their working lives. Other periodontal conditions that may be seen from time to time are also mentioned, as is the occurrence of non-carious tooth wear conditions, for the sake of completeness.

Gingivitis and periodontitis are discussed together as periodontal disease.

Dental caries

Dental caries (tooth decay) is a bacterial disease of the mineralised tissues of the tooth, where the strong crystal structure found in both enamel and dentine is **demineralised** (dissolved) by the action of acids. This allows the softer organic component of the tooth structure to be broken down to form cavities.

The acids involved are produced as a waste product by oral bacteria, as they digest the foods we eat for their own nutrition. Although the acids are relatively weak organic ones, such as **lactic acid** or **citric acid**, they are strong enough to attack enamel and dentine. Not all of the bacteria found in the oral cavity are associated with the production of these acids, and the usual ones involved are listed below:

- *Streptococcus mutans* (initial stages of cavity formation)
- *Streptococcus sanguis*
- Some **lactobacilli** (later stages of cavity formation)

427

Not all of the foods that we eat can be broken down into acids either, but those foods that can easily be formed into these damaging organic acids contain carbohydrates. Foods that consist of protein or fats are not relevant to the onset of dental caries. So, in summary, the relevant factors in the development of dental caries are:

- The presence of certain types of **bacteria**
- **Carbohydrate foods**
- The production of **weak organic acids** by these bacteria
- Adequate **time or frequency** for the acids to attack the tooth

The bacteria involved need to become attached to the tooth surface to be able to digest food debris and initiate dental caries, and they do this by forming themselves into a sticky layer called **bacterial plaque**.

Bacterial plaque

Millions of bacteria live in our mouths, flourishing on the food that we eat. Some of this food sticks to our teeth and attracts colonies of bacteria to the tooth surfaces concerned. This combination of bacteria and food debris on a tooth surface forms a thin, transparent, protein-containing, soft and sticky film called **plaque**. It tends to form and stick most readily in areas where it cannot be easily dislodged, such as at the **gingival margins** of the teeth (Figure 15.1), in the **fissures** of teeth, and around the edges of **dental restorations**. These are called **stagnation areas**.

The build-up of plaque at the gingival margins of the teeth is directly associated with the onset of **gingivitis** and **periodontal disease**. The plaque that sticks to the tooth surfaces allows the bacteria living within it to turn sugar into weak acids, which in turn dissolve enamel to produce **dental caries**.

The main microorganism which initiates the process of caries is ***Streptococcus mutans***. Large numbers of **lactobacilli** are then later able to thrive in the acid environment, and the presence of these two microorganisms is put to practical use as a test for caries activity. By periodically counting the number of mutans streptococci or lactobacilli in a patient's saliva, the level of caries activity and the effect of preventive measures can be monitored.

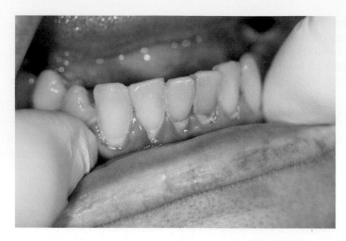

Figure 15.1   Gingival plaque.

Carbohydrates and sugars

All types of food are classified into three distinct groups:

- Protein – such as meats, fish, various dairy products and pulses
- Fat – such as animal fats and vegetable oils
- Carbohydrate – natural sugars and starches from fruit and vegetables, and artificial sugars from processed foods

Of these, only carbohydrates can be turned into acid by bacteria and thereby cause caries – so they are described as **cariogenic foods** because they are capable of causing caries. The most acid-producing carbohydrates are those that are artificially added during food preparation, and which therefore tend to be based on **non-milk extrinsic sugars (NMES)**.

As their name suggests, these types of sugar are not derived from milk and have been added artificially to the food during the manufacturing process, rather than being found naturally in the food product itself. The most damaging ones of all are the **refined sugars sucrose and glucose** (also called dextrose).

Naturally occurring sugars that produce so little organic acid that they are considered harmless to teeth include the following:

- **Intrinsic sugars** – found naturally in foods, such as **fructose** in fruits
- **Milk extrinsic sugars** – especially lactose

Refined sugars can be instantaneously turned into acid by the bacteria concerned, and the available types include table sugar, sugar used in cooking and sugar added to anything else taken by mouth, whether liquid or solid. Any food containing added sugar can cause caries; some obvious ones are:

- Cake, biscuits, jam and sweets
- Breakfast cereals
- Pastry, desserts, canned fruit, syrups and ice cream
- Soft drinks
- Hot beverages sweetened with sugar

Sugar is widely added to many savoury foods, too, in order to flavour or preserve them, but without making its taste apparent. Such foods can include soups, sauces, canned vegetables and breakfast cereals and are accordingly sources of **hidden sugar**. Medicines may also contain hidden sugar and can be a significant cause of caries in chronically sick children, those who are ill over long periods and require many courses of medication.

Sugar occurring naturally in milk, fruit and vegetables is not a significant cause of caries. Naturally starchy and fibrous vegetables such as potatoes, carrots, peas and beans are rich in carbohydrate but may be regarded as insignificant causes of caries as long as no sugar is added by producers or during cooking. The prime cause of dental caries is refined sugar (**sucrose**) processed from sugar beet and sugar cane, and commercial **glucose**, which together constitute such a large proportion of the manufactured and sweetened food in our diet. Unfortunately, foods containing these NMES tend to be a cheap and readily available food source in most developed countries, along with acidic drinks such as carbonated "fizzy pop".

Acid formation

As soon as the carbohydrate food source is eaten, the oral bacteria take the sugar component into the plaque structure and begin to digest it themselves. Within just a minute or two, it is turned into acid by the plaque bacteria and this then attacks the enamel surface beneath the plaque. Enough acid is produced to last for about 20 minutes, and in this initial acid attack a microscopic layer of enamel is dissolved away. This phase is called **demineralisation**.

At the end of the meal or snack, when the intake of sugar is over, the acid persists for a period of time ranging from 20 minutes to 2 hours before it is neutralised by the buffering action of saliva.

Saliva is the fluid bathing the oral cavity that is secreted from the salivary glands (see Chapter 13). Amongst its many roles, it maintains the mouth at a **neutral level**, being neither acidic nor alkaline. The measure of acidity/alkalinity of a solution is called its **pH level**, and the neutral level maintained by saliva is **pH 7**. When the weak organic acids are produced by the oral bacteria, the pH level starts to fall and, once it passes the **critical pH 5.5**, the environment is acidic enough to attack the enamel and dentine of teeth and produce cavities.

Once neutralisation has occurred, no further demineralisation can take place until such time as more sugar is consumed. In this phase where no more sugar is present in the plaque, some natural healing takes place; mineral constituents naturally present in saliva enter demineralised enamel and restore the part lost by the initial acid attack. This healing phase is called **remineralisation**.

What happens next is entirely dependent on the frequency of sugar intake. If it is confined to mealtimes only, e.g. breakfast, midday and early evening, there can only be three acid attacks a day on the teeth. The amount of time available for remineralisation will greatly exceed that of demineralisation and the initial phase of caries will be arrested. But if a series of snacks is eaten between meals throughout the day, the reverse will occur and there will be more episodes of demineralisation than there are of remineralisation. This is because most processed snacks contain some added sugar and the result is a rapid succession of acid attacks, with insufficient respite between them for saliva to neutralise the acid and allow the healing process of remineralisation to become dominant. Caries can then spread rapidly through affected teeth, as described later.

The longer the sugar stays on the teeth, the longer the duration of acid production. Thus sweet fluids, such as tea or coffee with sugar, which are rapidly washed off the teeth by saliva, are not normally a major cause of caries unless many drinks are taken throughout the day, whereas the much more frequent consumption of very sweet soft drinks by children is far more serious. But, overall, the most dangerous sources of sugar are those that have a sticky consistency when chewed, as it is far more difficult for the natural saliva flow to wash them away. The adherent nature of such foods allows them to cling to the teeth for a very long time, throughout which they are supplying plaque bacteria with the raw materials for prolonged acid formation and demineralisation.

Foremost among these sticky forms of sugar which cause caries are:

- Toffee and other sweets
- Cakes, biscuits, processed white bread and jam
- Puddings with syrup or treacle

Our modern diet is such that added sugar is consumed nearly every time something is eaten, and the teeth are attacked by acid on each of these occasions. If snacks containing such sugar are frequently taken between meals, there will be a corresponding increase in the number of acid attacks on the teeth. The delicate balance between the forces of destruction (demineralisation) and those of repair (remineralisation) will then be completely upset in favour of tooth destruction, and **irreversible** damage will occur.

Thus it is evident that the prime cause of caries is the frequent and unrestricted consumption of sweet snacks **between** meals. It is not the amount of sugar eaten but the **frequency** with which it is eaten that is all-important. This fundamental fact forms the basis of personal caries prevention and good dental health education.

Sites of caries

The parts of a tooth most prone to caries are those where food tends to collect easily during normal chewing movements and plaque bacteria can flourish. Such sites are known as **stagnation areas**. Occlusal fissures and the spaces between the mesial and distal surfaces of adjoining teeth (the inter-proximal areas, or contact points) are the commonest stagnation areas. That is why caries occurs most often on occlusal and proximal surfaces. However, any other part of the tooth where food debris can accumulate is a stagnation area where plaque will proliferate and caries is likely to occur. Such food traps are the necks of teeth covered by ill-fitting partial dentures, irregular teeth in the arch line, and unopposed teeth in either jaw, as food debris is not dislodged easily from these areas.

Minimal harm is caused by partial dentures that fit perfectly, but those that do not are a menace to dental health. They leave spaces between the necks of the teeth and the acrylic plate or between any metal clasps and the teeth, which are dangerous stagnation areas.

During mastication, the movement of saliva and the food bolus over the tooth surfaces as it is chewed actually helps to clean teeth that are in good occlusion. This does not prevent plaque formation, but does reduce the amount of retained food debris which is responsible for the harmful effects of plaque. Teeth that are not in good occlusion, such as irregularly positioned and unopposed teeth, are not so exposed to this beneficial cleansing effect of mastication. Consequently, food collects around these instanding or outstanding irregular teeth. It also covers the crown of any tooth that has lost its opposing tooth in the other jaw, and remains unopposed because the space has not been replaced artificially. To make the situation even worse, the sticky sweet food most likely to produce caries needs the minimum amount of mastication anyway, and therefore has a negligible cleansing effect – even on teeth in good occlusion.

Caries and cavity formation

Unrestricted consumption of carbohydrates and their sugar content produces an abundance of acid-forming bacteria in the plaque which collects in stagnation areas. The resultant series of continual acid attacks prevents remineralisation from occurring and allows acid to eat through the enamel until it reaches dentine, whereupon the caries spreads more rapidly through the hollow, more open structure of this inner tooth layer (Figure 15.2).

Microscopically, the process of cavity formation is as follows:

- Very early acid attacks will show as "white spot lesions" on the enamel surface
- Continued and frequent acid attacks will follow the prism structure of the enamel and eat into any exposed cementum on the tooth root

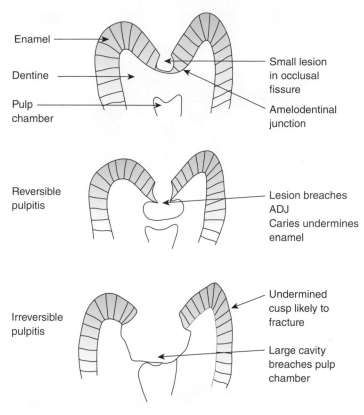

Figure 15.2   Cavity formation (ADJ, amelodentinal junction). Source: *Levison's Textbook for Dental Nurses*, 11th edition (Hollins), 2013. Reproduced with permission of Wiley-Blackwell.

- **Demineralisation** occurs, followed by episodes of **remineralisation** if the acid attacks are not too frequent – these areas of repair often appear as brown lesions on the teeth, especially at contact points (Figure 15.3)
- With frequent or prolonged acid attacks, the mineral structure of the enamel is eventually destroyed and caries enters the tooth
- Caries extends deep into the enamel and eventually reaches the **amelodentinal junction (ADJ)** – the point at which the enamel and dentine layers meet
- Up to this point, the patient will feel no pain, as enamel contains no nerve tissue
- Once past the ADJ, the caries enters dentine and can spread more rapidly because of the hollow structure of this tooth layer and its lower mineral content compared to enamel
- This undermines the overlying enamel, and normal occlusal forces are able to fracture off pieces of the tooth surface, leaving a hole in the tooth structure – this is called a **cavity** (Figure 15.4)
- Odontoblast cells (which form dentine) at the ADJ react to the bacterial attack by laying down **secondary dentine** in an attempt to protect the underlying pulp tissue
- The nerve fibrils lying within the dentine tubules will be stimulated as the caries progresses, and the patient will begin to feel sensitivity to temperature changes and to sweet foods
- The pulp tissue will also become irritated and inflamed; this is called **pulpitis**
- At this point, the caries can be removed by the dentist and the cavity restored with a **filling** (see later in this chapter and Chapter 8), the inflamed pulp will settle and the tooth will be restored to its normal function – the inflammation is then better described as **reversible pulpitis**

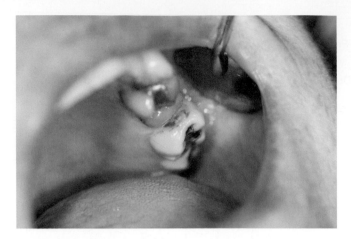

Figure 15.3   Brown spot lesion.

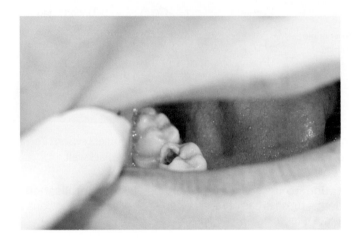

Figure 15.4   Tooth cavity.

- Otherwise, the cavity will continue to enlarge and the caries will progress towards the pulp chamber, as the production of secondary dentine is overrun by the speed of the bacterial attack
- The patient will be experiencing more severe pain of longer duration and will eventually be unable to bite with the affected tooth
- When the carious attack reaches the immediate surroundings of the pulp chamber, the level of inflammation is too great to be resolved simply by removing the caries – this condition is called **irreversible pulpitis**
- The pain will become constant and throbbing in nature, often disturbing the patient's sleep
- Once the pulp chamber itself is breached by the caries, a **carious exposure** of the contents occurs and the pulp will eventually die
- The tooth can now only be treated by undergoing an endodontic procedure (see later and Chapter 10) or by extraction (see Chapter 11)

Irreversible pulpitis

Pulpitis (inflammation of the pulp) occurs when caries extends through the dentine to reach the pulp. The pulp is then said to be **cariously exposed** and the sequence of events described under inflammation (see Chapter 12) follows:

- There is an increased blood flow through the apical foramen into the pulp
- Swelling cannot occur, however, as the pulp is confined within the rigid walls of the root canal and pulp chamber
- Pressure therefore builds up instead and causes intense pain
- Another effect of this increased pressure is the compression of blood vessels passing through the tiny apical foramen – this cuts off the blood supply to the tooth and causes death of the pulp
- When the pulp dies, its nerves die too, and the severe toothache stops abruptly
- The respite is short, however, as pulp death leads to another very painful condition called alveolar abscess

Pulpitis may be acute or chronic. It has many causes, apart from caries, but almost always ends in pulp death. Other causes of pulpitis are covered later and in Chapter 10.

Alveolar abscess

433

When pulpitis occurs, the pulp eventually dies as its blood supply is cut off by inflammatory pressure. The dead pulp decomposes and infected material passes out of the tooth through the apical foramen and into the alveolar bone surrounding the apex of the tooth. These irritant products give rise to another inflammatory reaction in the tissues surrounding the apex. Pus formation occurs and an **acute alveolar abscess** develops:

- This is an extremely painful condition
- The affected tooth becomes loose and very tender to the slightest pressure
- There is a continual throbbing pain and the surrounding gum is red and swollen
- Frequently, inflammatory swelling involves the whole side of the face and the patient may have a raised body temperature (pyrexia)
- Looseness is caused by swelling of the periodontal ligament
- Pain is caused by the increased pressure of blood within the rigid confines of the periodontal ligament and alveolar bone. The tooth is so tender that it cannot be used for eating
- Thus an acute alveolar abscess may show all of the cardinal signs of acute inflammation:
  - Pain
  - Swelling
  - Redness
  - Heat
  - Loss of function
  - Raised body temperature

Pulp death is sometimes followed by the development of a **chronic alveolar abscess** instead of an acute one. This usually gives rise to very little pain and most patients are quite unaware of its presence. It may often be detected by the dentist due to the presence of a small hole in the gum called a **sinus**, which is a track leading from the abscess cavity in the alveolar bone to the surface of the gum. Pus drains from the abscess through the sinus into the mouth. This outlet prevents a build-up of pressure inside the bone and explains the lack of pain. Patients often refer to this lesion as a "gum boil".

If an acute abscess is not treated, it eventually turns into a chronic abscess by the drainage of pus through a sinus (Figure 15.5). This relieves the pain and the features of acute inflammation

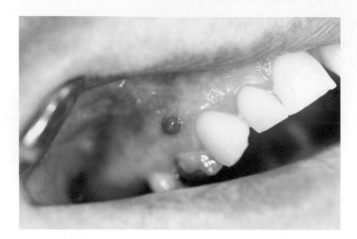

Figure 15.5 Chronic abscess with sinus.

largely disappear. The relative freedom from pain does not last indefinitely, however, as a chronic alveolar abscess is liable to revert into an acute abscess at any time.

It should now be clear that pulpitis is followed by pulp death, which eventually leads to an acute alveolar abscess, either directly or via a chronic abscess.

It was formerly taught that all carious dentine should be removed, but this is now considered unnecessary. Adequate preparation, filling and sealing of a cavity cuts it off from further plaque and acid formation and allows a vital pulp to remineralise the deeper underlying dentine. Removal of carious dentine should therefore stop short of exposing the pulp when possible.

Role of saliva in oral health

The oral soft tissues in health are constantly bathed in **saliva**, the watery secretion from the three pairs of major salivary glands as well as from the numerous minor salivary glands present in the cheeks and lips (see Chapter 13).

Saliva contains the following components:

- **Water**, as a transport agent for all of the other constituents
- **Inorganic ions and minerals**, such as calcium ions and phosphate
- **Ptyalin**, a digestive enzyme that acts on carbohydrates (also called **salivary amylase**)
- **Antibodies**, as part of the defensive immune system, and known as **immunoglobulins**
- **Leucocytes**, or white blood cells, also part of the body's defence system

These constituents all have important functions in the maintenance of a healthy oral environment, as described here:

- The **inorganic ions and minerals** are released as required to act as **buffering agents** to help control the pH of the oral environment, by neutralising the organic acids produced by bacteria
- A high inorganic ion/mineral content produces thick, stringy saliva which gives the teeth good protection against caries, but allows **dental calculus** (tartar) to form easily and in large amounts
- A low inorganic ion/mineral content produces watery saliva, which offers little protection to the teeth against caries, but prevents large amounts of calculus from forming
- Calculus formation is associated with **periodontal disease** (see later)

- **Water** forms the carrying agent for the other salivary constituents and allows self-cleansing of the oral environment to occur by dislodging food debris from the teeth before being swallowed
- The water also moistens the food bolus and the soft tissues, allowing **swallowing** (deglutition) and **speech** to occur
- It also **dissolves** food particles, so that the sensation of **taste** is produced – the taste buds on the tongue can only detect the taste of food when it is in solution (dissolved in water)
- Both **antibodies** and **leucocytes** help to protect and defend the oral environment from infection by microorganisms

Reduced salivary flow

The condition of a reduced salivary flow is called **xerostomia**, or **dry mouth**. There are many reasons why a patient can suffer from this, apart from it being the result of normal age-related changes of the salivary glands themselves. Other causes are as follows:

- Low fluid intake over a period of time, or even dehydration
- Some autoimmune disorders, especially **Sjögren's syndrome**, which specifically affects the salivary glands and the lacrimal glands of the eyes, which produce tears
- Several routinely prescribed drugs, including **diuretics** (prescribed to alleviate water retention in patients with heart failure), some **antidepressants** (prescribed to alleviate anxiety) and **beta-blockers** (prescribed to slow down the heart rate, especially in angina sufferers)

Reduced salivary flow has several important consequences for the patient and for the oral health team, as explained here:

- Reduced self-cleansing allows more food debris to accumulate around the teeth, increasing plaque production and the likelihood of caries and periodontal disease developing
- It will also allow food debris to stagnate in the mouth, causing **halitosis** (bad breath)
- Reduced buffering of the oral environment allows longer and more frequent acid attacks, increasing the likelihood of caries developing
- Poor lubrication of the oral soft tissues makes speech and swallowing more difficult
- Reduced amounts of water in the saliva affect the sensation of taste
- Reduced flow and amounts of saliva in the mouth will make the retention of dentures more difficult

The opposite condition of xerostomia, which is that of excessive saliva production, is called **ptyalism**, and is often seen in patients with periodontal disease. It can also occur in Parkinson's disease and temporarily in pregnancy.

Diagnosis of caries

Before caries is treated, it must first be detected. Early diagnosis is very important in controlling the extent of the damage done to a tooth, as well as reducing the level of discomfort experienced by the patient. The earlier a cavity is detected, the better the chance of saving the tooth. This is why regular dental examinations are recommended, and the frequency of attendance should be determined by the **caries experience** of the patient – those with a high caries incidence need to be examined more frequently than others. Unfortunately, these are often the very patients who do not attend regularly for dental examination, for various reasons.

Large cavities are obvious to the naked eye but it is easier to treat caries before cavities reach such a size. The dentist has various methods available for detecting smaller carious lesions, as follows:

- Close visible inspection under magnification (Figure 15.6), with the help of a bright examination light and a mouth mirror to reflect the light onto less visible areas

435

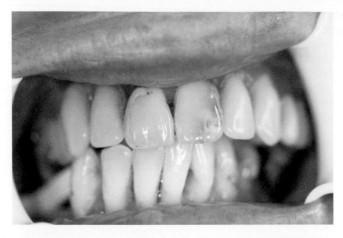

Figure 15.6   Enamel undermined by caries. Source: *Levison's Textbook for Dental Nurses*, 11th edition (Hollins), 2013. Reproduced with permission of Wiley-Blackwell.

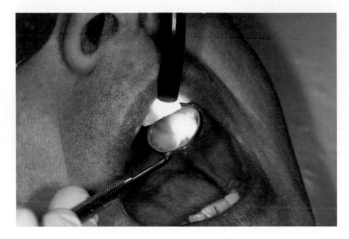

Figure 15.7   Transillumination technique.

- The use of various **blunt dental probes** to detect any stickiness in suspicious areas – particularly a **sickle probe** or **right-angle probe** for occlusal surfaces, and a special double-ended **Briault probe** for interproximal areas (see Figure 6.14)
- **Transillumination** of anterior teeth, using the curing light to shine through their contact points, and viewing from behind with a mouth mirror to detect any shadowing (Figure 15.7)
- **Caries dyes** wiped into prepared cavities to stain any residual bacteria to make them visible and allow their removal
- Periodical **horizontal bitewing radiographs** (see Chapter 14) to detect interproximal caries in posterior teeth
- These can also detect **recurrent caries** beneath existing restorations, as well as early caries beneath occlusal fissures

Although probes have traditionally been manufactured as sharp instruments, it is now realised that they may damage the enamel in the earliest stages of caries, if pressed hard into the tooth. For early detection of occlusal caries, the current advice is to thoroughly clean and dry the tooth surface, and carefully examine it with the aid of a very bright light and magnification. Early caries will then be indicated by loss of the normal shiny enamel surface and its transition to a dull white matt appearance. Early mesial and distal caries is detected with bitewing X-ray films, as already described.

The assessment methods used to diagnose and record the presence of carious lesions is discussed in detail in Chapter 13.

Periodontal disease

Periodontal disease is the oral disease that affects the supporting structures of the teeth. These supporting structures are the gingivae, the periodontal ligament (formerly called the periodontal membrane) and the alveolar bone. In addition, the intimate anatomical relationship between the cementum covering the tooth root and the periodontal ligament accounts for the cementum being included as a supporting structure, and therefore being affected by periodontal disease too.

Periodontal disease and caries are amongst the commonest diseases of civilisation. Caries is the major cause of tooth loss in children and young adults, while periodontal disease is the major cause in older people. This does not mean that periodontal disease starts much later in life, but that it takes so much longer than caries to cause tooth loss.

Indeed, there is a relatively uncommon, but specific, type of periodontal disease that begins in childhood rather than in adults, called **juvenile periodontitis**.

The earliest stage of periodontal disease is **chronic gingivitis** which is a chronic inflammation involving the gingivae alone. This can occur in a localised area and affect only a few teeth or it can occur generally and affect the majority of the dentition. Once present and if allowed to continue, the chronic inflammation spreads deep into the underlying cementum and periodontal ligament, and eventually to the alveolar bone. These structures are gradually destroyed and the teeth become very loose as their supporting tissues are lost. The name given to this late stage of the disease is **chronic periodontitis**. There is no obvious dividing line between the two stages, and untreated chronic gingivitis usually progresses into chronic periodontitis.

Although the disease process occurs gradually, there are usually intermittent episodes of disease activity alternating with quiescent phases of no activity in a sporadic manner.

Causes of periodontal disease

Periodontal disease is a bacterial infection of the supporting structures of the tooth, caused by an initial accumulation of **bacterial plaque** at the gingival margin of the tooth. Plaque is a tenacious transparent film of saliva, microorganisms and oral debris on the tooth surface (Figure 15.1). Food debris adheres to plaque, and the resultant paste of saliva and food remnants attracts far more microorganisms which feed and multiply on it.

It is the same plaque as that involved in the onset of dental caries. However, whereas caries can only occur when sugar is present in the plaque to form the acids that cause enamel demineralisation, the presence of sugar is not necessary for periodontal disease to occur. Any sort of food debris will allow plaque microbes to proliferate and cause it.

Plaque can be removed by adequate tooth brushing, but in the absence of this counter-measure, it thickens as its microbial population flourishes amid a permanent food supply. Toxic by-products of the plaque microorganisms then act as a continual source of bacterial irritation, which causes chronic inflammation of the gum margin (chronic gingivitis). The plaque extends above and below the gum margin, and wherever it is present **calculus** (tartar) formation can occur.

Calculus is the hard rock-like deposit commonly seen on the lingual surface of lower incisors (see Figure 13.34). Two factors are necessary for its formation: **plaque** and **saliva**. The interaction between these two factors allows mineralisation to occur within the plaque and produce a deposition of calculus, which may be defined as solidified plaque. It is most easily seen opposite the orifices of salivary gland ducts – on the lingual surface of lower incisors and the buccal surface of

437

upper molars. This visible calculus on the crowns of teeth has a yellowish colour and is called **supragingival calculus** as it forms above the gum margin. However, it also occurs in plaque beneath the gum margin on all teeth and in that situation it is known as **subgingival calculus**. This is harder and darker than supragingival calculus and its surface is covered with a layer of the soft microbial plaque from which it was formed.

Calculus plays only a **passive mechanical role** in periodontal disease. Its rough surface and ledges create food traps which are inaccessible to a toothbrush and thus allow even more food debris to fertilise the plaque. The **active role** in periodontal disease belongs to plaque microorganisms.

This description shows that supragingival plaque and calculus are associated with bad oral hygiene. If teeth are cleaned properly, the plaque and calculus are less able to accumulate. But if they are allowed to accumulate, they spread subgingivally and become inaccessible to tooth brushing.

Furthermore, there are some additional reasons for plaque formation which are not due to poor oral hygiene by the patient, but instead are caused by imperfect dentistry; these are known as **iatrogenic factors** and include:

- Fillings or crowns that have an overhanging edge at their cervical margin
- Fillings or crowns with loose contact points that allow food trapping to occur
- Ill-fitting or poorly designed partial dentures

These defects are all food traps which act as stagnation areas that the patient cannot keep clean. Plaque and calculus proliferate there and periodontal disease follows at these sites, even though the rest of the mouth may be perfectly healthy. Food stagnation also occurs on unopposed and irregular teeth, with consequent liability to periodontal disease as well as caries. The full microscopic sequence of events leading to periodontal disease will be described later in this chapter.

Periodontal tissues in health

To be able to recognise the presence of periodontal disease, the appearance of these tissues in health must first be identified. This is illustrated in Figure 15.8 and anatomically is as follows:

- The tooth sits in its socket within the alveolar bone
- It is attached to the bone by the fibres of the periodontal ligament, which run from the cementum of the root into the alveolar bone
- Other periodontal ligament fibres run from the alveolar bone crest to the neck of the tooth, and from the neck of the tooth into the gingival papilla
- The bone and the periodontal ligament are covered by the mucous membrane of the gingiva, which lines the alveolar ridges
- The gingiva is attached directly to the neck of the tooth itself at a specialised site called the **junctional epithelium**
- In health, a gingival crevice of up to 3 mm deep runs as a "gutter" around each tooth, the deepest part of which is the attachment of the junctional epithelium
- Looking at the tissues in the mouth, then, the gingiva is generally pink in colour with a stippled appearance like orange peel (there will be colour variations according to ethnicity)
- There is a tight gingival cuff around each tooth, then, with the gingival crevice no deeper than 3 mm
- The interdental papillae between the teeth are sharp, with a knife-edge appearance
- No bleeding occurs when the gingival crevice is gently probed during the dental examination
- Subgingivally, the periodontal ligament and alveolar bone are intact – this will only be visible on a radiograph

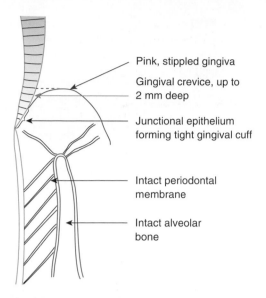

Pink, stippled gingiva

Gingival crevice, up to
2 mm deep

Junctional epithelium
forming tight gingival cuff

Intact periodontal
membrane

Intact alveolar
bone

Figure 15.8   Periodontium in health.

If plaque is allowed to accumulate around the gingival margins of the teeth, the gingiva will become inflamed and the first stage of periodontal disease, **gingivitis**, will develop. When this is a generalised condition affecting the oral cavity as a whole because of poor oral hygiene, it is called **chronic gingivitis**.

Chronic gingivitis

The sequence of events that occur microscopically and that lead to chronic gingivitis are as follows (see also Figure 15.9):

- The bacteria within the plaque at the gingival margins use food debris to nourish themselves, so that the colony grows in size
- They produce **toxins** (poisons) as a by-product during their own food digestion
- These toxins tend to accumulate in the gingival crevice, as they are not removed by oral hygiene measures or washed away by the normal cleansing action of saliva
- The gingiva in direct contact with the toxins becomes irritated, causing inflammation and the early signs of **chronic gingivitis**
- The inflamed gingiva becomes red in colour, and the swelling associated with the inflammation creates **false pockets** around the necks of the teeth – there appears to be a deepening of the gingival crevice but this is due to the swelling only, not to a loss of attachment between the junctional epithelium and the tooth; hence the name "false"
- The presence of these pockets allows more plaque to accumulate as cleansing becomes even more difficult, and the plaque now begins to extend below the gingival margin
- In this environment, there is little oxygen available for the initial bacteria to use, and the plaque becomes colonised by specialised bacteria that are able to survive without oxygen – these are called **anaerobic bacteria**
- Examples of these are ***Actinomyces*** and ***Porphyromonas gingivalis***, both of which are bacteria specifically associated with periodontal disease
- In the meantime, the inorganic ions within saliva are incorporated into the structure of the plaque so that it hardens and mineralises as **dental calculus** develops

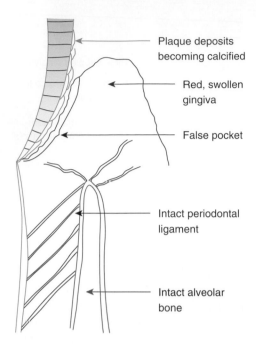

Plaque deposits
becoming calcified

Red, swollen
gingiva

False pocket

Intact periodontal
ligament

Intact alveolar
bone

Figure 15.9 Formation of chronic gingivitis.

- Calculus forming above the gingival margin is called **supragingival calculus** and is **yellow** in colour (see Figure 13.34)
- That forming below the gingival margin is called **subgingival calculus** and is **brown** in colour, due to the blood pigments incorporated into it from the bleeding gingival tissues
- The rough surface of the calculus irritates the gingiva further and allows more plaque to develop on it
- The rough calculus and the irritation of the bacterial toxins cause painless **micro-ulcers** to develop within the gingiva, so that they **bleed** on touch or gentle probing
- The red swollen gingiva and the presence of bleeding on probing are the classic visible signs of **chronic gingivitis**

Chronic gingivitis is fully reversible if the plaque and calculus are completely removed from above and below the gingival margins. This requires the intervention of the dental team by carrying out scaling of the teeth, after which the patient must maintain a good standard of oral hygiene.

Chronic periodontitis

If chronic gingivitis is not treated, microbial poisons from the plaque soak through the micro-ulcers in the gingival crevice and penetrate the deeper tissues. These poisons gradually destroy the periodontal ligament and alveolar bone, and while this is progressing, the gingival pocket deepens, thus further aggravating the condition. Whereas the false pockets of chronic gingivitis are caused by inflammatory swelling of the gum only, in chronic periodontitis they are **true pockets** caused by the destruction of the base of the gingival crevice and its attachment to the tooth. In other words, the attachment between the junctional epithelium and the tooth surface is lost.

At the same time, the gingival margin may recede, exposing the root of the tooth to view. This **gingival recession** is commonly known as being "long in the tooth". If no treatment is provided, so much bone is lost that the teeth eventually become too loose to be of any functional value.

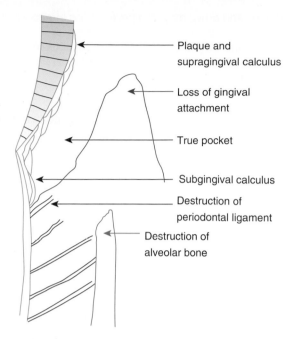

Plaque and
supragingival calculus

Loss of gingival
attachment

True pocket

Subgingival calculus

Destruction of
periodontal ligament

Destruction of
alveolar bone

Figure 15.10   Development of chronic periodontitis.

The sequence of events that occur microscopically in the development of chronic periodontitis are as follows (see also Figure 15.10):

- The bacterial toxins build up within the false pockets and eventually begin soaking into the gingival tissue itself, through the micro-ulcerated areas
- Here, they gradually destroy the periodontal ligament and the attachment of the tooth to its supporting tissues, and a **true pocket** forms
- The loss of attachment gradually moves down the tooth root, creating deeper pockets that allow even more plaque and calculus to develop within them
- The toxins eventually begin attacking the alveolar bone itself, destroying the walls of the tooth socket so that the tooth becomes loose
- This tooth loosening is often the first indication the patient has of the presence of their disease, as it is usually painless and often takes several years to reach this point
- Periodontitis also tends to have intermittent active phases where much tissue destruction occurs, interspersed with quiet phases of little bacterial activity, so in a sporadic fashion rather than occurring as a gradually progressive condition

This description of periodontal disease follows a slowly progressive but painless course of several years, but during that time pus and microorganisms in the pockets cause bad breath (**halitosis**) and may affect the patient's general health.

Once periodontal disease is established, it can be made worse by certain other factors, which do not in themselves cause the disease alone. Some of these aggravating factors are:

- Smoking
- Unbalanced or excessive masticatory stress
- Natural hormonal changes such as puberty and pregnancy
- Open lip posture (such as occurs during mouth breathing) which dries out the oral cavity and prevents the normal cleansing action of saliva to occur

Certain medical conditions and drugs may also have similar effects, such as:

- Diabetes, acquired immune deficiency syndrome (AIDS), leukaemia, and other blood disorders or diseases where resistance to infection is poor – these patients are referred to as being **immune-compromised**
- Epilepsy treated with phenytoin (Epanutin)
- Vitamin C deficiency
- Treatment with immunosuppressant drugs such as ciclosporin and cytotoxic agents (used to fight cancers)

Dental plaque forms in everyone's mouth in a short space of time after tooth brushing, but some factors exacerbate its accumulation in certain areas and in some patients' mouths. These are called **plaque retention factors**, some of which have already been mentioned:

- Poor oral hygiene due to apathy by the patient
- Poorly aligned teeth, a condition that increases the number of stagnation areas available for plaque to accumulate
- Incompetent lip seal, which allows the oral soft tissues to dry out and prevents the self-cleansing action of saliva to occur
- Small oral aperture, making effective tooth brushing difficult for the patient to achieve
- Iatrogenic causes (poor dentistry)

The rate of progress of periodontal disease depends on the balance between the patient's individual resistance to the bacterial attack and the toxic effects of plaque bacteria. Both these factors vary from time to time and in different parts of the mouth, and the predominant one will determine whether the disease appears dormant or progressive.

Diagnosis of periodontal disease

The diagnosis of periodontal disease is based on the medical history, appearance and recession of the gums, depth of gingival pockets, amount of bone loss, tooth mobility and the distribution of plaque.

Medical history

Periodontal disease affects the vast majority of the population, but most people are otherwise healthy and curable if they exercise adequate plaque control. However, patients with certain conditions are more at risk of severe periodontal disease and less likely to respond as favourably to treatment.

A regularly updated medical history is an essential feature of all patients' records, whatever their reason for attendance or the treatment required. As far as periodontal disease is concerned, the dentist will be particularly interested in:

- Past and present illnesses
- Drugs prescribed
- Hormonal changes, e.g. pregnancy
- Smoking habits

Relevant illnesses are those where resistance to infection is low, such as:

- Diabetes, leukaemia and other blood disorders
- Vitamin deficiencies
- AIDS
- Treatment with immunosuppressant drugs, e.g. ciclosporin (Sandimmun), used for some types of cancer and for organ transplant patients

Certain drugs can cause a severe, non-inflammatory enlargement of the gums called **gingival hyperplasia**, which requires surgical correction. Such drugs include:

- Phenytoin (Epanutin), used to control epilepsy
- Nifedipine (Adalat), used to control angina pectoris and reduce high blood pressure
- Ciclosporin, used to prevent organ rejection after transplant

Signs

There are many clinical signs that the dentist will look for during a routine dental examination to determine if periodontal disease is present. The signs of early onset chronic gingivitis are as follows:

- The gingiva bleed on brushing, or on gentle probing during the dental examination
- They appear visibly red and swollen
- Plaque is visible at the gingival margins of the teeth or can be shown using disclosing solution (see later)
- The patient has halitosis

With established gingivitis, pus can be expressed from the gingival crevice when the gingiva is gently pressed. The clinical signs of the presence of chronic periodontitis are as follows:

- Periodontal probing detects pockets > 3 mm
- Both supragingival and subgingival calculus will be present
- Some teeth may be mobile
- Radiographs will show destruction of the alveolar bone in long-standing cases, with associated deep periodontal pockets present

It can be seen that one of the early diagnostic signs of periodontal problems is bleeding of the gingiva. However, the nicotine from tobacco smoking acts on the gingival blood vessels to constrict them, causing less bleeding, if any. The resultant lack of bleeding on brushing or probing masks the presence of periodontal disease in smokers, so that the disease is not evident to either the patient or the dentist without other clinical signs being present.

The easiest assessment carried out by the dentist is to determine the presence of periodontal pockets, by using special **periodontal probes**, such as the basic periodontal examination (BPE) probe shown in Figure 6.21. The assessment methods used to diagnose and record the presence of periodontal disease are discussed in detail in Chapter 13.

Summary

As discussed previously, the presence of bacterial dental plaque is a prerequisite for the development of all three of the main dental diseases (dental caries, gingivitis and periodontitis), in addition to other causative factors as described in the following.

The causative factors of dental caries are:

- A diet containing a high proportion of NMES
- Poor oral hygiene allowing the accumulation of dental plaque and the bacteria it contains
- Stagnation areas of the teeth themselves, such as occlusal fissures, overhanging restorations and abutments with dentures and orthodontic appliances
- The action of the bacteria on the NMES to produce acid, which demineralises the tooth structure and allows cavities to develop

The causative factors of gingivitis and periodontitis are:

- Poor oral hygiene which allows the accumulation of dental plaque, specifically in the gingival crevice and periodontal pockets and on any pre-existing surface of tartar
- The existence of stagnation areas, including the gingival crevice, which allows the plaque to accumulate specifically around the necks of the teeth against the gingiva
- Failure to treat and eradicate the subsequent gingivitis allows inflammation of the periodontal supporting structures to occur, leading to periodontitis

Which of the two diseases (caries or periodontal disease) predominates depends on the following factors, but the plaque is the same whichever disease occurs:

- The site of the plaque
- The diet, and specifically the presence of NMES
- The age of the patient

If the plaque is in contact with a tooth surface, it will result in caries developing there unless the plaque is removed. If the plaque is in contact with the gingiva, it will result in gingivitis and then periodontitis developing unless the plaque is removed.

Caries is mainly a disease of children and young adults whereas periodontal disease predominates in later life. The difference is caused by the rate at which the two diseases progress. Caries can cause loss of teeth within a few years, whereas periodontal disease may take decades to have the same effect. By the time periodontal disease has reached an advanced stage, the earlier onslaught of caries has already been overcome and is often no longer a problem, as the teeth that were susceptible to caries have already been treated – by exposure to fluoride, fissure sealing, filling or other restoration, or extraction.

Another reason for the difference between which disease predominates in each age group is the diet they tend to follow. Consumption of sweets and sugary food and drinks is probably far greater, and far less controlled, in children and young people, and their teeth are consequently much more vulnerable to caries. However, it must not be assumed that adults and older people are immune to caries. It still occurs if childhood patterns of unrestricted, indiscriminate consumption of sweets persist. A typical example is the adult smoker who continually sucks mints after giving up the habit for health reasons – and then develops rampant caries affecting the buccal tooth surfaces, as the sugary mints dissolve and wash over the teeth.

The main method of preventing these diseases, then, or managing them when they are already present is to control the formation and build-up of bacterial plaque. When informing patients of the causes and prevention of oral diseases, it is referred to as oral health education, and when teaching them the main methods of achieving control of their oral diseases it is called oral hygiene instruction.

A huge part of the day-to-day work of the dental team is to educate patients in the risk factors of these three main oral diseases so that they can avoid their initial onset, or avoid their recurrence once treatment has resolved any diagnosed disease that was present.

The success of this oral health education depends on various factors, as outlined in the following and also discussed later, some of which are outside the control of the dental team:

- **Communication skills** – irrespective of how important the advice is to the patient, if it is delivered in a way that the patient cannot understand, it will not be followed
- **Age group** – the style of communication and the advice to be given will vary between age groups, and these groups are generally divided into the following:
  - Adults
  - Young people
  - Children

- **Patient motivation** – despite the best attempts by the dental team, some patients are simply not interested in their own oral health and are unwilling to participate in efforts to assist them in achieving good oral health
- **General health** – some medical and physical conditions (including old age) will affect the likelihood of oral disease development in some patients, while other conditions will affect patients' ability to carry out effective oral hygiene methods

Prevention and management of dental disease

As indicated previously, caries occurs due to a combination of certain types of bacteria being present within dental plaque that use NMES to produce acids that cause enamel demineralisation. There are therefore three main areas of caries prevention available to the patient and the dental team:

- **Control the build-up of bacterial plaque** – practise its regular removal by using good oral hygiene techniques
- **Increase the tooth resistance to acid attack** – by incorporating fluoride into the enamel structure
- **Modification of the diet** – to include fewer cariogenic foods and drinks and to reduce their frequency of intake

The main cause of periodontal disease is consistently poor oral hygiene, along with contributory factors such as smoking, and in some cases an unfortunate genetic predisposition to periodontal problems. So the prevention of periodontal disease can be achieved in most patients, whereas it can only be controlled in others:

- **Control the build-up of bacterial plaque** – practise its regular removal by using good oral hygiene techniques
- **Modify the contributory factors** – by giving advice on smoking cessation, for instance
- **Control the host response** – in patients predisposed to periodontal problems, by more frequent dental attendance for monitoring and evaluation, and intervention where necessary

Educating patients in how to successfully remove bacterial plaque, on a daily basis and for the rest of their lives, is the most important aim of the dental team to achieve in helping their patients maintain a good standard of oral health.

Control of bacterial plaque

Plaque forms within hours on newly cleaned tooth surfaces, due to the action of oral bacteria on foods. Unless removed from these areas, the plaque will allow dental caries to develop, while that formed around the gingival crevice will be involved in the onset of gingivitis and eventually periodontitis.

Controlling bacterial plaque on a daily basis is the main method available to patients to assist themselves in the protection of their oral health. It is the role of the dental team to ensure that the patients are taught the correct oral hygiene methods suitable to them and that they carry them out on a frequent enough basis to avoid damage to their oral health.

Plaque can be easily and regularly removed by the patient at home by carrying out a regular combination of the following oral hygiene techniques on a daily basis:

- **Tooth brushing**, using a recommended **toothpaste**
- **Interdental cleaning**
- **Using suitable mouthwashes**

445

Tooth brushing

Tooth brushing is the method used to remove supragingival plaque and food debris from the smooth surfaces of the teeth – that is, the buccal, labial, lingual, palatal and occlusal surfaces, as well as the gingival crevice. Unless the patient has widely spaced teeth, the interdental areas will require special techniques of cleaning to remove plaque efficiently. General advice on tooth brushing techniques is as follows:

- Toothbrushes with a small head and multi-tufted medium nylon bristles are probably the most effective for the vast majority of patients
- Good-quality, rechargeable electric toothbrushes take the need for consistently good manual techniques away from the patient, and are more likely to achieve prolonged high standards of oral hygiene (see Figure 5.6)
- The brush is rinsed to wet the bristles and a portion of the recommended toothpaste added (see later)
- Each dental arch is divided into three sections: left and right sides, and front
- Side sections are subdivided into buccal, lingual and occlusal surfaces; front sections into labial and lingual
- When instructing patients, these areas should be referred to in terms the patient can understand – such as "cheek side", "tongue side", "lip side" and so on
- This amounts to eight groups of surfaces in each jaw, and at least 5 seconds should be spent on each group
- Egg timers or similar devices are useful here so that the patient obtains an idea of how long the recommended "2 minute" brushing cycle actually is – some electric brushes may have a timer incorporated into their design
- Patients should be encouraged to develop their own start and end points within the oral cavity and then follow this systematically at each brushing session, so that a methodical routine is developed – e.g. it might be lower left side (all surfaces) followed by lower front (all surfaces) and then lower right side (all surfaces), before moving to the upper arch
- Each area is brushed in turn and the mouth is then cleared by spitting out the toothpaste and oral debris
- The patient should be instructed **not** to rinse the mouth out, as this will remove the residual toothpaste and prevent its chemical constituents from continuing to act in the mouth – this is particularly important advice with fluoridated toothpastes
- Parents will need to perform effective tooth brushing on children up to the age of around 8 years, to ensure that all plaque is removed and to teach the child how to brush correctly (see Figure 5.5)
- Brushes should be rinsed afterwards and allowed to dry – they only have a limited life and need replacement every few months, as the bristles curl down and render the brush ineffective (see Figure 5.9)

Toothpastes

A huge variety of toothpastes are available nowadays, from shops' own brands to specialised ones from oral health product suppliers, with ingredients to fight against all aspects of common oral disease. Individual recommendations should be given for any patient requesting advice from the dental team as to the most suitable product for their use (see Figure 5.10). This may vary from time to time as the patient may experience certain oral problems throughout life:

- Over 95% of toothpastes available in this country contain **fluoride**, as sodium monofluorophosphate and sodium fluoride at 1000 parts per million (ppm)
- **High-fluoride** toothpastes containing between 2800 and 5000 ppm, for use by adult patients with an existing high caries rate or an excessive risk to developing caries (see Figure 5.11)

- Several other toothpastes contain ingredients specifically to slow down **calculus** formation
- Many now contain the substance triclosan combined with zinc, which acts as an **antiseptic plaque suppressant**
- Some toothpastes are specifically formulated to help **relieve sensitivity**, and contain ingredients such as stannous fluoride (see Figure 5.12)
- Others are advertised as "**whitening toothpastes**" and act to remove surface tooth staining by the use of abrasives or, more recently, by the use of biological enzyme systems
- More recent developments have included toothpastes designed to help protect teeth against **acid erosion** (see Figure 5.13)

Interdental cleaning

However good the tooth brushing technique, it is still impossible to clean interdental spaces perfectly with a toothbrush alone, unless a specialist electric brush is used. Consequently, these mesial and distal contact areas between adjoining teeth are more prone to developing caries and periodontal disease. To clean the interdental areas adequately, several oral health aids are available to assist patients with removal of plaque that has formed here, as follows:

- **Dental floss** and **dental tape** are thread-like aids that are widely used by many patients to achieve interdental plaque removal; however, correct usage depends to some extent on the patient's manual dexterity and on receiving sound oral health instruction (see Figure 5.14)
- "**Flossette-style**" handles hold the length of floss in place for the patient so that they can floss with one hand, therefore making the procedure less cumbersome, especially for posterior teeth where access is difficult for the majority of patients (see Figure 5.15)
- **Interdental brushes** are of a typical "bottle-brush" design and are able to clean in spaced interdental areas, as well as around the individual brackets of fixed orthodontic appliances (see Figure 5.16)
- **Woodsticks** (although they may also be plastic!) are also available to dislodge solid pieces of food debris from interproximal areas, as well as to massage the gingivae here; however, their use should be restricted to competent adults whenever possible, as they can easily be stuck into the gum and cause problems if used incorrectly or by an inexperienced patient

The aim of all of these interdental aids is to dislodge food particles and accumulated plaque from the interdental areas of the teeth, so that the debris can be swallowed or removed from the oral cavity. As the plaque sticks to the tooth surface itself, the cleaning aids should be physically pulled across the mesial and distal tooth surfaces to remove this biofilm layer; the majority of patients will therefore require demonstrations in the correct technique by a member of the dental team. In particular, dental floss and tape need to be "wrapped around" the separate tooth surfaces for adequate cleaning, and this requires a certain level of manual dexterity by the patient (see Figure 5.18).

Even when used correctly, woodsticks are the least effective method of interdental cleaning available and other techniques should be recommended to the patient wherever possible.

Mouthwashes

A wide range of mouthwashes are currently available, ranging from shops' own brands to specialised products from dedicated oral health product suppliers (see Figure 5.19). Widely available types are as follows, and each patient should have specific products recommended for use by the dental team, once their particular oral health needs have been assessed:

- General-use mouthwashes contain various ingredients to promote good oral hygiene, including:
  - **Sodium fluoride** – to provide topical fluoride application to the teeth
  - **Triclosan** – a chemical that suppresses the formation of plaque in the oral cavity

- Others are specialised for use on sensitive teeth (see Figure 5.20)
- Some are used specifically in the presence of oral soft tissue inflammation as a first aid measure, or after oral surgery, and contain **hydrogen peroxide** which helps to eliminate anaerobic bacteria (see Figure 5.21)
- Specialised mouthwashes are also available for patients suffering from both acute and chronic periodontal infections, and contain chlorhexidine, an **antiseptic plaque suppressant** (see Figure 5.22)

Other methods of plaque removal

After eating a meal, tooth brushing may not always be possible until several hours later, by which time plaque will have formed and possibly started to cause damage. Obvious examples are after eating lunch at school or at work, or while out for a meal in the evening.

In these situations, loose food debris can be removed by using sugar-free chewing gum or finishing the meal with a **detergent food** and/or a piece of cheese. Detergent foods are raw, firm, fibrous fruits or vegetables, such as apples, pears, carrots and celery. By virtue of their tough fibrous consistency, they require much chewing and stimulate salivary flow, thereby helping to scour the teeth clean of food remnants. Although plaque is unaffected by detergent foods they can remove some of the food debris that nourishes all plaque bacteria and enables some of them to produce acid. Although cheese at the end of a meal has no direct detergent effect, it stimulates salivary flow, neutralises acid and enhances remineralisation of enamel, due to its calcium content. Hard cheeses are more beneficial than soft cheeses.

The excessive use of chewing gum should be discouraged in all patients in whom there is evidence of attrition or bruxing. Its use should be confined to immediately after a meal only, and not continually throughout the day.

Increase tooth resistance to acid attack

The outer layer of the tooth, the enamel, is made up of inorganic crystals of calcium hydroxyapatite arranged as prisms running from the ADJ to the tooth surface (see Chapter 13). It was discovered many years ago that the incorporation of fluoride into and onto the tooth structure resulted in the replacement of the hydroxyapatite crystals by **fluorapatite crystals**. This new chemical structure of the tooth was found to be much more resistant to the damage caused by the weak organic acids formed by plaque bacteria – in other words, the fluoride protected the teeth from developing caries so easily.

Fluoride is therefore the single most important chemical compound that is of use in the battle against dental caries. It occurs naturally in the water in some areas and is added artificially to water supplies in other areas during the process of water fluoridation (usually as a salt) as an oral health measure to aid in the reduction of caries incidence.

Fluoride can be taken into the enamel structure by the direct application of various oral health products to the teeth (this is called **topical fluoride application**), or by being taken **internally** with food and drink products (this is called **systemic fluoride application**).

In addition its action of reducing the solubility of enamel to acids, by the formation of fluorapatite, fluoride also has an inhibitory effect on the **feeding rate** of oral bacteria. This effect results in the production of lesser amounts of weak acids and polysaccharides to initiate the carious attack.

The protective effect of fluoride on the teeth is at its best after they have formed and recently erupted into the oral cavity, before any carious damage has begun. Many oral hygiene products are now available that contain fluoride to allow their regular use by the general public throughout their lifetime, so that the protective effect of fluoride on the teeth is constantly "topped up".

Topical fluorides

These are administered externally to the tooth surface, by either the patient or the dental team, to provide a continual source of fluoride directly onto the enamel.

- For use by the patient:
  - **Fluoride toothpastes** containing the current recommended dose for all patients of 1000 ppm, and up to 5000 ppm for use by adults at high risk of developing caries (see Figure 5.11)
  - A minimum of twice-daily brushing is advised to achieve maximum benefits
  - Patients should be advised **not to rinse out** after brushing, as it washes the fluoride away and is therefore less effective
  - **Fluoride mouthwashes** for regular use by those with a high caries risk and those under-going orthodontic treatment (see Figure 5.23)
  - **Dental floss** and tape impregnated with fluoride, for delivery directly to the interproximal areas
- For use by the dental team:
  - **Fluoride gels** applied in trays over all of the teeth for several minutes; they are administered at each examination appointment and are especially useful for patients with special needs and those who are a high caries risk:
    - Children with rampant caries
    - Patients with medical conditions such as haemophilia and heart defects which would make tooth extraction dangerous
    - Patients who are too disabled to achieve adequate oral hygiene on a regular basis
- The technique has two stages: first a thorough polish to remove any plaque present, after which the teeth are washed and dried; and second, the gel is applied in the special applicator tray for a few minutes. On removal of the tray, patients are instructed not to rinse, drink or eat for half-an-hour. The gels are pleasantly flavoured and the procedure is usually well tolerated
- **Fluoride varnish** (such as "Duraphat" products; see Figure 8.7) applied to individual teeth showing areas of previous acid attack or to roots exposed by gingival recession or periodontal surgery – registered dental nurses can undergo extended duties training to enable them to carry out this procedure on patients, under the prescription of the dentist

Systemic fluorides

These products are supplied in a form to be ingested and then taken from the digestive tract to be incorporated into the enamel structure, within the body:

- **Fluoridated water** supplies by the addition of the optimum concentration of 1 ppm to drinking water
- Naturally occurring fluoridated water supplies, in some parts of the world
- Addition of fluoride to table salt (but this does not happen in the UK)
- **Fluoride drops and tablets**, available on prescription for children, to be taken daily during the period of tooth development (up to 13 years); the doses required vary with the patient's age and the amount of fluoride in the local water supply
- Drops and tablets are usually reserved for those with medical or physical conditions that would make dental treatment difficult, or those whose general health would suffer if caries occurred

Water fluoridation is carried out as a public health measure in some areas of the UK, where fluoride at the optimum concentration of 1 ppm is added to the local water supply, is ingested by the local population and absorbed from their digestive tracts so that it can be incorporated into the enamel structure of their teeth.

449

Public health surveys have consistently proved the benefit of the use of systemic fluoride by water fluoridation, by comparing the number of **decayed, missing and filled teeth** (DMF count) in various populations. In areas where systemic fluoride is present at the 1 ppm concentration, the incidence of caries is reduced by 50% compared with areas where there is no water fluoridation. However, the technique remains controversial as some opponents consider it to be a form of "mass medication" of the population, carried out without necessarily having their approval, as they can only avoid ingesting the drinking water by using bottled water instead.

Fissure sealing

Topical fluorides exert most of their effect on mesial and distal (proximal) surfaces of the teeth. Occlusal fissures and pits are just as vulnerable to caries but are less well protected by fluorides. Fortunately they can receive extra, and even better, protection by the application of fissure sealants. These materials are composite fillings or glass ionomer cement, which are used to seal the naturally occurring stagnation areas of pits and fissures, therefore preventing damage from acid attacks and avoiding the onset of dental caries.

Successful fissure sealing should make an occlusal surface safe from caries. Like topical fluoridation, it can be carried out by hygienists and therapists as well as dentists and is of major importance in preventive dentistry as it can produce a significant reduction in the commonest disease of children.

Enamel fluorosis

This is a condition that occurs when excessive fluoride is ingested during enamel formation. The teeth erupt with mottled white areas in the enamel surface, which vary in severity but can be quite unsightly. Restorative techniques, such as veneers, are available to mask the areas but the condition is prevented by ensuring that parents receive the correct advice regarding fluoride:

- Children below the age of 8 years should have tooth brushing supervised by an adult, to prevent ingestion of the toothpaste
- The amount of toothpaste should be kept to a minimum and allowed just twice daily
- The parents must ensure that children spit the toothpaste out after use, rather than swallow it
- All fluoride supplements should only be prescribed as necessary, and at the correct dosage, which is dependent on the local water fluoridation levels
- The dental team must therefore have knowledge of any local water fluoridation levels

Modification of the diet

The single most important modification to the diet to reduce the incidence of dental caries is the reduction (or ideally the elimination) of NMES and dietary acids in the patient's daily food and drink intake.

It cannot be emphasised too strongly that even if teeth are thoroughly cleaned after meals, caries will still occur if NMES snacks and acidic drinks are taken between meals on a regular basis. This is because plaque persists in the inaccessible areas of fissures and tooth contact points after a meal, unless brushed away by the patient. Acid forms in this residual plaque within minutes of eating sugar, the pH of the oral environment is lowered, and the tooth enamel will be at risk of demineralisation until the pH balance is restored.

Then, as described previously in this chapter, a constant acid environment at the enamel surface allows demineralisation to proceed unchecked and leaves insufficient time between intakes of sugar for the natural defence mechanism of remineralisation to occur. Although adequate tooth brushing and twice-daily interdental cleaning may prevent supragingival periodontal disease, it cannot prevent caries unless accompanied by strict dietary discipline to eliminate NMES snacks between meals.

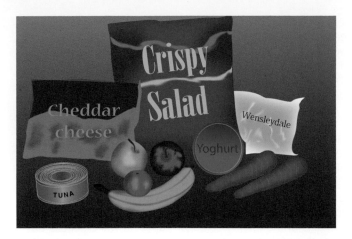

Figure 15.11   Examples of good snacks.

If NMES foods and acidic drinks (such as carbonated "pops" and fizzy flavoured waters) are confined to mealtimes only, the acids involved are neutralised to some extent by the buffering action of the increased volume of saliva released during the meal, thus reducing the extent of any demineralisation.

When giving dietary advice to patients, it helps if they are made aware of which food and drink products are safe or harmful in relation to dental caries. This is especially important with what are known as "**hidden sugars**" in foods – where NMES have been artificially added during the manufacturing and processing of foods for taste and preservation purposes, very often in foods that patients would not expect to be harmful to their teeth and which do not necessarily taste "sweet".

A simple list of "good" and "bad" foods and drinks can then be developed and referred to by the dental team when giving dietary advice to patients;

Good snacks (Figure 15.11) include:

- Non-citrus fruit, such as apples, pears and peaches
- Fibrous raw vegetables, such as carrots and celery
- Unflavoured crisps
- Low-fat cheese
- Unsweetened yoghurt

Bad snacks (see Figure 5.1) include:

- Sweets and other confectionery
- Biscuits and cakes
- Carbonated drinks
- Pure citrus fruit juices
- Tea and coffee with sugar
- Care should be taken with excessive intake of citrus fruits, such as oranges, lemons, grapefruits and limes between meals

Those foods containing "hidden sugars" can be identified by carefully reading the contents label of each product, and include the following (see also Figure 5.2):

- Cooking sauces, especially those with a tomato base
- Table sauces, including ketchup

- Flavoured crisps
- Fruits tinned in syrup
- Some tinned vegetables, including baked beans and sweetcorn
- Some breakfast cereals
- Jams, marmalades and chutneys
- Some low-fat products, as sugar is often added to improve their taste
- Tinned fish and meat in tomato sauce
- Soups
- Savoury crackers and biscuits
- Some processed ready meals
- Energy drinks

A universal system of clearly labelling food products so that contents such as hidden sugars are more readily identified is currently under discussion by politicians and food manufacturers. If enforced, bad snacks and unexpected sugar contents will be more obvious to the patient, and their ingestion can therefore be avoided or at least controlled more easily.

Although the incidence of caries is gradually reducing in this country, it remains a major health problem. It is most prevalent in younger age groups, so parental support is imperative if oral health messages are to be successful. The following general dietary advice should be given to patients:

- Eat a healthy diet with foods of low cariogenic (caries causing) potential
- Follow the "good snacks" list
- Limit any cariogenic foods to mealtimes, so that they can be neutralised by the increased flow of saliva that occurs while chewing
- Avoid carbonated drinks and confine fruit juices to mealtimes only
- Use diet sheets to determine if any hidden sugars are being taken
- Advise mothers on the damage caused by using cariogenic drinks in baby feeders
- Parents should be encouraged to request sugar-free medicines for their children whenever possible

Modify the contributory factors

In the management of periodontal disease, the contributory factors involved and to be discussed do not, in themselves, cause the disease – this is due to the presence of consistently poor levels of oral hygiene by the patient. The contributory factors merely **exacerbate** (make worse) the periodontal disease that is already in existence – they aggravate it so that the extent of the disease is worse than it would be otherwise, and/or it progresses more easily and quickly than it would do otherwise.

The most common contributory factors include the following:

- Smoking
- Unbalanced masticatory stress – such as when teeth have erupted out of alignment (especially when they are proclined) and normal chewing puts force on them in an abnormal direction
- Excessive masticatory stress – such as when several posterior teeth are missing and the patient then "nibbles" with the anterior teeth only, resulting in excessive chewing forces on them
- Hormonal imbalance that affects the reaction of gingival tissues to normal events such as plaque build-up – pregnancy and puberty are the usual examples
- Open lip posture that allows the gingival tissues to dry out readily – such as occurs in various malocclusions or in patients who routinely breathe through their mouth rather than their nose (this may be a habit or could be due to conditions such as large adenoid glands)

- A history of radiotherapy treatment for cancer in the head and neck region will result in reduced saliva flow (as the salivary glands are damaged by the treatment), so that plaque is able to build up more easily (these patients also tend to experience a higher rate of dental caries)
- Certain medical conditions that alter the patient's ability to fight infection or to self-heal when attacked by pathogens – these patients are referred to as being **immune-compromised**:
  - Diabetes
  - Leukaemia and other blood disorders
  - Vitamin C deficiency
  - AIDS
- Certain medicines that affect the normal reaction of the gingival tissues to the presence of plaque, often resulting in an overgrowth of tissue which makes plaque removal more difficult for the patient to achieve successfully – the resultant tissue overgrowth is called **gingival hyperplasia**:
  - Phenytoin (Epanutin), used in the control of epilepsy
  - Antihypertensive agents, such as nifedipine
  - Immunosuppressant drugs to prevent transplant rejection, such as ciclosporin
  - Cytotoxic drugs used to treat various cancers
- Certain medicines affect saliva production so that the patient suffers from xerostomia (dry mouth), resulting in the loss of the natural cleansing effect of the saliva and a greater build-up of plaque:
  - Diuretics used to treat various heart conditions
  - Some antidepressants
  - Some antihypertensive medicines
- Plaque retention factors that allow an increased local build-up of plaque and/or prevent its ready removal by normal oral hygiene methods:
  - Tooth crowding in malocclusion
  - Unopposed teeth in one arch, so that there is no normal contact and self-cleansing action by friction of food or other teeth
  - Iatrogenic factors – these are factors created by the dentist and include overhanging restorations, poor marginal fit of crowns and the like, and poorly designed dentures

453

Of this large list of contributory factors, the most obvious and relatively easiest ones for the dental team to overcome are those due to masticatory stress and those due to localised plaque retention factors. Among the remainder, patients can be informed of the effect of their various medications on their oral health and advised to discuss them with their doctor, who will be able to determine if alternative medications are available. Those patients suffering from medication-induced gingival hyperplasia can undergo a simple gingivectomy procedure to remove the excess tissue, so aiding plaque removal in the affected areas.

Little can be done for those patients suffering from hormonal imbalances and the various medical conditions that are an issue, except to ensure that they attend regularly for oral health assessment and treatment and that the relevant oral hygiene messages are reinforced at each attendance.

As smoking has such a huge detrimental effect on both general and oral health, many patients are likely to have been previously exposed to smoking cessation advice on numerous occasions by other healthcare workers. However, the dental team should still use every attendance by the patient as an opportunity to reinforce the health benefits of stopping smoking, and inform them of the various techniques that are currently available under the excellent NHS "quit smoking" referral scheme.

Dental treatment is one of the few areas of the NHS where many patients are expected to pay for their health services, and while it may be an unusual tactic, the cost of dental treatment may be highlighted as an additional good reason for advising those patients who smoke to give up, especially where it can be shown that smoking has contributed to their individual treatment costs. The dentist should advise and lead the team in this technique, as skilful communication methods are required to ensure that the patient is helpfully advised and supported, rather than insulted and humiliated.

Control the host response

Some patients are unfortunate enough to be prone to periodontal problems, often for genetic reasons. No matter how thorough their oral hygiene efforts might be, with help and support from the dental team, and even in the absence of any contributory factors, they may still go on to develop periodontal disease. As their genetic predisposition cannot be altered, the periodontal disease development is inevitable over time. These patients will require a high level of support and maintenance by the dental team to ensure that their disease does not spiral out of control and result in the loss of multiple teeth that could have been saved.

These patients may therefore require interventive dental treatment on a regular basis:

- Any calculus that has built up must be removed by **scaling** and **subgingival debridement**, by a suitable member of the dental team (see later)
- Advice should be given on suitable oral health products that act specifically to control calculus formation
- Patients taking drugs that cause **gingival hyperplasia** may require the overgrown tissue to be surgically removed as a gingivectomy procedure, thereby eliminating these plaque retention areas
- Once debrided, the periodontal pockets may have an antibiotic gel (Figure 15.12) inserted as an alternative to repeated courses of systemic antibiotics, in an effort to eradicate the bacteria involved in the disease process
- Areas of persistent periodontal infection that fail to respond to treatment may require the **extraction** of the individual tooth involved, to remove the associated periodontal pockets as a source of the anaerobic bacteria
- Patients that require a high level of periodontal maintenance are best referred to a **periodontal specialist** for their treatment

Non-surgical periodontal treatment

The prevention of periodontal disease is a far more desirable task for the dental team to have to carry out than attempting to cure it, so good oral hygiene instruction from an early age is the best course of action. Obviously, this is not possible for patients who are seen initially as

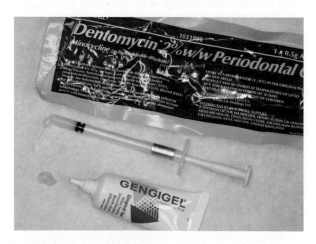

Figure 15.12   Periodontal pocket treatments.

adults, especially if they already have periodontal disease when they do attend. Oral hygiene instruction and methods of achieving a good standard of oral hygiene are discussed earlier in the chapter.

The oral health messages given by the dental team will need to be reinforced regularly if problems persist, and the advice given will vary for the different age groups. Removal of all plaque and its subsequent control by the patient will bring about a complete resolution of chronic gingivitis. Failure to achieve this will allow calculus to form, and the dental team will then have to intervene to remove it.

Accessible plaque is removed by the patient by efficient **tooth brushing** and **interdental cleaning**. Subgingival plaque and calculus are inaccessible to patients and are removed by members of the dental team during **scaling**. Once these aims have been achieved by the patient and the team and then routinely maintained, the sources of irritation that cause the disease are removed.

In chronic gingivitis, bleeding ceases, swollen gums return to their normal healthy condition and false pockets are thereby eliminated. The patient is then cured, but strict oral hygiene and regular dental checks are required thereafter to prevent recurrence of plaque and calculus formation.

In chronic periodontitis there is no regeneration of lost bone, but mild cases can be cured in the same way as chronic gingivitis. In the advanced stages of the disease, scaling alone cannot eliminate true pockets if they are too deep to be accessible. In such cases, they are treated surgically by repositioning and/or recontouring the gingival margin.

In this way, even advanced periodontal disease can be arrested, but a return of the condition is inevitable unless the patient follows the advice given and the instructions on supragingival plaque control, and also attends regularly for the team to check progress and continue subgingival plaque control.

Apart from scaling and gingival surgery, appropriate treatment is given for any other conditions facilitating plaque retention, e.g. the replacement of unsatisfactory fillings, crowns and dentures, or the treatment of unopposed and irregular teeth.

As periodontal disease is an infection by plaque bacteria and other microorganisms, one approach to treatment is the application of antimicrobial drugs directly into the gingival crevice and pockets, such as with Periochip, Dentomycin gel and Gengigel applications (Figure 15.12). The establishment of their long-term success in the battle against periodontal disease is an ongoing and exciting area of clinical research.

Supragingival plaque control

Supragingival calculus and any overhanging cervical margins of restorations are removed in the surgery. At home, thorough, twice-daily tooth brushing by the patient will then keep accessible plaque under control. Appropriate instruction in the surgery, and the use of disclosing agents at home, will show patients how well they are performing and indicate where improvement is required.

Areas of the oral cavity that are inaccessible to an ordinary toothbrush are the interdental spaces above or below the contact points of adjacent teeth (interproximal areas). They can be cleaned with dental floss, wood sticks and an interspace brush. The dentist or hygienist must give the patient special instruction in these methods as they can do more harm than good if done incorrectly or unnecessarily.

- **Dental floss** is thread or tape that is worked between the teeth to keep their contact areas clean (Figure 15.13). Where recession of the gum has occurred, or gingival surgery has been performed, the resulting interdental spaces may be too large for flossing
- **Wood sticks (al**so called interspace sticks) are used for these large spaces. They are soft wooden sticks that are passed through the spaces to keep them clear of food debris and reduce plaque formation

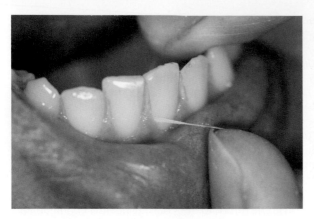

Figure 15.13 Flossing technique.

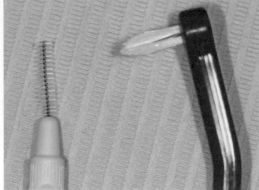

Figure 15.14 Interdental and interspace brushes.

- **Interspace brushes** and **interdental brushes** are special types of toothbrush designed to clean interdental spaces and the interproximal tooth surfaces in the same way as floss and wood sticks. The former have only one tuft of bristles, while the latter are similar in appearance to a bottle brush (Figure 15.14)

Any calculus present cannot be removed by the patient as it is hardened onto the tooth surface, and instead must be treated by regular scaling. This is done by a dentist, therapist or hygienist, and the patient's own efforts at supragingival plaque control are checked at the same time. Supragingival scaling removes plaque and calculus deposits from the enamel surface of the teeth down to the gingival crevice.

Scaling hand instruments come in various designs appropriate for the removal of calculus from any part of a tooth, and those used for supragingival calculus removal include the following:

- **Sickle scaler**
- **Cushing's push scaler**
- **Jaquette scaler**

Hand scaling is tiring for the operator to carry out but gives excellent tactile sensation, so specks of residual calculus are easily detectable and can be fully removed. Alternatively, an ultrasonic scaler may be used which is much faster and less tiring (see Figure 8.4). However, its action depends on the water spray produced during use, and this can be uncomfortable for patients with sensitive teeth unless performed under local anaesthesia.

Once scaling has been completed, the teeth are polished with prophylactic polishing paste using a rubber cup or bristle brush in the slow handpiece (see Figure 8.6). The paste is abrasive and removes any residual surface stains, leaving a smooth tooth surface that slows down the reaccumulation of plaque.

Subgingival plaque control

With chronic periodontitis, any alveolar bone loss is permanent, although research is ongoing into the use of synthetic bone in both humans and other animal species, to replace that lost due to natural resorption or periodontal disease. In the meantime, however, if subgingival calculus is thoroughly and regularly removed by the dental team and a good standard of oral hygiene is consistently maintained by the patient, there is every chance that the periodontal ligament will reattach and any periodontal pockets will heal.

The instruments used to remove subgingival calculus have to be long enough to reach the base of any periodontal pockets, and thin enough to do so without tearing the gingival tissues. In addition, they are used to scrape the tooth root surfaces and dislodge any contaminated cementum, which is then removed from the pockets by both aspiration and irrigation. This technique is called **subgingival debridement**.

The instruments used for subgingival scaling include the following (see also Figure 8.5):

- **Gracey curette**
- **Other subgingival curettes**
- **Periodontal hoe**
- **Ultrasonic scaler**

Once subgingival debridement is complete, the periodontal tissues can heal and the junctional epithelium can reattach to the tooth surface. In so doing, the periodontal pockets are eliminated.

Subgingival scaling entails much instrumentation within the gingival crevice and pockets. This, in addition to the gingivitis already present, produces considerable bleeding and trauma, and requires the use of local anaesthesia. Again, the scaling may be carried out more easily and quickly than by hand with the use of an ultrasonic scaler. This apparatus produces ultrasonic vibrations, which are transmitted through a cable to a special scaling instrument. When it is applied to a tooth, the vibrations help to loosen the plaque and calculus and they are flushed away by a water-cooling spray which is part of the apparatus. The scaling instrument consists of a special handpiece with a range of detachable scaling tips of various shapes. Use of a chlorhexidine mouthwash by the patient before scaling reduces any risk of cross-infection with staff. Patients are advised to take analgesic tablets, if required, as the area may feel rather sore for a day or two afterwards.

Scaling cannot always remove the deepest, hardest and most adherent layer of calculus from the root surface of teeth. The additional stage **of subgingival debridement** is then carried out using Gracey curettes. These are distinguished from other curettes by having only one cutting surface. Their planing action eliminates any residual plaque and calculus. as it scrapes away some of the root cementum to provide a smooth root surface.

Provided the patient achieves adequate supragingival plaque control while the dentist deals with any restoration overhangs, imperfect partial dentures or other hindrances to plaque removal, and the hygienist/therapist or dentist can maintain subgingival plaque control, most cases of straightforward chronic periodontitis can be cured. Continued periodontal health is dependent to a very large degree on the cooperation and motivation of the patient to maintain a consistently good standard of oral hygiene. Of all the exacerbating factors that can worsen the situation, smoking plays a large part in the failure of periodontal treatment and the ultimate loss of teeth by the patient.

Some cases will remain where non-surgical periodontal treatment alone cannot succeed. Patients with very deep pockets, for example, especially those involving multi-rooted teeth, may present a problem of inaccessible subgingival plaque and calculus that can only be removed by surgical procedures to gain and maintain access to it.

Non-carious tooth surface loss

The enamel surface of the tooth can be lost for reasons other than dental caries, specifically by the following processes:

- **Erosion**
- **Abrasion**
- **Attrition**
- **Abfraction**

Erosion occurs due to the action of extrinsic acid on the enamel. This is acid that has not been produced by oral bacteria – dietary acid that has been ingested in foods or drinks by the patient. The usual dietary sources of these extrinsic acids are as follows:

- Carbonated fizzy drinks – whether labelled as "diet" types or not
- Acidic fruits, such as lemons, oranges, limes and grapefruit, which are eaten raw in large quantities
- Pure fruit juice of acidic fruits, especially when consumed in large quantities and between meals
- Wines
- Excessive vinegar consumption

In a similar way, there are some medical conditions and eating disorders that involve the regular regurgitation, or actual vomiting, of the stomach contents into the mouth. As discussed in Chapter 13, the gastric juices of the stomach are very acidic (pH2) and have a similar erosive effect on the tooth enamel as extrinsic acids. Some medical conditions and disorders that are related to tooth erosion are as follows:

- Bulimia
- Reflux oesophagitis
- Hiatus hernia
- Stomach ulcers
- Some chemotherapy treatments for cancer

Unlike with tooth surface loss due to dental caries, no bacteria are involved in the enamel loss caused by erosion. The tooth surface appears pitted and worn but shiny and clean, with no plaque present. Erosion particularly affects the labial or palatal surfaces of the upper incisors, and the occlusal surfaces of the lower molars (Figure 15.15). The teeth affected are often hypersensitive to hot, cold and sweet stimulation as the underlying dentine is exposed. This therefore mimics the symptoms of caries, but no cavity is present.

Treatment of erosion does not necessarily involve restoration, but does involve all of the following:

- Dietary and/or medical advice
- Desensitisation of the dentine

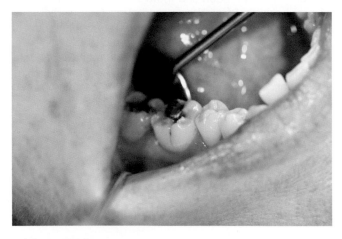

Figure 15.15   Erosion of the enamel.

- The use of high concentration fluoride toothpastes and mouthwashes to help to restore the pH balance of the oral cavity
- The use of "enamel repair" oral health products (see Figure 5.13)

Abrasion occurs when patients scrub their teeth clean using excessive side-to-side sawing forces, rather than brushing them correctly to remove plaque. The condition is especially seen in smokers with significant tar staining on their teeth, who either brush with a sawing action or use abrasive smokers' toothpastes to remove the stains.

Abrasion is seen at the cervical necks of the teeth, as a deep ridge on the buccal or labial surfaces (see Figure 5.8). The surface is shiny rather than carious, and sometimes the ridge is deep enough to see the pulp chamber within the tooth itself. Again, no bacteria are involved in the production of these lesions, and the patient often experiences hypersensitivity with temperature changes. As the ridges can be so deep, they are often restored with glass ionomer cements or composites (see later in this chapter and Chapter 8). In extreme cases, the pulp can be exposed, and endodontic treatment will be required to save the tooth from extraction.

Attrition is the loss of enamel specifically from the biting surfaces of the teeth and is caused by any of the following:

- Normal "wear and tear" of chewing, especially in older patients (Figure 15.16)
- Occlusion of natural teeth onto ceramic restorations, such as crowns and bridges
- **Bruxing** – the abnormal, and often subconscious, action of clenching and grinding the teeth

459

Bruxing is a very common condition, seen in many patients but especially in those under stress. It can also occur habitually while undertaking repetitive tasks, such as while exercising. Besides the obvious enamel loss and tooth fracture that occur as a result of bruxing, patients often experience face pain and disruption of the temporo-mandibular joint (TMJ). The joint and the muscles of mastication go into spasm in severe cases and can cause jaw clicks or even jaw locking. Various muscle relaxants, anti-inflammatory drugs and occlusal splints can be used to alleviate these symptoms, but the reason for the bruxing must also be investigated and mitigated or removed.

Abfraction is the specific loss of tooth in the cervical (neck) region, due to the shearing forces that occur by overloading single standing teeth. It appears visibly as an abrasion cavity, but can affect the buccal, lingual or palatal surfaces of a tooth and will occur suddenly rather than as a gradual loss of tooth structure, as happens with abrasion.

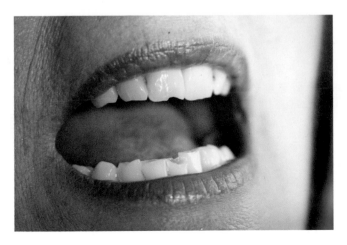

Figure 15.16   Tooth attrition.

The teeth affected are usually single standing premolars, especially where the molars have been lost in the same jaw (Figure 15.17). Treatment involves not only restoration of the affected tooth, but also replacement of any missing teeth to reduce the occlusal loading of the affected tooth and prevent a recurrence of the tooth loss.

Other periodontal conditions

Several other interesting periodontal conditions exist that may present from time to time in the dental workplace, although they are not as common as chronic gingivitis and periodontitis. They are summarised in the following sections.

Sub-acute pericoronitis

This is an infection of the gingival flap that lies over a partially erupted tooth, called the **operculum**, and sometimes affects the surrounding soft tissues too (Figure 15.18). It especially affects the lower third molars as they erupt, because these teeth are not only difficult to clean, allowing plaque bacteria to proliferate, but the operculum is often traumatised by the opposing tooth during normal mouth closure. The combination of infection and trauma produces inflammation of the operculum, which then swells and becomes more traumatised. It is treated in a number of ways, depending on the severity of the infection and the regularity of its occurrence, as follows:

- Irrigation of any food debris from under the operculum, ideally using a chlorhexidine-based disinfectant
- Oral hygiene instruction for the area, especially the use of hot salt water or disinfectant mouthwashes, or an oxygen-releasing mouthwash to remove the ideal conditions for the bacteria involved (see Figure 5.21)
- Antibiotics if the patient has a raised temperature (anaerobic bacteria are usually involved, so metronidazole is often prescribed)

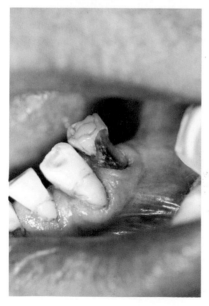

Figure 15.17   Abfraction with caries present.

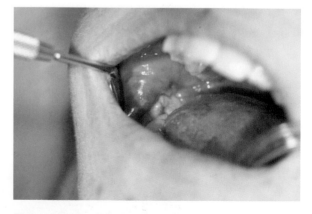

Figure 15.18   Pericoronitis around lower right third molar.

- Operculectomy if the condition recurs (the surgical removal of the operculum from over the tooth)
- Alternatively, the extraction of the opposing tooth to break the cycle of trauma and inflammation

Acute herpetic gingivitis

This condition is caused by the herpes simplex virus and most commonly affects infants. All the signs of acute inflammation are present and the rest of the oral mucous membrane may also be involved, in the form of tiny blisters that leave painful ulcers (**acute herpetic gingivo-stomatitis**). The condition is short-lived but uncomfortable; the patient feels unwell and may be unable to eat solids, but it resolves without treatment and the gingival condition returns to normal.

However, the virus remains dormant in the body and can be reactivated later by a common cold to produce a cold sore (herpes labialis) on the lip (see Figure 13.1). During the acute phase or the presence of a cold sore, the condition is highly infectious and dental treatment is best deferred until the condition has resolved.

Acute necrotising ulcerative gingivitis

This is abbreviated to ANUG and was formerly called acute ulcerative gingivitis (AUG) or Vincent's disease. It is an acute gingivitis characterised by pain and halitosis (bad breath). The affected gingiva appears bright red, with a covering layer of a yellow/grey sloughing membrane where the gum margin has been destroyed by bacterial action. The bacteria involved include **Bacillus fusiformis** and **Treponema vincenti**.

All the features of acute inflammation are present: red, swollen, painful gums; loss of function, because it is too painful to chew hard food; and frequently a raised temperature. It usually affects young adults and occurs in areas already affected by chronic gingivitis. In many cases, stress, heavy smoking and a lowered general resistance precipitate an attack. Thus it is more common in winter when colds, influenza and other infections are rife, but more importantly it may occur as the first presenting sign of a patient suffering from AIDS.

It is treated as follows:

- Antibiotic treatment that is specific for anaerobic bacteria, usually **metronidazole**
- If the patient is pregnant, this antibiotic cannot be used and so it is substituted by penicillin
- Use of a disinfectant mouthwash, such as those containing chlorhexidine, while the area is too painful to clean by brushing
- Thorough scaling and polishing once the symptoms have settled, followed by oral hygiene instruction
- Smoking cessation advice, where relevant
- Long-term use of a good-quality mouthwash and an adequate brushing technique

Acute lateral periodontal abscess

This is an occasional complication of chronic periodontitis in which pus formation in a deep pocket is unable to drain through the gingival crevice. The pus accumulates instead at the base of the pocket to form an abscess. This condition must not be confused with an acute alveolar abscess, which follows pulp death and occurs at the root apex. Acute lateral periodontal abscess occurs on a vital tooth at the side of the root (the lateral region of the root).

Treatment depends on the depth of the pocket and the probability of curing the underlying periodontal disease. The options are as follows:

- Drainage of the pus present
- Thorough subgingival scaling of the affected tooth

461

- Local administration of antibiotic into the pocket itself, especially metronidazole-containing gel products
- Oral hygiene instruction
- If all else fails, extraction of the affected tooth

Patient evaluation and motivation

Every patient's knowledge and skills in relation to their own oral health are evaluated by adequate communication with them, and the aim of good communication is to identify their level of motivation, and if poor, what the actual problems are for them – what is preventing them from achieving and then maintaining a good standard of oral health?

During consideration of the issues, all of the following points need to be looked at and taken into account:

- Do they just need direct advice, help and support to adequately achieve good oral health, such as one-to-one oral hygiene instruction with a member of the dental team?
- Are factors involved that prevent them from achieving good oral health, such as a disability or a diet- or habit-related problem?
- Are they simply uninterested in their oral health, or are they unaware that they have a problem?
- Are general health factors involved that either exacerbate or actually cause the oral health problem?
- Is a serious general health problem present that overrides their oral health problems?
- Are there barriers to good communication with certain groups, or do specific communication skills need to be applied?

Following the evaluation of each patient, their individual problems will have been identified and help can then be given by the dental team to aid the patient in achieving a better standard of oral health. The help offered by the dental team must be delivered in a way that individual patients are able to understand, and this can only be achieved by having good communication skills and the ability to recognise how to adapt those skills for the benefit of each patient.

Communication skills

Good communication between the dental team and their patients is crucial if they are to take an active role in managing their own oral health. Not only is it a necessity if any consent given for treatment is to be valid (see Chapter 13), but it will also lead to greater understanding between all parties, especially if the patient is unsure about treatment options or even refuses to have treatment as advised by the dentist.

An open relationship must exist at all times, so that patients feel they can ask for advice, query options given or explain why they do not wish to have certain treatments. All of this depends on the dental team showing good communication skills, and this is especially important for dental nurses as patients often prefer to discuss matters with them rather than with the dentist.

Communicating means "to give or exchange information", and this can be done both verbally and non-verbally, as follows:

- **Talking** – either directly with the patient face to face, or on the telephone
- **Written explanations** – which reiterate any verbal information given
- **Information leaflets or posters** – which can be read and then discussed verbally as necessary
- **Body language** – which can be open and friendly, or defensive and "stand-offish"
- **Eye contact** – maintaining eye contact shows attentiveness, while breaking eye contact indicates the patient is being dismissed by the listener
- **Facial expressions** – again, these can be friendly or not (smile, frown, querying, laughing, etc.)

- **Body position** – sitting to listen to the patient is more attentive than standing, especially if the body position of the listener is turned away from the speaker
- **Touching** – this is sometimes used to reinforce points, although it is not acceptable in some situations and with some patients, and should only be used where there is a friendly and well-established rapport between the patient and the team member concerned

A friendly staff member will obviously appear more approachable to patients than one who seems unfriendly, but often an unfriendly demeanour occurs without the staff member realising it. When unexpected situations arise, such as an equipment failure or a very busy appointments session, staff can seem abrupt, harried or even dismissive towards patients as they try to deal with the situation.

To continue to carry out tasks while being spoken to, especially if eye contact is not maintained, can appear extremely rude and dismissive to patients. On the other hand, standing too close to a patient ("invading their personal space") or making inappropriate physical contact, may be construed as threatening or offensive by the patient. Some individuals have naturally good communication skills, but for other dental staff a training course or "in house" experiential learning, by following the lead of good communicators, is vital in the development of their own skills.

Communicating with patients whose first language is not English

There are bound to be patients whose first language is not English, and communicating with them may present problems for the dental team, so in these cases, wherever possible, a family member or friend should be encouraged to attend to act as an interpreter. Full communication can then occur so that the patient is fully aware of the state of their oral health and is fully informed of all risks and benefits before undergoing any dental procedure.

Valid consent cannot be given for treatment if the patient does not understand the language being spoken and the relevant points have not been translated for them. The National Health Service issues patient information leaflets in various languages, and it would be advisable for practices with a large ethnic minority patient base to have them to hand as required. They are free and can be delivered to the workplace quite easily.

These multilingual patient leaflets are especially useful now that the UK has opened its borders to member states of the European Union, with the resultant influx of migrants. Fortunately, many EU countries have an excellent record of teaching English to their populace, and their communication skills are usually good, and sometimes better, than those of the local population.

Dental staff should also be aware of any cultural differences between ethnic groups, and accept and deal with them in an appropriate manner. Religious beliefs may prevent oral examination and dental treatment occurring at certain times, and these facts should be accommodated and handled sympathetically as far as possible, rather than being seen as an unnecessary hindrance to the running of the practice.

Religion probably plays the most important role in the differences encountered amongst many ethnic groups, both in their culture and in their daily lives, including their diet and eating habits. Several points of interest for dental staff around these cultural differences are summarised here.

Hindus:

- Many are vegetarian, some vegan, and they take no beef in their diet
- Fasting days for religious reasons are common
- Their diet tends to be very high in saturated fats and is often expensive

Sikhs:

- They eat more dairy products than many other ethnic groups
- They are often vegetarian
- If meats are eaten, they tend to avoid beef and pork

463

Muslims:

- They have strict food laws, even including the methods used for animal slaughter
- They avoid both alcohol and pork
- They celebrate Ramadan – a period of fasting during daylight hours for 1 month per year
- They tend to eat a diet rich in fish

All Asian groups tend to breast feed their babies for up to 2 years, and sugar is routinely added to feeds, especially as milk-based additions that are therefore cariogenic and have low nutritional value.

All these issues are of relevance to both the oral and general health of these patient groups, but are unlikely to be altered because of their religious basis. The dental team must accept this and respect the wishes of each patient, while also advising them of the likely consequences to their oral (and general) health.

Communicating with different age groups

Not only will variations be apparent in the communication methods that are suitable for different age groups during evaluation, but the factors that determine the level of oral health in these groups will also be different. Generally, the age groups are divided into the following:

- Adults
- Young people
- Children

Any risk factors identified during the evaluation need to be discussed with the patient or with their escort, and it will be seen that within these age groups the various risk factors are influenced by complex social attitudes and outside pressures.

Adults:

- Smoking and drinking habits should be discussed in relation to oral health, but in a non-judgmental manner. Information should be given on the links between these risk factors and both the general and oral health problems associated with them, especially periodontal disease and oral cancer
- Some patients may require referral to their dental or medical practitioner for individual advice on aids to stop smoking, such as nicotine patches and nicotine substitutes, and this is easier to arrange nowadays with the free NHS smoking cessation schemes available
- Similarly, excessive alcohol intake should be discussed in relation to oral cancer and general health problems, but it is the patient's choice whether or not to act on the advice given
- Diet should be discussed in detail, using accurate diet sheets filled in by the patient to identify any hidden dietary problems if necessary, such as a high NMES intake or frequent snacking episodes
- The patient's diet should also be assessed in relation to any general health effects

Young people:

This group of patients will require a quite different approach to support and motivation in relation to their oral health, for the following reasons:

- They have a different outlook on life and different priorities in their lives from adults – events that are important to adults are often of less concern to young people, and vice versa

- They are likely to have little, if any, experience of long-term oral and general health problems and will therefore require some convincing that a problem actually exists
- They are likely to require evidence of the existence of an oral health problem from the dental team, rather than just accepting their word for it, so the use of disclosing agents to stain bacterial plaque on their teeth is often an invaluable aid
- Some young people may already be experimenting with alcohol and tobacco usage because of peer pressure, and this may already be having an effect on their oral health (and ultimately on their general health)
- Some may not wish to accept responsibility for maintaining their own oral health as yet and prefer to rely on their parents for this
- Parental influence will be greater for some young people than others
- Parental support will differ similarly, but is therefore of great importance – well motivated parents tend to instil their attitudes and beliefs into their youngsters

Children:

The oral health of this group depends very much on their parental influence and support, especially for the younger patients of the group. Parents who have little interest in their own oral and general health are unlikely to instil their children with high levels of interest and motivation, although exceptions do occur.
   The following points are relevant:

- Wherever possible, parents should be included in their child's oral health education, and their support should be gained at an early stage
- The oral health messages given by the dental team can then be reinforced at home by the parent, and will usually revolve around brushing techniques and dietary advice
- A suitable vocabulary should be established for each child; if it is aimed too high they are unlikely to understand, but if it is too low they will be insulted as a result of being treated childishly
- A friendly, non-threatening approach is required so that their trust is gained
- Ideally, children should not be threatened by phrases such as, "If you don't brush your teeth you'll have to have a needle", as this will cause them to associate dental visits with fear and pain – unfortunately, the team may sometimes find that this has already been threatened by a parent or another family member
- The patient should also feel comfortable when asking questions, so the oral health team should develop an open, frank manner with each child
- Oral health messages need to be fun so that the interest of the child is maintained
- Consequently, the use of games, drawings and competitions should be considered wherever possible
- Again, the use of disclosing agents (either tablets or liquids) should be encouraged, both by the dental team and at home, to stain the bacterial plaque and make its removal easier

Motivation can be thought of as the act of persuading people to do something for their own benefit. When there is a lack of motivation by patients to take an interest in their oral health, it needs to be established whether this is due to lack of knowledge, disinterest or the presence of previously unrealised risk factors. Once these points have been understood, priorities and goals can be set out for each patient and the role of the dental team can be established.
   Having established the different groups requiring oral health advice and the factors that can affect their motivation in relation to both their oral and general health, the various methods available to the dental team to improve that motivation can be considered in detail for each patient. Using this information, a plan of action can be developed in relation to the relevant oral and general health advice that is to be delivered, and how the various oral health messages should be communicated, especially in relation to caries and periodontal disease.

Successful communication with **adult patients** can be achieved in various ways:

- The use of specific oral health leaflets from dental suppliers
- One-to-one discussions of relevant oral health issues with a member of the dental team, in a non-patronising manner
- The non-use of dental jargon unless it is appropriate, but without condescension
- The adoption of an attentive manner, so that the patient's own difficulties and problems relating to their oral health maintenance are listened to and understood
- Any queries raised need answering at a level that the patient will understand, and may require referral to another member of the dental team by less experienced staff members
- Eye contact should be maintained with the patient during the discussions, to ensure the correct level of attention is given
- Reflective replies to their queries and concerns should be given, which relate to the patient's individual experiences

The more mature **young people** can be approached in a similar fashion, but less mature patients will require an individual approach aimed at their level of understanding. Pubescent teenagers may even take offence at the implication that they have a "dirty" mouth, and act quite negatively during any sessions to discuss their oral health issues. This tends to be especially the case with boys.

A young person of a "rebellious" nature may well be determined not to make efforts to improve their oral health, enjoying the "shock tactic" approach that this has on both the dental team and their parents. Thankfully, most tend to grow out of this phase as they mature.

Oral health messages can be communicated to this group as follows:

- The use of relevant leaflets and dental literature, many of which are specifically aimed at this age group
- Definitely a one-to-one approach to give oral health messages for those who are easily embarrassed
- Some will tend to react better in small groups, especially with similarly aged siblings or friends
- Authority and control of the situation need to be maintained by the dental team throughout the session, but in a friendly manner
- The dental team should never lose patience with these individuals, no matter how obstreperous they become
- Good patient management by the dental team at this age should produce attentive and responsible adults in the future

Children tend to respond best to a group approach when learning new information, but their interest in a subject can soon be lost and they can be easily distracted. Consequently, short and interactive sessions are best, with plenty of opportunities for individual involvement by the children, such as:

- The use of disclosing tablets to show the presence and position of bacterial plaque
- Supervising individual attempts at tooth brushing, to determine how to improve plaque removal
- Developing relevant games to play, especially any involving current TV or film characters
- Encouraging parental involvement in the oral health sessions wherever possible, as the parents need to maintain and promote the oral health messages discussed at home

Having received all of the available oral health advice given by the dental team, patients should now be able to determine whether they are motivated and willing to improve their oral health.

466

A gentle and tactful reminder of the reasons why good oral health should be a personal goal to be achieved by the patient can be given at this stage:

- To avoid the embarrassment of having halitosis (bad breath)
- To avoid the embarrassment and pain of having carious teeth
- To avoid tooth loss due to periodontal disease or caries
- To avoid the need for (and expense of) fixed or removable prostheses

Review of patient progress

The patient will need to be seen on a regular basis to determine whether progress regarding the level of oral hygiene has been made or not. The success or failure of the dental team in promoting and maintaining oral health depends on an understanding of the determinants of oral health:

- Social factors
- Environmental factors
- Economic factors
- Patient's knowledge
- Patient's skills

Oral health education should aim to modify any damaging behaviour, rather than unrealistically trying to reverse this behaviour, and oral health educators need to have an understanding of why any damaging behaviour occurs. In particular, the effects of being in a low socioeconomic group need to be understood by the dental team, as many of these patients are entitled to free dental care under the NHS and yet often exhibit poor standards of oral health compared with other socioeconomic groups.

Some of the reasons identified for this anomaly are as follows:

- They are the least likely group of patients to attend for routine and regular dental examinations, so there is little advice and preventive input from the dental team
- Their associated poor diet, often high in carbohydrates, predisposes them to general poor health
- The high rate of smoking and alcohol use in this group of patients tends to predispose them to periodontal disease and oral cancer
- Dental ignorance, often compounded by low self-esteem, prevents their own oral health from being a high priority
- Their high carbohydrate input tends to be related to the expected high caries incidence and early tooth loss
- Some of these patients feel intimidated by professionals and are unlikely to seek dental advice, especially about information regarding lifestyle changes
- Some people may also have difficulty understanding oral health advice, and this highlights the need for the dental team to develop good communication skills that can be adapted for various patients and situations as necessary

Studies indicate that patients in lower socioeconomic groups tend to have poorer general health overall, and advice given by the dental team must be sympathetic to this, as it is often related to the financial situation of these patients. All oral and general health advice should be given sympathetically and targeted at realistic outcomes. For example, parents in these groups often use sweets for their children as treats, or even bribes, because sweets are often cheaper to buy than books, toys or other presents. The finances of these families cannot be changed, so it would be totally unrealistic to try and stop the parents buying sweets for their children under these circumstances, and the delivery of the oral health advice and its promotion would fail. It is more sensible in these circumstances to educate the parents to restrict consumption of sweets to mealtimes, so that the frequency of acid attacks on their children's teeth is minimised and hopefully their caries experience will be reduced or even eradicated.

Similarly, it would be unrealistic to expect older smokers to give up their nicotine habit without plenty of encouragement and support from a smoking cessation scheme, as nicotine is addictive and the longer the patient has smoked, the harder it usually is to stop. Advice about current aids to help to stop smoking, such as nicotine patches and chewing gum, can be given, or the patient can be referred to the local cessation scheme for professional help and support.

Teenage smokers may be easier to re-educate, as they often only smoke to appear socially acceptable to their friends, or because of peer pressure. Advice regarding the overall damage to health caused by smoking, given in an informed but friendly manner, is often the first step in their re-education.

With all the information collated during the assessment with regard to the level of the patient's oral health, the extent of their known risk factors to oral disease and their level of motivation to improve their oral health, the dental team is able to determine the outcome of their oral health promotion efforts on each patient at their review appointment. This will fall into one of the following categories:

- **Has progress been made, resulting in a higher standard of oral hygiene?**
- **Has the original oral hygiene status been maintained, but with no improvement?**
- **Has the oral hygiene status deteriorated, such that more damage has occurred?**

When progress has been made, the patient should be congratulated and encouraged to maintain this raised standard of oral hygiene. Children can be given stickers, badges or certificates – all of which are available from oral hygiene product distributors. Computer programs are also available that can be used to design and print out certificates exclusive to the dental practice.

It should be remembered that oral health promotion is a long-term process, so regular monitoring will still be required for some time, although if the higher standard of oral hygiene becomes consistent, review appointment intervals can gradually be lengthened.

When the oral health status has been maintained but with no improvement, the patient should still be congratulated on the fact that there has been no relapse, and encouraged to try harder still before the next review. These patients tend to have considered the financial and emotional costs and benefits to themselves of changing their oral hygiene status, and decided that the costs outweigh the benefits at the present time. All is not lost, as this decision may be transitory, due, say, to a particularly stressful period in their lives, which leaves them unable or unwilling to attempt change now. Once this period is over, however, they may be receptive to further attempts by the dental team to promote oral health.

If the goals set by the dental team are not achievable, or are felt to be unrealistic for now, these patients should be reviewed regularly and supported until they feel able to try again.

The patients whose oral health has deteriorated may need referral to the dentist or hygienist for specialist input and reinforcement. However, reflection still needs to determine whether the goals set were completely unrealistic and unachievable for that particular patient. If so, then new ones will need to be discussed and agreed upon with the dental team.

Alternatively, and frustrating though it is, some patients really do not wish to change their lifestyle, nor do they accept the consequences to their oral health that may occur, as advised by the dental team. Regular monitoring and review are all that the dental team can hope to achieve for these patients, although they should stay alert to any indication by the patient that they are willing to try again at any time.

The patient's right to choose not to accept the oral health advice given by the dental team should be respected and accepted by all.

With regard to oral health assessment recall intervals, these depend on various factors for each patient. Figure 15.19 shows the current National Institute for Health and Clinical Excellence (NICE) guidelines that are used to determine the appropriate recall frequency in each case dependent on the listed risk factors shown.

NHS

National Institute for
Clinical Excellence

Issue date: **October 2004**

Quick reference guide

Dental recall

Recall interval between routine dental examinations

Guidance

- The recommended interval between oral health reviews should be determined specifically for each patient, and tailored to meet his or her needs, on the basis of an assessment of disease levels and risk of or from dental disease.

- This assessment should integrate the evidence presented in this guideline with the clinical judgement and expertise of the dental team, and should be discussed with the patient (see pages 2 and 3).

- During an oral health review, the dental team (led by the dentist) should ensure that comprehensive histories are taken, examinations are conducted and initial preventive advice is given. This will allow the dental team and the patient (and/or his or her parent, guardian or carer) to discuss, where appropriate:
  - the effects of oral hygiene, diet, fluoride use, tobacco and alcohol on oral health
  - the risk factors (see the checklist on page 2) that may influence the patient's oral health, and their implications for deciding the appropriate recall interval
  - the outcome of previous care episodes and the suitability of previously recommended intervals
  - the patient's ability or desire to visit the dentist at the recommended interval
  - the financial costs to the patient of having the oral health review and any subsequent treatments.

- The interval before the next oral health review should be chosen, either at the end of an oral health review if no further treatment is indicated, or on completion of a specific treatment journey.

- The recommended shortest and longest intervals between oral health reviews are as follows.
  - The shortest interval between oral health reviews for all patients should be 3 months.
  - The longest interval between oral health reviews for patients younger than 18 years should be 12 months.
  - The longest interval between oral health reviews for patients aged 18 years and older should be 24 months.

- For practical reasons, the patient should be assigned a recall interval of 3, 6, 9 or 12 months if he or she is younger than 18 years, or 3, 6, 9, 12, 15, 18, 21 or 24 months if he or she is aged 18 years or older.

- The dentist should discuss the recommended recall interval with the patient and record this interval, and the patient's agreement or disagreement with it, in the current record-keeping system.

- The recall interval should be reviewed again at the next oral health review, in order to learn from the patient's responses to the oral care provided and the health outcomes achieved. This feedback and the findings of the oral health review should be used to adjust the next recall interval chosen. Patients should be informed that their recommended recall interval may vary over time.

469

Clinical Guideline 19

Developed by the National Collaborating Centre for Acute Care

Figure 15.19   National Institute for Health and Care Excellence (NICE) guidelines for dental recall. Source: National Institute for Clinical Excellence (2004) CG 19 *Dental Recall: Recall Interval Between Routine Dental Examinations*. London: NICE. Available from http://guidance.nice.org.uk/CG19 Reproduced with permission.

Checklist of modifying factors						
Name:		Date of birth:				
Oral health review date:						
Medical history	Yes	No	Yes	No	Yes	No
Conditions where dental disease could put the patient's general health at increased risk (such as cardiovascular disease, bleeding disorders, immunosuppression)	☐	☐	☐	☐	☐	☐
Conditions that increase a patient's risk of developing dental disease (such as diabetes, xerostomia)	☐	☐	☐	☐	☐	☐
Conditions that may complicate dental treatment or the patient's ability to maintain their oral health (such as special needs, anxious/nervous/phobic conditions)	☐	☐	☐	☐	☐	☐
Social history						
High caries in mother and siblings	☐	☐	☐	☐	☐	☐
Tobacco use	☐	☐	☐	☐	☐	☐
Excessive alcohol use	☐	☐	☐	☐	☐	☐
Family history of chronic or aggressive (early onset/juvenile) periodontitis	☐	☐	☐	☐	☐	☐
Dietary habits						
High and/or frequent sugar intake	☐	☐	☐	☐	☐	☐
High and/or frequent dietary acid intake	☐	☐	☐	☐	☐	☐
Exposure to fluoride						
Use of fluoride toothpaste	☐	☐	☐	☐	☐	☐
Other sources of fluoride (for example, the patient lives in a water-fluoridated area)	☐	☐	☐	☐	☐	☐
Clinical evidence and dental history						
Recent and previous caries experience						
New lesions since last check-up	☐	☐	☐	☐	☐	☐
Anterior caries or restorations	☐	☐	☐	☐	☐	☐
Premature extractions because of caries	☐	☐	☐	☐	☐	☐
Past root caries or large number of exposed roots	☐	☐	☐	☐	☐	☐
Heavily restored dentition	☐	☐	☐	☐	☐	☐
Recent and previous periodontal disease experience						
Previous history of periodontal disease	☐	☐	☐	☐	☐	☐
Evidence of gingivitis	☐	☐	☐	☐	☐	☐
Presence of periodontal pockets (BPE code 3 or 4) and/or bleeding on probing	☐	☐	☐	☐	☐	☐
Presence of furcation involvements or advanced attachment loss (BPE code *)	☐	☐	☐	☐	☐	☐
Mucosal lesions						
Mucosal lesion present	☐	☐	☐	☐	☐	☐
Plaque						
Poor level of oral hygiene	☐	☐	☐	☐	☐	☐
Plaque-retaining factors (such as orthodontic appliances)	☐	☐	☐	☐	☐	☐
Saliva						
Low saliva flow rate	☐	☐	☐	☐	☐	☐
Erosion and tooth surface loss						
Clinical evidence of tooth wear	☐	☐	☐	☐	☐	☐
Recommended recall interval for next oral health review:	months		months		months	
Does patient agree with recommended interval? If 'No', record reason for disagreement in notes	Yes	No	Yes	No	Yes	No
BPE code * is used when attachment loss is ≥7mm and/or furcation involvements are present						

Figure 15.19 *(continued)*

Effect of general health on oral health

It is essential that patients understand that the condition of their oral health is not a separate issue from that of their general health and that the two are very much linked together. The dietary and lifestyle advice that the dental team offers to ensure good oral health will also be relevant to maintaining an overall high level of general health, if patients choose to follow that advice.

There are numerous medically related examples of the links between oral health and general health, as outlined in the following:

- Several chronic diseases have the **same risk factors** as oral diseases:
  - The association of **smoking** and other tobacco habits with heart and respiratory disease, periodontal disease and cancers such as oral cancer
  - Diets high in **NMES** and those containing many processed meals are linked to dental caries, obesity and an increased risk of heart disease
  - **Excessive alcohol consumption** is associated with liver disease, periodontal disease, dental trauma (due to falls) and several cancers, including oral cancer
  - **Eating disorders**, such as anorexia nervosa and bulimia, are associated with general ill health and acid erosion of the enamel of teeth, respectively
  - **Diabetics** suffer from poor wound healing generally, which also affects the oral soft tissues and makes the patients prone to postoperative complications, as well as to a higher incidence of oral infections (including periodontal infections)
- Certain commonly prescribed medicines have the unwanted side-effect of **reducing saliva flow**:
  - Some antihypertensives
  - Some antidepressants
- Some medical conditions may also result in a reduced salivary flow, such as Sjögren's syndrome
- Other medicines have the unwanted side-effect of causing gingival overgrowth, or **gingival hyperplasia**, which makes effective oral hygiene techniques more difficult:
  - Phenytoin – used to prevent epileptic fits
  - Nifedipine – used to control heart problems
  - Ciclosporin – used in some autoimmune conditions, as well as to prevent organ rejection after transplant

In addition to these, the effects of patient disability (physical or mental) as well as that of old age have a huge influence on the dental team with regard to oral health advice and promotion, and oral disease prevention.

Patients with disabilities

Disability comes in many forms and can be either mental or physical in its effect on the patient. Mentally disabled patients range from those with minor learning disabilities, through the elderly suffering from various forms of senile dementia (such as Alzheimer's disease), to those with congenital problems, such as Down's syndrome sufferers. There are also some patients who have significant problems associated with learning and socialising with others, due to inherited disorders such as Down's syndrome, autism and Asperger's syndrome, or acquired but permanent disorders following severe head injury. Those with mild impairment are likely to access dental treatment via general practice, while the more severe cases are likely to be referred for specialist dental care in community-run special needs clinics.

The dental care of these patients can be very demanding and time-consuming for the dental team, but also professionally challenging and very rewarding, and those dental nurses with a particular interest in this area are advised to consider the post-registration qualification in special care dental nursing, run by the National Examining Board for Dental Nurses (NEBDN).

471

Sometimes, but not always (e.g. in the case of autistic patients), those with some learning disabilities may exhibit a reduced ability to understand generally, which presents the following problems to the dental team:

- They have a short attention span, so explaining treatment plans and gaining valid consent are often difficult
- Poor memory retention requires information and advice to be repeated many times
- Any reduced level of understanding may cause problems with gaining the trust of the patient before dental treatment can be provided
- Careful explanations of treatment must be given using basic and non-threatening terms – e.g. avoiding the use of words such as "pain" and "needle"
- The link between diet, oral hygiene and dental disease is often impossible to explain satisfactorily, making cooperation in the management of the patient's oral health very difficult
- Some dental staff may slip into a type of "baby talk" when communicating with these patients – this is particularly unnecessary and offensive to those with acquired learning disabilities

Those who have physical disabilities make up a wide-ranging group of patients, from those who are paralysed and wheelchair-bound, and those with visual or auditory impairments, to those who have acquired medical conditions that affect the level of dental care they are able to receive. Again, the more severely disabled patients tend to be treated in specialist units rather than general dental practice, the latter being able to accommodate the milder cases to varying levels of efficiency. Some of the more common problems that these patients present to the dental team are as follows:

- Hearing-impaired patients often rely on hearing aids or lip reading to understand when being spoken to by the team, so the lowering of personal protective equipment (PPE) masks in order to have face-to-face contact is very important in communicating with them
- Visually impaired patients like to touch and feel, or listen to the sound of, dental equipment before it is used on them, and the dental team should accede to these requests at all times
- Some physical disabilities will require the patient to be treated in downstairs surgeries only, with wheelchair access available too
- Any disabilities causing variations in muscle tone may restrict the patient's ability to sit comfortably in the dental chair and may also require the use of muscle relaxants to achieve adequate access to the oral cavity
- Stroke victims may have difficulty communicating if their speech has been affected, and may rely on family members or carers to make themselves understood
- Arthritic patients, and those with upper limb deformities (such as thalidomide victims or those with dwarfism), may find adequate oral hygiene impossible to achieve without special adaptations to toothbrushes, and so on.

Members of the dental team have a vital role to play in assisting disabled patients they come into contact with in their dental workplace, not only by adapting the level of oral health promotion given, but also in the oral hygiene techniques they teach. Effective oral hygiene measures may require adaptations to oral health products, such as adapting a toothbrush handle so that it can be gripped more firmly by an arthritic patient, for instance. The oral health of the patient may even be the responsibility of a carer, and it is vital that this person also attends the evaluation, support and review appointments with the patient, so that help, advice and support from the dental team can be given, as necessary.

Angled toothbrushes, or even children's rather than adult sizes, can make access to the teeth much easier for the patient or carer. Good-quality rechargeable electric toothbrushes, when used correctly, can ensure a good standard of oral hygiene, although battery-operated designs are not particularly recommended, as they can lose their charge with time and become quite inefficient at plaque control.

Several floss holders are now available to allow efficient interdental cleaning (see Figure 5.15), and even manually dextrous patients may find these less cumbersome than the traditional method of wrapping floss around the fingers.

Elderly patients

As discussed in Chapter 13, the oral tissue changes that occur during ageing have prompted the formation of a specialist discipline of dentistry which deals with elderly patients and their particular dental requirements – this is known as gerodontology (similarly to the equivalent specialised area of medicine, geriatrics). The provision of general dental treatment to the majority of elderly patients is often possible in the dental workplace, but in terms of communicating with them and assisting in the management of their oral health and hygiene, this group may also experience difficulties in accessing dental care for any of the following reasons:

- Immobility, or poor mobility, making regular attendance at a dental practice difficult or impossible
- Poor mobility may restrict access to ground floor surgeries only
- Complicated medical problems, which may limit the dental treatments available to them
- Complicated drug regimes, some of which may interact with dental anaesthesia and dental medicaments
- Various degrees of senile dementia, which may make explanations of dental treatment difficult for them to understand or remember
- Various degrees of visual impairment or hearing loss, which can again make explanations difficult

473

Summary

Overall, there are many factors for the dental team to consider in relation to oral health advice and promotion, and oral disease prevention, but in summary the key points of global dental health education for all patients can be condensed into four simple messages:

- Reduce the frequency of consumption of food and drink containing sugar, and avoid acid drinks
- Maintain adequate oral hygiene measures
- Brush twice daily with fluoride toothpaste
- Regular dental attendance, at least once a year

Manage and handle materials and instruments, and understand the purpose and stages of different dental procedures

It is unrealistic to expect patients to maintain a perfect level of plaque control throughout their lives, and from time to time they will therefore require some form of restorative treatment, as well as having to undergo plaque control measures. The various dental procedures that may be carried out are given in the following list, while the theory and underpinning knowledge of each one are discussed in subsequent main sections (the role of the dental nurse in the provision of chairside assistance for each procedure is further discussed in the relevant chapters shown).

The procedures are:

- Administration of local anaesthesia
- Cavity restoration with fillings (also see Chapter 8)

- Periodontal therapy (also see earlier and Chapter 8)
- Non-surgical endodontic treatment (also see Chapter 10)
- Fixed prostheses (temporary and permanent crowns, bridges and veneers) (also see Chapter 9)
- Removable prostheses (partial, full, and immediate dentures) (also see Chapter 9)
- Orthodontic treatment (also see Chapter 9)
- Extractions and minor oral surgery (also see Chapter 11)

Administration of local anaesthesia

As described in Chapter 13, the oral cavity has an excellent nerve supply to all areas and anyone who has suffered the misery of "toothache" or even minor mouth ulcers will vouch for just how well developed the pain reception in this area can be. To carry out any of the oral or dental surgical treatments listed in the preceding section without some form of pain control would be acutely painful for the patient, and the majority of procedures are therefore usually carried out under a technique of **local anaesthesia**.

Local anaesthesia

The term "anaesthesia" is defined as "the loss of all sensation", but in dentistry when local anaesthetics are administered, they produce the loss of pain sensation only – pressure can still be felt by the patient. These drugs used to produce the loss of pain sensation only are therefore more correctly termed "local analgesics".

Teeth and their support structures are particularly well innervated with a sensory nerve supply that responds to temperature, pressure and pain. Local anaesthetics must be given by injection before dental treatment begins, so that the patient is comfortable and pain-free throughout the procedure. All sensations felt by the body tissues are transmitted as electrical impulses along the length of the sensory neurones (nerve cells) to the brain, where the information is analysed and interpreted. Local anaesthetics act by blocking these electrical transmissions from the source of the stimulation (the tooth or its surroundings), so that the information that a painful procedure is being carried out does not reach the brain. The patient is conscious and fully aware of the treatment being carried out (unless sedated), but feels no unpleasant or painful stimuli.

In addition, the sensations of hot and cold are also blocked, as they would be interpreted as pain under these circumstances – the heat generated when a tooth is drilled with no cooling water spray is interpreted as pain by the brain, and similarly anyone with sensitive teeth will relate to the very uncomfortable sensation that occurs when cold drinks are taken.

The sensations of pressure and vibration will remain – so, for example, the patient will be aware of the pushing and wiggling sensations that occur during a tooth extraction procedure, but it should be completely painless if the local anaesthetic has been administered correctly.

Local anaesthetic drugs

Many local anaesthetics are now available for use in dentistry, and they are all supplied within glass or plastic cartridges for use in special dental syringes (Figure 15.20). The cartridges are available in either 2.2 or 1.8 mL sizes, and contain the following:

- **Anaesthetic** – to block the electrical nerve transmissions to the brain so that neither pain nor temperature changes can be felt
- **Sterile water** – acts as a carrying solution for the other constituents and makes up the bulk of the cartridge contents

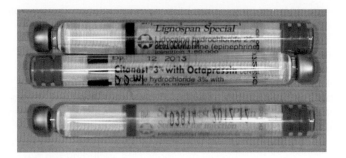

Figure 15.20   Local anaesthetic cartridges.

- **Buffering agents** – maintain the contents of the cartridge at a neutral pH of 7, so they are neither acidic nor alkaline and do not irritate the soft tissues when they are injected
- **Preservative** – to give an adequate shelf life to the contents
- **Vasoconstrictor** – present in some types of local anaesthetic (but not all) and acts to prolong the action of the anaesthetic by closing (constricting) local blood vessels so that the solution is not carried so quickly in the bloodstream

Both the anaesthetic agent and any vasoconstrictor present are classed as drugs, and are therefore subject to strict regulations with regard to their safe disposal from the dental workplace. Used local anaesthetic cartridges are now classified as "**infectious hazardous waste**", while unused but out-of-date cartridges are classified as "**non-hazardous waste**" as a medicine, although broken cartridges should be disposed of as sharps waste under the "infectious hazardous waste" category.

The more common local anaesthetics currently in use in dentistry are as follows:

- **Lidocaine** – 2% lignocaine hydrochloride as the local anaesthetic with 1:80 000 adrenaline (epinephrine) as a vasoconstrictor (known as Lignospan and xylocaine)
- **Articaine** - carticaine as the local anaesthetic with 1:100 000 adrenaline as a vasoconstrictor
- **Citanest** – 3% prilocaine hydrochloride as the local anaesthetic, with 0.03 units/mL felypressin (octapressin) as a vasoconstrictor
- **Citanest plain** – 4% prilocaine hydrochloride as the local anaesthetic, with no vasoconstrictor present
- **Mepivacaine** – 3% mepivacaine hydrochloride as the local anaesthetic, with no vasoconstrictor present (known as Scandonest)

Adrenaline (also called epinephrine) is the commonest vasoconstrictor used in dental local anaesthetics, but it is a potent cardiac stimulant which acts to increase the rate and depth of a patient's heart beat generally. This explains its usefulness as an emergency drug in various situations, such as during anaphylaxis when the blood pressure falls to such low levels that the heart can stop beating (see Chapter 13). Unfortunately, it also means that local anaesthetics containing it cannot be used safely on patients with certain medical conditions, including the following:

- **Hypertension** – high blood pressure
- **Cardiac disease** – poor functioning of the heart, whether due to valve defects or acquired problems such as coronary artery disease
- **Hyperthyroidism** – an overactive thyroid gland, which tends to increase the overall metabolic rate of the patient, including the heart rate

In addition, care should be taken with the following groups of patients or with those taking certain drugs:

- **Elderly patients** – as they may have complicated medical histories, be taking other drugs that could react with adrenaline, have undiagnosed diseases, or simply not be able to excrete drugs efficiently due to their age
- **Hormone replacement therapy (HRT)** – given to women to counteract the adverse effects of the menopause and prevent the development of osteoporosis (thinning of the bones), but may produce hypertension as a side-effect
- **Thyroxine** – a drug given to patients suffering from hypothyroidism (an underactive thyroid gland), which increases their overall metabolic rate, including the heart rate

Theoretical risks are also said to exist with patients taking certain antidepressants, including tricyclics and monoamine oxidase inhibitors (MAOIs).

The use of local anaesthetics containing no vasoconstrictor is an alternative in these groups of patients, but then the analgesic action would wear off more quickly and there is more risk of haemorrhage during surgical procedures. Alternatively, they can be given 3% Citanest – the only contraindications to its use being **pregnancy**, as felypressin is a potent drug used to induce labour due to its contractive action on the muscles of the uterus.

476

Local anaesthetic equipment

The equipment required to administer the local anaesthetic consists of the cartridge itself, the syringe and needle, and sometimes a topical anaesthetic is used.

The anaesthetic cartridge is a glass or plastic tube sealed at one end with a thin rubber diaphragm and at the other with a rubber bung. A special syringe and needle are required for use with dental cartridges. When a cartridge is inserted into the syringe, the double-ended needle pierces the diaphragm. Solution is injected when the syringe plunger engages the rubber bung and pushes it down the tube. As some patients are now known to have an allergy to latex, the rubber bung and diaphragm have been replaced with plastic alternatives in some types of specialised cartridges.

Various designs of local anaesthetic syringe are available, some of which are side-loading and some breech-loading (from the back) (see Figure 15.21). The majority are metallic so that they can be sterilised in an autoclave after each use, but single-use plastic disposable ones are also available.

In addition, the head of the plunger is adapted in some syringes so that the dentist can use an **aspirating technique** when administering the local anaesthetic, for patient safety reasons

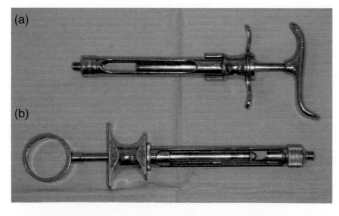

Figure 15.21   Local anaesthetic syringes: (a) side-loading; (b) breech-loading.

(Figure 15.22). The technique is designed to avoid the injection of the solution into a blood vessel, rather than around the nerve, as is required. Once the needle has been positioned, the plunger is drawn back or pressed slightly and released, before the injection of any solution occurs, so that if a blood vessel has been pierced, blood will flow visibly into the anaesthetic cartridge. The needle tip can then be repositioned, the cartridge aspirated to check again, and then the contents safely injected into the correct position around the nerve.

All syringes have a universal-sized thread end for the needle to be positioned and attached. The needles are provided in various lengths and sizes, or gauges, depending on the type of injection to be given (Figure 15.23). Smaller sizes are less painful to use, but are too fine to be used in some oral injection sites, especially where muscle tissue has to be penetrated to reach the target nerve.

Topical anaesthetics are used on the surface of the oral mucous membrane to provide localised anaesthesia in that area, so that a syringe needle can be inserted painlessly and the local anaesthetic can be administered. They are used in the form of a paste, solution or spray, which is applied to the appropriate site a few minutes before an injection is given. Commonly used surface anaesthetics are 5% lidocaine paste (Figure 15.24) or 20% benzocaine.

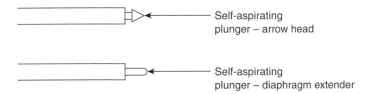

Self-aspirating
plunger – arrow head

Self-aspirating
plunger – diaphragm extender

Figure 15.22   Self-aspirating syringe plungers. Source: *Levison's Textbook for Dental Nurses*, 11th edition (Hollins), 2013. Reproduced with permission of Wiley-Blackwell.

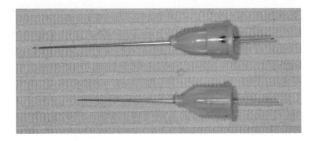

Figure 15.23   Local anaesthetic needles.

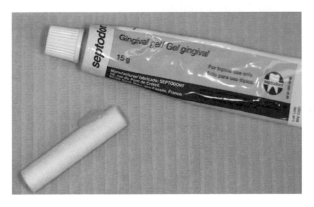

Figure 15.24   Topical anaesthetic gel.

These products are also used to minimise the discomfort of superficial scaling, for fitting matrix bands and for preventing stimulation of the gag reflex when taking impressions.

Local anaesthetic administration techniques

Due to the variable anatomy of the jaws, the administration technique required to anaesthetise teeth is dependent on whether the relevant sensory nerve is deep within the bone, or superficial to the surface. Other techniques can be used to anaesthetise individual teeth and their surroundings only, without causing any soft tissue effects. Generally, there are four basic methods of administering a dental local anaesthetic (Figure 15.25):

- Nerve block (regional anaesthesia)
- Local infiltration
- Intra-ligamentary injection
- Intra-osseous injection

Nerve block

A nerve block is an injection that anaesthetises the nerve trunk as it runs in soft tissue, either before it enters the jaw bone or after it leaves it to reach the teeth and associated parts. Pain sensations from every part supplied by the nerve are blocked at the site of injection and cannot reach the brain – so the technique is also referred to as regional anaesthesia. A nerve block is used when it is necessary to anaesthetise several teeth in one quadrant or where a local infiltration cannot work.

The commonest example of this type of injection is the **inferior dental block**. For this injection, the anaesthetic solution is injected over the mandibular foramen, on the inner surface of the ramus of the mandible (Figure 15.26). At this site, the inferior dental and lingual nerves are so close to each other that both nerves are anaesthetised together. Thus it has the effect of anaesthetising all the lower teeth and lingual gum on the side of the injection, together with that half of the tongue as well. Furthermore, it anaesthetises the lower lip and buccal gum of the incisors, canine and premolars, as these are supplied by the mental branch of the inferior dental nerve. So once the patient confirms the numbness of the lower lip, the dentist knows that all the lower teeth on that side will also be numb.

The only part unaffected by this injection is the buccal gum of the lower molars; this area of soft tissue is supplied by the long buccal nerve, which is too far from the injection site to be affected. The nerve supply of the oral cavity is covered in detail in Chapter 13.

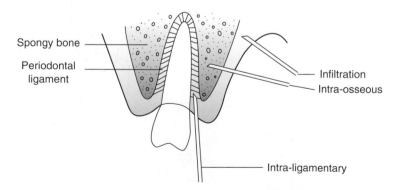

Figure 15.25   Types of local anaesthetic injection. Source: *Levison's Textbook for Dental Nurses*, 11th edition (Hollins), 2013. Reproduced with permission of Wiley-Blackwell.

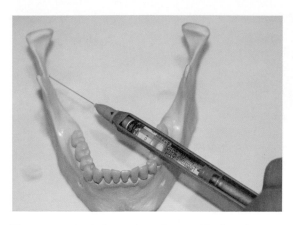

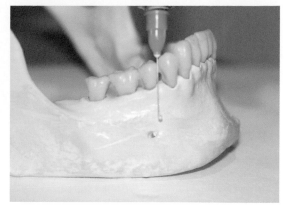

Figure 15.26   Inferior dental nerve block technique.   **Figure 15.27**   Mental nerve block technique.

Other nerve block injections that may be administered by the dentist are as follows:

- **Mental nerve block** – to anaesthetise the end portion only of the inferior dental nerve, as it leaves the mandible through the mental foramen, so that only the anterior teeth and their buccal or labial soft tissues are affected (Figure 15.27)
- **Posterior superior dental nerve block** – to anaesthetise this nerve before it enters the maxillary antrum, so that both the upper second and third molar teeth are affected

The nerve block technique is useful in situations where an infection is present around a tooth requiring dental treatment, as it can be anaesthetised without risking the spread of the infection by placing the injection at a distance from the tooth involved.

As stated previously, the nerves tend to run as neurovascular bundles and an aspirating technique should be used during a block injection, to prevent the inadvertent introduction of the cartridge contents into a blood vessel.

Local infiltration

A local infiltration injection is given over the apex of the tooth to be anaesthetised. The needle is inserted beneath the mucous membrane overlying the jaw bone. The anaesthetic soaks through pores in the bone and anaesthetises the nerves supplying the tooth and gum at the site of injection. Thus the difference between these two types of injection is that a nerve block applies the anaesthetic to the nerve trunk, whereas an infiltration applies it to the nerve endings.

A local infiltration injection can only be used where the compact bone is sufficiently thin and porous to allow the anaesthetic to penetrate into the inner spongy bone. Thus it is usually effective for all upper teeth, and for the lower incisor teeth. The compact bone overlying the mandibular premolars and molars is too thick, however, and an inferior dental and mental blocks, respectively, are necessary for these. A local infiltration can always be used to anaesthetise the local gingivae only, as will be required for procedures such as extractions.

Intra-ligamentary injection

The intra-ligamentary injection technique tends to be used in conjunction with either an infiltration or a nerve block, to produce deeper anaesthesia around hypersensitive teeth. Various specialised syringes are available, which hold the smaller 1.8 mL anaesthetic cartridge within a protective plastic sheath (Figure 15.28). The force required to administer the cartridge contents is

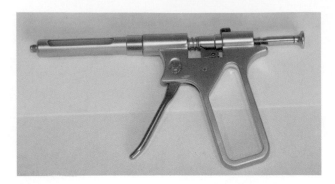

Figure 15.28   Ligmaject syringe. Source: *Levison's Textbook for Dental Nurses*, 11th edition (Hollins), 2013. Reproduced with permission of Wiley-Blackwell.

considerable, so a ratchet design of plunger is used to maintain the pressure, and the plastic sheath prevents injury if a glass cartridge shatters during use, as sometimes happens.

The anaesthetic is administered into the periodontal ligament of the tooth, and the surrounding gingivae can be seen to blanch (turn pale) as it takes effect. This technique is especially useful when a nerve block has failed to produce sufficient anaesthesia of the tooth, but it cannot be used in the presence of gingival infection unless the tooth is being extracted. The force required for administration may also cause some postoperative soreness for the patient.

Intra-osseous injection

An intra-osseous injection is given directly through the outer cortical plate of the jaw and into the spongy bone between two teeth. A few drops of anaesthetic are first injected into the overlying gum to permit painless drilling of a small hole through the compact bone, in order to allow a needle to be inserted directly into the spongy bone (Figure 15.29).

This injection provides a relatively short duration, but profound depth, of anaesthesia for the tooth, and buccal and lingual gum, on either side of the injection site, but it does not numb the cheek, lip or tongue. This makes it an excellent method for extractions. Other advantages are that it works immediately and rarely fails, thus making it useful where an infiltration or nerve block has been unsuccessful. The disadvantages are that it cannot be used where gingival (gum) infection is present, nor should it be used in the region of the mental foramen of the mandible, as the nerve could easily be damaged while the access hole is being drilled.

The technique is very old but has gained a new lease of life with the introduction of the Stabident kit, containing a special drill for perforating the compact bone, and a matching ultra-short needle for injecting directly into spongy bone.

Local anaesthesia for extractions

When a tooth requires extraction, it is necessary to anaesthetise the surrounding periodontium as well as the tooth itself, as the periodontal ligament will be severed during the procedure. The injections required for each tooth will be more readily understood by referring back to the nerve supply of the teeth.

Upper teeth

To anaesthetise any upper tooth for extraction, a local infiltration injection is given on both its buccal/labial and palatal sides. The buccal infiltration will anaesthetise the tooth and the buccal/labial

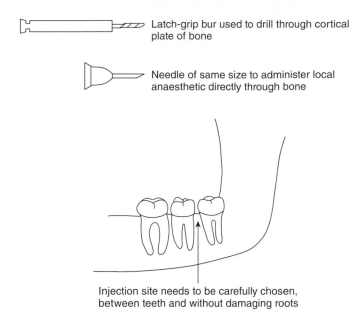

Latch-grip bur used to drill through cortical plate of bone

Needle of same size to administer local anaesthetic directly through bone

Injection site needs to be carefully chosen, between teeth and without damaging roots

Figure 15.29   Intra-osseous system. Source: *Levison's Textbook for Dental Nurses*, 11th edition (Hollins), 2013. Reproduced with permission of Wiley-Blackwell.

periodontium, and the palatal injection will anaesthetise the palatal periodontium. It also helps to ensure sufficient anaesthesia of the tooth by infiltrating the palatal root of the molars too.

For the second and third molars, some operators prefer to give a posterior superior dental block instead of a local infiltration on the buccal side. The nerve supply of the upper teeth and their gingivae is illustrated in Figure 15.30.

Lower teeth

An inferior dental block injection blocks the lingual as well as the inferior dental nerve. This single injection will therefore suffice for the extraction of premolars, canines and incisors, as their buccal/labial periodontium is supplied by the end section of the inferior dental nerve, the mental nerve.

For lower molars, whose buccal periodontium is supplied by the long buccal nerve, an additional local buccal infiltration is required for full anaesthesia.

The compact bone in the incisor region of the mandible is sufficiently thin to allow the use of a labial and lingual local infiltration, and many operators prefer this technique rather than an inferior dental block for anaesthetising lower incisors. The nerve supply of the lower teeth and their gingivae is illustrated in Figure 15.31.

Local anaesthesia for restorative treatments

It is unnecessary to anaesthetise the palatal or lingual gingivae in addition to the tooth and buccal/labial gingivae for restorative treatments, unless the gingivae in these areas need adjustment or removal as part of the restorative procedure. Examples of when this is necessary are:

- When a cavity has been present for some time and the gingiva has grown into the space present – its removal is necessary to ensure that the filling material is fully adapted to the cavity walls

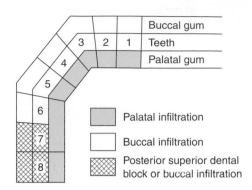

Figure 15.30 Injections for upper teeth. Source: *Levison's Textbook for Dental Nurses*, 11th edition (Hollins), 2013. Reproduced with permission of Wiley-Blackwell.

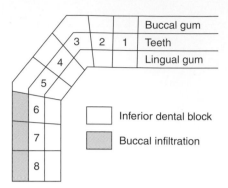

Figure 15.31 Injections for lower teeth. Source: *Levison's Textbook for Dental Nurses*, 11th edition (Hollins), 2013. Reproduced with permission of Wiley-Blackwell.

- When a crown lengthening technique is required during tooth preparation for a fixed prosthesis – its adjustment is necessary to allow for a lengthened tooth preparation so that adequate retention of the restoration is achieved, or to achieve good aesthetics
- When a crown has been lost and the remaining root face has been covered by gingival overgrowth – its removal is required to ensure an accurate impression is taken so that the new restoration fits the root face adequately

Upper teeth

A local buccal/labial infiltration is enough for routine restorative treatments, although a posterior superior dental block is sometimes preferred for the second and third molars.

Lower teeth

An inferior dental block will anaesthetise every lower tooth, while a mental block may be used when treatment involves any tooth other than the lower molars. For restorative treatment involving just the lower incisors, a local labial infiltration will suffice instead of a full mental nerve block technique.

Preparation for local anaesthesia

All cartridges and needles are supplied by their manufacturers pre-sterilised and ready for use. Reusable metal syringes are sterilised as usual in an autoclave.

A long needle of 27 gauge is used for a nerve block. For local infiltration, a short needle of 30 gauge is usually preferred. Although needles rarely break during an injection, precautions must still be taken to deal with such accidents immediately. A suitable pair of artery forceps (such as Spencer Wells or mosquito forceps) should always be available to grasp and remove the broken end.

A topical surface anaesthetic is applied for a few minutes on a cotton wool roll while the local anaesthetic equipment is prepared for use. The required cartridge is loaded into the syringe and then the smaller plastic guard at the syringe end of the needle is removed so that it can be screwed on to the syringe hub. When an aspirating technique is to be used, those syringes with a screw-type plunger will need the device to be screwed into the cartridge bung *before* the needle is attached; otherwise the cartridge contents will be partially ejected as it is screwed in with the needle already attached.

Injection of cold solutions can be painful, so cartridges should not be stored in a refrigerator but kept at room temperature. The injection site may be dried and disinfected by applying a suitable disinfectant, such as chlorhexidine or iodine, on a pledget of cotton wool for 15 seconds. This disinfection procedure is not routinely carried out before administering a local anaesthetic for general dental treatment, but is more likely to be done during large surgical procedures, such as implant insertion or maxillofacial treatments. The injection is now given and the needle guard refitted immediately, using a re-sheathing device. Ideally, this should be carried out by the team member who administered the local anaesthetic, while they are still holding the syringe. The alternative is for them to lay down the syringe with its unsheathed needle on the work surface, from where it then needs to be picked up by another team member for re-sheathing – increasing both the potential for a needle-stick injury to occur and the number of team members who may be injured during such an incident.

The used cartridge and needle are disposed of in accordance with the hazardous waste regulations – both are classed as infectious hazardous waste, subcategory "sharps", so they need to be deposited in the sharps bin.

The used needle is a very real source of cross-infection, as it has pierced the patient's tissues and will be contaminated with blood (and possibly microorganisms), no matter how small the amount. Re-sheathing of the needle is the commonest cause of needlestick injuries to the dental team, and various needle guard devices have been designed to lower their incidence. Whatever the design, the needle sheath needs to be held firmly upright in a container, so that the syringe can be safely held by its back end while the needle is re-sheathed (see Figure 1.29). In this way, fingers are kept away from the dirty needle and injury is unlikely. The team member who administered the local anaesthetic should also always take responsibility for re-sheathing the needle personally, to reduce the number of potential injured persons involved – this may be the dentist, the therapist or the hygienist. If a contaminated needlestick injury does occur, the following actions must be followed:

- Stop working immediately, so that the patient and other team members are not contaminated and the potential for cross-infection is minimised
- The pierced area should be squeezed immediately to encourage bleeding, ideally under running warm water to slow down clotting at the wound site and increase the volume of blood expressed
- Under no circumstances should the wound be sucked to encourage bleeding, as this will increase the chance of cross-infection by pathogens still further
- The wounded area should then be cleaned with disinfectant soap, dried and covered with a waterproof dressing
- The senior team member should be informed of the incident
- The patient's medical history form should be checked for known cross-infection risks, such as being HIV-positive
- If necessary, the matter should be reported to the local occupational health adviser (OHA) at the local hospital, and any advice given should be followed immediately
- The contact details of the OHA should be stored in the infection control policy documentation
- The incident should be recorded in either the accident book (low risk of serious infection) or a Reporting of Injuries, Diseases and Dangerous Occurrences Regulations (RIDDOR) report should be written (high risk of serious infection) and the RIDDOR process followed

Patient advice following local anaesthesia

Patients need to be informed of the effects they are likely to experience after receiving a local anaesthetic, especially if it is their first injection. Otherwise, they may be unduly

483

concerned at what they feel or they may even accidently injure themselves. The necessary advice is as follows:

- Sensation will be lost in the affected area for several hours – this varies between patients but is usually of at least 2 hours' duration when a local anaesthetic containing a vasoconstrictor has been used
- During this time, they should not attempt to eat, drink, or smoke, as they may bite or burn themselves without realising
- Chewing food directly onto the restored teeth should be avoided that day, to prevent damaging the new restoration (unless the dentist has said otherwise)
- When the anaesthetic is wearing off, they will feel a "pins and needles" sensation in the area – this is called **paraesthesia** and is perfectly normal
- They should wait for this "pins and needles" sensation to completely wear off before attempting to eat or drink
- Nerve block techniques may cause a localised tenderness of the soft tissues
- Intra-ligamentary techniques may cause soreness of the surrounding gingivae
- Contact the surgery if any problems persist

Cavity restoration with fillings

Cavities are caused by dental caries attacking the hard structure of the tooth, and if left untreated they will cause pain for the patient and develop into a more serious dental problem that may result in the loss of the tooth. A cavity will therefore require treatment, and once its presence has been determined, a treatment plan will be decided upon based on the following information:

- **Cavity size** – is restoration of the tooth feasible with a restorative filling alone, or should a fixed restoration (such as a crown) be considered?
- **Cavity position** – which tooth surface or surfaces are involved; do aesthetics need to be considered?
- **Tooth involved** – is a posterior chewing tooth involved, which will require a strong and long-lasting restoration, or is an anterior tooth involved where chewing forces are less, but aesthetics have to be considered?
- **Extent of caries** – is it possible that full caries removal will cause pulp exposure, so that endodontic treatment will also be required?
- **Patient's wishes** – is the patient amenable to restorative treatment, or are they likely to be unco-operative, as may occur especially with younger children and some patients with special needs?

Taking into consideration all of these points, restoration by filling may be on a temporary or a permanent basis as follows:

- **Temporary restoration** – in less co-operative patients, and if a fixed restoration is being considered as the final restoration in the short term; the usual materials used are:
  - Zinc oxide and eugenol cement
  - Zinc phosphate cement
  - Zinc polycarboxylate cement
- **Amalgam restoration** – in posterior teeth, where restoration strength and longevity are more of an issue than aesthetics
- **Composite restoration** – in anterior teeth for aesthetics, although more modern composite materials are suitable for use in restorations in posterior teeth too
- **Glass ionomer restoration** – in deciduous teeth (because of its fluoride release) and in certain cavity sites where retention of the restoration is difficult

The aims of good cavity preparation are the same no matter where the lesion has occurred and whatever restorative material is to be used – those that apply for the restoration of permanent teeth are as follows:

- To remove all caries from the cavity
- To remove the minimum amount of healthy tooth tissue while doing so
- To avoid accidental pulp exposure as a result of poor dental technique
- To protect the pulp after treatment by using linings or bases as necessary
- To produce a retentive cavity for restoration, if necessary (some materials are adhesive to tooth tissue – see later)
- To restore the tooth to its normal shape and prevent stagnation areas developing, as these would allow plaque retention and further carious attack to occur
- To restore the function of the tooth for adequate mastication
- To restore the retentive shape of the tooth if it acts as a bridge abutment or denture retainer
- To restore the aesthetics of the tooth (its correct appearance)
- To alleviate any discomfort or pain experienced by the patient, due to the initial presence of the cavity

The situation is a little different with deciduous teeth as they will be naturally exfoliated at some point as the child grows, and the permanence of their restoration is therefore of less importance. The aims of good cavity preparation in these cases are as follows:

485

- To alleviate any discomfort or pain experienced by the patient, due to the initial presence of the cavity
- To restore the function of the tooth for adequate mastication
- To allow the retention of the tooth until the time that it is naturally exfoliated, so that the eruption space for its permanent successor is retained – otherwise the permanent tooth may become crowded out of the arch, and orthodontic treatment may be necessary
- As the pulp chamber of deciduous teeth is large relative to the tooth, pulp exposure is more likely if attempts are made to remove all the caries in some cases, and it is sometimes necessary to leave some deep caries so that the pulp is not exposed – this is acceptable when the tooth will be lost naturally anyway
- Deciduous teeth are often restored with fluoride-releasing glass ionomer cements, or by the placement of a pre-formed metal crown on molars

Classification of cavities

Cavities are classified into five different types, depending on the site of the original caries attack. This is called **Black's classification**, after the American dentist who devised the system. In general usage, his classification of cavities also applies to the naming of the shape of the fillings inserted in each class of cavity:

- **Class I** cavities are those involving a **single** surface in a pit or fissure – e.g. a class I filling could be an occlusal, a buccal or a lingual filling
- **Class II** cavities involve at least **two** surfaces of a posterior tooth, the mesial or distal, and the occlusal surface of a **molar** or **premolar** – e.g. a class II filling could be a mesial-occlusal (MO) filling in a premolar, or a mesial-occlusal-distal (MOD) filling in a molar
- **Class III** cavities involve the mesial or distal surface of an **incisor** or **canine**
- **Class IV** cavities are the same as class III but extend to involve the **incisal edge** on the affected side
- **Class V** cavities involve the **cervical margin** of any tooth – e.g. a class V filling could be a labial cervical filling in an upper incisor or a lingual cervical filling in a lower molar

Tooth charting is discussed in detail in Chapter 13.

Cavity preparation

A permanent filling cannot be inserted directly into a carious cavity. Instead, careful preparation of the cavity is required to ensure that:

- All plaque and soft carious dentine is removed from the cavity margins, although the deepest layer of dentine may be conserved to avoid exposure of the pulp
- As much of the enamel as possible is also conserved
- The filling will be as much a permanent fixture as possible, although its longevity will also depend on the standard of plaque control and the quality of the patient's diet
- Caries will not recur at its margins due to any restoration overhang or other defect

Every dentist has personal preferences for the instruments used during restorative procedures, such as the placement of fillings, and the following table shows the more usual items and an explanation of their function. They are usually set out on a tray for use, which is often referred to as a "**conservation tray**" (see Figure 9.8).

Item	Function
Mouth mirror	To aid the dentist's vision To reflect light onto the tooth To retract and protect the soft tissues
Right-angle probe	To feel the cavity margins To feel softened dentine within the cavity To detect overhanging restorations
Excavators	Small and large spoon-shaped – used to scoop out softened dentine
Amalgam plugger	To push filling materials into the cavity and adapt them to the cavity shape, leaving no air spaces and forcing excess mercury to the surface of the filling for removal during carving
Burnisher	Ball-shaped or pear-shaped, to press and adapt the restoration margins fully against the cavity edges so that no leakage occurs under the restoration
Flat plastic	To remove excess filling material and mercury from the restoration surface and create a shaped surface that encourages food particles to flow off naturally, rather than becoming lodged around the restoration
College tweezers	To pick up, hold and carry various items such as cotton wool pledgets
(Gingival margin trimmer)	To trim the margin of the cavity to ensure no unsupported enamel nor soft dentine remains – their use is becoming obsolete with the wider range of burs available
(Enamel chisel)	To remove any unsupported enamel from the cavity edges – their use is becoming obsolete with the wider range of burs available

486

The vast majority of tooth restoration carried out using fillings will require the administration of a local anaesthetic before proceeding, so that the patient does not have a painful experience.

Retention of fillings

Permanent fillings are meant to stay in place permanently and the cavity must be specially prepared to provide maximum retention. Before explaining how this is done, it is necessary to consider the types of filling materials used. There are two types available: plastic and pre-constructed.

Plastic fillings are soft and plastic on insertion but set hard in the cavity. They include:

- All temporary cements
- Amalgam
- Glass ionomer cements
- Composites

Pre-constructed restorations are called **inlays**, and these are made in the laboratory, after the teeth have been prepared, and then cemented into place. They include:

- Gold
- Porcelain
- Other ceramic materials

Retention for plastic fillings is obtained by simply cutting tiny grooves in the cavity walls to make the entrance smaller than its inside dimensions, as shown in Figure 15.32. As the materials are initially soft, they can be packed into the cavity easily to fill all of the available space, but cannot drop out of the cavity once set because they have hardened and are locked into position. For fillings involving occlusal and mesial surfaces, or occlusal and distal, a **dovetail** effect is produced by grooving the cavity walls to prevent the filling coming out mesially or distally (Figure 15.32). Note that this diagram is deliberately exaggerated to show more clearly the principles of retention. In reality, sound tissue is not sacrificed for the sake of extensive undercuts. Tiny grooves in the cavity walls are often sufficient to provide adequate retention.

487

Sometimes it is not possible to prepare cavities that are sufficiently undercut to retain a plastic filling. In such cases they may be made retentive in other ways by the use of:

- Self-tapping dentine pins for amalgam restorations
- Acid etching for composites, to provide a microscopically rough surface on the enamel and allow mechanical locking of the material onto the enamel prisms
- Chemical bonding for glass ionomer cement onto the dentine surface

These methods are covered in the later in this chapter, for each filling material.

Inlays are hard and rigid when inserted into the cavity, so the dentist would not be able to place and seat them fully if undercuts were present. To prevent them coming out occlusally, they rely on parallel cavity walls to provide maximum retention and the use of adhesive cement to "glue" them into the prepared cavity. As with plastic fillings, a small dovetail effect may be used to prevent dislodgement mesially or distally.

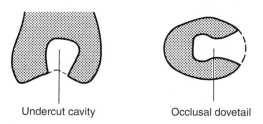

Undercut cavity   Occlusal dovetail

Figure 15.32   Undercutting of cavities to achieve retention. Source: *Levison's Textbook for Dental Nurses,* 11th edition (Hollins), 2013. Reproduced with permission of Wiley-Blackwell.

Cavity lining

Before a permanent filling is inserted, the cavity may need to be lined. A **lining** is an insulating layer of cement that is placed on the cavity floor and which has the following functions:

- Protects the pulp from temperature fluctuations that may be transmitted through metallic filling materials and that are experienced as sensitivity or even pain in the tooth
- Protects the pulp from chemical irritation of non-metallic materials
- Seals the pulp from any residual caries bacteria, allowing secondary dentine to be laid down

Depending on the depth of the cavity, pain – and possibly death of the tooth – may occur through failure to protect the pulp tissue by the insertion of an adequate lining.

The linings used are zinc oxide and eugenol cement, zinc phosphate cement, polycarboxylate cement and calcium hydroxide. The methods of insertion and techniques of finishing by polishing of fillings varies according to the material used, and this is discussed in detail later.

Moisture control

Adequate moisture control during restorative procedures is one of the most important duties of the dental nurse. Control of moisture – from saliva, blood or instrument cooling sprays – is necessary for the following reasons:

- To protect the patient's airway from fluid inhalation, especially as the majority of procedures are carried out with the patient lying back in the dental chair (supine position)
- To ensure patients are comfortable during treatment – so that they do not have a mouth full of fluids while lying in the supine position during dental treatment
- To allow the dentist good visibility to the treatment area, therefore avoiding inadvertent patient injury by catching the soft tissues or the wrong tooth with the drill
- To allow the restorative materials to set correctly, without moisture contamination
- To allow the adhesion of cements and linings to the tooth, without moisture contamination
- To avoid the uncontrolled loss of materials from the cavity during use, such as acid etchant which can burn the soft tissues

The following methods are used to control moisture:

- High-speed suction
- Low-speed suction
- Use of absorbent materials – cotton wool rolls, cotton wool pledgets and oral inserts such as a "dry guard"
- Use of rubber dam
- Compressed air drying, using the triple syringe (3 in 1) of the dental unit

High-speed and low-speed suction

This is provided by either high-speed aspiration (suction), for fast removal of moisture during drilling, or low-speed aspiration for continual moisture control without sucking at the soft tissues. In the case of high-speed suction, the dental nurse uses a wide-bore aspirator connected to the suction unit to rapidly remove fluids, blood and debris from the treatment area. This prevents the patient from choking, as well as emptying the oral cavity of volumes of fluid that would be uncomfortable for the patient to hold without feeling the need to spit out. With low-speed aspiration, the patient holds a **saliva ejector** attached to the suction unit or **aspirator** to slowly but continually remove any fluids that have pooled in the floor of the mouth, so that the patient does not have to constantly swallow during the treatment. Many different types of ejector are used but those with a flange to keep the tongue away from the treatment area are particularly helpful. The dental nurse may also use the high-speed aspirator tube as a soft tissue retractor. Examples of aspirators and ejectors are shown in Figure 8.21.

Absorbent materials

Cotton wool rolls or absorbent pads are placed in the buccal or lingual sulcus to absorb saliva and to keep the soft tissues away from the teeth. Cotton wool pledgets are used to dab the actual cavity dry, while excessive saliva contamination can be prevented by placing a "dry guard" over the parotid salivary gland duct. These pads contain an absorbent material similar to that used in babies' nappies, and considerable volumes of fluid can be retained by them. The cavity itself can be further dried by blowing it with compressed air from the triple syringe of the dental unit. Examples of some of these materials are shown in Figure 6.13.

Rubber dam equipment

This is the best method of moisture control of all and the various components are shown in Figure 9.9. Rubber dam is a thin sheet of latex rubber or vinyl material which is placed over a tooth to isolate it from the rest of the mouth. A **rubber dam punch** is used to punch a small hole in the rubber sheet, which is then fitted on so that the tooth projects through the hole (see Figure 9.25).

The rubber dam is kept in place by a **rubber dam clamp**, which is fixed on the tooth with **rubber dam clamp forceps**. Finally, a **rubber dam frame** is used to support the sheet while in use, so that it remains taut and maintains a clear visual field. A napkin is placed between the patient's chin and the rubber to make it more comfortable; and a saliva ejector may be provided to remove any pooled saliva. **Dental floss** or an additional piece of rubber dam material is used to work the sheet between the teeth.

Rubber dam may be applied to any number of teeth. It enables the operator to keep a tooth dry and maintain an uncontaminated field during dental treatment, and prevents pieces of filling material, debris or small instruments falling into the patient's mouth.

This moisture control technique is more comfortable for patients as it prevents water spray or irrigation fluids entering the mouth; and it is far better for the dentist, as it improves access and visibility by keeping the tongue, lips and cheek out of the way. It also helps prevent cross-infection of patients and chairside staff, by minimising the aerosol of infected debris spread by the use of compressed air and water spray.

The two main uses of rubber dam are:

- In root canal therapy (endodontic treatment), to maintain a sterile field and to prevent inhalation or the swallowing of small instruments
- During the insertion of fillings (especially composites and glass ionomers), to avoid their failure due to saliva contamination

Ideally, rubber dam should be used for all fillings, but most operators consider it too time-consuming for routine use in all procedures except endodontics. The technique is also not well tolerated by every patient.

Handpieces

Cavities are cut by the use of dental burs fitted into the head of a handpiece. The speed of cutting depends on the type of handpiece and the purpose for which it is used. They have a built-in water spray to counteract the heat generated when cutting hard tissue and may also have fibreoptic illumination to aid cavity preparation.

Air turbine handpieces run at very high speeds of up to 500 000 revolutions a minute, and use friction grip **diamond** or **tungsten carbide burs to cut easily through both enamel and**

489

dentine. There is a tiny air turbine motor in the head of the handpiece which is driven by compressed air. The advantages of air turbines are the ease and speed of cutting. The disadvantages are that they offer little tactile sensation to the dentist, so excessive tooth removal can occur, and their vibration may be associated with a condition called "vibration white finger" when used over many years.

Slow handpieces run at around 40 000 revolutions per minute, and are driven by air or electric motors at the base of the handpiece. These are much more versatile in their range of speed and uses, varying from low-speed root canal treatment and removal of carious dentine to high-speed conventional cavity preparation. They use latch grip stainless steel or tungsten carbide burs when employed on teeth or friction grip stainless steel acrylic trimming burs when used to trim dentures. They are more "user-friendly" for the dentist, as the tactile sensation provided is much better. Portable versions of the electric motors are particularly suitable for domiciliary dental treatment (that carried out away from the surgery, often in the patient's home).

An air turbine and a slow handpiece are shown in Figure 8.8.

All handpieces, however driven and of whatever age, are made in two basic designs: **contra-angled** and **straight**. A contra-angle is used most often in the mouth as it provides access to every tooth. A straight handpiece is used to trim acrylic denture items.

Burs

Burs for low-speed procedures are made of steel. They are used for removing caries, cutting dentine (but not enamel), trimming dentures and other laboratory work. Examples are shown in Figure 15.33.

Burs for high-speed handpieces have **diamond** or **tungsten carbide** cutting surfaces and are used for rapid removal of enamel, dentine and old fillings. Examples are shown in Figure 15.34.

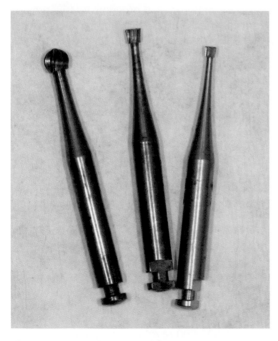

Figure 15.33   Slow-speed burs.

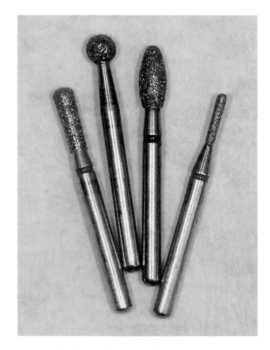

Figure 15.34   High-speed burs.

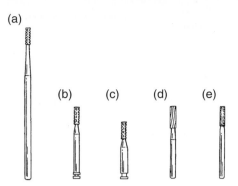

Figure 15.35 Burs: (a) steel for straight handpiece; (b) steel, latch grip, for low-speed contra-angle handpiece; (c) steel, latch grip, for miniature contra-angle handpiece; (d) tungsten carbide, friction grip, for air turbine handpiece; (e) diamond, friction grip, for air turbine handpiece. Source: *Levison's Textbook for Dental Nurses*, 11th edition (Hollins), 2013. Reproduced with permission of Wiley-Blackwell.

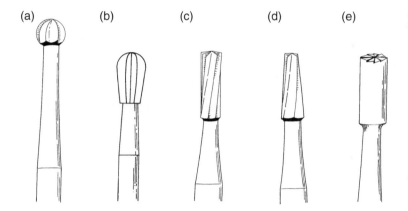

Figure 15.36 Bur shapes: (a) round; (b) pear; (c) flat fissure; (d) tapered fissure; (e) end-cutting. Source: *Levison's Textbook for Dental Nurses*, 11th edition (Hollins), 2013. Reproduced with permission of Wiley-Blackwell.

Straight handpiece burs have a long, plain shank. Burs for low-speed contra-angle handpieces are short and have a notch in the shank which fits by a **latch grip**. Short burs are also used for air turbine handpieces, but they have a plain shank which gives a **friction grip** (Figure 15.35).

Contra-angled low-speed handpieces with smaller heads, and using even shorter burs, are used on children. They are called **miniature** handpieces and burs.

The cutting ends of burs come in many different shapes depending on the dental treatment being carried out (Figure 15.36), but those most commonly used are as follows:

- Round – used for gaining access to cavities, and at low speed for removing caries
- Pear – used for shaping and smoothing cavities
- Fissure – used for shaping and outlining the cavity

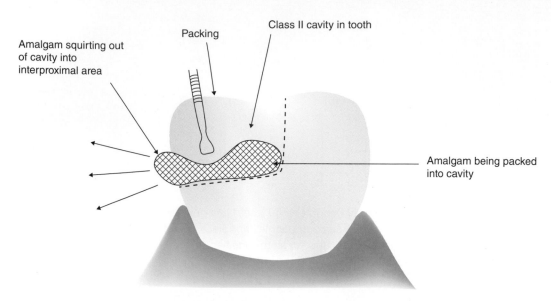

Amalgam squirting out
of cavity into
interproximal area

Packing

Class II cavity in tooth

Amalgam being packed
into cavity

492

Figure 15.37   Amalgam squirting out of a class II cavity.

Matrix systems

When a cavity is shaped to involve two or more surfaces of a tooth, the force used to push any plastic filling material into it from one direction will tend to squirt some out in the direction of the second surface. So, for example, amalgam pushed occlusally into a mesio-occlusal (class II) cavity will tend to squirt out from the mesial surface of the cavity (see Figure 15.37). The same will happen with class III and class IV cavities while being restored with composite, and with class V cavities with glass ionomer due to the rounded shape of the tooth in its cervical region.

The excess filling material will be difficult to remove from the interproximal areas, and once set will act as a stagnation area for plaque retention, allowing further caries and periodontal disease to occur here. The filling material within the cavity will also not have been fully condensed (packed, or compressed) into the tooth and will be weakened by air spaces and liable to fracture during normal occlusal loading.

To avoid these problems when restoring two-surface cavities, each permanent filling material is placed using a matrix system – a device that replaces the missing wall of the cavity so that no overspill occurs, and so that the material can be adequately packed into the tooth with no air spaces remaining. Those in use for each type of permanent filling material are as follows:

- **Amalgam** – metal strips held in a retainer device which can be tightened around the tooth, sometimes adapted further using a wooden or plastic wedge pushed interproximally during the filling procedure; two systems in use are the Siqveland (see Figure 8.10) and the Tofflemire
- **Composite** – transparent plastic strip to allow light curing to occur, which is held in place by hand during curing (see Figure 8.12)
- **Glass ionomer** – specially shaped cervical foil matrix which adapts to the shape of the tooth in this area (see Figure 8.15); it is held in place by hand and the inner foil layer produces a smooth surface to the glass ionomer as it sets – cannot be used with light-cured materials, as the matrix is opaque

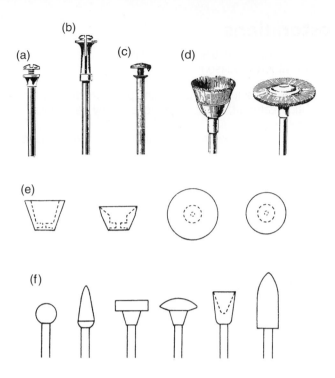

Figure 15.38   Mandrels and brushes: (a) Huey mandrel; (b) Moore mandrel; (c) pinhead mandrel; (d) polishing brushes; (e) abrasive rubber cups and discs for Huey mandrel; (f) mounted fine abrasives.

Polishing instruments

There is a great variety of polishing instruments but they generally comprise fine abrasive stones, wheels, discs and strips, finishing burs, brushes and polishing pastes. Apart from hand abrasive strips, they are all used with a handpiece. Finishing burs and stones are used for smoothing cavity margins and trimming fillings (see Figure 9.11). Abrasive discs and strips are used for fine trimming and polishing.

Small abrasive stones, wheels and brushes are manufactured with a shank that fits the appropriate handpiece. Larger wheels, stones and abrasive discs require an independent mounting shank called a **mandrel**. Wheels and metal discs are fitted on a "Huey" mandrel; sandpaper discs with a metal centre and Soflex discs use a "Moore" mandrel; and plain sandpaper discs a "pinhead" mandrel (Figure 15.38).

Care of instruments

All cutting instruments must be kept sharp, because blunt ones are inefficient and painful for the patient. Hand instruments such as chisels and excavators should be sharpened regularly on a small flat oilstone (**Arkansas stone**) or with an abrasive disc in a straight handpiece. Burs are cleaned in an ultrasonic cleaner and autoclaved after use, although any that become heavily contaminated during use or that are used on known high-risk patients are considered as single-use items and are discarded. These burs, along with all blunt burs, are discarded into the sharps container.

All handpieces must be lubricated regularly according to manufacturers' instructions before being decontaminated and sterilised.

493

Temporary restorations

These restorations, which are placed as a temporary measure before the tooth is restored permanently, are used for a variety of reasons:

- As an emergency measure to seal a cavity and prevent carious ingress
- During endodontic treatment, as repeated access may be required to the pulp chamber over several appointments
- During inlay construction to seal the preparation while the permanent inlay is constructed
- To allow a symptomatic tooth to settle and become symptom-free, before being permanently sealed

There are several materials available for use as a temporary restoration, some of which have other uses in dentistry – they are multi-purpose materials. Overall, they are unsuitable for use as a permanent restoration because they are too soft to chew on, are too soluble in saliva, and would not remain intact for long.

The key features of all temporary restorations are as follows:

- Quick mixing and placement
- Cheap compared with permanent restorative materials
- Easily removed from the cavity when required
- Not strong enough to be chewed on routinely
- Have varying degrees of adhesiveness to the tooth
- Some contain sedative ingredients to help settle inflamed pulps

A variety of materials are available, under many trade names, but temporary restorations can generally be categorised into one of the following groups of materials:

- Zinc oxide and eugenol cement – zinc oxide powder, eugenol liquid
- Zinc phosphate cement – zinc oxide powder, phosphoric acid liquid
- Zinc polycarboxylate cement – zinc oxide powder, polyacrylic acid liquid, or both as powder with sterile water as liquid
- (Gutta-percha) – greenstick compound, which is practically obsolete as a temporary filling

Details of their presentation and mixing are discussed in Chapter 8, while details of their uses, advantages, and disadvantages are given in the following table.

Cement	Uses	Advantages	Disadvantages
Zinc oxide and eugenol	<ul><li>Temporary filling</li><li>Non-irritant base for deep cavities</li><li>Sedative dressing for painful carious teeth and for dry sockets</li><li>Main constituent of some impression pastes, periodontal packs, and root filling materials</li></ul>	<ul><li>Sedative properties of eugenol, helps to settle hypersensitive pulp</li><li>Multi-use cement</li><li>Best base cement for use with amalgam fillings</li></ul>	<ul><li>Only modern cements set fast enough for use at filling visit</li><li>Incompatible with composite fillings</li><li>Should be avoided in patients who are sensitive to eugenol products</li><li>Not adhesive to tooth</li></ul>

Cement	Uses	Advantages	Disadvantages
Zinc phosphate	Uses of a thick mix of the cement are: • A temporary filling • Cavity base • Blocking out undercuts in inlay and crown preparations Uses of a thin mix of the cement are; • A luting cement to place inlays, crowns and bridges • A luting cement to place orthodontic bands	• Ability to control setting by varying the mix of the cement • Multi-use cement • Adhesive to dentine, so useful as a luting cement • Sets hard and quickly, so stronger base beneath fillings	• Acidic liquid with a pH of 2, so can be irritant to the pulp in deep cavities • May then need a lining placed beneath the zinc phosphate base • Moisture-sensitive and non-adhesive if the tooth is wet
Zinc polycar-boxylate	• Cavity base as a thick mix • Luting cement as a thin mix	• Alternative to zinc phosphate in most applications • Less acidic than zinc phosphate • More adhesive than zinc phosphate	• Adhesive to stainless steel instruments • Therefore can be difficult to manipulate • Must be removed from instruments before setting
(Gutta-percha)	• Practically obsolete as a temporary filling	• None over other materials	• Poor marginal adaptation

495

Linings

These are materials placed in the deepest part of the cavity, over the pulp chamber, before a restoration is placed.

Their aim is to protect the pulp from thermal and chemical shock, by providing a barrier between the permanent restoration and the living pulp tissue, so that temperature fluctuations in the mouth are not transmitted and there is no adverse chemical stimulation from restorations.

Technically, thin layers of the zinc oxide materials discussed previously can be said to be linings in cavities, although realistically they are more correctly termed as "bases", because they have to be of an adequate thickness to be placed, whereas a lining, by definition, is a very thin layer of a material used just to cover the inner surface of the cavity. The material universally referred to as a lining in dentistry is calcium hydroxide.

Details of its presentation and mixing are discussed in Chapter 8, while details of its uses, advantages, and disadvantages are given in the following table.

Liner	Uses	Advantages	Disadvantages
Calcium hydroxide	• Universal cavity lining • Pulp capping (see later) • Pulpotomy (see later) • Other root treatment procedures (see later)	• Non-irritant to the pulp • Alkalinity helps to kill caries bacteria • Compatible with all filling materials • Promotes secondary dentine formation at cavity base • Promotes enamel remineralisation due to its calcium content	• Too weak to use without a base in deep cavities • Soluble in water unless a light-cured product is used

Permanent restorations

These are the materials used to permanently restore the tooth to its full function and appearance, and they must all have the following properties:

- Set to a hard enough degree to allow normal masticatory function to occur, without fracture of the material
- Do not dissolve or otherwise deteriorate in saliva over time
- Are biologically safe, by not reacting with the body's tissues or giving off any harmful chemicals
- Can be applied to the tooth using normal conservation instruments, in a straightforward manner – some cavity shapes will require the use of a matrix system
- Have a reasonable working life span of years, rather than months
- Ideally they should be aesthetically acceptable, although this limits the use of amalgam

The three commonly used materials are:

- **Amalgam** – alloy powder (silver, copper, zinc, tin), liquid mercury
- **Composite** – inorganic filler (powdered glass, quartz, silica), liquid resin binder
- **Glass ionomer** – powder (aluminosilicate and polyacrylic acid particles), sterile water

Details of their presentation and mixing are discussed in Chapter 8, while details of their uses, advantages, and disadvantages are given in the following table.

Material	Uses	Advantages	Disadvantages
Amalgam	• Permanent filling material for posterior teeth	• Easy to use • Relatively cheap, compared with composites and glass ionomers • Good set strength • Able to withstand normal occlusal forces • Excellent longevity, lasting for many years under normal conditions in well maintained mouths	• Mercury is toxic • Not retentive to tooth, so cavities have to be undercut • Can transmit thermal shocks, so liners and bases are required in deeper cavities • Has to be mixed very accurately to be dimensionally stable • Aesthetics are poor, so its use is limited to posterior teeth

496

Material	Uses	Advantages	Disadvantages
Composite	• Permanent filling material for anterior teeth • Can be used as a posterior filling in smaller cavities • Restoration of fractured incisors, rather than a crown • Fissure sealant • Use of unfilled resin as a surface glaze	• Excellent aesthetics with a wide range of shade choice • Adhesive to tooth, using acid etch and bond • Little marginal leakage occurs, due to their adhesion to enamel • Sufficient strength in smaller posterior restorations • Usually only require lining of calcium hydroxide • Indirect inlay technique possible for larger restorations • Fast set with curing light • Available in pre-mixed compoules for easy insertion into cavity	• Technique-sensitive • Longer procedure than for amalgam restoration • More expensive material than amalgam • Not as strong and hard-wearing as amalgam in posterior teeth • Possible safety issue with resin bond • Can only use glass ionomer as a base, as composites react with other bases • Acid etchant can burn soft tissues if used carelessly • Safety issue with curing light causing eye damage, – orange safety shield must always be used
Glass ionomer	• Permanent filling material • Especially used to restore deciduous teeth • Fissure sealant • Cavity base • Luting cement for fixed restorations and orthodontic bands • Dentine substitute where excessive loss of tooth substance has occurred, avoiding the use of pinned amalgam restorations • Core build-ups	• Adhesive to enamel, dentine and cementum, so minimal cavity preparation is required • Ideal for use with class V abrasion cavities • Good marginal seal, preventing leakage • This can be improved further with the use of conditioners • Releases fluoride over time, so very useful when restoring deciduous teeth • Better aesthetics than amalgam • Addition of metals to some products produces cermets, which are strong enough for use as core build-ups • Addition of glass ionomer to composites produces compomers, which have better aesthetics plus fluoride release and better adhesion than composite alone	• Low strength compared with amalgam or composite • Very technique-sensitive • Exact proportions of material and liquid must be used to produce the ideal mix • Requires calcium hydroxide lining in deep cavities, to avoid pulpal damage by polyacrylic acid • Moisture contamination causes failure of restoration • Requires protection from moisture during full setting • Produces a chalky surface if any attempt at finishing occurs before the material has fully set, and then the restoration has to be replaced

497

Amalgam

Amalgam is probably still the most widely used permanent restorative material for posterior teeth in the UK and has been in use for over 150 years. Despite advances in dental material science, it is still often cheaper to buy, more durable and easier to use than its tooth-coloured competitors – composite and glass ionomer. Its safe use as a dental restorative is currently under review due to its mercury content and the potential hazard that waste amalgam poses to the environment if not disposed of safely.

Recommendations for providing the best long-term results of amalgam restorations are:

- In shallow cavities, a calcium hydroxide lining or three coats of cavity varnish will suffice as a lining and marginal seal
- Medium cavities are lined with either a zinc oxide and eugenol base or glass ionomer cement, and may also be sealed with three coats of varnish
- Calcium hydroxide is used as a sublining in deep cavities, especially where zinc phosphate cement is used as a base

Mercury poisoning

Despite the many advantages of amalgam over other permanent restorative materials, its one big disadvantage is the fact that it contains mercury, which is known to be toxic. It was formerly believed that mercury poisoning could only occur after several years of mishandling. However, it is now known that it can occur within a few months if a large quantity of mercury is spilled. There is also some debate about the safety of the material within the oral cavity (to patients) and in the dental workplace (to the dental team). The risks are considered high enough that some countries are currently considering a ban on the use of amalgam as a dental restorative material, although this does not include the UK yet. In the meantime, every dental nurse must understand the risks involved and the methods of preventing hazards associated with the use of mercury and amalgam.

Mercury poisoning can occur in the following ways:

- **Inhalation** of the vapours
- **Absorption** through the skin, the nail beds, the eyes and wounds on the hands
- **Ingestion** by being swallowed

Although the possibility of skin contamination is obvious when handling mercury or amalgam, the risk of inhaling mercury vapour is not. Both mercury and amalgam release mercury vapour at ordinary **room temperature** – and the higher the temperature, the more vapour is released. Mercury vapour is odourless and invisible, so it is of the utmost importance to keep all mercury and waste amalgam in sealed containers in a cool, well-ventilated place – not near a hot steriliser or radiator, or even in sunlight. In particular, amalgam carriers must be dismantled and fully emptied of any residual amalgam before they are autoclaved, not only to prevent the release of mercury vapour but also to prevent blockage of the carrier by hardened amalgam residue.

Another source of mercury poisoning is the removal of old amalgam fillings. This releases a cloud of minute amalgam particles which can be inhaled or contaminate eyes and skin. It can be prevented by combining the use of copious water spray and an efficient aspirator, which is sealed to prevent the release of vapour in the clinical area. The use of rubber dam and safety glasses are the best protection available for patients during filling removal.

Apart from very rare cases of allergy, there is currently no evidence of danger to patients from the presence of their amalgam fillings, as a well-placed restoration should have had all excess mercury removed during the procedure. However, it has been advised that removal or insertion of amalgam fillings in pregnant patients should be deferred until after the baby is born, if it is clinically reasonable to do so. Pregnant chairside staff involved in such procedures may also be concerned, but regular urine tests for mercury contamination of staff can be carried out to show if there is any risk.

The symptoms of mercury poisoning that may be experienced are as follows:

- Early symptoms may include headache, fatigue, irritability, nausea and diarrhoea – at this stage it is unlikely that mercury poisoning would be suspected
- Later symptoms are **hand tremors** and **visual defects** such as double vision
- The final stage is **kidney failure**, and then death

Precautions to be followed by all staff

The routine use of **PPE**, such as gloves, mask and safety glasses, or visors worn for protection against cross-infection, will also provide corresponding protection against mercury hazards. Dental nurses can be reassured that no danger exists if the following precautions are taken.

To avoid absorption of mercury through the skin, the basic rules of cross-infection control should be followed:

- Always wear disposable gloves when handling mercury, mixing amalgam and cleaning amalgam instruments
- Do not wear open-toed shoes in the clinical area, as the floor may be contaminated by spilled mercury or dropped amalgam
- Do not wear jewellery or a wristwatch as they may harbour particles of amalgam
- Incidentally, gold jewellery can be spoiled by contact with mercury or amalgam, due to a chemical reaction occurring between the two metals

To avoid pollution of the air by mercury vapour:

- Ideally, a pre-loaded capsule system should be in use, rather than the old-fashioned system of bottled mercury and alloy powder being manually loaded into the amalgamator
- If the latter system is still in use, containers of mercury must be tightly sealed, and stored in a cool well-ventilated place
- When transferring mercury from a stock bottle, great care must be taken not to spill any. It is very difficult to find and recover mercury that has dropped on the floor or working surface as it is a liquid metal and rolls away easily (see Figure 1.17)
- For removal of old amalgam fillings, the use of a high-speed handpiece with diamond or tungsten carbide burs, water spray and efficient aspiration helps to reduce the aerosol of amalgam dust and mercury vapour, while the use of rubber dam will protect the patient
- Surgery staff must wear full PPE throughout such procedures, as they should for all chairside procedures
- All traces of amalgam must be removed from instruments before autoclaving, otherwise vapour will be released as the autoclave heats up – this is especially pertinent with amalgam carriers
- Keep the surgery well ventilated
- Amalgamators and the capsules used therein should be checked after use, as cases have been reported of mercury leakage from capsules during mixing
- Amalgamators must be stood on a tray lined with aluminium foil so that any droplets can be easily collected and disposed of as hazardous waste, using a disposable syringe (see Figure 1.17)
- The machines must also have a lid over the capsule holder, so that leaking capsules do not throw their dangerous contents into the surgery
- All premises using amalgam must have a **mercury spillage kit** so that any accidents can be dealt with swiftly and correctly

499

Surgery hygiene

Much can be done to minimise any dangers of working with mercury by adopting the following rules, many of which would be common sense anyway:

- Smoking, eating, drinking and the application of cosmetics must not take place in the surgery. Any of these actions could permit absorption of mercury – from mercury vapour in the air or from contaminated hands
- The storage and handling of mercury must be confined to one particular part of the surgery, away from all sources of heat
- Any spillage of mercury **must** be reported to the dentist or other senior staff member
- Mercury spillage kits must be used for the safe recovery of all spillages greater than the a few droplets
- Vacuum cleaners must never be used for this purpose, as they vaporise any mercury they pick up and discharge it back into the surgery
- Floor coverings must not have any cracks or gaps in which mercury or amalgam can be trapped, and carpets must not be used as a surgery floor covering
- Surgery equipment and plumbing must have easily accessible filter traps to collect particles of waste amalgam flushed through spittoons, aspirators or other suction apparatus. This waste must be collected and transferred to the surgery waste amalgam containers
- Modern aspirators must be fitted with an amalgam trap, so that no waste material enters the drains (Figure 15.39)
- Waste amalgam must be saved in sealed tubs containing a mercury absorption chemical, and taken for collection by specialist waste contractors for recycling (see Figure 1.13)
- Efficient ventilation is essential at all times of the year, and high surgery temperatures should be avoided
- The Environmental Protection Agency must be notified of any large spillage that may result in mercury poisoning, under RIDDOR regulations

Safe disposal of waste amalgam

All amalgam waste and extracted teeth with amalgam fillings present must only be collected for disposal by authorised **hazardous waste contractors** (see Chapters 1 and 12). The reason for this is that most other hazardous waste is incinerated, and if that containing any amalgam waste

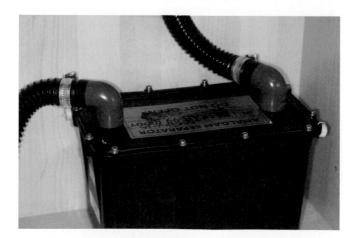

Figure 15.39 Waste amalgam separator trap.

500

was included, the incineration process would pollute the air with mercury vapour. Before collection by the authorised contractor, the amalgam waste must be stored in special containers, which they supply and which prevent the escape of mercury vapour (see Figure 1.13). The contractors may also arrange periodic testing of the workplace mercury vapour levels, and the checking of amalgamators for mercury leakage. If these tests show an unexpectedly high concentration of mercury vapour in a workplace with no report of a spillage occurring previously, expert advice can be sought from the Environmental Health Agency in tracing the source and resolving the problem. As stated previously, urine tests can also be carried out on staff to ensure that they have not been exposed to high levels of mercury vapour, although unfortunately these tests are not routinely carried out by occupational health departments at the moment.

Mercury spillage

Accidental spillage of mercury or waste amalgam must always be reported to the dentist or other senior staff member. If a spillage occurs, globules of mercury can be drawn up into a disposable intravenous **syringe** or **bulb aspirator** and transferred to a mercury container (see Figures 1.16 and 1.17), while small globules can be collected by adhering them to the **lead foil** from X-ray film packets. Waste amalgam can be gathered with a **damp paper towel**. For larger spillages, the following protocol should be followed:

- Stop work and report the incident to the dentist immediately
- Put on full PPE
- Globules of mercury or particles of amalgam must be smeared with a **mercury-absorbent paste** from the mercury spillage kit (see Figure 1.19)
- This consists of equal parts of **calcium hydroxide** and **flours of sulphur** mixed into a paste with **water**
- It should be left to dry and then removed with a wet disposable towel and placed in the storage container
- Risk-assess the incident to determine if protocols require amendment and change
- Larger spillages still require the evacuation of the premises, the sealing of the area and the involvement of **Environmental Health** to remove the contamination as a specialist procedure
- The **Health and Safety Executive** will be notified under RIDDOR regulations, so that an investigation can be carried out to determine if the practice procedure needs to be changed to prevent a recurrence of the spillage

Composite

Composites are tooth-coloured restorative materials that come in a wide range of shades, to match the darkest or lightest teeth. Modern systems are set quickly by exposure to a blue curing light, rather than the older systems that relied on a chemical reaction for setting to occur. They were initially developed for the aesthetic restoration of anterior teeth, but specialist products can also be used for restoring posterior teeth too, but they do not tend to wear as well here as amalgam fillings.

However, there is still a need for chemical curing in situations where metallic restorations (crowns, bridges and inlays) are cemented into, or on to, prepared teeth. The blue curing light cannot penetrate metal, so a special type of **dual-cure** composite material has been developed, which can be set at the margins by a curing light and then will set chemically beneath the metallic restoration.

There are so many different brands of composite materials, and so many different types of curing lights, that it is essential to strictly follow manufacturers' instructions for the curing time, light bulb life, and care and maintenance of this equipment. A simple test of the curing light's effectiveness is to cure a small measured portion of composite on a glass block or mixing pad and then check that it has set hard throughout its full thickness.

Safe handling and usage of composite

Great care is required when using the acid etch liquid or gel during the placement of a composite restoration, to prevent soft tissue damage to the patient or the dental team. It consists of a **33% concentration of phosphoric acid**, and this is more than sufficient to cause acid burns and permanent scarring of the patient's soft tissues, including their facial skin. Good handling and aspiration techniques should avoid any soft tissue contact with the etch gel, and any inadvertent contact must be immediately dealt with by removal with damp gauze and copious irrigation.

Also, the **blue curing light** used to fast-set the restoration can cause damage to the retina of the eyes if looked at directly, so the patient must wear correctly tinted safety glasses during treatment (orange tinted are best). An orange-tinted protective shield should also be held over the fibreoptic end of the light during use, to prevent the dental team from having to look at the light without eye protection.

Glass ionomer cements

Glass ionomers are tooth-coloured restorative materials that are adhesive to all of the hard tissues of the teeth, so they tend to be used in situations when little natural retention of the restoration is available, especially in class V cavities. Although they have a range of shades available, aesthetically they are inferior to composites. Some products set chemically, while others are set by exposure to the blue curing light, as for composites.

Safe use of glass ionomers

As with light-cured composite materials, suitable PPE must be provided for the patient during restorative procedures using glass ionomers, and the dental team should be protected from eye exposure to the blue light by the correct use of the orange shield device.

Periodontal therapy

Non-surgical periodontal treatment, involving supragingival and subgingival calculus removal by scaling, is discussed earlier in the chapter. Where there are deep periodontal pockets, especially where multi-rooted teeth and their furcation area are involved, conventional scaling alone is unlikely to achieve healing of the periodontal tissues. Surgical access to the pockets is required in these cases, so that the dentist can see the area more clearly and ensure that thorough calculus removal and debridement are achieved. In other cases, false pockets may persist and prevent adequate plaque removal, especially in patients who take medication which causes gingival overgrowth (hyperplasia).

The surgical periodontal therapy techniques that may be carried out are:

- **Flap surgery**
- **Gingivectomy and gingivoplasty**

Flap surgery

Periodontal flap procedures use techniques and instruments similar to some of those used for the surgical extraction of an unerupted tooth, but they do not involve the raising of a full mucoperiosteal flap. They cover a variety of procedures to remove inaccessible subgingival plaque and facilitate subsequent plaque control. Teeth with irregular gingival pocketing, a complex and uneven pattern of bone loss, or involvement of the **furcation** (the branching of roots of multi-rooted teeth), are those most likely to need such operations (Figure 15.40).

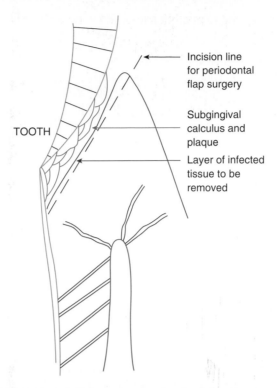

TOOTH

Incision line for periodontal flap surgery

Subgingival calculus and plaque

Layer of infected tissue to be removed

Figure 15.40 Periodontal flap incision. Source: *Levison's Textbook for Dental Nurses*, 11th edition (Hollins), 2013. Reproduced with permission of Wiley-Blackwell.

The surgical instruments required for the procedure are described in the following table.

Item	Function
Scalpel blade and handle (see Figure 11.8)	To make the initial incision through the full-thickness mucoperiosteum and around the necks of the teeth to create the flap
Austin and Kilner retractors	To protect and retract cheeks, lips and tongue from the surgical field, providing clear access for the dentist
Dissecting forceps (see Figure 11.11)	To hold the loose flap edges taut during suturing
Needle holders (see Figure 11.12)	To hold the pre-threaded needle firmly while suturing
Suture pack (see Figure 11.13)	Half-moon needle, pre-threaded with either black braided silk or a resorbable suture material, such as vicryl, to suture the flap back into position over the alveolar bone
Suture scissors (see Figure 11.14)	To cut the suture ends after each stitch

Once access has been gained to the root and/or furcation area, conventional periodontal instruments for subgingival calculus removal are used. The full procedure is described here:

- The incision is made through the gingival papilla of the tooth, down to the tooth surface, so that the layer of gingiva in contact with the tooth and forming the inner wall of the periodontal pocket is separated from the remainder of the gingival tissues
- This severed piece of tissue is removed from the area
- The remaining gingival flap is then reflected to expose the underlying bone, root surface and all the hidden subgingival calculus
- Alveolar bone surfaces may then be trimmed and contoured to eliminate bony pockets
- All subgingival plaque and calculus are removed, using curettes or an ultrasonic scaler
- In addition, all contaminated cementum and any toxin-impregnated granulation tissue are removed
- Local delivery antibiotic systems such as Gengigel, Dentomycin or Periochip may then be placed in these inaccessible areas to help the healing process (see Figure 15.12)
- The flap is then sutured back into place
- There is no removal of full-thickness gingival tissue, but the gingival margin may be repositioned more apically, thus permanently exposing more of the root to make cleaning easier in future

Gingivectomy and gingivoplasty

Sometimes, successful treatment of periodontal disease is hindered by the failure of established false pockets to be eliminated, and they can be surgically removed by the technique of gingivectomy.

This is the removal of a strip of gingival margin level with the point of the epithelial attachment (Figure 15.41). It is mainly confined to cases with excessive overgrowth of gum (**gingival hyperplasia**) caused by certain drugs used for medical conditions. The drugs involved include phenytoin (for epilepsy), nifedipine (for hypertension) and ciclosporin (following organ transplant).

The excess gum is removed with a **gingivectomy knife** or one used for periodontal flap surgery. There are many different types of gingivectomy knife available with various angled handles and blades for ease of access, the most common being Blake's gingivectomy knife (Figure 15.41). The strip of incised gum is removed with tweezers and the raw area is covered with a zinc

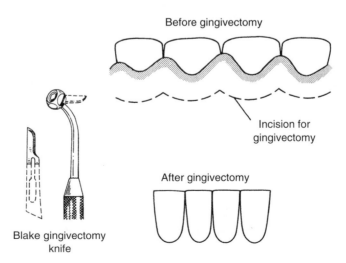

Figure 15.41   Gingivectomy procedure and Blake knife. Source: *Levison's Textbook for Dental Nurses*, 11th edition (Hollins), 2013. Reproduced with permission of Wiley-Blackwell.

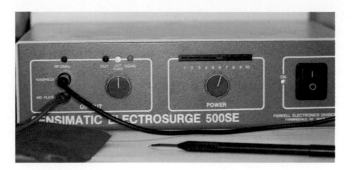

Figure 15.42   An electrosurgery unit.

oxide/eugenol **periodontal pack**, such as Coe-Pak, to protect the gum and promote rapid, pain-less healing. The pack is removed about a week later and thorough scaling is then performed.

A technique similar to gingivectomy may also be necessary for exposing more root surface prior to crown preparation, in cases where there would otherwise be insufficient retention for a crown. This procedure is called **crown lengthening**.

Surgical re-contouring of the gingiva can also be carried out once periodontal health has been established, to help the patient cleanse the area thoroughly. This technique is called **gingivo-plasty** and is often carried out using an electrosurgical cautery unit, which cuts and coagulates bleeding tissues at the same time (Figure 15.42).

Following gingival surgery, patients are given or prescribed analgesic drugs to relieve after-pain; given an appointment for removal of sutures or pack a week later; and instructed to avoid smoking, eating hard food and using a toothbrush on the operative area in the meantime. A soft diet and chlorhexidine mouthwashes are advised instead.

Non-surgical endodontics

Once caries has progressed deep inside a cavity so that the pulp is involved, the tooth cannot be saved by caries removal and filling alone, but must undergo some form of root canal therapy or **endodontic treatment**. The only other alternative is extraction.

Endodontics is the term used for all forms of root canal therapy. Non-surgical endodontics includes all of the following procedures:

- **Pulpectomy** – conventional root filling, also called root canal therapy
- **Pulpotomy** (and open apex root filling)
- **Pulp capping**

The procedure of surgical endodontics is correctly called **apicectomy**.

Caries is not the only reason why endodontic treatment might be required – any event that causes significant inflammation of the pulpal tissues or a breach of the pulp chamber is likely to result in the need for some form of endodontic treatment. Other reasons for endodontic treatment are as follows:

- **Thermal injury**, by heat transmission through unlined restorations or inadequate cooling of the air turbine during restorative treatment
- **Chemical irritation** from restorative materials
- **Tooth fracture** following trauma, possibly causing pulp exposure
- **Severe impact injury** without causing tooth fracture

505

- **Irritation** from very deep fillings over time
- **Accidental pulp exposure** during restorative procedures, especially during restoration of deep cavities

Any of these events will result in inflammation of the pulp tissue, and as it is confined within the closed root canal chamber of the tooth, any swelling that occurs will squeeze the pulp contents, cutting off the blood supply to the tooth and ultimately resulting in its death.

The correct term for inflammation of the pulp is **pulpitis**, and this can occur as either of the following events:

- **Reversible pulpitis** – not causing pulp death and treated by a restorative filling of the tooth only
- **Irreversible pulpitis** – causing partial or full pulp death and requiring one of the non-surgical endodontic techniques to save it

Any tooth can be affected by irreversible pulpitis at any age, and the tooth involved and when it erupted, as well as the severity of the pulpitis, will determine which of the three non-surgical techniques is used to try to save it.

Deciduous teeth will eventually be resorbed and exfoliate, as a natural progression to the eruption and development of the permanent dentition, so full root canal therapy is not required to treat them, and either pulp capping or pulpotomy are adequate. When permanent teeth erupt, it can take up to 3 years for the root apex to close, so these teeth will have a good blood supply during this time and can also be maintained by either a pulp capping or pulpotomy procedure. Once the root end has closed, and in the full adult dentition, pulpectomy is required to treat the tooth in an attempt to save it from extraction.

Diagnosis of irreversible pulpitis

The dentist's decision on whether to treat a carious tooth by an ordinary filling, endodontics or extraction depends on the state of the pulp. If it is dead, endodontics or extraction is necessary. If it is alive and unexposed, an ordinary filling will suffice.

The state of the pulp is not always apparent and vitality tests are often required to determine whether it is alive, dying or dead. These tests depend on the painful response of the pulp to temperature extremes or electrical stimulation and are fully discussed in Chapter 13. If the pulp responds to these stimuli, it is vital or dying; if not, it is probably dead.

In addition, a periapical radiograph can also be used as an indicator of the health of the tooth, as follows:

- A widened periodontal ligament space indicates some level of inflammatory response present, although it may not always result in tooth death
- A crown fracture or deep cavity may be seen to be in contact with the pulp chamber or very close to it
- A root fracture will be visible as a black line across the root
- A periapical abscess will appear as a radiolucent area around the apex of the tooth (Figure 15.43)

Often, a tooth will have been giving symptoms for some time before deteriorating into irreversible pulpitis, and this is especially true when caries is the cause, as it is a progressive infection of the dental hard tissues, rather than a sudden event such as trauma.

The patient usually experiences symptoms that gradually increase in severity until the tooth dies, as follows:

- Occasional sensitivity to cold, then to hot and sweet stimulation
- Develops into spontaneous intermittent spasms of pain
- Becomes a continuous throbbing pain with time, which prevents use of the tooth

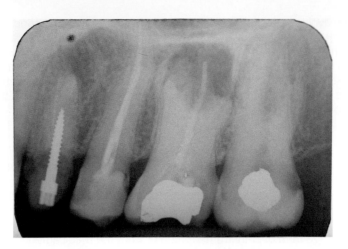

Figure 15.43   Radiograph showing periapical areas.

- Eventually not affected by hot, cold or sweet stimulation
- Becomes hypersensitive to vitality testing as the pulp is dying, and then becomes unresponsive as it dies
- No longer tender to percussion (TTP) when tapped

Treatment option considerations

There are many factors to be considered by both the dentist and the patient (or their guardian) when discussing treatment involving non-surgical endodontics, as summarised here:

- **Usefulness of the tooth in occlusion** – if the tooth stands alone and is not routinely used for mastication or involved in the retention of a prosthesis, then it could be argued that there is little point in trying to save it from extraction
- **Tooth restoration possibilities** – if the tooth is badly broken down with little structure remaining for restoration, the feasibility of restoring it to full function is less likely
- **Dental health of the patient** – if this is poor generally, with a lack of good oral hygiene and poor diet control, the tooth is unlikely to survive for any reasonable length of time
- **Patient co-operation** – both child and adult patients may refuse the treatment offered for whatever reason, and their right to do so has to be respected by the dental team
- **Medical history of the patient** – some medical conditions contraindicate endodontic treatment due to the risk of a residual infection:
  - Diabetes
  - Acquired valvular heart disease and other heart conditions
  - Congenital heart defects
- Other medical conditions contraindicate extraction:
  - Epilepsy – dentures should be avoided in these patients if possible, to avoid their fracture and choking risk during a seizure
  - Bleeding disorders – especially haemophilia where haemostasis may be difficult to achieve
  - Cleft palate
- **Cost of treatment** – successful endodontic treatment usually culminates in the tooth being crowned eventually to preserve it for as long as possible, and both treatments can be too expensive for some patients to consider

All these considerations need to be fully and clearly discussed with the patient, or their guardian in the case of children, before the decision can be made as to whether to proceed. Dental terminology may have to be avoided with some patients, and the necessary explanations adapted to their level of understanding or language. However, this must never result in full information not being given or the patient being patronised. It is possible to issue patient leaflets in various languages nowadays to help explain dental treatment, and their availability should be investigated in each locality.

In addition, some specific information about possible complications and procedure details must be given to the patient or guardian to enable them to be fully informed and therefore to give consent to endodontic treatment.

Complications

- The procedure carries a 70–80% chance of success, so extraction may still ultimately be necessary in some cases
- Teeth that have undergone endodontic treatment become brittle with time, so long-term restoration is likely to involve a crown to protect the tooth and prevent future fracture
- If the root apices are close to underlying nerves (especially lower molars), there is a possibility of nerve damage from over-instrumentation or from the medicaments used
- If the root apices of upper molars are close to the floor of the maxillary antrum, there is a risk of creating an oro-antral fistula

Pulpectomy – conventional root canal therapy

508

This is the non-surgical endodontic procedure carried out in an attempt to save a fully formed permanent tooth from extraction, once it has suffered from irreversible pulpitis. The aim of the treatment is to:

- **Remove all of the pulpal tissue from the pulp chamber and root canal**
- **Replace it with a sterile root filling material**.

The sterile root filling must be placed to fully seal the whole root canal system and prevent any contamination from causing a recurrent infection at the root apex, so the material used must be insoluble in saliva and tissue fluids.

The same procedure provides drainage and complete cure of an existing abscess. The root-filled tooth will then function just as well as one with a normal pulp. Success depends on achieving a leak-proof seal at each end of the root canal, and thereby preventing microorganisims from entering or leaving it.

Pulpectomy is often carried out in two stages: the first is to remove the infective material and prepare the canal; the second is to insert the root filling. However, if no difficulties arise during the first stage, the dentist may choose to complete both stages in one visit.

Although the dentist will use many dental hand instruments during the endodontic procedure that are multi-functional and used in other dental disciplines, there are several instruments used exclusively for root canal therapy, as outlined in the following table. Their functions are similar whether used as hand instruments or as rotary instruments in the dental handpiece.

Item	Function
Broach	Plain broach to help locate the entrance to each root canal Barbed broach (see Figure 10.1a) to remove (extirpate) the pulpal contents from the canal
Reamer (see Figure 10.1b)	Hand or rotary – to enlarge the root canals in a circular shape laterally, down to the root apex

Item	Function
File (see Figure 10.1c)	Hand or rotary – to enlarge the canal in its actual shape laterally, smooth the root canal walls and remove any residual debris from them
Irrigation syringe (see Figure 10.3)	Blunt-ended with a side bevel, to irrigate and wash out debris from the root canal without injecting the syringe contents through the root apex Solutions used include chlorhexidine, sodium hypochlorite, local anaesthetic solution
Metal ruler	Used with a file in place, to work out the full length of each root canal by comparing with a periapical radiograph view of the tooth to the established working length
Apex locater (see Figure 10.4)	To determine the working length electronically
Spiral paste filler (see Figure 10.1d)	Used with the slow dental handpiece to spin sealant material into the root canal
Lateral condenser, or finger spreader (see Figure 10.5)	Used to condense the root filling points laterally into each root canal, so that no space remains for microorganisms to return. It is not required if root-filling material used is inserted while hot and flowable

509

Instrument details

Barbed broaches are single-use disposable hand instruments for removing the pulp. They consist of a fine wire with multiple barbs. When the broach is inserted into a root canal and rotated, its barbs snag into the pulp tissue and pull it out of the canal as the broach is removed.

Root reamers resemble wood drills and are used for enlarging root canals in a circular fashion so that a filling can be inserted. They are made in standardised sets – all of the same length, but with an increasing range of widths. Each reamer is numbered or colour-coded to indicate its size. The reamer is inserted into the canal and advanced by hand or by specially adapted handpieces for use with rotary endodontic instruments. As very few root canals are exactly circular in shape, reamers have largely been superseded by files.

Root canal files are hand or handpiece instruments that are similar to reamers but are flexible, and can be engaged around the walls of any canal shape present in the tooth. They are also made in the same standardised range of sizes and colours as reamers. Their function is to smooth and clean the walls of enlarged root canals and remove debris, and their flexibility allows them to negotiate curved root canals as well as the more typical oval shape of root canals (rather than circular). They are inserted into the canal and used with a down-twist-and-up filing action against the canal walls. Many practitioners use files exclusively instead of reamers, but in the same sequence of sizes.

Reaming and filing root canals by hand are laborious and time-consuming tasks. However, the introduction of flexible nickel-titanium root canal instruments used with modern variable-speed handpieces now allows dentists to undertake these procedures far more easily and precisely. They are particularly useful for the curved canals of multi-rooted teeth.

In addition, some of these specialised handpieces are also electronic apex locators, and can be set to give an audible alarm when the tooth apex has been reached – this is called the working length. Once determined, all other files used can then be pre-measured to this length so that the root canal is fully obturated. When used correctly, the apex locator is far more reliable at determining the accurate working length of the tooth, and this can be confirmed with a postoperative periapical radiograph.

Root canal pluggers or **spreaders** have a long, tapered smooth point used to condense the gutta-percha filling points against the canal walls and obliterate any gaps. These may also be referred to as lateral condensers, but they all have the same function.

Rotary paste fillers are engine instruments for inserting pastes into a root canal. They consist of a spiral wire which fits in a slow-running handpiece and propels the required material to the full length of the root canal.

As with the use of some specific instruments for endodontic treatment only, there are materials and medicaments used exclusively in non-surgical endodontic treatment too, all of which will have been risk-assessed before their use in accordance with Control of Substances Hazardous to Health Regulations (COSHH). Their potential to cause both the patient and dental personnel harm if misused must be fully appreciated and understood by the whole dental team. Consequently, working safely as a member of the dental team throughout chairside procedures should be second nature to the dental nurse, ensuring that there is no potential for accidents or mistakes during any treatment session.

The materials and medicaments used throughout root canal therapy treatments are as follows:

- **Irrigation solution** – used during root canal preparation to lubricate the instruments and wash out any debris; the solution used is an individual choice of sodium hypochlorite (bleach), chlorhexidine (although some patients may be allergic to this product) or local anaesthetic solution
- **Antiseptic paste** – non-setting and containing antiseptic anti-inflammatories, and used to dress infected root canals for a time before root filling, e.g. Ledermix paste (see Figure 10.7)
- **Cresophene** – medical-grade creosote used to dress infected root canals for a time, soaked onto paper points before insertion (see Figure 10.9)
- **Lubricating gel** – for use with engine files and reamers (those used with a handpiece) to ensure the instruments do not snag on the canal walls and snap during use, e.g. Glyde (see Figure 10.10)
- **Gutta-percha points (GP points)** –tapered rubber points of various diameters used to fill (obturate) the root canal system, and following the same colour-coded width system as files and reamers (see Figure 10.11) – so if a "red" (size 25) file or reamer is used as the final canal preparation instrument, then a red gutta-percha point must be used to obturate the root canal
- **Sealing cement** – setting cement used to aid the insertion of the gutta-percha points and to seal off any residual spaces in the root canal; some contain antiseptics and anti-inflammatories
- **Restorative materials** – used to restore the tooth to full function and appearance after root filling, and as discussed earlier

Pulpotomy

In adults, the conservative treatment of an exposed vital pulp in a permanent tooth is by conventional root filling, as described earlier. But in the permanent teeth of children, growth of the root is not complete until up to 3 years after eruption, so an exposed tooth may still have a wide open apex, instead of the minute apical foramen. Root filling is unnecessary for these teeth, as pulp death does not always occur, because the wide open apex allows blood circulation through the pulp to continue, without being cut off by a build-up of inflammatory pressure. Instead of total removal of the pulp from the chamber and the root, followed by root filling, it is only necessary to remove the infected part of the pulp in the pulp chamber itself – a procedure known as **pulpotomy**. The very rich blood supply through an open apex allows healing to occur. The radicular pulp (that within the root) survives and root growth continues to its natural completion. In fully grown teeth, such healing is rarely possible and that is why the entire pulp must be removed and a root filling inserted.

The procedure in pulpotomy is similar to root filling only in so far as a sterile technique is necessary. The pulp tissue is removed from the pulp chamber within the crown of the tooth only. The amputated pulp stump at the entrance to the root canal is then covered with a calcium hydroxide dressing. This stimulates the radicular pulp in the root canal to form a layer of secondary dentine over itself. The pulp is thereby completely sealed off again, as it was before the exposure occurred, and normal growth continues until apical formation is complete. In some cases, it may still then be necessary to do a full root filling.

Open apex root filling

The technique of pulpotomy is only successful if the exposed radicular pulp is vital and can separate itself from the exposure site by laying down a secondary dentine bridge. A dead tooth with an open apex must be root-filled as no secondary dentine will form, but this cannot be done in the same way as one with a closed apex, because the gutta-percha points will be too small to seal the open apex and will perforate the apical foramen and pass through it instead. In these cases of an open apex, an endodontic technique is used that seals the open apex over time, before filling the rest of the root canal conventionally at a later date.

Pulp capping

This can be carried out in either deciduous or permanent teeth, as a temporary measure before tooth exfoliation in the former, or before pulpotomy or pulpectomy in the latter. It is a procedure carried out in the following instances:

- When routine restorative treatment produces a small, unexpected pulp exposure in an otherwise healthy tooth
- When a patient attends as an emergency with a small pulp exposure following trauma

The aim is to **seal the exposed pulp** from the oral cavity so that no oral microorgansms contaminate the tooth and cause an infection. This buys time for either the tooth to exfoliate naturally or for the patient to be reappointed so that either pulpotomy or pulpectomy can be carried out without them developing pain and/or an infection in the interim.

Prosthodontics

Prosthodontics is the branch of dentistry that involves the restoration or replacement of damaged or missing teeth by the use of artificially constructed devices. In this speciality, teeth that have been damaged (whether by dental caries, trauma or some other means) are restored by dental techniques other than fillings – namely, those of inlays, crowns and veneers – or they are extracted and replaced. Missing teeth are replaced by the use of dentures, bridges or implants.

Tooth restorations or replacements that are permanently cemented to existing teeth are also referred to as **fixed prostheses**, while those that are able to be removed from the mouth by the patient are referred to as **removable prostheses**. Implants are a stand-alone category of tooth replacement that are provided by dentists who have undergone additional training in their use

All the artificial devices used to restore or replace the teeth are constructed outside of the oral cavity by a technician, rather than within it by the dentist or therapist, as for fillings. For this reason, accurate copies of the prepared teeth and/or the dental arches must be taken and provided to the technician for them to create the artificial restoration or replacement. This is then returned to the dentist for placement or fitting in the patient's mouth at a later date. These accurate copies are made by taking **impressions** of the teeth, after the necessary tooth preparation has been carried out by the dentist beforehand.

In addition, the occlusion of the individual patient's dental arches must also be recorded accurately, as any disruption to the normal occlusion will be uncomfortable to the point of painful for the patient. This is because the musculature surrounding the temporo-mandibular joint, especially the lateral pterygoid muscles, will become strained as the teeth attempt to bite in their correct positions, and the patient will experience facial pain as the muscles are stretched, as well as dental pain due to premature contacts on the teeth.

The skill of the dental technician involved in fixed prosthetic dentistry is to construct the restorations with the same tooth morphology as the original tooth, and to fit the restoration into the occlusion of that individual patient. So each restoration is consequently constructed by hand as a unique artificial device. An inlay or crown made for one specific tooth in one dental arch would therefore not fit any other tooth in any other patient. Although the teeth used in denture construction are pre-formed, the technician involved in removable prosthetic dentistry is equally skilled in constructing prostheses that accurately fit the individual oral anatomy of the patient and sit comfortably in the correct occlusion. Again, each removable artificial device is handmade and unique to that patient.

Impression materials used in prosthodontics

As mentioned earlier, all prosthodontic devices are constructed outside the patient's mouth and impression materials are used to record an accurate copy for that construction to take place. An impression is also taken of the opposing arch of the patient (the dental arch that does **not** contain the tooth to be restored or replaced), and this may involve a different impression material too.

The variety of impression materials available for use in dentistry is vast, but they must all have the following properties:

- Easily mixed – if their correct mixing is too difficult to achieve by the average member of staff, their use will be limited
- Cost-effective – certainly within the National Health Service, where treatment costs are fixed, materials that are overly expensive for routine use will not be cost-effective to the workplace and are likely to be avoided by the profession
- Have an adequate working time before setting – the working time is that available to correctly mix the material before it begins to set; if this is too short then the impression will not be in place before it begins to set, and the mix will be unusable
- Have a relatively short setting time – the setting time is that taken for the material to fully set so that it can be removed from the mouth without any tearing or distortion; it needs to be as short as possible for the patient's comfort
- Able to record the tooth details accurately – a high level of accuracy must be achieved with every impression, so that tooth morphology, tooth preparation and occlusion can be reproduced correctly
- Stable when set – models cast from the impression must be accurate and not distorted, so the material must not deteriorate at normal room temperature and conditions before it has arrived with the technician and the models cast up
- Elastic – this property ensures that tearing of the impression on removal from the mouth does not occur, while any distortion that does occur as the impression is pulled out of any undercuts is not permanent, and the impression "bounces back" into its original shape and maintains the recorded details accurately
- Able to be disinfected without affecting the accuracy of the details recorded – this is to avoid cross-infection from the patient to the dental staff and the technician, and the impression must be able to withstand the use and concentrations of any recommended disinfectants

Where no undercuts are present in the mouth, such as in some edentulous patients (those with no remaining teeth), non-elastic impression materials may be used, but they have been largely superseded by more modern elastic materials. The more commonly used elastic types of impression materials fall into one of the following categories:

- **Irreversible hydrocolloids** – alginate
- **Addition silicones**, from heavy-bodied putty to light=bodied paste
- **Polyethers** – similar applications to addition silicones

Details of the more common materials available are shown in the following table, but some of the more modern ones can be mixed automatically in special machines, rather than by hand. However, mixing of impression materials is a daily task of the dental nurse in the vast majority of dental workplaces, and all should be proficient in the hand mixing of all commonly used materials. The techniques and skills required should be covered in all good training courses.

Name	Type of material	Mixing components and technique
Alginate	Irreversible hydrocolloid	Powder and room temperature water in equal portions, mixed by spatulating in a bowl
Addition Silicone	Elastomer	Base and catalyst, as putty and liquid or two pastes, mixed in equal portions by spatulation, or in pre-loaded tubes, or in a mixing machine
Polyether	Elastomer	Base and catalyst pastes, mixed in equal portions by spatulation, then loaded into a syringe for direct application

Alginate impression material

This is the most commonly used impression material in the dental workplace, as it is easy to mix and relatively cheap. It is suitable for producing impressions for models for the following:

- Opposing arch models for crown, bridge, inlay and veneer construction
- Models for the construction of full and partial acrylic dentures
- Models for the construction of removable orthodontic appliances
- Study models, for any purpose
- Models for the construction of special trays, bleaching trays, orthodontic retainers
- Reproduction of models, as more than one cast can be made from a single impression

However, the set material is not accurate enough to be used in taking the working model for crown, bridge, veneer or inlay construction.

The powder and water mix is loaded into an impression tray before insertion into the patient's mouth. A set impression is shown in Figure 15.44.

The working time of alginate (the time available to load the mixed material into the tray and insert it into the patient's mouth) is affected by the temperature of the mixing water used, and the

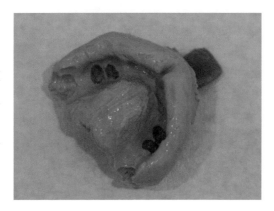

Figure 15.44   An alginate impression.

setting time is affected by the room temperature. In both cases, the higher the temperature, the less time is required. Room temperature water and surroundings provide the optimum conditions for use, but are not always possible, such as on cold winter days and hot summer days. Some alginates are presented as "chromogenic" materials, which change colour during the mixing and setting stages, so that the tray can be loaded and the impression taken at the optimal points of the procedure. Thus an initial white powder changes to pink during the working time, when the tray is loaded and inserted into the patient's mouth. Once the material has changed to a purple colour, it is set, and the impression can be removed from the patient's mouth.

The uses and advantages of alginate were listed earlier. Its disadvantages are as follows:

- Can undergo dimensional changes in the presence or absence of water:
  - If left immersed in water, the impression expands
  - If allowed to dry out, the impression shrinks
- Ideally, then, the model should be cast immediately
- When this is not possible, the impression should be wrapped in a damp gauze and sealed in an airtight plastic bag before sending to the laboratory

Addition silicone impression material

These are one of the elastomer impression materials and are highly accurate when set. They are used specifically for all fixed prosthetic work and some removable prosthetic work. They have a variety of presentations:

- Tubs of heavy-bodied putty with liquid or paste activator – a chemical that starts the reaction to produce the impression material (e.g. Express – Figure 15.45)
- Tubes of light-bodied paste with liquid or paste activator (e.g. Xantopren – Figure 15.46)
- More recent pre-loaded gun syringes that mix the constituents automatically (e.g. Express – Figure 15.47)

The putty base materials can also be measured and mixed by hand, and it is possible for the mixing and setting times to be affected by some types of rubber PPE gloves used. If mixing is to occur by hand, then, it is advisable that vinyl gloves are worn, as other types may affect the setting of the silicone impression.

The silicones can be used in either a one-stage technique (the most widely available, and using addition cured silicones) or a two-stage technique (using condensation cured silicones). With the former, both the heavy-bodied putty and the light-bodied paste are mixed at the same time. The putty is loaded into the impression tray while the paste is either syringed on to the prepared tooth or placed on it using a flat plastic instrument. Both materials then set and are removed together.

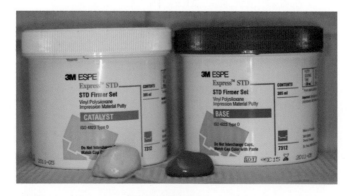

Figure 15.45 Express putty.

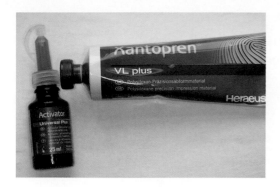

Figure 15.46   Xantopren paste.

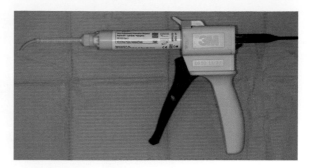

Figure 15.47   Express soft body material in delivery gun.

For the two-stage technique, the putty is first mixed, loaded into the tray, inserted into the mouth and allowed to set. It is then carefully removed and spaced in the area of the preparation, while the mixed paste is syringed or wiped onto the tooth. The set putty and tray are reinserted and the whole is removed when the paste has set.

While the one-stage technique is obviously quicker, the two-stage technique ensures that adequate paste remains around the prepared tooth during tray insertion and gives a very accurate impression – it can be displaced by the putty during tray insertion in the one-stage method. Adhesive is usually supplied by the manufacturer, but perforated trays can also be used.

Setting time for the silicones is usually 4 minutes or more, so adequate moisture control to maintain patient comfort is of great importance during this period.

The advantages of silicones are as follows:

- They are dimensionally stable in the presence of moisture
- They have excellent elasticity, strength and accuracy that allows for:
  - Use in deep undercuts, without tearing of the impression
  - Undistorted final impression for model casting, as their elasticity allows the material to "bounce back" to its original shape once it has been removed from the mouth
  - Strength of the set material allows several tooth preparations to be recorded accurately in one impression, without tearing
- They are suitable for use in all types of denture construction, as well as for fixed prostheses

The disadvantages of silicones are as follows:

- A more complicated and time-consuming technique of impression taking than for alginate
- More expensive materials
- Longer setting time may be too uncomfortable for some patients to tolerate
- Paste materials are particularly sticky before setting and need to be carefully handled to avoid causing an unnecessary mess

Polyethers

These are also highly accurate impression materials, used specifically for fixed prosthetic work and certain removable prosthetic work. An example of this type of impression material is Impregum (Figure 15.48).

The bulk of the mixed material is loaded into the impression tray, and the remainder is syringed around the prepared teeth. Tray adhesive is supplied by the manufacturer. Polyether materials have a similar setting time to silicones, and set more stiffly than other elastomers. They therefore need to be removed with a sharp displacing action from the mouth, otherwise they can be difficult

515

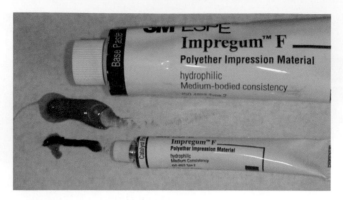

Figure 15.48   Impregum paste.

to remove. Their advantages and disadvantages are as for silicones, except that they are slightly less dimensionally stable when moist.

Impression handling

As all of the impressions taken have been inside the patient's mouth, they will obviously be contaminated by their saliva and perhaps even their blood. To avoid cross-infection from the patient to either staff or the technician, the impressions (and bite records – see later) must be disinfected immediately after their removal from the mouth. This is done as follows:

- Rinsed under cold running water to remove any visible debris
- Fully immersed in a disinfectant bath of a recommended impression disinfectant, such as a solution of up to **10% sodium hypochlorite** (bleach)
- Immersed in this disinfectant solution for up to 10 minutes
- Rinsed under cold running water again, to remove the disinfectant solution
- Alginate impressions – covered with wet gauze and sealed in an air-tight bag
- Elastomer impressions – blown dry using the triple syringe and then sealed in an air-tight bag
- All stored at room temperature or below (in the fridge) before transportation to the laboratory
- Work ticket enclosed – detailing dentist, patient name and age, prosthesis to be constructed, material to be used, shade, additional features, date of delivery for fitting, disinfection details

The work ticket details should also be recorded on the patient's record card or computer notes.

As indicated, the majority of impressions are sent away to a laboratory and this can take some considerable time, especially if they are posted. During this period, they must remain stable so that the cast models produced are accurate; otherwise the fixed prostheses will not fit properly on the patient's tooth or in the mouth. For this reason, they should not be exposed to any heat sources nor chemicals, and alginate impressions must be kept moist and not be allowed to dry out; otherwise they will distort and any models cast from them will be useless.

Impression trays

Impression trays are the devices used to hold the semi-solid impression material in the shape of a dental arch, so that it can be inserted into the patient's mouth and held in place without dripping, while it sets over the teeth and the other oral structures. The tray then holds the set impression in a horseshoe shape while it is removed from the mouth, inspected and disinfected, before being sent to the laboratory for model casting.

The trays are available for use with edentulous patients (Figure 15.49) and dentate patients (Figure 15.50), the latter being referred to as "box trays". They can be plastic and single use, or metal and autoclavable for reuse. As many impression materials are not adhesive to plastic or metal, the trays are either perforated so the set material locks itself into the tray, or unperforated, requiring the use of an adhesive so that the impression sticks to the tray. Obviously, the shape of upper and lower trays differs by the inclusion of the palatal coverage required in the upper trays.

Impression trays that are available in a variety of child and adult sizes and pre-formed by the manufacturers are called "stock trays", while those that are handmade in acrylic by the technician from an initial study model are called "special trays" (see Figure 9.15). These are therefore custom-made and individual to the patient, and are used when a high level of accuracy is required, such as when chrome-cobalt dentures are being constructed.

A final type of tray is that used for fixed prosthodontic work, which records a partial section of both dental arches and the occlusion of the area in one impression. Examples of these are "triple trays", as shown in Figure 15.51.

517

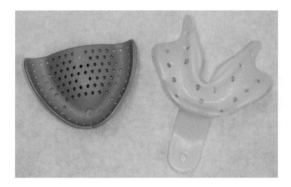

Figure 15.49   Edentulous impression trays.

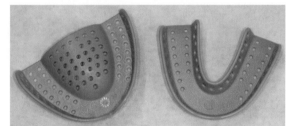

Figure 15.50   A boxed impression tray.

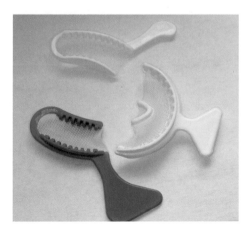

Figure 15.51   Triple trays.

Fixed prosthodontics

These are tooth restorations or replacements that are cemented within, or onto, a tooth and include the following prostheses:

- **Temporary or permanent crown** – a cap or shell-like device made to cover three-quarters to the whole surface of a single tooth
- **Temporary or permanent bridge** – two or more crown-like units joined together as a single device, at least one of which is to replace a missing tooth
- **Veneer** – a facing made to fully cover the labial surface of a tooth
- **Inlay** – an insert into a tooth cavity that has been constructed in a laboratory

All are provided for varying reasons but involve the use of similar impression and cementation materials, and similar instruments. They are constructed from various materials (see the following table), the choice of which depends on the following considerations:

- Tooth involved – are high chewing forces likely to occur?
- Aesthetics – is an anterior tooth involved?
- Longevity – is the prosthesis temporary or permanent?
- Occlusion – is the patient's bite unusual in any way?

518

Fixed prosthesis	Purpose of prosthesis	Construction materials
Temporary crown (see Figure 9.4)	To cover the prepared tooth while awaiting a permanent crown As an emergency restoration	Preformed acrylic or polycarbonate Cold cure acrylic
Permanent crown (Figure 15.52)	To protect a heavily filled or root-filled tooth from fracture during chewing Aesthetics Tooth shape change	Porcelain ceramic Bonded porcelain to metal Precious metal alloy Non-precious metal alloy
Temporary bridge	To cover prepared teeth and replace missing teeth while awaiting the permanent bridge To replace missing teeth after extraction while resorption occurs	Acrylic Resin-based materials
Permanent bridge (Figure 15.53)	To replace missing teeth Aesthetics	Ceramic Bonded porcelain to metal Precious metal alloy Non-precious metal alloy
Veneer (Figure 15.54)	Aesthetics, to cover the labial surface of an anterior tooth when it is discoloured or misshapen	Porcelain
Inlay (Figure 15.55)	To restore a cavity in a tooth with a material stronger than conventional filling materials	Porcelain Precious metal alloy Non-precious metal Alloy

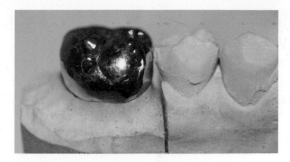

Figure 15.52   A full gold crown on a model.
Source: *Levison's Textbook for Dental Nurses*, 11th edition (Hollins), 2013. Reproduced with permission of Wiley-Blackwell.

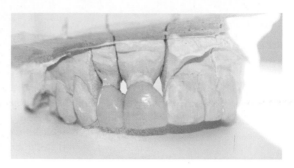

Figure 15.53   A permanent bridge on a model.

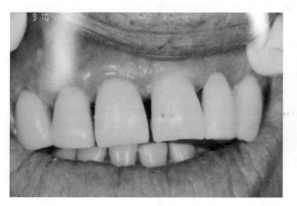

Figure 15.54   Porcelain veneers.

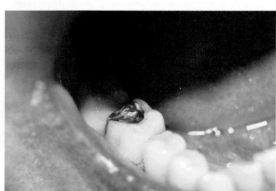

Figure 15.55   A cemented gold inlay.

Although some temporary crowns and bridges can be constructed at the chairside, using either stock crown forms or preoperative impressions, all other fixed prostheses are sent to a laboratory for construction by the technician.

Crowns

A crown is a laboratory-constructed artificial restoration which replaces at least three-quarters of the natural crown surface of the tooth. There are various types, made of various materials, and they require at least two visits for the tooth preparation, crown construction and fitting to be completed. After tooth preparation and impressions have been completed, a temporary crown is fitted while the permanent crown is constructed in the laboratory.

Instruments and materials required

The majority of dentists have a normal "conservation tray" set up as the basic instruments required for crown preparation and fitting, and some may work under rubber dam as well. The additional equipment and materials specifically required are shown in the following table. Luting cements, used to permanently cement the crown to the prepared tooth, are also shown.

Item	Function
Diamond burs (see Figure 9.1)	Tapered so that no undercuts are produced on the prepared tooth or teeth, otherwise the fixed prosthesis will not sit fully onto the tooth
Retraction cord	Cord soaked in an astringent solution (adrenaline or alum) that is then packed into the gingival crevice to cause shrinkage of the gingiva away from the prepared tooth This provides a definitive tooth margin which is reproduced in the impression and also in the cast model
Impression trays (Figures 15.50 and 9.15)	Variety of plastic or metal boxed trays, sized to fit fully over the dental arch – upper and lower styles Also the triple tray system
Crown former (see Figure 9.4)	Pre-formed plastic or polycarbonate tooth-shaped formers, in a variety of sizes and available for each tooth shape
Beebee crown shears (see Figure 9.5)	Short beaked shears for cutting and shaping the margins of temporary crowns
Shade guide (see Figure 9.6)	Shaded teeth in holder – to determine the required shade of the prosthesis by comparing each example against the adjacent teeth and arriving at the best match available

The fixed prosthesis is permanently cemented to the prepared tooth using a luting cement. These are **adhesive to the dentine** of the tooth, and are mixed to a **creamy consistency** so that the prosthesis can be seated fully on to the tooth before the cement sets. The types of luting cement available, discussed earlier in the chapter, are summarised in the following table.

Type	Action	Mixing
Zinc phosphate	Mechanically adhesive to rough inner surface of prosthesis and surface of tooth	Glass slab and spatula
Zinc polycarboxylate	Chemically adhesive to tooth and inner surface of prosthesis	Glass slab and spatula
Glass ionomer	Chemically adhesive to tooth and inner surface of prosthesis	Waxed pad and spatula
Polyester resin	Chemically adhesive and inert in saliva	Waxed pad and spatula
Self-cure resin	Chemical bonding between tooth and prosthesis	Double-syringe mix
Light-cure resin	Light-cure bonding between tooth and prosthesis	Double-syringe mix
Dual-cure resin	Combination of self-cure and light-cure bonding between tooth and prosthesis	Double-syringe mix

Modern types of cement tend to be provided in double-syringe form with no mixing necessary, but older types (such as phosphate, polycarboxylate and glass ionomer cements) require correct proportioning and thorough mixing before use.

The types of permanent crown available for use can therefore be summarised as follows:

- Porcelain jacket crown (PJC) – an early type of all-porcelain crown used for anterior teeth only, to provide good aesthetics when the only other alternatives were metal crowns
- Ceramic crown – the modern successor to PJCs, constructed of stronger ceramic materials than porcelain alone (such as zirconia) and therefore able to be used both anteriorly and posteriorly to give a more "tooth-like" appearance than other crowns
- Porcelain bonded crown (PBC) – these consist of a substructure of metal for strength with a buccal or labial face of porcelain for better aesthetics than an all-metal crown (Figure 15.56); these crowns are currently popular although the porcelain can be cracked off the underlying metal in patients with a heavy bite
- Full gold crown (FGC) – these can be made of yellow gold (Figure 15.52) or a mixture of precious or non-precious metals to give a silvery appearance, and are the strongest of all crowns available, making them ideal for posterior teeth, especially in patients with a heavy bite
- These can be made as full coverage crowns, or as three-quarter crowns which leave the buccal or labial surface of the tooth intact but cover the rest of the tooth – this gives better aesthetics while still providing adequate coverage of the tooth cusps, so providing strength to the device
- Three-quarter crowns have tended to be superseded by bonded crowns, which provide both good aesthetics and strength in the same situations

521

Post crowns

As discussed earlier, when teeth die and are preserved by root filling and restoration, the remaining tooth structure often becomes brittle with time and fractures. Sometimes the fracture is so extensive that there is not enough tooth structure left to restore it without the use of additional support. This support is often achieved by the placement of a metallic post and core structure, which is then shaped to hold a conventional crown – these restorations are called post crowns (Figure 15.57).

The metallic post and core system can be constructed from pre-formed posts (see Figure 9.7), such as Paraposts or Dentatus posts, with a core constructed at the chairside. Alternatively, the

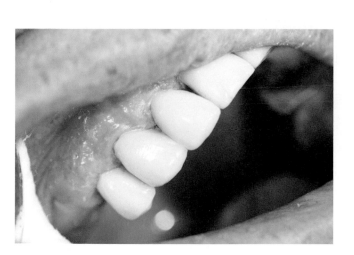

Figure 15.56   Porcelain bonded crowns.

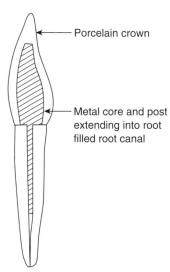

Porcelain crown

Metal core and post extending into root filled root canal

Figure 15.57   A post crown.

prepared root forms part of the crown preparation impression, and the post and core are hand-made by the technician, along with the crown.

Temporary crowns

Temporary crowns are placed for a limited time only while the permanent crown is being constructed and are used for the following reasons:

- To maintain the appearance
- To prevent sensitivity of the prepared teeth between the preparation and fitting visits
- To maintain the correct space between adjacent teeth so that the permanent crown fits – sometimes the adjacent teeth tend to tip into the space once the crown preparation has been carried out, as the contact points between the teeth are removed during the procedure
- To maintain the correct occlusion between opposing teeth – the opposing tooth to the prepared tooth will have no occlusal contact after the crown preparation procedure and may therefore tend to over erupt

Temporary crowns are made by fitting a **crown form** over the prepared tooth.

For anterior teeth, a clear plastic crown form, such as an **Odus Pella** (Figure 15.58), may be used. It is trimmed with crown shears and filled with a material that matches the teeth, such as composite. Alternatively, tough tooth-coloured **polycarbonate** crown forms are used, such as **Directa** (see Figure 9.4), and these only need trimming with slow burs. Metal crown forms made of aluminium, nickel-chromium or stainless steel (Figure 15.59) are used on posterior teeth.

Trimmed temporary crowns are cemented with a material that is adhesive, but easily and cleanly removed for fitting the permanent crown, e.g. Temp Bond or ProTemp. Stainless steel crown forms, cemented with glass ionomer cement, are also used as the best restoration for large cavities in deciduous molars instead of a conventional filling. Alternatively, temporary crowns can be handmade at the chairside on the day of the crown preparation, using a material such as Pro Temp in an alginate impression of the original tooth.

Bridges

A bridge is a laboratory-constructed artificial device that is composed of two or more units, one of which will replace a missing tooth. Essentially, bridges consist of one or more units, each of

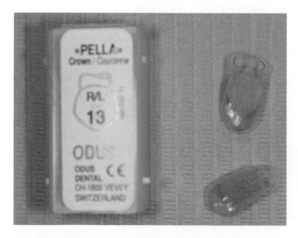

Figure 15.58   Odus Pella crown forms.

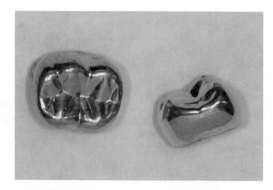

Figure 15.59   Metal temporary crowns.

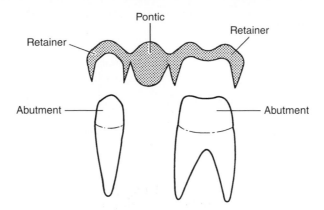

Figure 15.60   Bridge components.

which is exactly the same as a single crown, but which are joined together to make one structure. Within that structure will be one or more units that lie over the dental ridge where a tooth is missing, while the other units sit over the prepared teeth that will hold the bridge in place.

The unit replacing the missing tooth is called a **pontic**, the units holding the bridge in place are called **retainers**, and the teeth they are cemented onto are called **abutments**. A conventional bridge is illustrated in Figure 15.60.

Bridges have several advantages over removable prostheses (dentures), which may also be used to replace missing teeth:

- There is no embarrassment of a loose prosthesis falling out, as bridges are fixed to the teeth permanently
- On the whole, they are aesthetically superior to dentures
- They are more hygienic than dentures, because there is no involvement of any teeth except the retainers and therefore fewer stagnation areas
- Usually only two appointments are required for their provision, while denture construction may require up to five visits
- The materials used in their construction are better able to resist occlusal forces than the acrylic used to construct many dentures
- The shades available can be customised in any way by the laboratory technician to mimic the patient's other teeth, whereas those available for dentures are mass-produced and unalterable
- They solve the problem of patients with a strong gag reflex who require tooth replacement, and who usually cannot cope with a denture
- They are also better tolerated because of the minimal amount of soft tissue coverage involved

However, the need for good oral hygiene control postoperatively is of paramount importance with bridges, as they produce stagnation areas unlike any others in the mouth (i.e. **under the pontics**), and therefore require special techniques for effective cleaning to be carried out. Due to the complexity of their design and construction, as well as the cost of the materials used in their manufacture, bridges also tend to be far more expensive than dentures.

Several different types of bridge have been developed, but all designs rely on retaining teeth (abutments) to hold the bridge permanently in place, and they are joined to the missing teeth (pontics) in one structure as follows:

- **Fixed–fixed bridge**, where retaining teeth are on either side of the missing teeth, as one solid design (Figure 15.61)
- **Fixed–moveable bridge**, where a joint is incorporated in the design to allow the bridge some degree of flexibility (Figure 15.62)

523

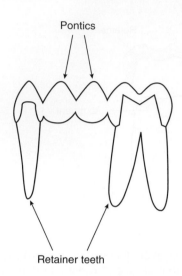

Figure 15.61   A fixed–fixed bridge.

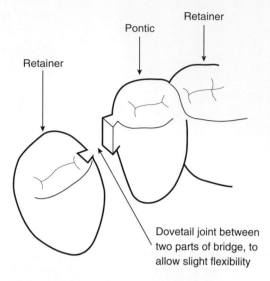

Figure 15.62   A fixed–moveable bridge.

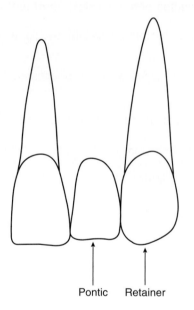

Figure 15.63   A simple cantilever bridge.

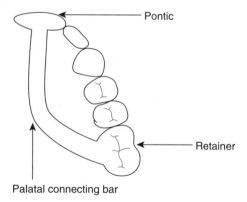

Figure 15.64   A spring cantilever bridge.

- **Cantilever bridge**, where the retaining tooth or teeth are to one side of the pontic only:
  - **Simple cantilever** design, where retaining teeth are those immediately to one side of the pontic only (Figure 15.63)
  - **Spring cantilever** design, where the retaining teeth are to one side but several teeth away from the pontic (Figure 15.64)
- **Adhesive bridge**, where the retaining teeth undergo minimal tooth preparation and retention is provided by lingual or palatal metal wings only (Figure 15.65)

Pontic

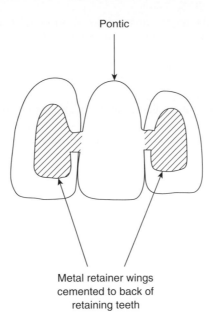

Metal retainer wings
cemented to back of
retaining teeth

Figure 15.65   An adhesive bridge.

The choice of bridge depends on several factors:

● Whether an anterior or a posterior tooth is being replaced, as the latter usually undergoes heavier occlusal forces, so full crown retainers are generally required
● Like crowns, bridges can be constructed of all-metal or ceramic materials, and obviously the former would not be provided anteriorly
● Fixed–fixed bridges tend not to be used so frequently nowadays, as their inflexibility during use has been seen to cause damage to retaining teeth – their solid structure, especially with long bridge spans, allows occlusal forces on one end of the bridge to gradually loosen the other end from the abutment tooth; if undetected this would allow caries to seep under the retainer and eventually destroy the abutment tooth
● Wherever possible, adhesive bridges are used, as they involve minimal tooth preparation
● If a patient has natural spaces between the teeth, only a spring cantilever design can be used so as to maintain the spaces and give good aesthetics
● The health of the abutment teeth is of paramount importance to the success of the bridge, and if there is any cause for concern, an adhesive type of bridge is advisable so that any problems would result in its dislodgement rather than causing damage to the abutments

All types of bridge, except for adhesive ones, rely on the retaining teeth being of full crown coverage. Indeed, the tooth preparation is exactly the same as for a single crown, as are the instruments and the impression materials used. Some additional procedures and techniques are used when constructing and fitting a bridge, and these are summarised here:

● While radiographs are always taken to determine the health of any tooth involved in fixed prosthodontics, study models are often also taken before bridge construction, so that:
   ○ The occlusion can be checked from all angles
   ○ The bridge design can be visualised and decided upon
   ○ Any potential undercuts of adjacent teeth can be identified

- With bonded bridges, the metal substructure is often tried out on the abutment teeth before proceeding with the porcelain work; if the fit is found to be incorrect, a full remake will not be required
- Ensuring the correct occlusion is present with a multi-unit bridge is a complicated process, and needs to be checked and finalised before the bridge is cemented onto the abutments. It is best carried out as follows:
  - High spots are identified by the patient closing onto a fine film of articulating foil or Mylar (shim stock)
  - Alternatively, fine, coloured articulating paper may be used – that used for removable prosthodontics is generally too thick
  - The foil or paper can be held in place using Miller forceps (see Figure 9.10), which can be slid gently into the buccal or labial sulcus without compromising the occlusion

Adhesive bridges

These bridges are used to replace just one or two front teeth. The pontic has a porcelain-bonded facing while the metal backing has wing-like flanges that rest against the palatal or lingual surface of the abutments, and are bonded directly to their acid-etched enamel.

These Maryland-type bridges (Figure 15.65) conserve tooth tissue, as the only preparation required is to roughen the palatal/lingual enamel to which the flanges will adhere, and possibly prepare a defining ridge in the enamel to help the technician to determine the margins of the flanges. Adhesive bridges are accordingly ideal for younger patients, who are more likely to have few if any restorations present. They are far quicker to make and can be replaced much more easily than conventional bridgework, as they do not have to be cut off the abutment teeth. However, they will not withstand heavy occlusal forces without becoming dislodged, so suitable cases have to be chosen carefully. The ideal cases are younger patients with a minimal overbite, or even an open bite, where the pontic is unlikely to experience little if any occlusal loading.

The adhesive bridge requires special dual-curing resin cements with primers, to provide a strong chemical bond between the retaining teeth and the metal wings of the bridge. The fitting surface of the flanges is made retentive by acid etching and sand blasting; a chemical-cure adhesive resin, such as Panavia Ex, which bonds to both metal and enamel, is used as a luting cement.

Temporary bridges

A temporary bridge is necessary between the bridge preparation and fitting visits to prevent tooth sensitivity, space closure and tipping or over-eruption of the abutment teeth. It may be made directly in a similar fashion to that of a chairside-constructed temporary crown. Alternatively, temporary bridges may be used as tooth replacements for up to 6 months after the extraction of a tooth, to allow bone resorption to occur before a permanent bridge is constructed. The abutment teeth are prepared in the same way and the impression is taken and sent to the technician. The abutment teeth have a temporary crown-like covering placed. The technician then removes the tooth to be extracted from the working model and constructs the temporary bridge to replace it, using composite-type resin materials or acrylics.

Once the temporary bridge is returned, the abutment covers are removed, the tooth is extracted and the prosthesis cemented to the abutment teeth. Bone resorption can then progress without leaving unsightly gaps beneath the pontic of a permanent bridge. Any gaps that do become apparent under the temporary bridge can be closed using composite materials, until the risk of further resorption is over – usually around 6 months post-extraction. The permanent bridge can then be constructed to replace the temporary bridge.

Oral hygiene instruction for crowns and bridges

No matter how well -fitting the crown or bridge is to the tooth, microscopically the junction between the two is a potential stagnation area for plaque to gather. Thorough brushing at the margins of the crown will ensure that plaque does not accumulate and cause recurrent caries or periodontal problems.

The general oral health messages to be relayed to the patient following crown or bridge cementation are:

- Regular and thorough tooth brushing daily
- Use of fluoride toothpaste and a medium-textured toothbrush
- Regular flossing to clean crown margins interproximally
- Careful use of floss so as not to dislodge crown
- Attend for dental examinations so that margins can be checked professionally
- Sensible diet, low in NMES
- Regular use of good-quality mouthwash, to reinforce plaque control

In addition, bridges provide a challenge to the patient with regard to adequate oral hygiene, as they are fixed prostheses producing stagnation areas beneath the pontics. As well as the oral hygiene instructions for crowns, patients with bridges need to be instructed in the use of "**Superfloss**" (see Figure 9.31).

This is a type of dental floss with a stiff end, which can be threaded under the pontic by the patient, and then drawn through to a sponge part, which is used to clean beneath the pontic. When used regularly, it keeps this region of the bridge plaque-free and prevents caries from undermining the retainers, with catastrophic consequences.

More recently, sonic toothbrushes have been shown to provide excellent cleaning in these areas, without dislodging the bridge, and these are being recommended more frequently in these cases.

527

Veneers

Conventional crown preparation requires the removal of a significant amount of enamel and dentine from the tooth, involving all the tooth surfaces. While this may be harmless in fully developed adult teeth, it could result in pulpal damage in younger patients as the pulp chambers are larger in recently erupted teeth. In other cases, it may be felt that labial enamel defects in incisors that require a restoration to improve appearance do not justify a full jacket crown preparation, and the teeth are more suitable for restoration by veneers.

Veneers are either a composite or porcelain facing made to cover the labial surface of anterior teeth, following minimal tooth preparation (Figure 15.66). Where composite is used, the dentist carries out the restorative procedure at the chairside, as for a routine filling with this material. Porcelain veneers require the input of a technician to construct each one by hand in the laboratory.

They are used in the following situations:

- To mask a **discoloured tooth** (such as with tetracycline staining)
- To mask a root-filled tooth that has become darkened with time
- To **close diastemas** between teeth and improve the appearance
- To **change the shape** of rotated teeth so that they appear aligned
- To change the shape of malaligned teeth so that they appear aligned
- To **correct poorly shaped teeth**, such as peg laterals
- As a **cosmetic procedure**, to lighten the whole labial segment, although this has been largely superseded by the use of tooth-whitening techniques

Porcelain veneers are fragile once constructed and can break if the patient is careless with them. Ideally, they are only fitted to patients with low incisal edge forces and they are sometimes constructed so as not to cover the incisal edge of the tooth at all, but finish just in line with it.

The instruments and impression materials used for porcelain veneer construction are the same as for crowns and bridges, but often no opposing arch impression is required, as veneers rarely encroach on the occlusion.

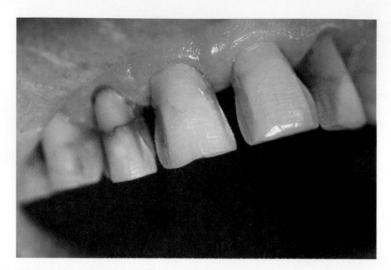

Figure 15.66   Veneer tooth preparations.

As with all other fixed prostheses, veneers are also custom made in the laboratory by a highly skilled technician. The shades taken in the surgery will be accurately replicated, as the veneer is constructed by hand from porcelain before having the final firing in an oven to produce the surface glaze. The fitting surface of the veneer will be abraded and chemically roughened using hydrofluoric acid in the laboratory to produce a rough surface for cement adhesion. The finished product is then carefully returned to the surgery for fitting.

Inlays

These are fixed prostheses that are used to restore a cavity in a tooth, rather than covering the whole or part of the surface of a tooth, as do other fixed prostheses. Unlike fillings, though, which are also used to restore cavities, inlays are constructed indirectly in a laboratory by a technician rather than being placed directly into the tooth.

They are constructed of gold alloy, porcelain or a special type of composite that contains more filler than usual and is therefore stronger than conventional composite filling materials that are placed at the chairside.

The purpose of using an inlay rather than a filling is to produce a restoration of higher strength than is possible with plastic materials, and of a more permanent nature – although with the continual improvement of filling materials, gold alloy inlays are being provided less frequently nowadays. They are generally confined to teeth that have lost cusps, undergo heavy occlusal forces or are otherwise too weak to be satisfactorily restored with amalgam. Small uncomplicated cavities do not usually warrant the extra time and expense of restoring them with inlays. Their use in anterior cavities has also declined with the development of better aesthetic anterior filling materials.

As the inlay is inserted into the tooth rather than cemented on to it, less tooth preparation is necessary than if the tooth were restored using a conventional crown. The equipment, materials and impression techniques are the same as for other fixed prostheses.

Inlay preparation is as for a conventional filling, with the full removal of all carious tooth tissue to sound dentine, but then the resultant cavity preparation is adjusted to ensure that the sides are not undercut but **parallel** (Figure 15.67). This may involve any undercut walls being filled in with plastic materials, such as glass ionomer cements.

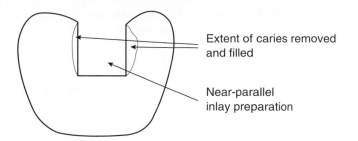

Figure 15.67   An inlay preparation.

This allows the following:

- The inlay to be inserted fully, without becoming stuck on an undercut
- The maximum retention possible is produced by ensuring that the inlay fits snugly against all the cavity walls
- Only a fine cement layer will then be required, which reduces the risk of cement dissolution in saliva with time and the gradual loosening of the inlay

Once the cavity has been prepared suitably, the necessary impressions and occlusal registrations are taken. Gingival retraction cord may be used to ensure that deep cavity margins are sufficiently exposed for an accurate impression to be taken. The tooth is restored with a temporary filling while the inlay is being constructed.

Removable prosthodontics

Removable prostheses are all types of dentures – appliances that are made in the laboratory in various stages to replace missing teeth. They can be removed from the mouth by the patient, e.g. for cleaning, and reinserted again easily without the use of cements. Generally, removable prostheses are made to replace several missing teeth rather than just one or two, as bridges do, or even, in some patients, to replace all their teeth.

When there are no teeth left in a jaw, it is said to be **edentulous** (edentate) and the artificial replacement is called a **full** or **complete denture**; if some teeth are still present, the replacement is called a **partial denture**. The majority of dentures are made completely of acrylic, although many may also be constructed with a base of chrome-cobalt metal.

The reasons why teeth should be replaced by a removable prosthesis (or indeed by a bridge or an implant) are as follows:

- To prevent excessive masticatory forces on the remaining teeth, which may cause their eventual fracture
- To prevent over-eruption of the opposing teeth, which may cause occlusal problems
- To prevent tilting of the adjacent teeth into the edentulous spaces, causing stagnation areas
- To prevent soft tissue trauma of the alveolar ridges during mastication
- To allow adequate mastication and avoid digestive problems and malnutrition, especially in the elderly
- To provide good aesthetics, especially if anterior teeth are missing

Not all patients are suitable for tooth replacement with dentures, and the following points are considered for every case before treatment commences:

- Is there any previous denture experience? If so, was it successful?
- If not, is there a cause which can be remedied?
- Is the shape of the patient's mouth naturally retentive for full dentures, with good ridges and a high palate, or might pre-prosthetic surgery be necessary?
- Are there any potential retention problems for partial dentures? If so, can they be remedied by tooth shape adjustment?
- Might the patient's occlusion cause problems with the provision of a denture? Is there enough clearance without premature contact onto the denture?
- Are there any medical contraindications to dentures, such as epilepsy or an adverse reaction to the acrylic material?
- Are there other dental problems that need addressing first, such as caries or periodontal disease?
- If the teeth have been lost within the previous 6 months, bone resorption is likely to occur and this will affect the fit of a denture adversely
- Good co-operation and perseverance by the patient are paramount to the success of dentures; if there is any doubt about these, the treatment is likely to fail
- Is the treatment affordable to the patient?

Full and partial acrylic dentures

These are the commonest types of denture produced – full ones (Figure 15.68) for edentulous patients and partial ones (Figure 15.69) for patients with any number of missing teeth, up to one tooth short of being edentulous. The material used for their construction, and that of removable orthodontic appliances as well, is either pink or transparent acrylic.

Acrylic consists of a powder called **polymer** and a liquid called **monomer**. When mixed together, they form a plastic mass with the consistency of dough. This sets into a hard acrylic by a process called **curing**. Curing is effected by heating the dough slowly in a special flask in an oven, or by adding a catalyst which allows it to cure at room temperature. These two methods of curing are known as **heat-curing** and **cold-curing**, respectively.

Heat-cured acrylic is used for dentures and orthodontic appliances, and the curing process is carried out by a technician in the laboratory. Cold-cured acrylic (also called self-cured or autopolymerised acrylic) can be used by the dentist at the chairside to make temporary crowns and to carry out denture repairs. It is also used by the technician for the construction of special trays to take accurate second impressions.

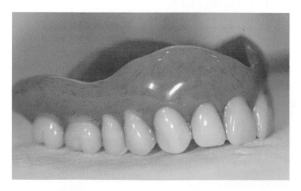

Figure 15.68   A full acrylic denture.

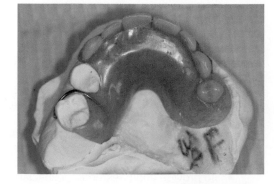

Figure 15.69   A partial denture on a model.

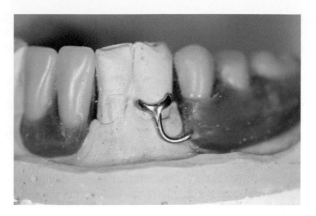

Figure 15.70   An example of a denture clasp.

As dentures are removable prostheses, their retention must be adequate to keep them in position in the mouth during speech and chewing, but weak enough so that patients can easily remove the device from their mouth as they wish, e.g. for cleaning purposes. The level of retention achieved relies on the following factors:

- A **suction film** of saliva developing between the denture and the patient's soft tissues
- A **post-dam** along the back border of the denture, to help the suction film to develop
- An **accurate design and fit** of denture, to allow the film to develop adequately
- Use of any **natural undercuts** in the patient's mouth, such as the alveolar ridges or any suitably shaped natural teeth
- Use of **stainless steel clasps** around standing teeth with partial dentures, to increase the retention of the denture by the clasps gripping the teeth and preventing it from being dislodged by normal soft tissue movements (Figure 15.70)

Sometimes no natural undercuts are present so the patient's own teeth are adjusted to provide them, in the following ways:

- Use of a crown to change the overall shape of the tooth
- Use of composite build-ups to provide a retentive area for clasps to engage
- Shape change of an existing restoration for similar reasons

With edentulous patients, the shape of the alveolar ridges can be changed surgically to improve retention and comfort:

- **Alveoplasty** – changing the shape of the existing ridge, such as by the removal of gross undercuts which would prevent the denture from being seated
- Flat ridges can be built up by the addition of **artificial bone substitutes** under the mucoperiosteum, to increase natural retention by creating a ridge on which the denture can sit
- **Alveolectomy** – the surgical removal and smoothing of sharp ridges to allow comfortable wearing of the denture

Denture construction

Usually, acrylic dentures are made in four or five stages, with each stage being returned to the technician at the laboratory between patient appointments. The dentist prepares and records the

531

details of the patient's oral cavity, and the technician uses these records to construct the dentures to fit that patient's mouth. Each laboratory stage is returned to the dentist for the next clinical stage to be recorded in the patient's mouth, until the end result – the acrylic dentures, with or without clasps – are produced for fitting.

The stages are as follows, although not every stage is required in every case:

- **First impressions** – using stock trays and alginate impression material (Figure 15.44), the tooth shade and shape (mould) are often decided at this stage too
- The impressions are correctly disinfected, as described previously, and suitably wrapped for dispatch to the laboratory
- **Laboratory** – study models are cast in plaster of Paris from the impressions, and special acrylic impression trays are custom-made from them if required – in simple cases, the first impression may be accurate enough on its own for denture construction to proceed
- **Second impression** – using special trays and either alginate or elastomer impression material to produce a very accurate impression; the tooth shade and mould may be chosen at this stage if not already recorded
- **Laboratory** – working models are cast in dental stone, and wax occlusal rims are constructed on them
- **Bite registration** – the existing, or required, occlusal face height of the patient is measured using a Willis bite gauge (see Figure 9.18) and recorded on the occlusal rims by warming or using bite registration paste to stick them together – the rims then hold the models in the correct position and angulation for the dentures to be constructed (see Figure 9.16)
- **Laboratory** – models in their recorded face height positions are mounted on to an articulator, so the technician can construct the wax try-in dentures in these correct horizontal and vertical positions (an articulator mimics the mandibular jaw movements)
- **Try-in** – wax try-ins with the actual acrylic teeth mounted in them (Figure 15.71) are inserted and checked for accuracy of fit and occlusion, as well as shade; any major inaccuracies will result in new records being taken and a retry being requested
- **Laboratory** – stainless steel clasps are added as necessary, and then the try-ins on their models are sealed into flasks and the wax is replaced by heat-cured acrylic to form the final dentures, which are then cleaned and polished to provide a shiny outer surface to the denture
- **Fit** – acrylic dentures are inserted into the patient's mouth and checked for comfort, fit and aesthetics, and then specific denture care information is given

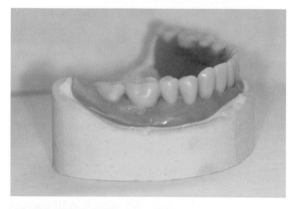

Figure 15.71 Try-in stage of a lower full denture.

Each stage of the denture construction in the surgery involves the use of specific instruments, materials and equipment which the dental nurse must be able to recognise and lay out at each appointment. These are summarised in the following tables.

First impressions:

Item	Function
Stock impression trays	To be sized and used to take the initial impressions, so that special trays can be constructed – they may be upper and/or lower, and edentulous or dentate
Alginate impression material and room temperature water	To be mixed, loaded into the trays and inserted to produce the initial impressions
Shade and mould guides	To determine the colour and shape of the denture teeth, to be as close in appearance to any remaining teeth as possible
Work ticket or docket (see Figure 9.14)	To record the patient and dentist details, the denture design and base material to be used, the tooth shade and mould, the type and position of any clasps, and the return date

The work ticket information must be duplicated on the patient record card or in the computerised notes, so that if the ticket itself is ever lost or misplaced, the relevant details are still available.

The handling and aftercare of the impressions is as for fixed prostheses.

Second impressions:

Item	Function
Study models and special trays	To take the more accurate second impressions where required, to produce the working models
Alginate or elastomer impression material	To take the more accurate second impressions
Work ticket	To record the next stage request and the return date

Bite registration:

Item	Function
Wax bite rims	Adjusted in height so that correct face height of the patient can be recorded
Heat source (see Figure 9.17)	To warm the hand instruments and rims for adjustment
Wax knife (see Figure 9.17)	To remove or add additional wax to the rims, as necessary
Bite registration paste (optional)	To be mixed and applied to the rims, so that they are held in the correct position once set
Pink sheet wax (see Figure 9.17)	For addition to the rims, as necessary
Willis bite gauge (see Figure 9.18)	To record the desired occlusal face height in edentulous patients, where no natural teeth remain as a guide
Work ticket	To record the next stage request and return date

Try-in:

Item	Function
Try-in prostheses	To determine if fit, occlusion and aesthetics are correct before finishing the dentures
Heat source	To warm the wax and make adjustments, as necessary
Le Cron carver (see Figure 9.19)	To make fine adjustments to the try-in, as necessary
Wax knife	To warm and smooth the wax after adjustments, as necessary
Shade and mould guides	To check or alter the shade or mould, as necessary
Pink sheet wax	For addition to the try-in, as necessary
Patient mirror	To allow the patient to view the try-ins and decide if they are happy with the appearance, before completion of the dentures
Work ticket	To record any changes required for a retry, or to record the fit return date

If changes are required to the prostheses, they must be requested at this point, as once the flasking process has been carried out, no further changes can be made and the whole construction process would have to be started again.

Any concerns that the patient may have must be identified and discussed at this point, and resolved to the satisfaction of both the patient and the dentist.

Fitting:

Item	Function
Completed removable prostheses	To fit to the patient and dentist's satisfaction
Straight handpiece and selection of trimming burs and carborundum polishing stones (see Figure 9.20)	To remove any acrylic pearls or occlusal high spots before polishing and smoothing the adjusted area for comfort
Patient mirror	To allow the patient to view the completed prostheses
Articulating paper	To identify occlusal high spots, for adjustment as necessary
Pressure relief paste	To identify high spots on the denture fitting surface, for removal as necessary

Aftercare instructions and advice

Instructions are given on the wear, care and cleaning of the new dentures, as follows:

- A demonstration of how to insert and remove the dentures is given, with the patient then practising the techniques in front of the mirror and under the dentist's supervision
- Avoid wearing them overnight if possible, to avoid the development of oral fungal infections (thrush)

- Store them overnight in a denture pot containing water, or ideally a soaking agent such as Steradent or Dentural
- Clean after each meal, if possible, using a denture brush and denture toothpaste – some ordinary toothpastes may be too abrasive for use on the acrylic teeth
- Clean over a bowl of water to avoid damage to the denture if it is dropped
- Avoid soaking in bleach-based cleansers if any metal components are included in the design
- Eat soft foods initially, while the oral soft tissues acclimatise to the prostheses
- Take time to chew foods thoroughly, to avoid causing indigestion by swallowing large food particles
- Harden oral soft tissues by carrying out hot salt water mouthwashes initially: otherwise the new dentures are likely to rub the soft tissues and make them sore
- Return to the surgery if any ulceration occurs beneath the dentures, as further adjustments are likely to be required to remove high spots and deep flange edges
- Dentate patients must continue to attend for oral health assessment at their regular recall interval, and edentulous patients are advised to attend at least once every 2 years, but ideally annually

Patients are also told that new dentures do not last forever, and their fit and appearance will be checked at each recall. Alveolar bone gradually changes its shape following the loss of teeth, and the denture will eventually become too loose as resorption spaces develop beneath the fitting surface. By that time, most patients will have learned how to control a loose denture using a combination of their soft tissues and denture adhesive products such as Polygrip and Fixodent (Figure 15.72), but the alveolar bone changes can adversely affect appearance as the loose denture may no longer provide adequate support for the lips and cheeks. It is consequently necessary to **re-line** the fitting surface of a denture from time to time and perhaps make other adjustments (see later). Ultimately, the denture will need to be replaced.

If the denture cleaning advice is not followed, the soft tissues covered by a denture may become inflamed and develop into a condition called **denture stomatitis.** This is treated with antifungal drugs, such as nystatin or fluconazole, and the reiteration of suitable oral hygiene instructions. Similarly, the dentures may become stained by products such as tea and coffee, and calculus may form on them in the same regions as for natural teeth. Patients with these problems are advised to clean the dentures by soaking in hypochlorite (e.g. Milton solution) for 20 minutes, rinsing thoroughly and then immersing in water overnight. Dentures with metallic components should be soaked in non-hypochlorite disinfectants instead (such as Dentural); otherwise the bleach-based products will cause metal corrosion.

Full and partial chrome-cobalt dentures

The metallic alloy chrome cobalt can be used as the base of the denture, rather than acrylic, but the teeth still need to be attached to this metal base by acrylic on the ridges. Chrome cobalt can form the base of both edentulous and partial dentures. Metal-based dentures are more difficult to construct than acrylic ones, as the metal is rigid and provides no room for adjustment once made, so the impression and working model must be perfectly accurate. They also cost more than acrylic dentures to construct, but still have several advantages over them, as follows:

- A much **thinner palatal covering** is possible with chrome-cobalt, which makes the whole denture more tolerable to patients, especially those with a strong gag reflex
- Overcomes any tissue reaction to acrylic monomer, as some patients are sensitive to it
- The denture base is **far stronger** and less likely to break, even in thin section
- Allows patients with deep overbites onto their palate to be able to wear a denture, as the bite point can be completely avoided or have just a very thin metal coverage

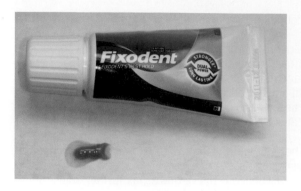

Figure 15.72   A denture adhesive.

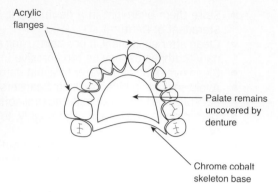

Acrylic flanges

Palate remains uncovered by denture

Chrome cobalt skeleton base

Figure 15.73   A chrome skeleton denture design.

- Can design partial dentures as "**skeletons**", giving minimal tissue coverage and making the denture more tolerable for the patients (Figure 15.73)
- As less tissue coverage is involved, especially around the teeth, chrome dentures tend to be more hygienic than acrylic ones

If the whole palate is covered by a chrome base, then retention is provided by the saliva suction film, as for acrylic dentures. However, if a skeleton design is used then chrome cobalt clasps must be incorporated into the design of the denture for retention, so an adequate number of healthy and well positioned teeth are required for this purpose.

The clasps will be part of the chrome base, and tooth adjustments can be carried out to provide undercuts, as for stainless clasps on acrylic dentures.

Denture construction

The surgery stages are as for acrylic dentures, with the following exceptions:

- Final impressions are often taken in a highly accurate **elastomer** material, rather than alginate, to ensure a good working model is produced for the metal casting
- The chrome-cobalt base is then made on the final model as a wax pattern by the technician, before being cast in a special furnace
- The casting of the metal base is sometimes carried out at specialised laboratories, so extra time between appointments may be necessary
- A try-in of the metal base on its own is often carried out, to ensure it is accurate before proceeding to add the teeth to the design
- A second try-in is then performed, with the teeth added and held by wax to the metal base
- No adjustment of the metal base can be made in the surgery once it has been constructed, except for minimal easing using a pink stone in the slow handpiece

Aftercare instructions and advice

Additional instructions are given to the patient at the fitting stage to ensure that they never use bleach-based denture cleaning products, because these will corrode the metal. A suitable alternative is the cleaning solution Dentural. Otherwise, the same post-fitting instructions are given to the patient.

Some designs of partial chrome-cobalt dentures can be quite intricate, and adequate time must be spent ensuring that the patient is competent in both fitting and removing the denture before leaving the premises.

Immediate replacement dentures

Dentures are usually made some months after the teeth have been extracted, as this allows time for completion of the initial alveolar bone resorption and gum healing to occur. Many patients, however, are not prepared to wait that long for the replacement of missing front teeth, and do not wish to have unsightly extraction gaps present, even for a few days. In such cases, the patient can be provided with an **immediate replacement denture,** which is made before the anterior teeth are extracted and fitted on the day of extraction – immediately after haemostasis has been achieved in the extraction sockets.

Obviously, there can be no try-in stage for this technique, but otherwise the procedure for construction is the same as for conventional dentures, until the final stage when the technician removes the teeth to be extracted from the model and replaces them with the new denture teeth. The construction procedure is as follows:

- The dentist provides the technician with final impressions, the occlusal registration, and the required shade for the new teeth, before any anterior extractions are carried out
- In the laboratory, the anterior teeth to be extracted are cut off the working model by the technician, and the artificial ones are fitted in their place as a wax-up on the model
- This cannot be tried in the patient's mouth, as their own teeth are still present, so the technician proceeds to tidy the wax-up and then processes it as a heat-cured acrylic
- The final denture is trimmed and polished, and then returned to the dentist
- In the surgery, the anterior teeth are extracted and the denture is fitted at the same visit
- Only minimal adjustments are made at this stage, as the oral soft tissues will be swollen from the local anaesthetic injections and the accuracy of the fit will not be obvious
- The patient is given an appointment to attend for a review the next day and is instructed not to remove the denture before then

The patient must be made aware that following the fitting of the immediate denture, alveolar bone resorption will occur and this could result in the prosthesis becoming loose quite quickly. Patients tend to accept this phenomenon readily, as the alternative is to have extraction spaces visible for months before a conventional denture is provided.

As chrome-cobalt cannot be adjusted once cast, immediate dentures are always constructed from acrylic only, although the replacement denture made after resorption has occurred can then be a metal-based one.

If just one anterior tooth is to be replaced, the denture is usually designed in a "spoon" shape, so that the gingival margins of other teeth are not covered by the denture, making it less likely to retain food debris around the teeth, and therefore more hygienic (Figure 15.74).

Aftercare instructions and advice

The aftercare instructions that should be given to the patient on the day of extraction and fitting are as follows:

- Leave the denture in place overnight, to protect all the extraction sockets from food debris and the loss of any blood clots

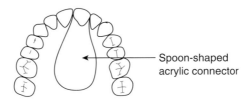

Figure 15.74 A spoon denture.

- Return to the surgery the following day, when the local anaesthetic has worn off and any high spots will be obvious – any adjustments necessary can then be carried out
- From then on, remove the denture after meals and carry out hot salt water mouthwashes to help heal the extraction sockets
- Return to the surgery when bone resorption has caused significant loss of retention, so that adjustments can be made or a permanent denture provided – this may take between 3 and 6 months to occur in some patients

Other removable prosthetic procedures

From time to time, other procedures may be carried out to existing removable prostheses to improve their fit or extend their period of wear, without having to resort to the construction of a new denture. These procedures are:

- Relines or rebases
- Additions of teeth or clasps
- Use of tissue conditioners as:
  - Soft linings
  - Functional impression materials

Relines and rebases

These may be required as alveolar bone resorption occurs beneath the denture with time, and the retentive fit is lost as a space develops beneath the fitting surface of the denture and it becomes loose. The bone lost during this natural process can be replaced with the addition of a new layer of acrylic within the fitting surface of the denture, as follows:

- The denture is thoroughly cleaned at the surgery, ensuring that no food debris is present
- The patient is asked to carry out a vigorous mouthwash at the surgery, and tooth brushing if necessary, to also remove any food debris from the mouth
- An accurate impression (**wash impression**) is taken within the denture itself, using an elastomer impression material
- Alternatively, an alginate impression is taken of the mouth itself (without the denture in place)
- The impression and the denture are sent to the technician
- The technician makes a cast within the denture, so that the alveolar bone is recorded where a wash impression has been taken, or casts a model of the arch from the alginate impression
- The wash impression is removed from the denture, and the space present between it and the model is filled with acrylic, or the denture is placed over the new model and the space between the two is filled with acrylic
- This creates a new base-fitting surface to the denture, which will then sit accurately against the oral soft tissues again and improve the retention of the denture

Additions

The addition of either a tooth or a clasp to an existing denture may be necessary from time to time, as the patient loses a natural tooth or the retention of the prosthesis deteriorates with time. The procedure is very straightforward and can often be completed by the technician within the day, as follows:

- An alginate impression is taken over the denture while in place in the mouth
- The impression and denture are sent to the technician
- The technician casts the model with the denture in situ
- The position of the denture is then accurately recorded on the model
- The denture can now be removed and repositioned exactly in place on the model, so that the new tooth or clasp can be fitted accurately to the existing denture, and will then fit perfectly into place when returned to the patient

Tissue conditioners

These are special materials used in two circumstances:

- As a **soft lining** when the soft tissues beneath the denture are continually sore, for whatever reason, so that the denture cannot be worn routinely without causing great discomfort to the patient
- As a **functional impression** material which sets over several hours and therefore records the soft tissues and denture extremities more accurately than conventional impression techniques

Persistent soreness beneath a denture is often a problem with elderly patients, and can cause medical problems as a result of their being unable to eat sufficiently well. The soft lining construction procedure is similar to that used to place a hard reline into a denture, in that an impression is taken inside it using an elastomer material, so that the technician can cast up a working model. The base of the denture is then cut out by the technician and replaced by a soft tissue conditioner which acts as a cushion between the alveolar ridge and the denture. When the patient bites with the revamped denture, the cushioning "bounces" and dissipates the occlusal force so that it is not transmitted to the alveolar ridge as pain and discomfort. The conditioner requires regular replacement every 12–18 months, though, as it deteriorates in saliva over time, gradually becoming hardened and losing its "bounce".

Functional impressions are required in complicated cases of removable prosthesis construction, where conventional impression techniques fail to record the oral anatomy in sufficient detail to produce an adequately retentive denture.

Normal impressions record the hard alveolar ridge and any standing teeth, with the soft tissues pushed out of the way and held stationary while the impression is setting. The real and natural situation in the mouth is one of continual movement and change. Recording this real situation in an impression requires a material that takes hours to set while the denture is being worn and used. The oldest functional impression material is black gutta-percha, but this has been superseded by modern materials that are a type of slow-curing acrylic resin, e.g. Visco-gel and Coe Comfort.

They usually consist of a powder and liquid, which are mixed together and applied to the fitting surface of the denture, reinserted into the patient's mouth and worn for up to 6 hours. The patient must take no food or drink during this time. When found to provide a comfortable and satisfactory fit, the denture and its incorporated impression are sent to the laboratory for the casting of a working model. The impression material is then removed and replaced with heat-cured acrylic, producing a well-fitting and functional prosthesis.

Obturators

These are a specialist removable prosthesis that will be provided to a patient via a hospital dental department, rather than from a general dental workplace.

They are appliances used to seal off an abnormal cavity in the maxilla, such as that due to a cleft palate or the space left after significant oral surgery for tumour or cyst removal. The abnormal cavity requires sealing off from the oral cavity to allow proper speech, as well as to prevent food and drink collecting in the maxilla. The denture area of the obturator is constructed in the usual way, but an elastomer material is also used to record the cavity accurately, before being incorporated into the denture design. As elastomers can record undercuts accurately, the impression material can be inserted into the cavity, allowed to set, then withdrawn without tearing and distorting.

Where large abnormal cavities require closing over, the extension area is made hollow so that the obturator is not too heavy to wear.

Overdentures

An overdenture is a full denture that is fitted on top of standing teeth or retained roots in the dental arch. The advantage of an overdenture is the presence of natural roots remaining in the alveolar bone. These have the effect of greatly reducing the absorption and shrinkage of alveolar ridges that normally occur after tooth extraction. When teeth are extracted, the alveolar bone becomes redundant, as it has lost its natural function of providing support for the teeth, and consequently diminishes in size as the bone resorbs. This loss of bone may be so great that it becomes very difficult to make a denture which is not perpetually loose, and lower dentures pose the most awkward problems in this respect.

As long as any roots remain, there is hardly any loss of alveolar bone and these problems of difficult lower dentures are far less common. However, dentures cannot be fitted directly on top of retained roots or teeth. In most cases, a certain amount of preparation of these abutment teeth is required to remove undercuts and prevent caries.

Retained roots are root-filled and ground to a dome shape level with the gum. If the root surface is irregular because of previous caries, the dome shape can be restored by fitting an appropriately shaped post crown. Teeth that still have intact crowns are usually treated by reducing the crown to a small tapered stump and fitting a full gold veneer thimble over the top. Having prepared the remaining teeth or roots, the overdenture is then made as a full denture in the usual way.

Overdentures are usually made as full dentures but they can be used as partial dentures in rare cases where some of the remaining teeth are unsuitable for the partial denture design. They may also be used for patients with cleft palates and for those who have undergone surgical removal of part of their jaw, as part of their treatment for oral cancer. In such cases, the alveolar ridges may be so misshapen that properly fitting conventional dentures cannot be made.

More recently, or where there are no remaining roots anyway, **dental implants** can be used to support an overdenture. These are covered later in the chapter.

Orthodontics

Orthodontic appliances share many common features with fixed and removable prosthodontics, especially in the materials used to construct and fit them. They are used to align (straighten) crooked teeth, so that the patient is able to carry out effective oral hygiene techniques and prevent caries or periodontal disease from developing.

Two basic types of appliance are used:

- **Fixed appliance** – composed of individual metal or ceramic components bonded onto each tooth and connected by an archwire; they cannot be removed from the mouth by the patient and are therefore similar to fixed prostheses
- **Removable appliance** – composed of an acrylic base with stainless steel clasps and springs, and able to be removed from the mouth for cleaning, eating and adjustment, these appliances are therefore similar to removable prostheses. Specialised removable appliances worn in both jaws together are called **functional appliances**

Greater and more complicated forces can be applied to the teeth using fixed appliances, and the range possible for both types of appliance is as follows:

- Movement of teeth forwards or backwards in each arch – removable and fixed
- Movement of jaws in relation to each other – functional and fixed
- Alignment of slightly misplaced teeth in arch – removable and fixed
- Alignment of severely misplaced teeth in arch – fixed
- Derotation of teeth – fixed
- Guided eruption of unerupted teeth – fixed
- Guided reduction of deep overbite – removable and fixed

Fixed orthodontic appliances

These consist of separate stainless steel or ceramic components called brackets that are individually bonded to each tooth, using an orthodontic light-cured resin material. Molar teeth often

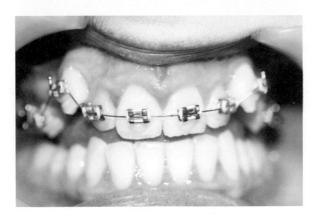

Figure 15.75 A fixed appliance – bonded arch with metal brackets.

have a circular metal device, called an orthodontic band, placed instead and these can be cemented with any type of luting cement.

The fitting procedure, called bonding, is carried out in the surgery with no laboratory input required except to cast up the preoperative and postoperative study models required. A bonded arch using metal brackets is shown in Figure 15.75. Bonding of the components causes no tooth damage and they are harmlessly "snapped off" at the end of the treatment, using special orthodontic instruments.

The equipment and instruments required for the monitoring and adjustment of the fixed appliance once it has been initially bonded are shown in the following table.

Item	Function
Archwire (see Figure 9.23)	Flexible nickel titanium or stainless steel wires, to fasten into the brackets or bands
End cutters	Right-angled cutters to trim the ends of the archwire after replacement
Alastiks	Rubber bands to hold the archwire into the slots of each bracket
Alastik holders	Ratcheted holders (similar to artery forceps) to apply the alastiks to the brackets
Brackets (see Figure 9.23)	Metal or ceramic components to attach to each tooth, if any have been lost since last appointment
Bands (see Figure 9.23)	Metal rings to attach to molars, in particular, although bands are available for all teeth and were the only attachments available before brackets were developed
Bracket holders	To hold and position each bracket to the centre of the tooth, if any replacements are required
Bracket and band removers (see Figure 9.24)	To remove brackets, bands and any residual bond material before replacing, if necessary
Bonding materials	Acid etch and orthodontic resin bond material, to hold brackets onto the tooth
Band cement	Any luting cement material, to hold bands onto the molar teeth

Patient advice for fixed appliances

Every tooth is incorporated into a fixed appliance, so the number of stagnation areas, and the potential for oral damage to occur, is far greater than for individual fixed prostheses. Routine twice-daily tooth brushing alone is insufficient to maintain adequate standards of good oral hygiene, and special instructions and techniques are recommended for patients undergoing fixed orthodontic therapy:

- Careful manual tooth brushing should be carried out after each meal
- Good-quality electric toothbrushes, such as Sonicare and Oral B, may be safely used instead
- Use of fluoridated toothpaste
- Daily use of **interdental brushes** to clean around each bracket individually
- Avoidance of cariogenic and acidic food and drinks for the full period of treatment
- Avoidance of sticky foods for the full period of treatment
- Use of **fluoride mouthwash** daily to minimise the risk of decalcification
- Regular use of **disclosing tablets** to highlight problematic areas where plaque is being retained, in order to minimise the risk of decalcification

Removable orthodontic appliances

These are similar to dentures in construction, in that alginate impressions of both arches and a wax bite registration are taken and sent to the laboratory, along with a work ticket detailing the exact design of appliance required. Usually, the technician involved in the appliance construction is one who specialises in orthodontic devices, as various of the components used are specific to this dental discipline and are not used with other prostheses.

A set of both study models and working models are cast from the impressions, and the latter set are used to construct the acrylic bases for each appliance, or just one appliance if treatment is being carried out in one arch only. The additional components that can then be added to the acrylic base are as follows:

- **Adams cribs** to retain the appliance in the mouth, usually to fit on to molar or premolar teeth and made of stainless steel (see Figure 13.15)
- **Springs** in a variety of designs, to move the teeth along the arch as required (see Figure 13.16)
- **Retractors** to push one or several teeth backwards (see Figure 13.17)
- **Expansion screws** to move several teeth or each half of the upper arch outwards

The equipment and instruments required for the monitoring and adjusting of the appliance are shown in the following table.

Item	Function
Adams crib pliers (see Figure 9.21)	To adjust all metal springs and retractors, as necessary
Straight handpiece and acrylic trimming bur (see Figure 9.22)	To adjust all acrylic areas of the appliance, as necessary
Measuring ruler	To record any measurable tooth movement, such as the overjet
Expansion screw key	To count the number of turns applied to the screw between visits, to ensure compliance by the patient

Patient advice for removable appliances

As with removable prostheses, orthodontic appliances are capable of acting as stagnation areas and holding food debris and plaque against the teeth and gingivae, unless a good standard of oral hygiene is maintained.

Although some dentists prefer patients to wear appliances during meals, it is possible that more acrylic breakages will occur if this is the case. The instructions necessary for patients wearing removable appliances are as follows:

- Wear as directed by the dentist
- Clean the appliance and teeth after each meal, using a toothbrush and toothpaste
- Avoid cariogenic and acidic foods and drinks, as advised
- Attend all dental appointments for the necessary adjustments
- Contact the surgery immediately if there are any breakages or if the appliance is lost
- Expect the appliance to feel tight initially after each adjustment
- Contact the surgery if there are any prolonged or excessive symptoms
- If the appliance is to be removed for meals, ensure it is placed safely in a rigid container to avoid breakages during mealtimes

Functional appliances

543

These are a specialised type of removable orthodontic appliance made of acrylic and stainless steel components, and worn in both arches at the same time, the commonest one currently being a "**Twinblock**" (see Figure 13.18)

They are used to correct skeletal class II discrepancies, where the mandible is further back from the ideal position, and work by holding the mandible forwards in the ideal class I position and allowing mandibular growth to occur and correct the malocclusion naturally. As their success depends on the growth of the mandible, they can only be used while the patient is still growing but after the premolars have erupted (these teeth are required for retention of the appliance), so the ideal age is up to 14 years.

The materials, instruments and patient advice are as for removable orthodontic appliances.

Dental implants

The use of dental implants over the last 20 years or so has seen the development of a technique for improving the life and masticatory efficiency of many patients. Previously, when a tooth had to be extracted, it could only be replaced by a denture or a bridge. Both these techniques have their own advantages and disadvantages, as discussed earlier in the chapter, but the main disadvantages of each are summarised here as a reminder:

- **Dentures** – poor retention, making chewing and successful wear very difficult
- **Bridges** – permanent loss of tooth tissue while preparing abutment teeth, and overloading of remaining teeth causing the eventual failure of the bridge

The development and use of dental implants as an alternative to the replacement of missing teeth has helped to overcome these disadvantages.

An implant is effectively a titanium double-screw cylinder that is inserted into a hole drilled into the alveolar bone of either jaw to replace one or several teeth. Unlike when posts are cemented into tooth roots when placing post crowns, the implant is not "glued" into place – instead, the alveolar bone gradually grows around it and into its hollow screw structure so that it is eventually locked into the bone itself. This is called **osseointegration** and takes several months to occur.

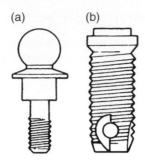

Figure 15.76   Dental implant components: (a) ball abutment for overdenture; (b) implant fixture.

Once the implant is firm within the bone structure, the top section can have the tooth replacement screwed onto it – this can be any of the following devices:

- Single crown tooth
- Multiple crowns to form a bridge
- Metal bar to act as a locking device beneath a denture
- Metal ball to act as a locking device beneath a denture (Figure 15.76)

The successful use of implants depends on many factors, as follows:

- **Bone** – there must be a deep enough section of alveolar bone into which to screw the implant, without it damaging other structures such as dental nerves or the maxillary antrum (although techniques are being developed to replace bone using synthetic alternatives, and an operation can be performed to "raise" the floor of the antrum to provide more space)
- **Patient selection** – not all patients will be suitable for such an extensive surgical procedure; some medical conditions may also contraindicate the use of implants (e.g. osteoporosis, haemophilia, diabetes due to poor wound healing)
- **Oral health** – patients with poor oral health are unsuitable for implants, as their success depends very much on being kept clean of dental plaque. The presence of plaque allows periodontal disease to develop around the implant, and the resultant pocketing will allow the titanium cylinder to become loose and the implant will fail – this condition is called **perimplantitis**
- **Lifestyle factors** – factors such as smoking and poor dental attendance may lead to failure of an implant in the same way that they are associated with higher levels of dental disease (especially periodontal disease) in dentate patients without implants

Implant and prosthesis placement procedures

- A team consisting of an implantologist, a specialist technician, and a hygienist examine and assess the patient, helped by study models, radiographs or even three-dimensional computer scans
- They can then plan the preparation, construction and maintenance of an implant procedure for the patient
- Depending on where the placement procedure is carried out, local anaesthetic (with or without conscious sedation) or general anaesthetic is given to the patient
- The oral surgery procedure of inserting the titanium implants into the alveolar bone is carried out under the usual surgical conditions as other minor oral surgery procedures (see the next section)

- A mucoperiosteal flap is raised to expose the bone, and special low-speed drills are used to prepare holes for the implants, or the extraction socket of the tooth itself is used and prepared in a similar fashion
- The implants are screwed into the prepared holes and the tissue flap is then sutured back into place to completely bury the implant (Figure 15.77)
- After a suitable time period, which can be up to several months long, the implants become firmly embedded in the bone by osseointegration, and the prosthesis can be placed
- Under local anaesthetic, a small incision is made in the overlying gingiva to expose the top of each implant, and the artificial abutments are then screwed into the inner surface of the implants
- Abutments may be in the form of stumps for fitting single crowns or bridge pontics (Figure 15.78), or a ball or bar for clipping on a removable overdenture

Obviously, the successful placement of implants in dentistry depends on the surgical skill of the dentist or oral surgeon involved. The training available ranges from weekend courses, to module type diplomas, to full surgical speciality and qualification. The more complicated cases should only ever be handled by those with an adequate training in the more complicated techniques or by specialist implantologists.

In addition, the laboratory stages of the top section of the appliance have to be carried out by specialist technicians, although the chairside preparation stage is no different from that for a conventional crown or bridge preparation. The use of denture locking devices requires special impression techniques to be employed.

The need for specialist training in dental implants, in addition to all the equipment required, means that implants are very expensive to place. The simplest case of a single tooth implant

545

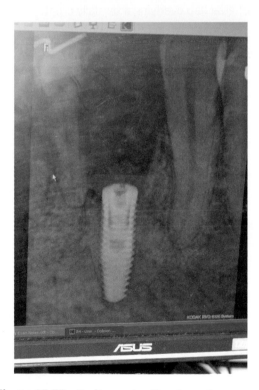

Figure 15.77   Radiograph of implant placement.

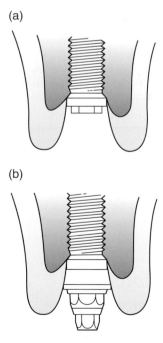

Figure 15.78   An implant procedure: (a) stage 1 – implant fixture in bone; (b) stage 2 – crown or bridge abutment fitted.

is usually in the region of £1500–£2000, and the more complicated cases will run into tens of thousands of pounds each. Their only availability on the NHS is as teaching cases in dental hospitals.

However, their use is on the increase as they provide successful dental treatment options to patients who were previously untreatable, as well as offering less invasive techniques in simpler cases, such as single tooth replacements. Training courses are currently being developed for qualified dental nurses to undertake, so that they are able to assist in specialist implant clinics and hospital departments.

In the meantime, dental nurses have an important role in helping to provide oral hygiene instruction and reinforcement for implant patients, similarly to that given for crowns, dentures and bridges.

Extractions and minor oral surgery

Many procedures carried out daily in the vast majority of dental workplaces can be collectively termed as "minor oral surgery" (MOS), as opposed to major oral surgery procedures such as treatment and reconstructive surgery for oral cancer, orthognathic surgery to correct skeletal problems, and head and neck trauma surgery. The most frequent minor surgical procedures carried out are the following:

- **Simple extractions** – of roots or whole teeth, where no soft tissue or bone removal is required
- **Surgical extractions** – of roots or whole teeth, where soft tissue, alone or with bone, has to be removed to gain access to the root or tooth
- **Operculectomy** – the surgical removal of the gingival flap overlying a partially erupted tooth, especially a lower third molar
- **Alveolectomy** – the surgical adjustment and removal of bone spicules from the alveolar ridge after tooth extraction, to produce a smooth base for denture seating (see earlier)
- **Gingivectomy and gingivoplasty** – periodontal soft tissue surgery to adjust the shape of the gingivae to aid oral hygiene measures (see earlier)
- **Periodontal flap surgery** – the surgical raising and replacing of surgical flaps to enable sub-gingival debridement to be carried out (see earlier)
- **Soft tissue biopsies** – the partial or complete removal of soft tissue oral lesions for pathological investigation and diagnosis

Arguably, these surgical procedures are among those most worrying to the patient, as bleeding and possible postoperative pain are quite likely to occur. The dental nurse has a very important role in the reassurance and monitoring of the patient during these procedures, so that the patient remains less anxious and cooperative throughout.

As always, health and safety and infection control procedures must be strictly adhered to before, during and after the surgical procedure.

Extractions

These procedures involve the removal of teeth, or their roots if the crown of the tooth has disintegrated, to leave a section of the alveolar ridge bare and ready for tooth replacement by:

- The pontic of a bridge
- A denture
- An implant

Reasons for tooth extraction

Both deciduous and permanent teeth may require extraction at some point. This is usually due to infection and pain being present following caries, periodontal disease or trauma, but may also be for the following reasons:

- The tooth is unrestorable, whether pain and infection are present or not
- The position of the tooth prevents the placement of a fixed or removable prosthesis
- The tooth is too poorly positioned to be aligned orthodontically
- The tooth may be selectively extracted to provide space in a crowded dental arch
- Attempts to save the tooth by root filling have failed
- The tooth may be partially erupted and impacted, and suffer from recurrent painful infections (pericoronitis) due to trapping of food
- Deciduous teeth can be selectively extracted to encourage the timely eruption of their permanent successors into more favourable positions
- The patient's choice, where attempting to save the tooth by root filling is not the preferred option

To ensure that any tooth is extracted painlessly and successfully, the dentist has an in-depth knowledge of the anatomy and physiology of the head and neck region, as well as the oral cavity and its nerve supply. An efficient and supportive dental nurse must also have a background knowledge of these subjects to be able to provide the level of preparation, chairside support and help required during any likely complication that may arise.

When the dentist has no choice and decides that a tooth has to be extracted, it will be for one or more of the following reasons:

- Unless successful treatment to save it can be carried out, as a carious or periodontally involved tooth is a continual source of infection in the patient's oral cavity
- Any infection may be intermittent, but often there are acute and very painful episodes that may require analgesic and antibiotic treatment
- Infection can spread into the bloodstream (**bacteraemia**) and the patient can become generally unwell – this can be a serious event in elderly and medically compromised patients
- Repeat prescriptions of antibiotics to treat infection without tooth removal are considered poor practice
- No replacement of the tooth can be carried out to restore oral health until the tooth has been extracted

Once it has been determined that a tooth or root requires extraction, the complexity of the procedure depends mainly on which tooth is involved, how much tooth or root is present, and its position in the jaw bone. The options available for the extraction procedure will then fall into one of the following categories:

- Simple extraction
- Surgical extraction involving soft tissue removal to expose an unerupted tooth or buried root
- Surgical extraction involving dissection of the tooth in its socket and removal in sections
- Surgical extraction involving the raising of a mucoperiosteal flap and bone removal to gain full access to a tooth or root

If the tooth involved is a deciduous one, the following points need to be considered:

- **Resorption** – has root resorption occurred so that effectively just the crown of the tooth remains, attached merely to the gingivae?
- **Permanent successor** – is the underlying permanent tooth present and likely to be damaged during the extraction procedure?

- **Infection** – is any dental infection present that may make the procedure unnecessarily painful?
- **Age and cooperation** – younger patients are usually less willing to undergo extraction procedures than older patients, and along with some of those with special needs are less able to understand the need for the procedure and the consequences if it is not carried out
- **Medical history of the patient** – some medical conditions contraindicate extraction
- **Tooth status** – a grossly carious deciduous tooth may be difficult to extract simply and quickly, but a surgical procedure is not usually feasible in conscious younger patients, so some form of anxiety control will have to be considered

If the tooth involved is a permanent one, the following points need to be considered:

- **Infection** – is any dental infection present that may make the procedure unnecessarily painful?
- **Medical history of the patient** – some medical conditions contraindicate extraction
- **Medications** – some adult medications will mean hospitalisation for extractions or MOS, because of possible serious side-effects
- **Cooperation** – some adults and some patients with special needs will require some form of anxiety control to undergo these types of procedure
- **Age** – older patients have more friable soft tissues, which are more easily traumatised during surgical procedures, and their jaw bones will be more brittle and more easily fractured
- **Tooth status** – a grossly carious tooth is more likely to require a full surgical procedure to complete its removal
- **Post-extraction** – will the missing tooth require replacement, and if so what are the options and cost implications?

Simple extractions

Simple extractions are so called because the tooth or root is removed whole from the dental arch without involving tooth sectioning, flap raising or bone removal. Any or all of these additional techniques may be required during a surgical extraction. Whether the tooth is still vital or has died from any associated infection, local anaesthesia will always be required to numb the surrounding gingivae at least, even for a simple extraction.

The specific instruments, equipment and medicaments that may be required for a simple extraction are shown in the following table.

Item	Function
Forceps	Range of sterile hand instruments used to grip a tooth or root at its neck before applying appropriate wrist actions to loosen the tooth/root in its socket during the extraction procedure. Various designs are available for use on upper or lower teeth, and for each individual tooth
Luxators	Sterile hand instruments used to widen the socket and sever the periodontal ligament attachment
Elevators	Sterile hand instruments used to prise the tooth/root out of the socket. Various patterns are available – Cryer's, Warwick James' and Winter's elevators (see later)
Fine-bore aspirator	Disposable suction tip used to suck away all blood and maintain good moisture control during the procedure – also useful for sucking and holding tooth debris so that it can be removed from the mouth safely
Haemostats	Gelatine sponges or oxidised cellulose packs, which are inserted into the socket after extraction to aid blood clotting and achieve haemostasis – can be used with or without a suture

548

Forceps are the instruments most frequently used to extract a tooth and are handled by being pushed along the sides of the root to sever the periodontal membrane. Once a reasonable position has been achieved, the root is gripped and gentle wrist movements are employed to gradually loosen the tooth in the socket. The forceps are gradually worked further towards the apex of the tooth until it is loose enough in the socket to be removed. In effect, then, a tooth is actually extracted by being **pushed out** of the socket, rather than being pulled out of it, as most people would assume.

Unnecessary force during extractions often results in tooth or root fracture, although this can also occur anyway with grossly carious or root-filled teeth.

Forceps are designed in various patterns, to be used individually for each type of tooth. Upper tooth forceps tend to have their handles and blades roughly in line with each other, whereas lower tooth forceps tend to be at right angles to each other for ease of access to the lower arch (Figure 15.79).

Multi-rooted molar tooth forceps have blades, which are shaped as beaks so that they can grip the **furcation** area between the roots, but single-rooted tooth forceps are smooth (Figure 15.80).

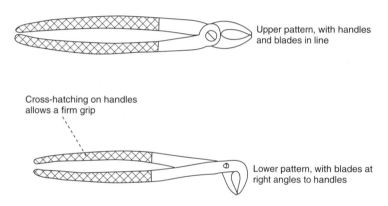

Figure 15.79   Upper and lower patterns of forceps.

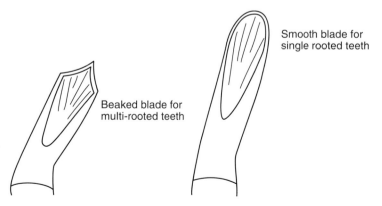

Figure 15.80   Blade details of forceps. Source: *Levison's Textbook for Dental Nurses*, 11th edition (Hollins), 2013. Reproduced with permission of Wiley-Blackwell.

The commonest patterns of forceps used are shown in Figure 11.3. They are as follows:

- **Upper incisor and canine forceps** are straight with single, rounded blades and have both wide and narrow patterns
- **Upper root forceps** are similar in appearance, with narrow, straight blades
- **Upper premolar forceps** have slightly curved handles and single, rounded blades
- **Upper left molar forceps** have curved handles and a beaked blade to the right of the instrument, and a rounded blade to the left to grip the buccal roots and the palatal root, respectively (many dental nurses identify upper molar forceps by the mantra "beak to cheek")
- **Upper right molar forceps** have curved handles and the beaked blade is to the left of the instrument
- **Upper bayonet forceps** have extended handles and angled blades to gain access to third molars, or have angled pointed blades to gain access to fractured roots
- **Lower anterior forceps** have single, rounded blades at right angles to the handle that are particularly useful for extracting lower premolars
- **Lower root forceps** are similar, with narrow and straight blades that are also particularly useful for extracting small or crowded incisors
- **Lower molar forceps** have beaked blades at right angles to the handles, to grip the furcation of the two roots
- **Lower "cowhorn" forceps** have curved and pointed blades at right angles to the handles, to grip the furcation of lower molar teeth
- **Smaller versions** of most patterns exist for deciduous tooth extractions

Similarly, elevators are available in a variety of patterns and are used to gradually sever the periodontal membrane and loosen the tooth in the socket (see Figure 11.5). They are specifically used to elevate retained roots and impacted teeth, where adequate access to the root or tooth is not possible with conventional forceps, or where the angle of elevation required to loosen the root or tooth is not possible with forceps.

The more common types are as follows:

- **Cryer's elevators** – available as left and right patterns, but can be used on either side of the mouth, depending whether they are engaged mesially or distally; the tips are triangular shaped and pointed
- **Winter's elevators** – have a similar blade design as Cryer's, but have a corkscrew style handle to give more leverage
- **Warwick James' elevators** – available as left, right and straight patterns; the tips are of a similar shape to the round blade of forceps

Alternatively, the dentist may choose to use one of a variety of **luxators** (see Figure 11.4) that are available and are used in a similar fashion to an elevator but with greater effect, as the tips are sharper and finer and therefore more easily pushed into the periodontal space between the root and the bony socket. It is possible to extract practically any tooth using a luxator alone, and many dentists are able to do so.

A single-bladed chisel is also available for splitting multi-rooted teeth; this is called a **Coupland chisel** and is available in sizes 1, 2 and 3 (see Figure 11.7).

Once the tooth has been extracted the patient is supervised while haemostasis is achieved, usually by biting on a bite pack (see Figure 11.1).

Preoperative and postoperative instructions

Often, patients will request information regarding the procedure itself in advance, and the dental nurse is ideally suited to allay their fears by giving advice beforehand as follows:

- Local anaesthesia will always be necessary for an extraction
- The procedure will not be painful, as adequate local anaesthesia will be given

- If a surgical procedure is being undertaken, sutures will be necessary
- The patient must take all medication as normal before the procedure unless the dentist informs them otherwise, except for aspirin, which prevents blood clotting and could cause postoperative bleeding – the patient must therefore avoid taking aspirin the day before and on the day of the procedure
- The patient must have a light snack 2 hours before the procedure to avoid fainting
- Full postoperative instructions will be given in writing, so the patient does not have to remember them
- If the patient is a nervous adult or child, they should be escorted by a reassuring and competent adult

Similarly, after the procedure, a full list of postoperative instructions should be given verbally and in writing (Figure 11.19). It is important that the patient understands that most postoperative complications occur because of disturbance to the blood clot which forms in the area, and that they should avoid this happening wherever possible. Postoperative instructions should include the following points:

- Pain, swelling or bruising may occur after the procedure
- Analgesics (**except aspirin**) may be taken as required
- Alcohol, hot drinks and exercise should be avoided for 24 hours after the procedure
- No mouth rinsing should be carried out on the day of the procedure
- Hot salt water mouthwashes should be carried out after each meal, from the day after the procedure for up to 1 week
- If bleeding does occur, bite onto a cotton pack for up to 30 minutes
- Give an emergency telephone number for care and advice if problems occur
- Give details of further appointments if necessary, including suture removal

Surgical extractions

Under certain circumstances, a simple extraction cannot be carried out to remove a tooth, and either soft tissue alone or soft tissue and alveolar bone must be removed so that the dentist can gain access to a tooth or root. These procedures are referred to as surgical extractions and may be necessary for any of the following reasons:

- When previous attempts at tooth extraction have left a significant section of retained root in the alveolar bone – very small apical sections are often left in situ, as they cause no problems and sometimes rise naturally to the surface of the alveolar bone some time later, when they can be simply extracted without having to carry out any bone removal to do so
- When a tooth is so grossly carious that attempts at simple extraction are impossible, as the tooth is too rotten to be held by forceps
- When the morphology of the roots makes it unlikely that the whole tooth can be removed simply, especially when the roots are curved so that the tooth cannot be pushed out of the socket in one direction alone
- When the tooth is only partially erupted and impacted, so that full eruption cannot occur and the tooth becomes a stagnation area
- When the tooth is unerupted and has associated pathology, such as a cyst
- When the tooth is unerupted and likely to cause future problems with either prostheses or orthodontic treatment
- When a deciduous tooth has failed to exfoliate because the root has become cemented to the alveolar bone and natural exfoliation cannot occur – the tooth is said to be ankylosed

551

Consequently, surgical extractions will fall into one of the following categories:

- Extraction involving tooth sectioning
- Extraction involving the raising of a mucoperiosteal flap

The preoperative and postoperative instructions given to the patient have been outlined earlier (see previous section). What differs from simple extractions is the list of instruments that may be necessary to allow the dentist to gain access to the tooth or root.

Extraction involving tooth sectioning

Tooth sectioning is effectively a variation on the simple extraction technique for multi-rooted teeth that cannot be extracted whole. This is often due to unfavourable root curvature or gross root caries that prevents a simple forceps removal of the roots. The dentist can cut the tooth into a number of sections equal to the number of roots present, and then effectively extract each one as a separate root in the usual way, using forceps, elevators or luxators.

Sometimes, it may be necessary to remove some of the septal bone that lies between the roots and forms the individual socket walls. The only differences in the tooth sectioning technique from that of simple extractions are as follows:

- Use of high-speed turbine and a suitable diamond bur (usually a crown preparation bur, for their greater length) to cut the tooth into sections down towards the furcation area
- Use of a Coupland chisel to achieve the final separation of the roots, by inserting the chisel into the drilled slot between the tooth sections and twisting to snap them apart
- Use of a surgical handpiece and bone burs to remove any septal bone
- Use of high-speed suction to remove the water coolant of the handpieces
- Careful retraction and protection of the patient's soft tissues during the cutting and sectioning procedures

Extractions involving mucoperiosteal flaps

There are certain cases when successful extraction cannot be carried out without gaining full access to a tooth or root by raising a mucoperiosteal flap, as follows:

- Unerupted or impacted tooth
- Buried retained root
- Root curvature is excessive and requires extensive bone removal
- Gross root caries prevents adequate instrumentation to extract the tooth in any other way

Teeth lie in sockets of alveolar bone, with a covering of mucoperiosteum over the bone which runs into the gingivae around each tooth (see Chapter 13). The mucoperiosteum is tightly held onto the bone and has to be cut and separated to its full thickness before bone removal can be carried out – this is the **mucoperiosteal flap**.

The flap thus raised has to have a wide base to ensure a good blood supply, so that full healing occurs once the procedure has been completed. It then has to be sutured accurately back into place for long enough so that reattachment can occur.

This is a full surgical technique, so all of the surgery and instrument preparation applies as described for simple extractions, but far more specific surgical instruments are required. These are detailed in the following table.

The principle of the sterile field and the maintenance of thorough infection control are of great importance in preventing any contamination complications during the procedure. Depending on the patient, those with a compromised medical history may require the surgical procedure to be carried out in a hospital or dental clinic environment.

Surgical instruments for flap procedures

Item	Function
Scalpel blade and handle (see Figure 11.8)	To make the initial incision through the full-thickness mucoperiosteum and around the necks of the teeth to create the flap
Osteotrimmer (see Figure 11.9)	To raise the corners of the flap off the underlying alveolar bone
Periosteal elevator (see Figure 11.10)	To complete the elevation of the flap off the bone, by pushing the instrument over the bone surface beneath the flap and effectively peeling it off the bone
Handpiece and surgical burs	To remove any alveolar bone necessary to gain access to the tooth or root
Irrigation syringe	To irrigate the surgical field with sterile saline or sterile water, although the handpiece often has its own irrigation supply from the bracket table bottle
Austin and Kilner retractors	To protect and retract cheeks, lips and tongue from the surgical field, providing clear access for the dentist
Rake retractor	To retract the mucoperiosteal flap itself
Bone rongeurs	To nibble away bony spicules and produce a smooth bone surface for healing
Dissecting forceps (see Figure 11.11)	To hold the loose flap edges taut during suturing
Needle holders (see Figure 11.12)	To hold the pre-threaded needle firmly while suturing
Suture pack (see Figure 11.13)	Half-moon needle, pre-threaded with either black braided silk or a resorbable suture material such as vicryl, to suture the flap back into position over the alveolar bone
Suture scissors (see Figure 11.14)	To cut the suture ends after each stitch

Again, full verbal and written postoperative instructions are given before the patient is discharged, and then the surgery is decontaminated. While the records are being written, the number of sutures used is specifically recorded so that all can be accounted for, if they are of the non-resorbable type, at the suture removal appointment.

Tooth impaction

The most usual teeth to become impacted are the lower third molars, or "wisdom" teeth. These are the last permanent teeth to erupt and are often short of space to do so. The type of impaction that occurs will affect the difficulty of the removal of the tooth, as follows:

- **Vertical impaction** – the tooth is upright but impacted into the ramus of the mandible
- **Horizontal impaction** – the tooth is lying on its side, facing forwards, backwards or across the dental ridge
- **Mesioangular impaction** – the tooth is tilted forwards into the second molar tooth (Figure 15.81)
- **Distoangular impaction** – the tooth is tilted backwards into the ramus of the mandible

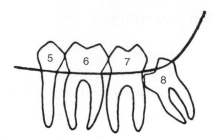

Figure 15.81   Mesioangular impaction.

Some dentists will refer patients with the more difficult types of impaction to a specialist oral sur-geon for extraction, if the teeth are persistently infected or are causing trapping of food and caries in adjacent teeth. However, if the impacted tooth is causing no problems (i.e. it is **asymptomatic**) then it is usual for it to be left in situ rather than extracted, as there are risks involved in having the tooth surgically extracted, as follows:

- Extensive bone removal can weaken the mandible
- Postoperative pain and swelling are very likely to occur after a full surgical procedure
- The inferior dental nerve and lingual nerve lie close to the operation site, and temporary or even permanent damage can occur to them if they become traumatised or severed during the surgical procedure
- Limited mouth opening (**trismus**) can occur temporarily after surgery, and this will make eating and talking difficult

Patients must be warned of all these possible complications before undergoing the surgical extraction procedure.

Complications of extractions

Complications that may occur during extraction are damage to adjacent nerves, fracture of the tooth, perforation of the maxillary sinus and loss of a tooth. Complications that may occur after extraction are bleeding and infection of the bony socket.

Some complications can be highlighted as potential risks that may occur during the extraction procedure, the commonest one being the possibility of damage to one of the trigeminal nerve branches during the procedure. This risk can be identified by good preoperative dental radiog-raphy and accurate planning of the procedure beforehand. Where there is a potential for nerve damage, such as when the roots of lower molars lie very close to the inferior dental nerve, the patient should be referred to a specialist for the procedure and warned of the possibility of it happening beforehand, so that informed consent may be given.

Similarly, those medically compromised patients with conditions that may cause problems dur-ing extractions (such as haemophiliacs) should also be referred to specialist clinics or hospitals for treatment. Of the other possible complications described that may occur during the extraction, reasons for their occurrence are as follows:

- Unexpected tooth fracture – especially if the tooth is heavily filled or root-filled; this may result in a simple extraction becoming a more complicated one
- Oral-antral fistulas – due to a perforation of the maxillary sinus, this can occur while extracting the upper premolar or molar teeth, as the maxillary sinus lies over their roots and is often only separated by a membrane, so perforation of the sinus is a real possibility in some cases
- Loss of the tooth – either into the respiratory or digestive tracts, or out of the mouth, and due to it slipping out of the dentist's grip while pushing the tooth out of the socket or lifting it out of the mouth

554

Reasons for the occurrence of those complications after the patient has left the surgery are as follows:

- Bleeding – either within hours of the extraction (**reactionary haemorrhage**) due to the blood clot being disturbed and reopening torn blood vessels, or after 24 hours (**secondary haemorrhage**) due to an infection developing at the surgical site
- Infection – between 2 and 4 days after the procedure and following loss of the blood clot from the socket, the bony socket walls become infected; this condition is called **localised osteitis** (dry socket)

Tooth fracture

A grossly carious or heavily filled tooth is likely to fracture during extraction attempts, and the dentist should be aware of the possibility and warn the patient regarding progression to a surgical procedure if necessary. This particular progression is likely to occur when the tooth fracture extends subgingivally, as adequate access to the roots may then be difficult without bone removal. Alternatively, root fracture may occur during extraction, especially where the roots are fine or curved, and then require a surgical procedure to remove them.

However, if small apical pieces of root fracture off during extraction, they can be left in situ, either to rise to the alveolar ridge surface themselves over time and be more easily removed, or to remain buried and cause no further problems.

Whichever occurs, the patient must always be informed and a full explanation given.

555

Oro-antral fistula

This is a complication of the extraction of upper premolar and molar teeth only, as the maxillary sinus lies over and between their roots. An inappropriate extraction technique can sometimes push the root into the sinus, where it will act as a foreign body and cause infection. The patient is best referred to a specialist oral surgeon for its removal.

Long-rooted upper molar and premolar teeth sometimes impinge into the sinus naturally, and when they are extracted, an opening will be created between the antrum and the oral cavity. This is called an oro-antral fistula, and if small it will close naturally within a week, although patients should be instructed not to blow their nose during this healing period. Indeed, the presence of a fistula can be confirmed by the appearance of air bubbles in the socket when a patient pinches the nose and blows.

Large openings require surgical repair either by direct suturing or by raising a gingival flap off the palate and swinging it across to seal the fistula.

Loss of the tooth

The tooth can be dropped during its removal from the mouth, or the force exerted during extraction can cause it to dislodge rapidly from the socket before a firm grip has been achieved with the forceps.

If the tooth is swallowed, it poses no problem and should be allowed to pass naturally. However, if the tooth is likely to have been inhaled (especially likely if the patient has a coughing fit as the tooth disappears), the patient should be sent to hospital immediately for chest and abdominal radiographs to locate the tooth, as it could cause a serious respiratory infection. It may be removed using a bronchoscope if lodged in the main bronchi, but if the tooth has descended further into the respiratory tract, thoracic surgery may be necessary to remove it.

Bleeding

Haemorrhage during extraction is a natural occurrence, as blood vessels in the periodontium are torn during the procedure. This usually stops within 5 minutes of completion of the extraction with the use of a bite pack, and is called **primary haemorrhage**.

When there is no history of previous haemorrhage, sutures may still be required if excessive bleeding occurs. This may even be carried out in elderly patients and those with hypertension as a precautionary measure. In all cases, however, the patient must not be dismissed from the premises until bleeding has ceased.

The blood clots in the following way:

- Torn blood vessels constrict to slow the blood flow
- **Platelets** circulating in the blood are exposed to air at the wound site
- This causes them to become sticky and clump together
- Two complicated **clotting mechanisms** ensue, resulting in the protein fibrinogen being converted to fibrin
- **Fibrin** chemically seals the cut vessels, and the haemorrhage ends

Bleeding that occurs several hours after the extraction is called **reactionary haemorrhage** and is usually caused by the patient not following the postoperative instructions accurately and disturbing the blood clot, either by using a mouthwash or taking alcohol or exercise.

In healthy patients, it is easily controlled by reapplication of pressure to the socket, reiteration of the postoperative instructions or suturing of the socket to compress the wound edges and promote clotting again, possibly also with the insertion of a haemostatic sponge.

An additional cause of primary haemorrhage is failure of the blood-clotting process so that uncontrolled bleeding occurs. This is an uncommon but very serious matter, occurring in patients taking anticoagulant drugs and those with liver disease, and with some rare blood diseases such as haemophilia. Patients with such conditions should have been identified by the completion of a thorough medical history beforehand, or they may carry a warning card for presentation to any practitioner they attend. In particular, patients with certain heart conditions may be prescribed the anticoagulant drug **warfarin.** The effectiveness of their blood clotting will be regularly monitored by undergoing a blood test to determine their international normalised ratio score (**INR score**), which will indicate whether extractions can be safely carried out in dental practice or whether the patient will require a hospital referral. Current practice is for patients with an INR score > 4 to be treated in hospital for surgical procedures, including extractions.

Patients taking aspirin to prevent a stroke should be treated carefully when undergoing surgical procedures in the practice. The use of a haemostatic sponge and suture may be required as a matter of routine to avoid complications.

The third type of bleeding complication is **secondary haemorrhage**, where the blood clot is lost early and the socket subsequently becomes infected, with breakdown of the healing mechanism. This occurs after 24 hours of the extraction being carried out. Cleansing of the socket, then pressure and the insertion of a haemostatic sponge should solve the problem.

Infection

The condition of infection of the extraction socket is called localised osteitis (dry socket); it is a very painful condition which develops 2–3 days after extraction. It is an acute inflammation of the bone (osteitis) lining the socket and is caused by a microbial invasion. The natural protective barrier against such an invasion is the blood clot that fills the socket immediately after an extraction, so anything that prevents formation of an adequate blood clot can give rise to a dry socket – for example:

- Infection of the blood clot
- Failure of formation of a blood clot
- Disturbance of the blood clot

Infection of the blood clot may occur in neglected mouths where gingival or periodontal infection is already present, and is also particularly likely to occur in patients who smoke. Hordes of microorganisms invade the socket, overwhelm the defending white cells, disintegrate the blood clot and set up an acute inflammation of the unprotected bare bone of the socket. Pre-extraction scaling of the teeth reduces gingival infection and may prevent a dry socket. Alternatively, application of chlorhexidine to the gingival crevice just before extraction helps to reduce the risk of infection.

Failure to form a blood clot may occur in difficult extractions, as pressure on the bone during such an extraction crushes the blood vessels and results in insufficient bleeding to produce a protective blood clot. It is more common in the mandible than in the maxilla as the former has a thicker layer of compact bone.

Disturbance of the blood clot is caused by too much mouthwashing soon after extraction, or by the patient poking and fiddling at the extraction socket, especially with dirty fingers. This breaks away the blood clot and leaves the socket bare, allowing microorganisms to be introduced to the immediate vicinity.

To treat the condition, any food debris or necrotic clot tissue is removed with gentle irrigation and the use of tweezers, and then a sedative dressing (such as Alvogyl) is carefully placed in the socket. The pain experienced by the patient can be relieved with the usual anti-inflammatory analgesics, and it is best if the postoperative instructions are reiterated, in particular the use of hot salt water mouthwashes.

Accidental extraction

This is the term used to describe the unplanned situation where a tooth is lost from its socket unexpectedly, and can occur for several reasons. One example is the removal of an unerupted premolar while extracting its deciduous predecessor. As a premolar crown is surrounded by the deciduous molar roots (Figure 15.82) it can be dislodged or completely extracted together with the deciduous tooth.

Fortunately the accidentally extracted premolar can be saved by immediately replanting it in its socket. The periodontal membrane and pulp should retain their vitality and the tooth subsequently erupts normally. Success is accomplished by immediate replacement, which gives no time for the periodontal membrane to become infected or dried out.

The same procedure can be adopted if a child's tooth – usually an incisor – is knocked out by a fall or a blow. Such a tooth is said to be **avulsed**. As long as the periodontal membrane remains vital, the tooth can be pushed back into its socket, with complete success in many cases. This type of accident constitutes a dental emergency and it is essential that correct first-aid treatment

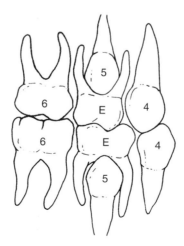

Figure 15.82   Position of deciduous second molar and premolar.

is applied before the child reaches the dental workplace. The following advice should be given to the person reporting the accident:

- Reassure the child (and the parent) that successful treatment is possible
- Retrieve the tooth and, holding it by its crown, rinse it gently in warm water
- Instruct them not to use any type of disinfectant or mouthwash solution to rinse the tooth
- Put the tooth back into its socket, it they feel able to do so
- If that is not possible, let the tooth lie loose in the child's own mouth to keep it moist in saliva, although care should be taken with younger patients to avoid choking
- If that is impracticable, immerse the tooth in a container of milk
- The tooth must not be wrapped in anything, but should be left bathing in the milk
- Come to the surgery immediately

Once the tooth has been replanted in its socket and an X-ray taken, no further treatment may be necessary, but a splint is sometimes required to immobilise it for a week or so, followed by root filling if the tooth becomes non-vital.

Use of antibiotics with MOS

As previously stated, many extractions are carried out because the patient presents with the pain of an acute infection. Previously, antibiotics were often prescribed for these patients as the first line of treatment (especially if the patient attended without an appointment), and the dental problem would be dealt with at a later date.

The current thinking is that antibiotics:

- Are an adjunct to treatment only – so they are to be used as a backup to treatment, not as a replacement for it
- Should only be given if there is evidence that the infection is spreading locally
- Should only be given if there is evidence of systemic involvement (raised body temperature is a good indicator)
- Should be given if the patient has a predisposing medical condition that necessitates antibiotics during treatment

The routine use of antibiotics is contraindicated for the following reasons:

- The source of the infection is better removed by extracting the tooth or by lancing any abscess present and draining as much pus as possible from the area
- Resistant strains of bacteria are more likely to develop if antibiotics are over-prescribed
- The long-term consequences to the normal bacterial flora in the body, from a single course of antibiotics, can last for months
- The dangerous potentiating action that antibiotics have on several drugs, especially oral anticoagulants – they increase the blood-thinning effect of the anticoagulants so that haemostasis cannot be achieved
- The possibility of other drug interactions, especially with oral contraceptives and alcohol
- The development of hypersensitivity to the antibiotics by the patient, preventing their use in future
- All drugs should be avoided wherever possible during pregnancy

If antibiotics do need to be prescribed, the following regimes are the current recommended choices:

- First choice – amoxicillin 250 mg, four times daily for 5 days
- Second choice – metronidazole 200 mg three times daily for 3 days
- Third choice – erythromycin 250 mg four times daily for 5 days, for patients who are allergic to penicillin and its derivatives

In severe infections and where more than one type of microorganism may be involved, the first and second choices can be given together.

Other MOS procedures

Operculectomy

This procedure is the surgical removal of the gingival flap (operculum) overlying a partially erupted tooth, especially a lower third molar.

As teeth begin to erupt, the overlying gingiva is pushed up into the mouth and bulges over the tooth until its incisal or occlusal surface breaks through into the oral cavity. However, in some patients, this gingival bulging over the lower third molars means that the area is constantly bitten and traumatised by the upper teeth when the mouth is closed, causing pain and inflammation in some cases.

As the area becomes more painful, the patient often reduces their oral hygiene efforts, which then compounds the issue by allowing plaque and food debris to collect further, and eventually an infection will develop – this is called **pericoronitis**. In severe cases, patients develop **trismus** and are unable to open their mouths fully.

Treatment is as follows, in order of lesser to greater severity of the symptoms:

- Oral hygiene instruction to ensure the removal of food debris and plaque
- Irrigation of the underside of the flap to remove debris, using chlorhexidine or an oxygen-releasing solution, such as Peroxyl mouthwash
- The use of anti-inflammatory analgesics, such as ibuprofen, to reduce the inflammation and ease the symptoms
- The surgical removal of the operculum if the problem recurs, ideally using an electrosurgical cautery unit (Figure 15.42) rather than conventional techniques, as the control of haemorrhage is far superior
- A 3-day course of metronidazole antibiotics to destroy the anaerobic bacteria involved

559

Alveolectomy and alveoplasty

These are procedures carried out to remove pieces of the alveolar ridge or smooth and alter its shape, respectively.

When teeth have been extracted, the edges of the sockets can sometimes remain as sharp spicules of bone, which make the wearing of dentures impossible, without discomfort to the patient. The quality of the alveolar ridge can easily be seen on a radiograph, and where appropriate the spicules and sharp edges can be removed, so that dentures can be worn. A mucoperiosteal flap must be raised to gain access to the ridge, and then bone rongeurs (Figure 15.83) or surgical burs are used to remove all the bony projections.

Alveoplasty is carried out to alter the shape of the ridge so that deep undercuts are removed and dentures can seat correctly and comfortably.

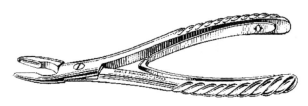

Figure 15.83   Bone rongeurs.

Gingivectomy and gingivoplasty

These are periodontal surgery techniques that are carried out to adjust the shape of the gingivae and aid oral hygiene measures, so that more effective plaque removal is possible. Both are described in detail earlier in this chapter under the main heading "Periodontal therapy".

Periodontal flap surgery

Periodontal conditions that do not respond to plaque control procedures, such as meticulous oral hygiene by the patient and subgingival scaling by a dental operator, may require treatment by MOS procedures. They are performed under local anaesthesia and may be undertaken by the patient's own dentist or by referral to a periodontal specialist.

Periodontal flap procedures are described in detail earlier in this chapter under the main heading "Periodontal therapy".

Soft tissue biopsies

These are procedures carried out to remove a soft tissue lesion from the mouth, so that it can be sent away for pathological examination and diagnosis. Large lesions may have just a section of tissue removed, and these are referred to as **incisional biopsies**. Ideally, and certainly with smaller lesions, the whole of the tissue lesion is removed – these are referred to as **excisional biopsies**.

It is usual for the patient to be referred to a hospital dental department for these types of procedure to be carried out by an oral surgery specialist, as incomplete removal of a sinister lesion (such as oral cancer) may make its treatment ultimately more difficult or even risk spreading cancerous cells more widely.

Cyst removal

A cyst is a fluid-filled sac confined within a soft tissue lining. There are many different types found in various parts of the body. In dental practice, they are most commonly seen as an abnormal cavity in the bone, at the apex of a dead tooth (**dental** or **apical cyst**), or surrounding and preventing eruption of an unerupted tooth (**dentigerous** or **follicular cyst** – see Figure 14.1). If left untreated, a cyst gradually enlarges, causing swelling of the jaw and displacement of other teeth. Whenever possible they are removed, complete with their lining, and invariably by a specialist oral surgeon in hospital.

Frenectomy

This means the removal of a frenum, which is a band of fibrous tissue covered with a mucous membrane that attaches the tongue and lips to the underlying bone. If the lingual frenum restricts the movement of the tongue so that speech is affected, a lingual frenectomy is performed. If the upper labial frenum is too large, it may allow a wide gap to persist between the upper central incisors – this gap is called a **median diastema**. It can also affect the fit of an upper denture. In such cases, an upper labial frenectomy is often undertaken.

560

Index

Note: Page numbers in *italics* refer to Figures; those in **bold** to Tables.

Diploma in Dental Nursing, Level 3, Third Edition. Carole Hollins.
© 2014 John Wiley & Sons, Ltd. Published 2014 by John Wiley & Sons, Ltd.
Companion website: www.wiley.com/go/hollins/dentalnursinglevel3